Comparative Effectiveness Review
Number 124

Meditation Programs for Psychological Stress and Well-Being

Prepared for:
Agency for Healthcare Research and Quality
U.S. Department of Health and Human Services
540 Gaither Road
Rockville, MD 20850
www.ahrq.gov

Contract No. 290-2007-10061-I

Prepared by:
Johns Hopkins University Evidence-based Practice Center
Baltimore, MD

Investigators:
Madhav Goyal, M.D., M.P.H.
Sonal Singh, M.D., M.P.H.
Erica M.S. Sibinga, M.D., M.H.S.
Neda F. Gould, Ph.D.
Anastasia Rowland-Seymour, M.D.
Ritu Sharma, B.Sc.
Zackary Berger, M.D., Ph.D.
Dana Sleicher, M.S., M.P.H.
David D. Maron, M.H.S.
Hasan M. Shihab, M.B.Ch.B., M.P.H.
Padmini D. Ranasinghe, M.D., M.P.H.
Shauna Linn, B.A.
Shonali Saha, M.D.
Eric B. Bass, M.D., M.P.H.
Jennifer A. Haythornthwaite, Ph.D.

AHRQ Publication No. 13(14)-EHC116-EF
January 2014

Addendum

In June 2013, we ran an updated search for the review from our last update in November 2012. We used the same search criteria across the electronic databases, and after removal of duplicate citations we identified 952 new citations. These citations underwent title-abstract review, and 27 trials were pulled for full article review. Of these, six new trials met criteria for inclusion in our review. Further details can be found online at: Goyal M, Singh S. Sibinga EMS, et al. Meditation programs for psychological stress and well-being: a systematic review and meta-analysis. JAMA Intern Med. Epub Jan 6 2014. doi:10.1001/jamainternmed.2013.13018.

Of the six new trials, one was a transcendental meditation trial among patients with HIV, involving nonspecific active controls. Of the remaining five mindfulness trials, two used a nonspecific active control among patients with anxiety or sleep disturbance, and three used a specific active control among patients with anxiety, depression or stress. Three trials contributed to the outcome of anxiety, four trials to the outcome of depression, three trials to the outcome of stress/distress, one trial to the outcome of positive affect, and two trials to the outcome of sleep.

The addition of these trials did not change the overall conclusions or the strength of evidence for any of the outcomes. While the meta-analytic effect sizes for the outcomes where the new trials contributed data changed slightly, the statistical significance did not change and the confidence intervals changed only slightly. Thus only the effect sizes are reported here. For the outcome of anxiety, the effect size changed from 0.40 to 0.38 for mindfulness programs compared with a nonspecific active control, and from 0.06 to 0.07 for mindfulness programs compared with specific active controls. For the outcome of depression, the effect size changed from 0.32 to 0.30 for mindfulness programs compared with nonspecific active controls, from 0.16 to 0.11 for mindfulness programs compared with specific active controls and from 0.24 to 0.27 for Mantra programs compared with nonspecific active controls. For the outcome of negative affect, the effect size changed from 0.34 to 0.33 for mindfulness programs compared with a nonspecific active control. For the outcome of positive affect, the effect size changed from 0.31 to 0.28 for mindfulness programs compared with a nonspecific active control. For the outcome of sleep, the effect size changed from 0.12 to 0.14 for mindfulness programs compared with a nonspecific active control.

This report is based on research conducted by the Johns Hopkins University Evidence-based Practice Center (EPC) under contract to the Agency for Healthcare Research and Quality (AHRQ), Rockville, MD (Contract No. 290-2007-10061-I). The findings and conclusions in this document are those of the authors, who are responsible for its contents; the findings and conclusions do not necessarily represent the views of AHRQ. Therefore, no statement in this report should be construed as an official position of AHRQ or of the U.S. Department of Health and Human Services.

The information in this report is intended to help health care decisionmakers—patients and clinicians, health system leaders, and policymakers, among others—make well-informed decisions and thereby improve the quality of health care services. This report is not intended to be a substitute for the application of clinical judgment. Anyone who makes decisions concerning the provision of clinical care should consider this report in the same way as any medical reference and in conjunction with all other pertinent information, i.e., in the context of available resources and circumstances presented by individual patients.

This report may be used, in whole or in part, as the basis for development of clinical practice guidelines and other quality enhancement tools, or as a basis for reimbursement and coverage policies. AHRQ or U.S. Department of Health and Human Services endorsement of such derivative products may not be stated or implied.

This report may periodically be assessed for the urgency to update. If an assessment is done, the resulting surveillance report describing the methodology and findings will be found on the Effective Health Care Program Web site at: www.effectivehealthcare.ahrq.gov. Search on the title of the report.

This document is in the public domain and may be used and reprinted without special permission. Citation of the source is appreciated.

Persons using assistive technology may not be able to fully access information in this report. For assistance contact EffectiveHealthCare@ahrq.hhs.gov.

> None of the investigators have any affiliations or financial involvement that conflicts with the material presented in this report.

Suggested citation: Goyal M, Singh S, Sibinga EMS, Gould NF, Rowland-Seymour A, Sharma R, Berger Z, Sleicher D, Maron DD, Shihab HM, Ranasinghe PD, Linn S, Saha S, Bass EB, Haythornthwaite JA. Meditation Programs for Psychological Stress and Well-Being. Comparative Effectiveness Review No. 124. (Prepared by Johns Hopkins University Evidence-based Practice Center under Contract No. 290-2007-10061–I.) AHRQ Publication No. 13(14)-EHC116-EF. Rockville, MD: Agency for Healthcare Research and Quality; January 2014. www.effectivehealthcare.ahrq.gov/reports/final.cfm.

Preface

The Agency for Healthcare Research and Quality (AHRQ), through its Evidence-based Practice Centers (EPCs), sponsors the development of systematic reviews to assist public- and private-sector organizations in their efforts to improve the quality of health care in the United States. These reviews provide comprehensive, science-based information on common, costly medical conditions, and new health care technologies and strategies.

Systematic reviews are the building blocks underlying evidence-based practice; they focus attention on the strength and limits of evidence from research studies about the effectiveness and safety of a clinical intervention. In the context of developing recommendations for practice, systematic reviews can help clarify whether assertions about the value of the intervention are based on strong evidence from clinical studies. For more information about AHRQ EPC systematic reviews, see www.effectivehealthcare.ahrq.gov/reference/purpose.cfm.

AHRQ expects that these systematic reviews will be helpful to health plans, providers, purchasers, government programs, and the health care system as a whole. Transparency and stakeholder input are essential to the Effective Health Care Program. Please visit the Web site (www.effectivehealthcare.ahrq.gov) to see draft research questions and reports or to join an email list to learn about new program products and opportunities for input.

We welcome comments on this systematic review. They may be sent by mail to the Task Order Officer named below at: Agency for Healthcare Research and Quality, 540 Gaither Road, Rockville, MD 20850, or by email to epc@ahrq.hhs.gov.

Richard G. Kronick, Ph.D.
Director
Agency for Healthcare Research and Quality

Stephanie Chang, M.D., M.P.H.
Director, EPC Program
Center for Outcomes and Evidence
Agency for Healthcare Research and Quality

Jean Slutsky, P.A., M.S.P.H.
Director, Center for Outcomes and Evidence
Agency for Healthcare Research and Quality

Shilpa H. Amin, M.D., M.Bsc., FAAFP
Task Order Officer
Center for Outcomes and Evidence
Agency for Healthcare Research and Quality

Acknowledgments

The authors gratefully acknowledge the continuing support of our AHRQ Task Order Officer, Shilpa H. Amin. We extend our appreciation to our Key Informants and members of our Technical Expert Panel (listed below), all of whom provided thoughtful advice and input during our research process.

The EPC thanks Swaroop Vedula for conducting meta-analyses and assisting with their interpretation. The EPC also thanks Manisha Reuben, Deepa Pawar, Oluwaseun Shogbesan, and Yohalakshmi Chelladurai for their contributions to this project and Eric Vohr for his editorial contribution.

Key Informants

In designing the study questions, the EPC consulted several Key Informants who represent the end-users of research. The EPC sought the Key Informant input on the priority areas for research and synthesis. Key Informants are not involved in the analysis of the evidence or the writing of the report. Therefore, in the end, study questions, design, methodological approaches, and/or conclusions do not necessarily represent the views of individual Key Informants.

Key Informants must disclose any financial conflicts of interest greater than $10,000 and any other relevant business or professional conflicts of interest. Because of their role as end-users, individuals with potential conflicts may be retained. The TOO and the EPC work to balance, manage, or mitigate any conflicts of interest.

The list of Key Informants who participated in developing this report follows:

Richard J. Davidson, Ph.D.
University of Wisconsin
Madison, WI

John R. Glowa, Ph.D.
National Center for Complementary and Alternative Medicine
Bethesda, MD

Barbara L. Niles, Ph.D.
National Center for PTSD
Boston University School of Medicine
Boston, MA

Dr. David Orme-Johnson, Ph.D.
Consultant
Seagrove Beach, FL

Robert Schneider, M.D., FACC, FABMR
Professor and Director
Institute for Natural Medicine and Prevention
Dean, Maharishi College of Perfect Health
Maharishi University of Management
Maharishi Vedic City, IA

Technical Expert Panel

In designing the study questions and methodology at the outset of this report, the EPC consulted several technical and content experts. Broad expertise and perspectives were sought. Divergent and conflicted opinions are common and perceived as healthy scientific discourse that results in a thoughtful, relevant systematic review. Therefore, in the end, study questions, design, methodologic approaches, and/or conclusions do not necessarily represent the views of individual technical and content experts.

Technical Experts must disclose any financial conflicts of interest greater than $10,000 and any other relevant business or professional conflicts of interest. Because of their unique clinical or content expertise, individuals with potential conflicts may be retained. The TOO and the EPC work to balance, manage, or mitigate any potential conflicts of interest identified.

The list of Technical Experts who participated in developing this report follows:

Kevin W. Chen, Ph.D., M.P.H.
University of Maryland School of Medicine
Baltimore, MD

Margaret Chesney, Ph.D.
UCSF School of Medicine
San Francisco, CA

Susan Gould-Fogerite
University of Medicine and Dentistry of New Jersey
Newark, NJ

Edward Mills. Ph.D.
University of Ottawa
Ottawa, Ontario, Canada

Karen J. Sherman, Ph.D., M.P.H.
Group Health Research Institute
Seattle, WA

Bonnie Tarantino
University of Maryland School of Medicine
Baltimore, MD

Peer Reviewers

Prior to publication of the final evidence report, EPCs sought input from independent Peer Reviewers without financial conflicts of interest. However, the conclusions and synthesis of the scientific literature presented in this report does not necessarily represent the views of individual reviewers.

Peer Reviewers must disclose any financial conflicts of interest greater than $10,000 and any other relevant business or professional conflicts of interest. Because of their unique clinical or content expertise, individuals with potential nonfinancial conflicts may be retained. The TOO and the EPC work to balance, manage, or mitigate any potential nonfinancial conflicts of interest identified.

The list of Peer Reviewers follows:

Vernon Barnes, Ph.D.
Georgia Prevention Center
Institute of Public and Preventive Health
Georgia Regents University
Augusta, GA

David S. Black, Ph.D., M.P.H.
Assistant Professor of Preventive Medicine
Institute for Prevention Research
Keck School of Medicine
University of Southern California
Los Angeles, CA

Mary Butler, Ph.D., M.B.A.
Associate Director, Minnesota EPC
University of Minnesota School of Public Health
Minneapolis, MN

Amparo Castillo, M.D., M.S.
Training Coordinator and Researcher
Midwest Latino Health Research Training and Policy Center at the
Jane Addams College of Social Work and
Institute for Health Research and Policy
University of Illinois at Chicago
Chicago, IL

Vinjar Fonnebo, M.D., Ph.D.
National Research Centre in Complementary and Alternative Medicine (NAFKAM)
University of Tromso
Tromso, Norway

Robert Kane, M.D.
University of Minnesota School of Public Health
Minneapolis, MN

Kathleen Kemper, M.D.
Ohio State College of Medicine
Center for Integrative Health and Wellness
Columbus, OH

Mary Jo Kreitzer, Ph.D., R.N.
Center for Spirituality & Healing
University of Minnesota
Minneapolis, MN

Meditation Programs for Psychological Stress and Well-Being

Structured Abstract

Objectives. Meditation, a mind-body method, employs a variety of techniques designed to facilitate the mind's capacity to affect bodily function and symptoms. An increasing number of patients are using meditation programs despite uncertainty about the evidence supporting the health benefits of meditation. We aimed to determine the efficacy and safety of meditation programs on stress-related outcomes (e.g., anxiety, depression, stress, distress, well-being, positive mood, quality of life, attention, health-related behaviors affected by stress, pain, and weight) compared with an active control in diverse adult clinical populations

Data sources. We searched MEDLINE®, PsycINFO®, Embase®, PsycArticles, SCOPUS, CINAHL, AMED, and the Cochrane Library in November 2012. We also performed manual searches.

Review methods. We included randomized controlled trials with an active control that reported on the stress outcomes of interest. Two reviewers independently screened titles to find trials that reported on outcomes, and then extracted data on trial characteristics and effect modifiers (amount of training or teacher qualifications). We graded the strength of evidence (SOE) using four domains (risk of bias, precision, directness, and consistency). To assess the direction and magnitude of reported effects of the interventions, we calculated the relative difference between groups in how each outcome measure changed from baseline. We conducted meta-analysis using standardized mean differences to obtain aggregate estimates of effects with 95-percent confidence intervals (CIs). We analyzed efficacy trials separately from comparative effectiveness trials.

Results. After a review of 17,801 citations, we included 41 trials with 2,993 participants. Most trials were short term, but they ranged from 4 weeks to 9 years in duration. Trials conducted against nonspecific active controls provided efficacy data. Mindfulness meditation programs had moderate SOE for improvement in anxiety (effect size [ES], 0.40; CI, 0.08 to 0.71 at 8 weeks; ES, 0.22; CI, 0.02 to 0.43 at 3–6 months), depression (ES, 0.32; CI, −0.01 to 0.66 at 8 weeks; ES, 0.23; CI, 0.05 to 0.42 at 3–6 months); and pain (ES, 0.33; CI, 0.03 to 0.62); and low SOE for improvement in stress/distress and mental health–related quality of life. We found either low SOE of no effect or insufficient SOE of an effect of meditation programs on positive mood, attention, substance use, eating, sleep, and weight. In our comparative effectiveness analyses, we did not find any evidence to suggest that these meditation programs were superior to any specific therapies they were compared with. Only 10 trials had a low risk of bias. Limitations included clinical heterogeneity, variability in the types of controls, and heterogeneity of the interventions (e.g., dosing, frequency, duration, technique).

Conclusions. Meditation programs, in particular mindfulness programs, reduce multiple negative dimensions of psychological stress. Stronger study designs are needed to determine the effects of meditation programs in improving the positive dimensions of mental health as well as stress-related behavioral outcomes.

Contents

Executive Summary ES-1
Introduction 1
    Definition of Meditation 1
    Current Practice and Prevalence of Use 1
    Forms of Meditation 1
    Psychological Stress and Well-Being 3
    Evidence to Date 4
    Clinical and Policy Relevance 4
    Objectives 5
    Scope and Key Questions 5
    Analytic Framework 5
Methods 7
    Topic Development 7
    Search Strategy 7
    Study Selection 8
    Data Abstraction and Data Management 10
    Data Synthesis 12
    Assessment of Methodological Quality of Individual Studies 15
    Assessment of Potential Publication Bias 16
    Strength of the Body of Evidence 16
    Applicability 19
    Peer Review and Public Commentary 19
Results 20
    Results of the Search 20
    Description of Types of Trials Retrieved 21
    Key Question Results 34
    Key Question 1. What are the efficacy and harms of meditation programs on negative affect (e.g., anxiety, stress) and positive affect (e.g., well-being) among those with a clinical condition (medical or psychiatric)? 47
        Key Points and Evidence Grades 47
        Trial Characteristics 49
        Population Characteristics 49
        Intervention Characteristics 50
        Outcomes 51
        Applicability 102
    Key Question 2. What are the efficacy and harms of meditation programs on attention among those with a clinical condition (medical or psychiatric)? 102
        Key Points and Evidence Grades 102
        Trial Characteristics 102
        Population Characteristics 103
        Intervention Characteristics 103
        Outcomes 103
        Applicability 104

Key Question 3. What are the efficacy and harms of meditation programs on health-related behaviors affected by stress, specifically substance use, sleep, and eating, among those with a clinical condition (medical or psychiatric)?..104
    Key Points and Evidence Grades 104
    Trial Characteristics 105
    Population Characteristics...105
    Intervention Characteristics...105
    Outcomes...106
    Applicability..114
Key Question 4. What are the efficacy and harms of meditation programs on pain and weight among those with a clinical condition (medical or psychiatric)? 116
    Key Points and Evidence Grades 116
    Trial Characteristics 116
    Population Characteristics...116
    Intervention Characteristics...117
    Outcomes...118
    Assessment of Potential Publication Bias 126
    Applicability..126

Discussion..129
    Key Question 1. What are the efficacy and harms of meditation programs on negative affect (e.g., anxiety, stress) and positive affect (e.g., well-being) among those with a clinical condition (medical or psychiatric)? 130
    Key Question 2. What are the efficacy and harms of meditation programs on attention among those with a clinical condition (medical or psychiatric)? 132
    Key Question 3. What are the efficacy and harms of meditation programs on health-related behaviors affected by stress, specifically substance use, sleep, and eating, among those with a clinical condition (medical or psychiatric)?...132
    Key Question 4. What are the efficacy and harms of meditation programs on pain and weight among those with a clinical condition (medical or psychiatric)? 133
    Harm Outcomes for All Key Questions...134
    Limitations of the Primary Studies 134
    Limitations of the Review...134
    Future Directions 136
    Conclusions...138

References..140

Tables
Table A. Study inclusion and exclusion criteria ES-6
Table B. List of major and minor criteria in assessing risk of bias ES-8
Table 1. Study inclusion and exclusion criteria 9
Table 2. Organization of various scales (instruments or measurement tools) for each Key Question 11
Table 3. List of major and minor criteria in assessing risk of bias 16
Table 4. Characteristics of included trials...22
Table 5. Training dose for included trials over duration of training period (numbers are calculated from information provided in trials)..30
Table 6. Teacher qualifications for included trials 31

Table 7. Risk of bias for included trials 32
Table 8. Synthesis summary for anxiety 38
Table 9. Synthesis summary for depression 39
Table 10. Synthesis summary for stress/distress 40
Table 11. Synthesis summary for negative affect 41
Table 12. Synthesis summary for positive affect (well being and positive mood) 42
Table 13. Synthesis summary for quality of life/mental component of health-related quality of life 43
Table 14. Synthesis summary for substance use, eating, sleep 44
Table 15. Synthesis summary for pain 45
Table 16. Synthesis summary for weight 46
Table 17. Grade of trials addressing the efficacy of mindfulness meditation program on anxiety compared with nonspecific active controls among various populations 53
Table 18. Grade of trials addressing the efficacy of mantra meditation programs on anxiety compared with nonspecific active controls among various populations 57
Table 19. Grade of trials addressing the efficacy of mindfulness meditation programs on symptoms of depression compared with nonspecific active controls among clinical populations 60
Table 20. Grade of trials addressing the efficacy of mantra meditation program on symptoms of depression compared with nonspecific active controls among cardiac and HIV populations ..64
Table 21. Grade of trials assessing the efficacy of mindfulness programs on stress and distress compared with nonspecific active controls among various populations 67
Table 22. Grade of trials addressing the efficacy of mantra meditation programs on stress compared with nonspecific active controls among cardiac and HIV patients 70
Table 23. Grade of trials addressing the efficacy of mindfulness meditation programs on negative affect compared with nonspecific active controls among diverse populations 72
Table 24. Grade of trials addressing the efficacy of mantra meditation programs on negative affect compared with nonspecific active controls among diverse populations 77
Table 25. Grade of trials addressing the efficacy of mindfulness meditation programs on positive affect compared with nonspecific active controls among organ transplant recipients and breast cancer patients 81
Table 26. Grade of trials addressing the efficacy of transcendental meditation on positive affect compared with nonspecific active controls among cardiac patients 84
Table 27. Grade of trials addressing the efficacy of mindfulness meditation programs on the mental component of health-related quality of life compared with nonspecific active controls among various patients 86
Table 28. Grade of trials addressing the efficacy of mindfulness meditation programs on anxiety compared with specific active controls among diverse populations 89
Table 29. Grade of trials addressing the efficacy of clinically standardized meditation programs on anxiety compared with progressive muscle relaxation among anxious participants 91
Table 30. Grade of trials addressing the efficacy of mindfulness meditation programs on depressive symptoms compared with specific active controls among diverse populations 93
Table 31. Grade of trials addressing the efficacy of clinically standardized meditation programs on depression compared with progressive muscle relaxation among anxious participants 95
Table 32. Grade of trials addressing the efficacy of mindfulness meditation programs on distress compared with specific active controls among populations with emotional distress 96

Table 33. Grade of trials addressing the efficacy of mindfulness meditation programs on positive affect compared with progressive muscle relaxation or spirituality among various patients 99
Table 34. Grade of trials addressing the efficacy of mindfulness meditation programs on the mental component of health-related quality of life compared with specific active controls among various populations 100
Table 35. Grade of trials addressing the efficacy of a meditation program on a measure of attention compared with a nonspecific active control among older caregivers 104
Table 36. Grade of trials addressing the efficacy of mindfulness meditation program on sleep quality among various populations compared with a nonspecific active control 107
Table 37. Grade of trials addressing the efficacy of mindfulness meditation programs on sleep quality compared with specific active controls in various populations 110
Table 38. Grade of trials addressing the efficacy of mindfulness meditation programs on eating compared with specific active controls in diabetic and breast cancer populations 111
Table 39. Grade of trials addressing the efficacy of mindfulness meditation programs on substance use compared with specific active controls in smoking and alcoholic populations....112
Table 40. Grade of trials addressing the efficacy and harms of mantra meditation programs on alcohol use among heavy alcohol drinkers compared with intensive running program or biofeedback 114
Table 41. Grade of trials addressing the efficacy of mindfulness-based stress reduction on pain severity compared with nonspecific active controls among visceral pain, musculoskeletal pain, and organ transplant patients 119
Table 42. Grade of trials addressing the efficacy of transcendental meditation on pain severity compared with nonspecific active controls among cardiac patients 122
Table 43. Grade of trials addressing the efficacy of mindfulness-based stress reduction on pain severity compared with specific active controls among chronic pain and mood disturbance patients 123
Table 44. Grade of trials addressing the efficacy of mindfulness-based stress reduction on weight among breast cancer and chronic pain patients compared with a specific active control 125
Table 45. Grade of trials addressing the efficacy of meditation programs on weight among those with a clinical condition 126

Figures
Figure A. Analytic framework for meditation programs conducted in clinical and psychiatric populations ES-4
Figure B1. Summary across measurement domains of comparisons of meditation with nonspecific active controls ES-12
Figure B2. Summary across measurement domains of comparisons of meditation with specific active controls ES-13
Figure 1. Analytic framework for meditation programs conducted in clinical and psychiatric populations 6
Figure 2. Algorithm for rating the strength of evidence 18
Figure 3. Summary of the literature search 20
Figure 4a. Summary across measurement domains of comparisons of meditation with nonspecific active controls 35
Figure 4b. Summary across measurement domains of comparisons of meditation with specific active controls 36

Figure 5. Relative difference between groups in the changes in measures of general anxiety, in the mindfulness versus nonspecific active control studies 54

Figure 6. Meta-analysis of the effects of meditation programs on anxiety with up to 12 weeks of followup 55

Figure 7. Meta-analysis of the effects of meditation programs on anxiety after 3–6 months of followup 56

Figure 8. Relative difference between groups in the changes in measures of general anxiety, in the mantra versus nonspecific active control/specific active control studies 58

Figure 9. Relative difference between groups in the changes in measures of depression, in the mindfulness versus nonspecific active control studies 61

Figure 10. Meta-analysis of the effects of meditation programs on depression with up to 3 months of followup 62

Figure 11. Meta-analysis of the effects of meditation programs on depression after 3–6 months of followup 63

Figure 12. Relative difference between groups in the changes in measures of depression, in the mantra versus nonspecific active control/specific active control studies 65

Figure 13. Relative difference between groups in the changes in measures of stress/distress, in the mindfulness versus nonspecific active control studies 68

Figure 14. Meta-analysis of the effects of meditation programs on stress/distress with up to 16 weeks of followup 69

Figure 15. Relative difference between groups in the changes in measures of stress, in the mantra versus nonspecific active control studies 71

Figure 16. Relative difference between groups in the changes in negative affect, in the mindfulness versus nonspecific active control studies 73

Figure 17. Meta-analysis of the effects of meditation programs on negative affect—main analysis (mindfulness meditation versus nonspecific active control interventions) 74

Figure 18. Relative difference between groups in the changes in measures of negative affect, in the mindfulness versus nonspecific active control studies (sensitivity analysis) 75

Figure 19. Meta-analysis of the effects of meditation programs on negative affect—sensitivity analysis (mindfulness meditation versus nonspecific active control interventions) 76

Figure 20. Relative difference between groups in the changes in measures of negative affect, in the mantra versus nonspecific active control studies 78

Figure 21. Relative difference between groups in the changes in measures of negative affect, in the mantra versus nonspecific active control studies (sensitivity analysis) 79

Figure 22. Meta-analysis of the effects of mantra meditation programs on negative affect—sensitivity analysis (mantra vs. nonspecific active control interventions) 80

Figure 23. Relative difference between groups in the changes in measures of positive affect, in the mindfulness versus nonspecific active control/specific active control studies 82

Figure 24. Meta-analysis of the effects of meditation programs on positive affect with up to 4 months of followup 83

Figure 25. Relative difference between groups in the changes in measures of positive affect, in the mantra versus nonspecific active control studies 85

Figure 26. Relative difference between groups in the changes in measures of mental component of health-related quality of life, in the mindfulness versus nonspecific active control/specific active control studies 87

Figure 27. Relative difference between groups in the changes in measures of general anxiety, in the mindfulness versus specific active control studies 90

Figure 28. Relative difference between groups in the changes in measures of depression, in the mindfulness versus specific active control studies 94

Figure 29. Relative difference between groups in the changes in measures of distress, in the mindfulness versus specific active control studies 97

Figure 30. Meta-analysis of the effects of meditation programs on the mental health component of health-related quality of life with up to 3 months of followup...101

Figure 31. Relative difference between groups in the changes in measures of sleep, in the mindfulness versus nonspecific/specific active control studies...108

Figure 32. Meta-analysis of the effects of meditation programs on sleep with up to 3 months of followup...109

Figure 33. Relative difference between groups in the changes in measures of substance use/eating, in the mindfulness versus specific active control studies 113

Figure 34. Relative difference between groups in the changes in measures of substance use, in the mantra versus nonspecific/specific active control studies 115

Figure 35. Relative difference between groups in the changes in measures of pain, in the mindfulness versus nonspecific active control studies 120

Figure 36. Meta-analysis of the effects of meditation programs on pain severity with 8–12 weeks of followup...121

Figure 37. Relative difference between groups in the changes in measures of pain, in the mindfulness versus specific active control studies 124

Figure 38. Relative difference between groups in the changes in measures of weight, in the mindfulness/transcendental meditation versus specific/nonspecific active control studies 128

Appendixes
Appendix A. Abbreviations and Glossary of Terms
Appendix B. Detailed Search Strategies
Appendix C. Screening Forms
Appendix D. Excluded Studies
Appendix E. Evidence Tables

Executive Summary

Introduction

Definition of Meditation

The National Center for Complementary and Alternative Medicine defines meditation as a "mind-body" method. This category of complementary and alternative medicine includes interventions that employ a variety of techniques that facilitate the mind's capacity to affect bodily function and symptoms. In meditation, a person learns to focus attention. Some forms of meditation instruct the student to become mindful of thoughts, feelings, and sensations, and to observe them in a nonjudgmental way. Many believe this practice evokes a state of greater calmness, physical relaxation, and psychological balance.[1]

Current Practice and Prevalence of Use

Many people use meditation to treat stress and stress-related conditions, as well as to promote general health.[2,3] A national survey in 2008 found that the number of people meditating is increasing, with approximately 10 percent of the population having some experience with meditation.[2] A number of hospitals and programs offer courses in meditation to patients seeking alternative or additional methods to relieve symptoms or to promote health.

Forms of Meditation

Meditation training programs vary in several ways, including the emphasis on religion or spirituality, the type of mental activity promoted, the nature and amount of training, the use of an instructor, and the qualifications of an instructor, which may all affect the level and nature of the meditative skills learned. Some meditative techniques are integrated into a broader alternative approach that includes dietary and/or movement therapies (e.g., ayurveda or yoga).

Researchers have categorized meditative techniques as emphasizing "mindfulness," "concentration," and "automatic self-transcendence." Popular techniques such as transcendental meditation (TM) emphasize the use of a mantra in such a way that one "transcends" to an effortless state where there is no focused attention. Other popular techniques, such as mindfulness-based stress reduction (MBSR), are classified as "mindfulness" and emphasize training in present-focused awareness. Uncertainty remains about the extent to which these distinctions actually influence psychosocial stress outcomes.

Psychological Stress and Well-Being

Researchers have postulated that meditation programs may affect a range of outcomes related to psychological stress and well-being. The research ranges from the rare examination of positive outcomes, such as increased well-being, to the more common approach of examining reductions in negative outcomes, such as anxiety or sleep disturbance. Some studies address symptoms related to the primary condition (e.g., pain in patients with low back pain or anxiety in patients with social phobia), whereas others address similar emotional symptoms in clinical groups of people who may or may not have clinically significant symptoms (e.g., anxiety or depression in individuals with cancer).

Evidence to Date

Reviews to date have demonstrated that both "mindfulness" and "mantra" meditation techniques reduce emotional symptoms (e.g., anxiety and depression, stress) and improve physical symptoms (e.g., pain) from a small to moderate degree.[4-23] These reviews have largely included uncontrolled studies or studies that used control groups that did not receive additional treatment (i.e., usual care or wait list). In wait-list controlled studies, the control group receives usual care while "waiting" to receive the intervention at some time in the future, providing a usual-care control for the purposes of the study. Thus, it is unclear whether the apparently beneficial effects of meditation training are a result of the expectations for improvement that participants naturally form when obtaining this type of treatment. Additionally, many programs involve lengthy and sustained efforts on the part of participants and trainers, possibly yielding beneficial effects from the added attention, group participation, and support participants receive, as well as the suggestion that symptoms will likely improve with these increased efforts.[24,25]

The meditation literature has significant limitations related to inadequate control comparisons. An informative analogy is the use of placebos in pharmaceutical trials. The placebo is typically designed to match the "active intervention" in order to elicit the same expectations of benefit on the part of both provider and patient, but not contain the "active" ingredient. Additionally, placebo treatment includes all components of care received by the active group, including office visits and patient-provider interactions. These nonspecific factors are particularly important to control when the evaluation of outcome relies on patient reporting. In this situation, in which double-blinding has not been feasible, the challenge to execute studies that are not biased by these nonspecific factors is more pressing.[25] Thus, there is a clear need to examine the specific effects of meditation in randomized controlled trials (RCTs) in which expectations for outcome and attentional support are controlled.

Clinical and Policy Relevance

There is much uncertainty regarding the differences and similarities between the effects of different types of meditation.[26,27] Given the increasing use of meditation across a large number of conditions, it is important for patients, clinicians, and policymakers to understand the effects of meditation, types and duration of meditation, and settings and conditions for which meditation is efficacious. While some reviews have focused on RCTs, many, if not most, of the included studies involved wait-list or usual-care controls. Thus, there is a need to examine the specific effects of meditation interventions relative to conditions in which expectations for outcome and attentional support are controlled.

Objectives

The objectives of this systematic review are to evaluate the effects of meditation programs on affect, attention, and health-related behaviors affected by stress, pain, and weight among people with a medical or psychiatric condition in RCTs with appropriate comparators.

Scope and Key Questions

This report reviews the efficacy of meditation programs on psychological stress and well-being among those with a clinical condition. "Affect" refers to emotion or mood. It can be positive, such as the feeling of well-being, or negative, such as anxiety, depression, or stress. Studies usually measure affect through self-reported questionnaires designed to gauge how much someone experiences a particular affect. "Attention" refers to the ability to maintain focus on particular stimuli; clinicians measure this directly. Studies measure substance use as the amount consumed or smoked over a period of time, and include alcohol consumption, cigarette smoking, and use of other drugs such as cocaine. They measure sleep as the amount of time spent asleep versus awake or as overall sleep quality. Studies measure sleep time through either polysomnography or actigraphy, and sleep quality through self-reported questionnaires. They measure eating using food diaries to calculate how much energy or fat a person has consumed over a particular period of time. They measure pain similarly to affect, by a self-reported questionnaire to assess how much pain an individual is experiencing. Studies measure pain severity on a numerical rating scale from 0 to 10 or by using other self-reported questionnaires. The studies measure weight in pounds or kilograms.

The Key Questions are as follows:

Key Question 1. What are the efficacy and harms of meditation programs on negative affect (e.g., anxiety, stress) and positive affect (e.g., well-being) among those with a clinical condition (medical or psychiatric)?

Key Question 2. What are the efficacy and harms of meditation programs on attention among those with a clinical condition (medical or psychiatric)?

Key Question 3. What are the efficacy and harms of meditation programs on health-related behaviors affected by stress, specifically substance use, sleep, and eating, among those with a clinical condition (medical or psychiatric)?

Key Question 4. What are the efficacy and harms of meditation programs on pain and weight among those with a clinical condition (medical or psychiatric)?

Analytic Framework

Figure A illustrates our analytic framework for the systematic review. The figure indicates the populations of interest, the meditation programs, and the outcomes that we reviewed. This figure depicts the Key Questions (KQs) within the context of the population, intervention, comparator, outcomes, timing, and setting (PICOTS) framework described in Table A. Adverse events may occur at any point after the meditation program has begun.

Figure A. Analytic framework for meditation programs conducted in clinical and psychiatric populations

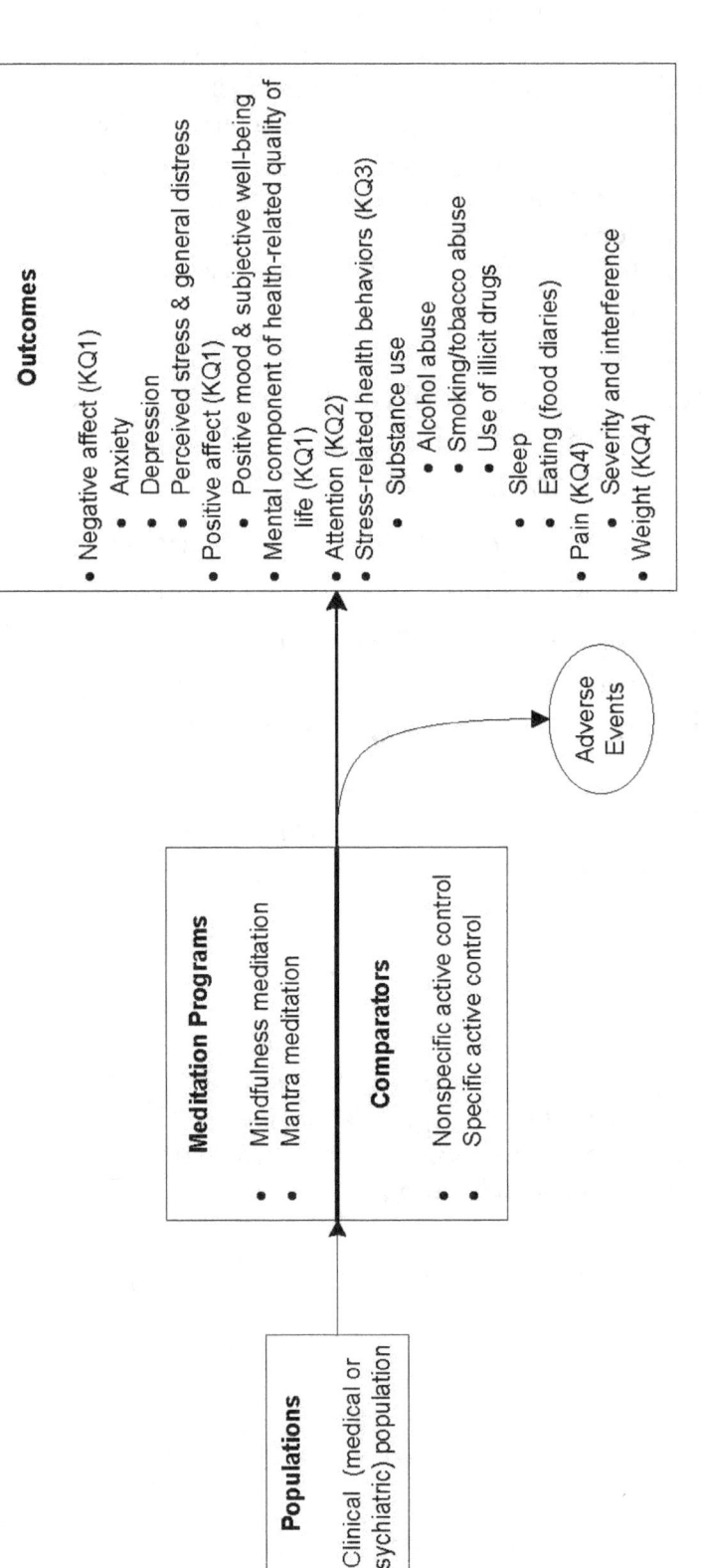

KQ = Key Question

Methods

Literature Search Strategy

We searched the following databases for primary studies through November 2012: MEDLINE®, PsycINFO®, Embase®, PsycArticles, SCOPUS, CINAHL, AMED, and the Cochrane Library. We developed a search strategy for MEDLINE, accessed via PubMed®, based on medical subject headings (MeSH®) terms and text words of key articles that we identified a priori. We used a similar strategy in the other electronic sources. We reviewed the reference lists of included articles, relevant review articles, and related systematic reviews (n=20) to identify articles that the database searches might have missed. We did not impose any limits based on language or date of publication.

Study Selection

Two trained investigators independently screened articles at the title-and-abstract level and excluded them if both investigators agreed that the article met one or more of the exclusion criteria (Table A). We resolved differences between investigators regarding abstract eligibility through consensus.

Paired investigators conducted a second independent review of the full-text article for all citations that we promoted on the basis of title and abstract. We resolved differences regarding article inclusion through consensus.

Paired investigators conducted an additional independent review of full-text articles to determine if they adequately addressed the KQs and should be included in this review.

We included RCTs in which the control group was matched in time and attention to the intervention group for the purpose of matching expectations of benefit. The inclusion of such trials allowed us to evaluate the specific effects of meditation programs separately from the nonspecific effects of attention and expectation. Our team thought this was the most rigorous way to determine the efficacy of the interventions. We did not include observational studies because they are likely to have a high risk of bias due to problems such as self-selection of interventions (since people who believe in the benefits of meditation or who have prior experience with meditation are more likely to enroll in a meditation program) and use of outcome measures that can be easily biased by participants' beliefs in the benefits of meditation.

For inclusion in this review, we required that studies reported on participants with a clinical condition such as medical or psychiatric populations. Although meditation programs may have an impact on healthy populations, we limited our evaluation of these meditation programs to clinical populations. Since trials study meditation programs in diverse populations, we have defined clinical conditions broadly to include mental health/psychiatric conditions (e.g., anxiety or stress) and physical conditions (e.g., low back pain, heart disease, or advanced age). Additionally, since stress was of particular interest in meditation studies, we also included trials that studied stressed populations even though they may not have a defined medical or psychiatric diagnosis. We excluded studies among otherwise healthy populations.

Table A. Study inclusion and exclusion criteria

PICOTS Element	Inclusion	Exclusion
Population and Condition of Interest	• Adult populations (18 years or older) • Clinical (medical or psychiatric) diagnosis, defined as any condition (e.g., high blood pressure, anxiety) including a stressor	• Studies of children (The type and nature of meditation children receive are significantly different from those for adults.) • Studies of otherwise healthy individuals
Interventions	Structured meditation programs (any systematic or protocolized meditation programs that follow predetermined curricula) consisting of at least 4 hours of training with instructions to practice outside the training session These include: Mindfulness-based: • MBSR • MBCT • Vipassana • Zen • Other mindfulness meditation Mantra-based: • TM • Other mantra meditation Other meditation	Meditation programs in which the meditation is not the foundation and majority of the intervention These include: • DBT • ACT • Any of the movement-based meditations, such as yoga (e.g., Iyengar, hatha, shavasana), tai chi, and qi gong (chi kung) • Aromatherapy • Biofeedback • Neurofeedback • Hypnosis • Autogenic training • Psychotherapy • Laughter therapy • Therapeutic touch • Eye movement desensitization reprocessing • Relaxation therapy • Spiritual therapy • Breathing exercise, pranayama • Exercise • Any intervention that is given remotely or only by video or audio to an individual without the involvement of a meditation teacher physically present
Comparisons of Interest	Active control is defined as a program that is matched in time and attention to the intervention group for the purpose of matching expectations of benefit. Examples include "attention control," "educational control," or another therapy, such as progressive muscle relaxation, that the study compares with the intervention. • A nonspecific active control matches only time and attention and is not a known therapy. • A specific active control compares the intervention with another known therapy, such as progressive muscle relaxation.	Studies that evaluate only a wait-list/usual-care control or do not include a comparison group
Outcomes	See Figure A	All other outcomes
Study Design	RCTs with an active control	Nonrandomized designs, such as observational studies
Timing and Setting	Longitudinal studies that occur in general and clinical settings	None

We excluded articles with no original data (reviews, editorials, and comments), studies published in abstract form only, and dissertations.

ACT = acceptance and commitment therapy; DBT = dialectical behavioral therapy; MBCT = mindfulness-based cognitive therapy; MBSR = mindfulness-based stress reduction; PICOTS = population, intervention, comparison, outcome, timing, and setting; RCT = randomized controlled trial; TM = transcendental meditation

Data Abstraction and Data Management

We used DistillerSR (Evidence Partners, 2010) to manage the screening process. DistillerSR is a Web-based database management program that manages all levels of the review process. We uploaded all the citations our search identified to this system.

We created standardized forms for data extraction and pilot tested them. Reviewers extracted information on general study characteristics, study participants, eligibility criteria, interventions, and outcomes. Two investigators reviewed each article for data abstraction. For study characteristics, participant characteristics, and intervention characteristics, the second reviewer confirmed the first reviewer's data abstraction for completeness and accuracy. For outcome data and risk-of-bias scoring, we used dual and independent review. Reviewer pairs included personnel with both clinical and methodological expertise. We resolved differences between investigators regarding data through consensus.

For each meditation program, we extracted information on measures of intervention fidelity, including dose, training, and receipt of intervention. We measured duration and maximal hours of structured training in meditation, amount of home practice recommended, description of instructor qualifications, and description of participant adherence, if any.

Data Synthesis

For each KQ, we created a detailed set of evidence tables containing all information abstracted from eligible studies.

To display the outcome data, we calculated relative difference-in-change scores (i.e., the change from baseline in an outcome measure in the treatment group minus the change from baseline in the outcome measure in the control group, divided by the baseline score in the treatment group). However, many studies did not report enough information to calculate confidence intervals for the relative difference-in-change scores. When we evaluated point estimates and confidence intervals for just the postintervention or end-of-study differences between groups and compared these with the point estimates for the relative difference-in-change scores for those time points, some of the estimates that did not account for baseline differences appeared to favor a different group (e.g., treatment or control) when compared with the estimates that accounted for baseline differences. We therefore used the relative difference-in-change scores to estimate the direction and approximate magnitude of effect for all outcomes. For the purpose of generating an aggregate quantitative estimate of the effect of an intervention and the associated 95-percent confidence interval, we performed meta-analysis using standardized mean differences (effect sizes) calculated by Cohen's method (Cohen's d). We also used these to assess the precision of individual studies, which we factored into the overall strength of evidence (SOE). For each outcome, we displayed the resulting effect-size estimate according to the type of control group and duration of followup. Some studies did not report enough information to be included in meta-analysis. For that reason, we decided to display the relative difference-in-change scores along with the effect-size estimates from meta-analysis so that readers can see the full extent of the available data.

We considered a 5-percent relative difference-in-change score to be potentially clinically significant, since these studies were looking at short interventions and relatively low doses of meditation. In synthesizing the results of these trials, we considered both statistical and clinical significance. Statistical significance is determined according to study-specific criteria; we reported p-values and confidence intervals for these where present.

Trials used either nonspecific active controls or specific active controls (Table A, Figure A). Nonspecific active controls (e.g., education control or attention control) are used to control for the nonspecific effects of time, attention, and expectation. Comparisons against these controls allow for assessments of the specific effectiveness of the meditation program above and beyond the nonspecific effects of time, attention, and expectation. Such a comparison is similar to a comparison against a placebo pill in a drug trial, where one is concerned with the nonspecific effects of interacting with a provider, taking a pill, and expecting the pill to work. Specific active controls are therapies (e.g., exercise or progressive muscle relaxation) known or expected to change clinical outcomes. Comparisons against these controls allow for assessments of comparative effectiveness and are similar to comparing one drug against another known drug in a drug trial. Since these study designs using different types of controls are expected to yield quite different conclusions (effectiveness vs. comparative effectiveness), we separated them in our analyses.

Assessment of Methodological Quality of Individual Trials

We assessed the risk of bias in studies independently and in duplicate based on the recommendations in the Evidence-based Practice Center "Methods Guide for Effectiveness and Comparative Effectiveness Reviews" (Methods Guide).[28] We supplemented these tools with additional assessment questions based on the Cochrane Collaboration's risk-of-bias tool.[29,30] While many of the tools to evaluate risk of bias are common to behavioral as well as pharmacologic interventions, some items are more specific to behavioral interventions. After discussion with experts in meditation programs and clinical trials, we emphasized four major and four minor criteria. We assigned 2 points each to the major criteria, weighting them more than the minor criteria in assessing risk of bias. We assigned 1 point each to the minor criteria. Studies could therefore receive a total of 12 points. If studies met a minimum of three major criteria and three minor criteria (9–12 points), we classified them as having "low risk of bias." We classified studies receiving 6–8 points as having "medium risk of bias," and studies receiving 5 or fewer points as having "high risk of bias" (Table B).

Table B. List of major and minor criteria in assessing risk of bias

Major Criteria[a]	Minor Criteria[a]
• Was the control matched for time and attention by the instructors? • Was there a description of withdrawals and dropouts? • Was attrition <20% at the end of treatment? As several studies did not calculate attrition starting from the original number randomized, we recalculated the attrition from the original number randomized. • Were those who collected data on the participants blind to the allocation?	• Was the method of randomization described in the article? To answer yes for this question, the trials had to give some description of the randomization procedure. • Was allocation concealed? • Was intent-to-treat analysis used? To answer yes for this question, the trial must impute noncompleter or other missing data, and it must do this from the original number randomized. • Did the trial evaluate the credibility, and if so, was it comparable? If the trial did not evaluate credibility, or if it evaluated credibility but did not find it comparable, then we did not give the trial a point.

[a]We assigned 2 points each to the major criteria in assessing risk of bias, and 1 point each to the minor criteria.

Assessment of Potential Publication Bias

We planned to use funnel plots to assess potential publication bias if numerous studies reported on an outcome of interest. We also searched for any trials on clinicaltrials.gov that completed recruitment 3 or more years ago and did not publish results, or listed outcomes for which they did not report results.

Strength of the Body of Evidence

Two reviewers graded the strength of evidence for each outcome for each of the KQs using the grading scheme recommended by the Methods Guide. In assigning evidence grades, we considered four domains: risk of bias; directness, consistency, and precision. We classified evidence into four basic categories: (1) "high" grade, indicating high confidence that the evidence reflects the true effect, and further research is very unlikely to change our confidence in the estimate of the effect; (2) "moderate" grade, indicating moderate confidence that the evidence reflects the true effect, and further research may change our confidence in the estimate of the effect and may change the estimate; (3) "low" grade, indicating low confidence that the evidence reflects the true effect, and further research is likely to change our confidence in the estimate of the effect and is likely to change the estimate; and (4) "insufficient" grade, indicating that evidence is unavailable or inadequate to draw a conclusion.

Applicability

We assessed applicability separately for the different outcomes of benefit and harm for the entire body of evidence guided by the PICOTS framework, as recommended in the Methods Guide.[28] We assessed whether findings were applicable to various ethnic groups, and whether race, ethnicity, or education limited the applicability of the evidence.

Results

Literature Search Results

The literature search identified 17,801 unique citations. During the title-and-abstract screening, we excluded 16,177 citations. During the article screening, we excluded 1,447 citations. During KQ applicability screening, we excluded an additional 136 articles that did not meet one or more of the inclusion criteria. We included 41 articles in the review.[31-71]

Most trials were short term, but they ranged from 4 weeks to 9 years in duration. Since the amount of training and practice in any meditation program may affect its results, we collected this information and found a fair range in the quality of information. Not all trials reported on amount of training and home practice recommended. MBSR programs typically provided 20–27.5 hours of training over 8 weeks. The mindfulness meditation trials typically provided about half this amount. TM trials provided 16–39 hours over 3–12 months, while other mantra meditation programs provided about half this amount. Only five of the trials reported the trainers' actual meditation experience (ranging from 4 months to 25 years), and six reported the trainers' actual teaching experience (ranging from 0 to 15.7 years).

Findings

Of the 41 trials we reviewed, 15 studied psychiatric populations, including those with anxiety, depression, stress, chronic worry, and insomnia. Five trials studied substance-abusing populations such as smokers and alcoholics, 5 studied chronic pain populations, and 16 studied diverse medical populations, including those with heart disease, lung disease, breast cancer, diabetes, hypertension, and HIV.

The strength of evidence on the outcomes of our review is shown in Figures B1 and B2. Since there were numerous scales for the different measures of affect, we organized the scales to best represent the clinically relevant aspects of each affect. For this review, the comparisons with nonspecific active controls provided efficacy data, whereas comparisons with specific active controls provided comparative effectiveness data. We found it difficult to draw comparative effectiveness conclusions from comparisons with specific active controls due to the large heterogeneity of type and strength of control groups. Therefore, we presented our results first for all the comparisons with nonspecific active controls in Figure B1 (efficacy), and then for the specific active controls in Figure B2 (comparative effectiveness).

The direction and magnitude of effect are derived from the relative difference between groups in the change score. In our efficacy analysis (Figure B1) we found low SOE of no effect or insufficient evidence that mantra meditation programs had an effect on any of the psychological stress and well-being outcomes we examined in these diverse adult clinical conditions.

Mindfulness meditation programs had moderate SOE for improvement in anxiety (effect size [ES], 0.40; confidence interval [CI], 0.08 to 0.71 at 8 weeks; ES, 0.22; CI, .02 to .43 at 3–6 months); depression (ES, 0.32; CI, −.01 to +0.66 at 8 weeks; ES, 0.23; CI, .05 to .42 at 3–6 months); and pain (ES, 0.33; CI, .03 to .62); and they had low SOE for improvement in stress/distress and mental health–related quality of life. We found either low SOE of no effect or insufficient SOE of an effect of meditation programs on positive mood, attention, and weight. We also found insufficient evidence that meditation programs had an effect on health-related behaviors affected by stress, including substance use and sleep.

In our comparative effectiveness analyses (Figure B2), we found low SOE of no effect or insufficient SOE that meditation programs were more effective than exercise, progressive muscle relaxation, cognitive-behavioral group therapy, or other specific comparators in changing any outcomes of interest.

Harm Outcomes for All Key Questions

Few trials reported on potential harms of meditation programs. Of the nine trials that reported on harms, none reported any harms of the intervention. One trial specified that the researchers looked for toxicities of meditation to hematologic, renal, and liver markers and found none. The remaining eight trials did not specify the type of adverse event they were looking for. Seven reported that they found no significant adverse events, while one did not comment on adverse events. The remaining 32 trials did not report whether they monitored for adverse events.

Assessment of Potential Publication Bias

We could not conduct any reliable quantitative tests for publication bias since few studies were available for most outcomes, and we were unable to include all eligible studies in the meta-analysis due to missing data. Consequently, funnel plots were unlikely to provide much useful information regarding the possibility of publication bias. We reviewed the clinicaltrials.gov registration database to assess the number of trials that had been completed 3 or more years ago and that prespecified our outcomes but did not publish at all, or published but did not publish all outcomes that were prespecified. We found five trials on clinicaltrials.gov that appeared to have been completed before January 1, 2010, and were published but did not publish the results of all outcomes they had prespecified on the registration Web site. We also found nine trials that appeared to have been completed before January 1, 2010, and had prespecified at least one of our outcomes but for which we could not find any publication. Ten registered trials had prespecified one or more KQ1 outcomes but did not publish them, two registered trials had prespecified attention as an outcome but did not publish, five registered trials prespecified one or more KQ3 outcomes but did not publish, and five registered trials prespecified one or more KQ4 outcomes but did not publish. It was not possible to determine whether eight of the nine registered trials for which we could not find a publication had actually been conducted or completed. Among 109 outcomes in 41 trials, trials did not give enough information to calculate a relative difference-in-change score (our primary analysis) for 6 outcomes due to statistically insignificant findings. Trials did not give enough information to conduct a meta-analysis on 16 outcomes. Our findings from the primary analysis are therefore less likely to be affected by publication bias than those from the meta-analysis.

Figure B1. Summary across measurement domains of comparisons of meditation with nonspecific active controls
[See combined legend for Figures B1 and B2 following the figures for further information, including explanations of symbols and definitions of lettered footnotes]

Outcome	Meditation Program	Population	Direction[a] (Magnitude[b]) of Effect	Number of Trials— Total [PO]: PA (MA);[c] Total N	SOE[d]
Anxiety (KQ1)	Mindfulness	Various	↑ (0% to +44%)	7 [3]: 6 (6); N = 558	Moderate for ↑
	Mantra	Various	Ø (−3% to +6%)	3 [2]: 3 (3); N = 237	Low for Ø
Depression (KQ1)	Mindfulness	Various	↑ (0% to +52%)	9 [4]: 8 (8); N = 768	Moderate for ↑
	Mantra	Various	↑↓ (−19% to +46%)	4 [1]: 4 (2); N = 420	Insufficient
Stress/Distress (KQ1)	Mindfulness	Various	↑ (+1% to +21%)	8 [3]: 6 (6*); N = 697	Low for ↑
	Mantra	Selected	Ø (−6% to +1%)	3 [1]: 3 (2); N = 219	Low for Ø
Negative Affect (KQ1)	Mindfulness	Various	↑ (0% to +44%)	13 [5]:11 (11**); N = 1,102	Low for ↑
	Mantra	Various	↑↓ (−3% to +46%)	5 [2]: 5 (0***); N = 438	Insufficient
Positive Affect (KQ1)	Mindfulness	Various	↑ (+1% to +55%)	3 [0]: 3 (3); N = 255	Insufficient
	TM (mantra)	CHF	Ø (+2%)	1 [0]: 1 (0); N = 23	Insufficient
Quality of Life (KQ1)	Mindfulness	Various	↑ (+5% to +28%)	4 [2]: 4 (3); N = 346	Low for ↑
Attention (KQ2)	Mindfulness	Caregivers	↑ (+15% to +81%)	1 [0]: 1 (0); N = 21	Insufficient
Sleep (KQ3)	Mindfulness	Various	↑↓ (−3% to +24%)	4 [1]: 3 (3); N = 451	Insufficient
Substance Use (KQ3)	TM (mantra)	CAD	Ø	1 [2]: 0 (0); N = 201	Insufficient
Pain (KQ4)	Mindfulness	Selected	↑ (+5% to +31%)	4 [2]: 4 (4); N = 341	Moderate for ↑
	TM (mantra)	CHF	Ø (−2%)	1 [2]: 1 (0); N = 23	Low for Ø
Weight (KQ4)	TM (mantra)	Selected	Ø (−1% to +2%)	3 [0]: 2 (0); N = 297	Low for Ø

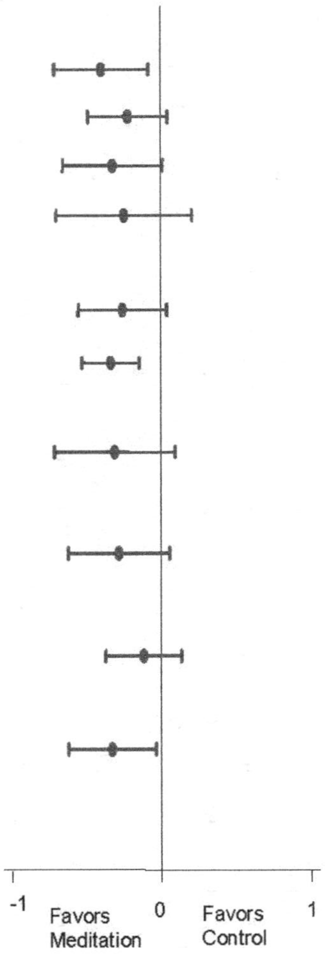

CAD = coronary artery disease; CHF = congestive heart failure; KQ = Key Question; MA = meta-analysis; PA = primary analysis;
PO = number of trials in which this was a primary outcome for the trial; SOE = strength of evidence; TM = transcendental meditation
Meta-analysis figure shows Cohen's d with the 95% confidence interval.
* Summary effect size not shown due to concern about publication bias for this outcome.
**Negative affect combines the outcomes of anxiety, depression, and stress/distress, and is thus duplicative of those outcomes.
***We did not perform meta-analysis on this outcome, since it would duplicate the anxiety meta-analysis for mantra. Two additional trials could be added (on depression) but did not have usable data that could be added to the anxiety meta-analysis. Anxiety and depression are indirect measures of negative affect, and therefore resulted in a lower strength of evidence than for the outcome of mantra on anxiety.

Figure B2. Summary across measurement domains of comparisons of meditation with specific active controls
[See combined legend for Figures B1 and B2 following the figures for further information, including explanations of symbols and definitions of lettered footnotes]

Outcome	Meditation Program	Population	Direction[a] (Magnitude[b]) of Effect	Number of Trials—Total [PO]: PA (MA);[c] Total N	SOE[d]
Anxiety (KQ1)	Mindfulness	Various	↑↓ (−39% to +8%)	9 [5]: 9 (8); N = 526	Insufficient
	CSM (mantra)	Anxiety	↓ (−6%)	1 [1]: 1 (0); N = 42	Insufficient
Depression (KQ1)	Mindfulness	Various	↑↓ (−32% to +23%)	11 [5]:11 (9); N = 821	Insufficient
	CSM (mantra)	Anxiety	↓ (−28%)	1 [1]: 1 (0); N = 42	Insufficient
Stress/Distress (KQ1)	Mindfulness	Various	↑↓ (−24% to +18%)	6 [4]: 6 (6); N = 508	Insufficient
Positive Affect (KQ1)	Mindfulness	Various	↑↓ (−45% to +10%)	4 [2]: 4 (4); N = 297	Insufficient
Quality of Life (KQ1)	Mindfulness	Various	↑↓ (−23% to +9%)	6 [1]: 6 (5); N = 472	Insufficient
Sleep (KQ3)	Mindfulness	Various	↑↓ (−2% to +15%)	3 [1]: 3 (2); N = 311	Insufficient
Eating (KQ3)	Mindfulness	Selected	↓ (−6% to −15%)	2 [1]: 2 (0); N = 158	Insufficient
Smoking/Alcohol (KQ3)	Mindfulness	Substance abuse	↑ (Ø to +21%)	2 [2]: 1 (0); N = 95	Insufficient
Alcohol Only (KQ3)	Mantra	Alcohol abuse	Ø (−5% to −36%)	2 [2]: 2 (0); N = 145	Low for Ø
Pain (KQ4)	Mindfulness	Selected	Ø (−1% to −32%)	4 [2]: 4 (4); N = 410	Low for Ø
Weight (KQ4)	Mindfulness	Selected	Ø (−2% to +1%)	2 [2]: 2 (0); N = 151	Low for Ø

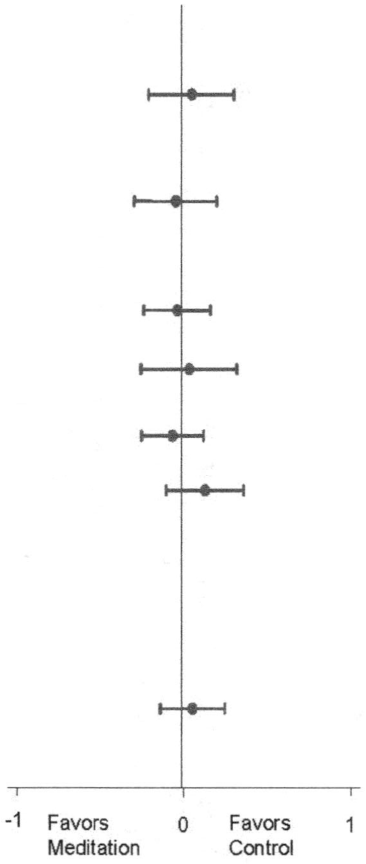

CSM = Clinically Standardized Meditation, a mantra meditation program; KQ = Key Question; MA = meta-analysis; PA = Primary Analysis; PO = Number of trials in which this was a primary outcome for the trial; SOE = strength of evidence

ES-13

Combined Legend for Figures B1 and B2

The figure on the far right shows the effect-size estimates using Cohen's d (in standard deviation units with the associated 95% confidence interval) for every outcome for which sufficient data were available to perform a meta-analysis. For comparisons with nonspecific active control, we included all eligible studies in the analysis for the outcomes of pain and positive affect for mindfulness trials, and for the outcome of anxiety for mantra trials. For comparisons with specific active control, we included all eligible studies in the analysis for the outcome of stress/distress, positive affect, and pain for mindfulness trials. For all other meta-analyses, we included only a subset of eligible studies because data were missing in some studies. One should interpret the meta-analysis results with caution because the inconsistent reporting of data suggests a possible reporting bias.

Footnote a: *Direction* —This is the direction of change in the outcome across trials based on the relative difference between groups in how the outcome measure changed from baseline in each trial. We calculate it as the difference between the change over time in the meditation group and the change over time in the control group, divided by the baseline mean for the meditation group.

- ↑ indicates that the meditation group improved relative to the control group (with a relative difference generally greater than or equal to 5% across trials).
- ↓ indicates the meditation group worsened relative to the control group (with a relative difference generally greater than or equal to 5% across trials).
- Ø indicates a null effect (with a relative difference generally less than 5% across trials).
- ↑↓ indicates inconsistent findings. Some trials reported improvement with meditation relative to control, while others showed no improvement or improvement in the control group relative to meditation.

Footnote b: *Magnitude* —This is the range of estimates across all trials in a particular domain based on the relative difference between groups in how the outcome measure changed from baseline in each trial. It is a relative percentage difference calculated as: {# (Meditation T2 - Meditation T1) - (Control T2 - Control T1)}/ (Meditation T1), where T1 = baseline mean and T2 = followup mean (after intervention or at the end of the study). This is a simple range of estimates, not a meta-analysis.

Footnote c: *Total number* —This is the number of trials that measured the outcome: primary outcome (PO), the number of trials for which this outcome was a primary outcome; primary analysis (PA), the number of trials that reported information that allowed us to calculate the relative difference between groups in the change score; and meta analysis (MA), the number of trials reporting sufficient information to be included in a meta-analysis. N refers to total sample size.

Footnote d: *Strength of evidence (SOE)* —We based SOE on the aggregate risk of bias, consistency across studies, directness of measures, and precision of estimates. We gave an SOE rating for the direction of effect in most cases.

Discussion

Forty-one RCTs included in this review tested the effects of meditation programs in clinical conditions relative to active controls. Ten programs tested mantra meditation, and 31 programs tested mindfulness meditation. Active control groups included nonspecific controls, as well as specific controls that offer an opportunity to examine the comparative effectiveness of meditation programs.

Our review finds that the mantra meditation programs do not appear to improve any of the outcomes we examined, but the strength of this evidence varies from low to insufficient. We find that, compared with nonspecific active controls, the mindfulness meditation programs show small improvements in anxiety, depression, and pain with moderate SOE, and small improvements in stress/distress, negative affect, and the mental health component of health-related quality of life with low SOE. The remaining outcomes had insufficient SOE to draw any level of conclusion for mindfulness meditation programs. We were unable to draw a high-grade SOE for either type of meditation program for any of the psychological stress and well-being outcomes. We also found no evidence for any harms, although few trials reported on this.

We found 32 trials for KQ1: 4 evaluating TM, 2 evaluating other mantra meditation, and 26 evaluating mindfulness meditation. In general, we found no evidence that mantra meditation programs improve psychological stress and well-being. Compared with a nonspecific active control, mindfulness meditation programs improve multiple dimensions of negative affect, including anxiety, depression, and perceived stress/general distress, and the mental health component of quality of life, with a low to moderate SOE. Well-being and positive mood are positive dimensions of mental health. While meditation programs generally seek to improve the positive dimensions of health, the available evidence from a very small number of studies did not show any effects on positive affect or well-being. Both analytic methods—the difference-in-change estimates (which accounted for baseline differences between groups) and the meta-analyses (which compared only end-line differences)—generally showed consistent but small effects for anxiety, depression, and stress/distress. However, there are a number of observations that help in interpreting and giving context to our conclusions.

First, very few mantra meditation programs were included in our review, significantly limiting our ability to draw inferences about the effects of mantra meditation programs on psychological stress-related outcomes. These conclusions did not change when we evaluated TM separately from other mantra meditation programs. Apart from the paucity of trials, another reason for seeing null results may be the type of populations studied; for example, three TM trials enrolled cardiac patients, while only one enrolled anxiety patients. In addition, it is not known whether these study participants had high levels of a particular negative affect to begin with.

Second, among mindfulness trials, the effects were significant for anxiety and marginally significant for depression at the end of treatment, and these effects continued to be significant at 3–6 months for both anxiety and depression.

Third, when we combine each outcome that is a subdomain of negative affect (anxiety, depression, and stress/distress), we see a small and consistent signal that any domain of negative affect is improved in mindfulness programs when compared with a nonspecific active control.

Fourth, the effect sizes are small. Over the course of 2–6 months, mindfulness meditation program effect-size estimates ranged from 0.22 to 0.40 for anxiety symptoms and 0.23 to 0.32 for depressive symptoms, and were statistically significant.

Fifth, there may be differences between trials for which these outcomes are a primary versus secondary focus, although we did not find any evidence for this. Some trials that had an outcome as a primary focus did not recruit based on high symptom levels of that outcome. Thus, the samples included in these trials more closely resemble a general primary care population, and there may not be room to measure an effect if symptom levels were low to start with (i.e., a "floor" effect).

Sixth, studies found an improvement in outcomes among the mindfulness groups (compared with control) only when they made comparisons against a nonspecific active control. In each comparison against a known treatment or therapy, mindfulness did not outperform the control for any outcome. This was true for all comparisons for any form of meditation for any KQ. Out of 53 comparisons with a specific active control, we found only 2 that showed a statistically significant improvement: mindfulness-based cognitive therapy improved quality of life in comparison with use of antidepressant drugs among depressed patients, and mindfulness therapy reduced cigarette consumption in comparison with the Freedom from Smoking program. However, we also found five comparisons for which the specific active control performed better, with statistically significant results, than the meditation programs. The comparisons with specific therapies led to highly inconsistent results for most outcomes (Figure B2) and indicated that meditative therapies were no better than the specific therapies they were being compared with. These include such therapies as exercise, yoga, progressive muscle relaxation, cognitive behavioral therapy, and medications.

One RCT compared a meditation program with active control on the outcome of attention. There were no statistically significant differences between groups on the Attentional Network Test. Trends suggested that the meditation program performed better than the nonspecific active control on this measure, although the difference did not reach statistical significance. These findings indicate the need for more comprehensive trials with a variety of clinical populations (e.g., people with disorders in which attention may be compromised) to provide a clearer understanding of the impact of meditation programs on attention.

Among the 13 trials evaluating the effects of meditation programs on health-related behaviors affected by stress, 4 evaluated the effect of meditation on substance use,[33,34,54,67] 2 evaluated eating,[43,50] and 7 evaluated sleep.[31,41,42,49,55,61,70] Overall, there is insufficient evidence to indicate that meditation programs alter health-related behaviors affected by stress. Our findings are consistent with those of previous reviews in this area, in which uncontrolled studies have usually found a benefit for the effects of meditation programs on health-related behaviors affected by stress, while very few controlled studies have found a similar benefit.[14-16]

Among the 14 RCTs evaluating the effect on pain and weight, we found moderate SOE that MBSR reduces pain severity to a small degree when compared with a nonspecific active control. This finding is based on four trials, of which two were conducted in musculoskeletal pain patients, one in patients with irritable bowel syndrome, and one in a nonpain population. Visceral pain had a large and statistically significant relative 30-percent improvement in pain severity, while musculoskeletal pain showed 5- to 8-percent improvements that were considered nonsignificant. We also found low SOE that MBSR was not superior in reducing pain severity when compared with various specific active controls (including massage). Two mindfulness trials evaluated weight as an outcome, and it was a primary outcome for both. Three TM trials evaluated weight as a secondary outcome. Due to consistently null results, there was low SOE to suggest that TM and MBSR do not have an effect on weight.

The comparative effectiveness of an intervention obviously depends heavily on what is done for the comparison group. A strength of our review is our focus on RCTs with nonspecific active controls, which should give us greater confidence that the reported benefits are not due to having a flawed comparison group that does not control for nonspecific effects, as seen in trials using a wait-list or usual-care control.

Limitations of the Primary Studies

Although we collected information on amount of training provided, the trials did not provide enough information to make use of the data. We could not draw definitive conclusions about effect modifiers, such as dose and duration, because of the limited amount of data.

It may be that specific outcome measurement scales may be more relevant for a particular form of meditation than for others. Many studies assessed only certain measures, and the scales may have been limited in their ability to detect an effect.

We intended to evaluate the effects of meditation programs on a broad range of medical and psychiatric conditions, since psychological stress outcomes are not limited to any particular medical or psychiatric condition. Despite our focus on active RCTs, we were unable to detect a specific effect of meditation on most outcomes, with the majority of our evidence grades being insufficient or low. This was mostly driven by two important evaluation criteria: risk of bias and inconsistencies in the body of evidence. The reasons for such inconsistencies may include differences in the particular clinical conditions, as well as the type of control groups that studies used. We could not easily compare studies in which a meditation program was compared with a specific active control versus trials that used a nonspecific active control. We therefore separated these comparisons in order to be able to evaluate the effects against a relatively homogeneous nonspecific active control group. In general, comparing trials that used one specific active control with trials that used another specific active control led to large inconsistencies that could be explained by differences in the control groups.

Another possibility is that programs had no real effect on many of the outcomes that had inconsistent findings. While some of the outcomes were primary outcomes, many were secondary outcomes, and the studies may not have been appropriately powered to detect changes in secondary outcomes.

Limitations of the Review

Our assessment of a 5-percent relative difference between groups in change scores as being potentially clinically significant needs to be interpreted in the context of heterogeneous scales reporting on various measures. The literature does not clearly define the appropriate threshold for what is clinically significant on many of these scales. Some may consider a higher threshold as being clinically relevant.

While this review sought to assess the effectiveness of meditation programs above and beyond the nonspecific effects of expectation and attention, it did not assess the preferences of patients. Even though one therapy may not be better than another, many patients may still prefer it for personal or philosophical reasons.

We were limited in our ability to determine the overall applicability of the body of evidence to the broad population of patients who could benefit from mindfulness meditation because the studies varied so much in many ways other than just the specific targeted population; that is, they also varied in characteristics of the intervention, comparator, outcomes, timing, and setting. Also, the studies generally did not provide enough information to be able to determine whether the effectiveness of mindfulness meditation varied by race, ethnicity, or education.

Future Directions

Further research in meditation would benefit by addressing several remaining methodological and conceptual issues. First, all forms of meditation, including both mindfulness and mantra, imply that more time spent meditating will yield larger effects. Most forms, but not all, also present meditation as a skill that requires expert instruction and time dedicated to practice. Thus, more training with an expert and practice in daily life should lead to greater competency in the skill or practice, and greater competency or practice would presumably lead to better outcomes. When compared with other skills that require training, the amount of training afforded in the trials included in our review was quite small, and generally the training was offered over a fairly short period of time. Researchers should account for or consider the level of skill in meditation and how variation in skill may affect the effectiveness of meditation when designing studies, collecting data, and interpreting data. To facilitate this, better measurement tools are needed. Research has not adequately validated currently available mindfulness scales, and the scales do not appear to distinguish between different forms of meditation.[26] Thus, we need further work on the operationalization and measurement of the particular meditative skill. For meditation programs that do not consider themselves to be training students in a skill, such as TM and certain mindfulness programs, there is still a need to transparently assess whether a student has attained a certain mental state or is correctly executing the recommended mental activities (or absence of activities).

Second, trials need to document the amount of training instructors provide and patients receive, along with the amount of home practice patients complete. This information gives an indication of how effective the program is at delivering training and how adherent participants were. This will allow us to address questions around "dosing."

Third, studies should report on teacher qualifications in detail. The range of experience in meditation and competence as a teacher of the skill or practice likely plays a role in outcomes.

Fourth, when using a specific active control, if one finds no statistically significant superiority over the control, one is left with the issue of whether the meditation is equivalent to or not inferior to the control, or whether the trial was just underpowered to detect any difference. Conducting comparative effectiveness trials requires prior specification of the hypothesis (superiority, equivalence, noninferiority) and appropriate determination of the margins of clinical significance and minimum importance difference.[72] In the case of equivalence and noninferiority, trials also need to have appropriate assay sensitivity. None of the trials showed statistically significant effects against a specific active control, nor did they appear adequately powered to assess noninferiority or equivalence. These issues leave a lot of uncertainty in such trial designs.

Fifth, positive outcomes are a key focus of meditative practices. However, most trials did not include positive outcomes as primary or even secondary outcomes. Future studies should expand on these domains.

Sixth, we were unable to review biological markers of stress for meditation programs. A comprehensive review would benefit meditation research and also allow for a cross-validation of psychological and biological outcomes.

Future trials should appropriately report key design characteristics so we can accurately assess risk of bias. Future trials should register the trial on a national register, standardize training using trainers who meet specified criteria, specify primary and secondary outcomes a priori, power the trial based on the primary outcomes, use CONSORT (CONsolidated Standards of Reporting Trials) recommendations for reporting results, and operationalize and measure the practice of meditation by study participants.

Conclusions

Our review found moderate SOE that mindfulness meditation programs are beneficial for reducing anxiety, depression, and pain severity, and low SOE that they may lead to improvement in any dimension of negative affect when compared with nonspecific active controls. There was no advantage of meditation programs over specific therapies they were compared with. Otherwise, much of the evidence was insufficient to address the comparisons for most of the questions.

There are reasons why a large number of outcomes lacked sufficient evidence. While we sought to review the highest standards of behavioral RCTs that controlled for nonspecific factors, there was wide variation in risk of bias among these trials. Another reason for a lack of sufficient evidence is that we found a limited number of trials for most outcomes, resulting in limited data available for meta-analysis or descriptive synthesis. For example, there were so few trials of TM that we could not draw meaningful conclusions from them. In addition, the reasons for a lack of significant reduction of stress-related outcomes may be related to the way the research community conceptualizes meditation programs, the difficulties of acquiring meditation skills or meditative states, and the limited duration of RCTs. Historically, the general public has not conceptualized meditation as a quick fix toward anything. It is a skill or state one learns and practices over time to increase one's awareness, and through this awareness gain insight and understanding into the various subtleties of one's existence. Training the mind in awareness, nonjudgmentalness, and the ability to become completely free of thoughts or other activity are daunting accomplishments. While some meditators may feel these tasks are easy, they likely overestimate their own skills due to a lack of awareness of the different degrees to which these tasks can be done or the ability to objectively measure their own progress. Since becoming an expert at simple skills such as swimming, reading, or writing (which can be objectively measured by others) takes a considerable amount of time, it follows that meditation would also take a long period of time to master. However many of the studies included in this review were short term (e.g., 2.5 hours a week for 8 weeks), and the participants likely did not achieve a level of expertise needed to improve outcomes that depend on a mastery of mental and emotional processes. The short-term nature of the studies, combined with the lack of an adequate way to measure meditation competency, could have significantly contributed to results.

References

1. National Center for Complementary and Alternative Medicine (NCCAM) [Web Page]. http://nccam.nih.gov. Accessed January 2012.

2. Barnes PM, Bloom B, Nahin RL. Complementary and alternative medicine use among adults and children: United States, 2007. Natl Health Stat Rep. 2008;(12):1-23.

3. Goyal M, Haythornthwaite J, Levine D, et al. Intensive meditation for refractory pain and symptoms. J Altern Complement Med. 2010;16(6):627-31.

4. Bohlmeijer E, Prenger R, Taal E, et al. The effects of mindfulness-based stress reduction therapy on mental health of adults with a chronic medical disease: a meta-analysis. J Psychosom Res. 2010;68(6):539-44.

5. Chambers R, Gallone E, Allen NB. Mindful emotion regulation: an integrative review. Clin Psychol Rev. 2009;29(6):560-72.

6. Chiesa A, Serretti A. Mindfulness-based stress reduction for stress management in healthy people: a review and meta-analysis. J Altern Complement Med. 2009;15(5):593-600.

7. Chiesa A, Calati R, Serretti A. Does mindfulness training improve cognitive abilities? A systematic review of neuropsychological findings. Clin Psychol Rev. 2011;31(3):449-64.

8. Chiesa A, Serretti A. Mindfulness based cognitive therapy for psychiatric disorders: a systematic review and meta-analysis. Psychiatry Res. 2011;187(3):441-53.

9. Hofmann SG, Sawyer SG, Wilt AA, et al. The effect of mindfulness-based therapy on anxiety and depression: a meta-analytic review. J Consult Clin Psychol. 2010;78(2):169-83.

10. Krisanaprakornkit T, Ngamjarus C, Witoonchart C, et al. Meditation therapies for attention-deficit/hyperactivity disorder (ADHD). Cochrane Database Syst Rev. 2010; (6):CD006507.

11. Ledesma D, Kumano H. Mindfulness-based stress reduction and cancer: a meta-analysis. Psychooncology. 2009;18(6):571-9.

12. Matchim Y, Armer JM, Stewart BR. Mindfulness-based stress reduction among breast cancer survivors: a literature review and discussion. Oncol Nurs Forum. 2011;38(2):E61-71.

13. Piet J, Hougaard E. The effect of mindfulness-based cognitive therapy for prevention of relapse in recurrent major depressive disorder: a systematic review and meta-analysis. Clin Psychol Rev. 2011;31(6):1032-40.

14. Wanden-Berghe RG, Sanz-Valero J, Wanden-Berghe C. The application of mindfulness to eating disorders treatment: a systematic review. Eat Disord. 2011;19(1):34-48.

15. Winbush NY, Gross CR, Kreitzer MJ. The effects of mindfulness-based stress reduction on sleep disturbance: a systematic review. Explore (NY). 2007;3(6):585-91.

16. Zgierska A, Rabago D, Chawla N, et al. Mindfulness meditation for substance use disorders: a systematic review. Subst Abus. 2009;30(4):266-94.

17. Bernardy K, Fuber N, Kollner V, et al. Efficacy of cognitive-behavioral therapies in fibromyalgia syndrome—a systematic review and metaanalysis of randomized controlled trials. J Rheumatol. 2010;37(10):1991-2005.

18. Rainforth MV, Schneider RH, Nidich SI, et al. Stress reduction programs in patients with elevated blood pressure: a systematic review and meta-analysis. Curr Hypertens Rep. 2007;9(6):520-8.

19. Anderson JW, Liu C, Kryscio RJ. Blood pressure response to transcendental meditation: a meta-analysis. Am J Hypertens. 2008;21(3):310-6.

20. Canter PH, Ernst E. The cumulative effects of Transcendental Meditation on cognitive function—a systematic review of randomised controlled trials. Wien Klin Wochenschr. 2003;115(21-22):758-66.

21. So KT, Orme-Johnson DW. Three randomized experiments on the longitudinal effects of the Transcendental Meditation technique on cognition. Intelligence. 2001;419-40.

22. Travis F GS, Stixrud W. ADHD, brain functioning, and Transcendental Meditation practice. Mind Brain J Psychiatry. 2011;73-81.

23. Chen KW, Berger CC, Manheimer E, et al. Meditative therapies for reducing anxiety: a systematic review and meta-analysis of randomized controlled trials. Depress Anxiety. 2012; 29(7):545-62.

24. Chambless DL, Hollon SD. Defining empirically supported therapies. J Consult Clin Psychol. 1998;66(1):7-18.

25. Hollon SD, Ponniah K. A review of empirically supported psychological therapies for mood disorders in adults. Depress Anxiety. 2010;27(10):891-932.

26. Chiesa A, Malinowski P. Mindfulness-based approaches: are they all the same? J Clin Psychol. 2011;67(4):404-24.

27. Rapgay L, Bystrisky A. Classical mindfulness: an introduction to its theory and practice for clinical application. Ann N Y Acad Sci. 2009;1172:148-62.

28. Methods Guide for Effectiveness and Comparative Effectiveness Reviews. AHRQ Publication No. 10(11)-EHC063-EF. Rockville, MD: Agency for Healthcare Research and Quality; 2011. Chapters available at www.effectivehealthcare.ahrq.gov.

29. Higgins JP, Altman DG, Gotzsche PC, et al. The Cochrane Collaboration's tool for assessing risk of bias in randomised trials. BMJ. 2011;343:d5928.

30. Higgins JPT, Green S, eds. Cochrane Handbook for Systematic Reviews of Interventions, Version 5.1.0. London: The Cochrane Collaboration; updated March 2011. www.cochrane.org/training/cochrane-handbook. Accessed February 17, 2012.

31. Barrett B, Hayney MS, Muller D, et al. Meditation or exercise for preventing acute respiratory infection: a randomized controlled trial. Ann Fam Med. 2012;10(4):337-46.

32. Bormann JE, Gifford AL, Shively M, et al. Effects of spiritual mantram repetition on HIV outcomes: a randomized controlled trial. J Behav Med. 2006;29(4):359-76.

33. Brewer JA, Sinha R, Chen JA, et al. Mindfulness training and stress reactivity in substance abuse: results from a randomized, controlled stage I pilot study. Subst Abus. 2009;30(4):306-17.

34. Brewer JA, Mallik S, Babuscio TA, et al. Mindfulness training for smoking cessation: results from a randomized controlled trial. Drug Alcohol Depend. 2011 Dec 11;19(1-2):72-80.

35. Castillo-Richmond A, Schneider RH, Alexander CN, et al. Effects of stress reduction on carotid atherosclerosis in hypertensive African Americans. Stroke. 2000;31(3):568-73.

36. Chiesa A, Mandelli L, Serretti A. Mindfulness-based cognitive therapy versus psycho-education for patients with major depression who did not achieve remission following antidepressant treatment: a preliminary analysis. J Altern Complement Med. 2012;18(8):756-60.

37. Delgado LC, Guerra P, Perakakis P, et al. Treating chronic worry: psychological and physiological effects of a training programme based on mindfulness. Behav Res Ther. 2010;48(9):873-82.

38. Elder C, Aickin M, Bauer V, et al. Randomized trial of a whole-system ayurvedic protocol for type 2 diabetes. Altern Ther Health Med. 2006;12(5):24-30.

39. Garland EL, Gaylord SA, Boettiger CA, et al. Mindfulness training modifies cognitive, affective, and physiological mechanisms implicated in alcohol dependence: results of a randomized controlled pilot trial. J Psychoactive Drugs. 2010;42(2):177-92.

40. Gaylord SA, Palsson OS, Garland EL, et al. Mindfulness training reduces the severity of irritable bowel syndrome in women: results of a randomized controlled trial. Am J Gastroenterol. 2011;106(9):1678-88.

41. Gross CR, Kreitzer MJ, Thomas W, et al. Mindfulness-based stress reduction for solid organ transplant recipients: a randomized controlled trial. Altern Ther Health Med. 2010;16(5):30-8.

42. Gross CR, Kreitzer MJ, Reilly-Spong M, et al. Mindfulness-based stress reduction versus pharmacotherapy for chronic primary insomnia: a randomized controlled clinical trial. Explore (NY). 2011;7(2):76-87.

43. Hebert JR, Ebbeling CB, Olendzki BC, et al. Change in women's diet and body mass following intensive intervention for early-stage breast cancer. J Am Diet Assoc. 2001;101(4):421-31.

44. Jayadevappa R, Johnson JC, Bloom BS, et al. Effectiveness of transcendental meditation on functional capacity and quality of life of African Americans with congestive heart failure: a randomized control study. Ethn Dis. 2007 Winter;17(1):72-77. Erratum in Ethn Dis. 2007 Summer;7(3):595.

45. Jazaieri H, Goldin PR, Werner K, et al. A randomized trial of MBSR versus aerobic exercise for social anxiety disorder. J Clin Psychol. 2012 May 23. Epub ahead of print.

46. Kuyken W, Byford S, Taylor RS, et al. Mindfulness-based cognitive therapy to prevent relapse in recurrent depression. J Consult Clin Psychol. 2008;76(6):966-78.

47. Lee SH, Ahn SC, Lee YJ, et al. Effectiveness of a meditation-based stress management program as an adjunct to pharmacotherapy in patients with anxiety disorder. J Psychosom Res. 2007;62(2):189-95.

48. Lehrer PM. Progressive relaxation and meditation: a study of psychophysiological and therapeutic differences between two techniques. Behav Res Ther. 1983;21(6):651-62.

49. Malarkey WB, Jarjoura D, Klatt M. Workplace based mindfulness practice and inflammation: a randomized trial. Brain Behav Immun. 2013 Jan;27(1):145-54.

50. Miller CK, Kristeller JL, Headings A, et al. Comparative effectiveness of a mindful eating intervention to a diabetes self-management intervention among adults with type 2 diabetes: a pilot study. J Acad Nutr Diet. 2012;112(11):1835-42.

51. Moritz S, Quan H, Rickhi B, et al. A home study-based spirituality education program decreases emotional distress and increases quality of life—a randomized, controlled trial. Altern Ther Health Med. 2006;12(6):26-35.

52. Morone NE, Rollman BL, Moore CG, et al. A mind-body program for older adults with chronic low back pain: results of a pilot study. Pain Med. 2009;10(8):1395-407.

53. Mularski RA, Munjas BA, Lorenz KA, et al. Randomized controlled trial of mindfulness-based therapy for dyspnea in chronic obstructive lung disease. J Altern Complement Med. 2009;15(10):1083-90.

54. Murphy TJ, Pagano RR, Marlatt GA. Lifestyle modification with heavy alcohol drinkers: effects of aerobic exercise and meditation. Addict Behav. 1986;11(2):175-86.

55. Oken BS, Fonareva I, Haas M, et al. Pilot controlled trial of mindfulness meditation and education for dementia caregivers. J Altern Complement Med. 2010;16(10):1031-8.

56. Paul-Labrador M, Polk D, Dwyer JH, et al. Effects of a randomized controlled trial of transcendental meditation on components of the metabolic syndrome in subjects with coronary heart disease. Arch Intern Med. 2006;166(11):1218-24.

57. Pbert L, Madison JM, Druker S, et al. Effect of mindfulness training on asthma quality of life and lung function: a randomised controlled trial. Thorax. 2012; 67(9):769-76.

58. Philippot P, Nef F, Clauw L, et al. A randomized controlled trial of mindfulness-based cognitive therapy for treating tinnitus. Clin Psychol Psychother. 2012 Sep;19(5):411-9.

59. Piet J, Hougaard E, Hecksher MS, et al. A randomized pilot study of mindfulness-based cognitive therapy and group cognitive-behavioral therapy for young adults with social phobia. Scand J Psychol. 2010;51(5):403-10.

60. Plews-Ogan M, Owens JE, Goodman M, et al. A pilot study evaluating mindfulness-based stress reduction and massage for the management of chronic pain. J Gen Intern Med. 2005;20(12):1136-8.

61. Schmidt S, Grossman P, Schwarzer B, et al. Treating fibromyalgia with mindfulness-based stress reduction: results from a 3-armed randomized controlled trial. Pain. 2011; 152(2):361-9.

62. Schneider RH, Grim CE, Rainforth MV, et al. Stress reduction in the secondary prevention of cardiovascular disease: randomized, controlled trial of transcendental meditation and health education in Blacks. Circ Cardiovasc Qual Outcomes. 2012 Nov;5(6):750-8.

63. Segal ZV, Bieling P, Young T, et al. Antidepressant monotherapy vs sequential pharmacotherapy and mindfulness-based cognitive therapy, or placebo, for relapse prophylaxis in recurrent depression. Arch Gen Psychiatry. 2010;67(12):1256-64.

64. SeyedAlinaghi S, Jam S, Foroughi M, et al. Randomized controlled trial of mindfulness-based stress reduction delivered to human immunodeficiency virus-positive patients in Iran: effects on CD4^{+} T lymphocyte count and medical and psychological symptoms. Psychosom Med. 2012;74(6):620-7.

65. Henderson VP, Clemow L, Massion AO, et al. The effects of mindfulness-based stress reduction on psychosocial outcomes and quality of life in early-stage breast cancer patients: a randomized trial. Breast Cancer Res Treat. 2012 Jan;131(1):99-109.

66. Smith JC. Psychotherapeutic effects of transcendental meditation with controls for expectation of relief and daily sitting. J Consult Clin Psychol. 1976;44(4):630-7.

67. Taub E, Steiner SS, Weingarten E, et al. Effectiveness of broad spectrum approaches to relapse prevention in severe alcoholism: a long-term, randomized, controlled trial of Transcendental Meditation, EMG biofeedback and electronic neurotherapy. Alcoholism Treatment Q. 1994;11(1-2):187-220.

68. Koszycki D, Benger M, Shlik J, et al. Randomized trial of a meditation-based stress reduction program and cognitive behavior therapy in generalized social anxiety disorder. Behav Res Ther. 2007;45(10):2518-26.

69. Whitebird RR, Kreitzer M, Crain AL, et al. Mindfulness-based stress reduction for family caregivers: a randomized controlled trial. Gerontologist. 2013;53(4):676-86.

70. Wolever RQ, Bobinet KJ, McCabe K, et al. Effective and viable mind-body stress reduction in the workplace: a randomized controlled trial. J Occup Health Psychol. 2012;17(2):246-58.

71. Wong SY, Chan FW, Wong RL, et al. Comparing the effectiveness of mindfulness-based stress reduction and multidisciplinary intervention programs for chronic pain: a randomized comparative trial. Clin J Pain. 2011;27(8):724-34.

72. Treadwell JR, Singh S, Talati R, et al. A Framework for "Best Evidence" Approaches in Systematic Reviews. Methods Research Report. (Prepared by the ECRI Institute Evidence-based Practice Center under Contract No. HHSA 290-2007-10063-I). AHRQ Publication No. 11-EHC046-EF. Rockville, MD: Agency for Healthcare Research and Quality; June 2011.

Introduction

Definition of Meditation

The National Center for Complementary and Alternative Medicine defines meditation as a mind-body method. This category includes interventions that employ a variety of techniques designed to facilitate the mind's capacity to affect bodily function and symptoms. In meditation, a person learns to focus attention. Some forms of meditation instruct the student to become mindful of thoughts, feelings, and sensations and to observe them in a nonjudgmental way. Practitioners generally believe these results in a state of greater calmness, physical relaxation, and psychological balance.[1]

Current Practice and Prevalence of Use

A national survey in 2008 shows a marked increase in the number of people meditating, with approximately 10 percent of the population having some experience with meditation.[2] Many people use meditation to treat stress and stress-related conditions, as well as to promote health.[2,3] In the United States, most meditation training and support has been provided through community resources, and in recent years a number of hospitals and programs offer courses in meditation to patients seeking alternative or additional methods to relieve symptoms or to promote health.

Forms of Meditation

Researchers have categorized meditative techniques into two forms, those that emphasize "concentration," such as transcendental meditation (TM) and other mantra-based meditation programs, and those that emphasize "mindfulness," such as mindfulness-based stress reduction (MBSR) and mindfulness-based cognitive therapy (MBCT). However this distinction is overly simplistic and may not adequately differentiate the effects of the techniques or the particular skills they teach.[4,5] Both forms appear to involve concentration or focused attention at some point in the training, although the object of attention may differ. Both forms prescribe a mental activity, or non-activity (which itself may be considered an activity by some), associated with the focused attention. Both forms appear to describe an attitude or intention associated with these practices. Furthermore, both forms appear to be dynamic. That is, as a student gains experience, understanding, and/or skill in the practice, their state of awareness and approach to the meditation may evolve. That being said, most descriptions of meditation do not account for this dynamic nature of meditation, and, in fact, some practitioners and instructors may not feel their particular form of meditation has an evolutionary component.

Meditation training is rarely manualized and there are challenges to knowing whether teachers within a practice tradition differ in their understanding of the practice, or whether they emphasize different aspects of the practice. Since meditation is within the mind, and there is not an established way to measure precisely what is being done, there are also significant challenges to knowing what exactly a student is doing when practicing.

The mantra-based techniques practiced in the United States primarily consist of TM, a program established by Maharishi Mahesh Yogi around 1955, and a few others that use a mantra as part of their meditative technique. Many consider TM instruction to be a standardized program that generally consists of daily 1–1.5 hour meetings for 1 week, then periodic meetings, roughly weekly, after the first week for the first month or so, and less frequently after that. Students also receive instructions for home practice and are expected to practice daily. While a mantra is given to each student, there is a dynamic nature to the practice in that the mantra is used as a vehicle to transcend mental activity.[6] This process has been referred to as "automatic self-transcending"—a process of meditation where one attempts to reach a state of being through meditation. In spite of TM having previously been labeled as a "concentration" form of meditation, some TM experts believe "proper" technique should not teach one to focus attention on the mantra. Rather, one should use the mantra in such a way that the mantra is "innocently" transcended. However, it is not clear how a practitioner can use mantra without focusing attention on it at least initially, nor what other mental activities or attitudes one needs to innocently transcend the mantra. Experts maintain that TM is different from all other forms of mantra meditation, but it is not clear specifically how one transcends the mantra in TM but not in other mantra-style meditations. However, emphasis is placed on the effortlessness of the technique, and electroencephalography has indicated a difference between automatic self-transcendence, and mindful focused attention/nonjudgmental awareness of the present moment.[6] While some meditative techniques require the ongoing development of skills, some experts feel this is not the case with TM. That is, the technique does not take long to learn, and once learned there is no further skill set to develop.

Mindfulness-based programs include MBSR and its adaptation MBCT. Most consider MBSR and MBCT to be standardized programs. However, instructors vary somewhat in how they teach the programs, partly depending on the clientele. Typically, the programs consist of weekly meetings for 8 weeks, each lasting 2 to 2.5 hours, with an additional 6–8 hour retreat on a weekend day in the middle of the 8-week training. In addition, students receive instructions for daily home practice. MBCT maintains an 8-week course length, similar to MBSR, but instructors modified MBCT for the particular condition of depression. Other adaptations have tried (usually) shorter versions of the program lasting 4 or more weeks targeting different conditions and providing varying amounts of meditation training during that time. Vipassana and Zen are the original practices from which MBSR and other mindfulness-based techniques are derived.[4]

Despite its growing popularity, there remains uncertainty as to what mindfulness exactly is and inconsistency as to how it is taught.[4] Mindfulness has been described as self-regulating attention toward the immediate present moment and adopting an orientation marked by curiosity, openness, and acceptance.[7] Others have described mindfulness as including five key components: nonreactivity, observing, acting with awareness, describing, and non-judging.[8-10] Still others have criticized these descriptions, noting that originally the practice emphasized qualities of awareness, which are not adequately captured by these definitions.[11,12] The number of mindfulness-based practices that have been created to target particular conditions, such as MBCT for depression, appear to be more focused on solving problems related to particular conditions rather than cultivating the general qualities of awareness. Thus, the conceptual and practical heterogeneity of mindfulness programs further complicates an understanding of what mindfulness is and how it differs both between and within different programs.

Some "mindfulness" approaches, such as dialectical behavioral therapy and acceptance and commitment therapy, do not use mindfulness as the foundation but rather as an ancillary component. Others, such as yoga and tai chi, involve a significant amount of movement. And although these techniques also contain a meditative component, it is often difficult to ascertain the effects of meditation itself on various outcomes separate from the physiological effects of the exercise component.[13,14] Many of the yoga interventions, in particular, do not clearly indicate how much meditation is involved in the intervention. Qi gong is a broad term encompassing both meditation and movement, as such, we're faced with similar difficulties parsing the effects of movement from the effects of meditation.

It should be noted that although this report evaluates the health effects of meditation programs, meditation historically was not necessarily practiced for a specific health benefit. For many the goal was either philosophical or spiritual enlightenment, a sense of mental and physical peace and calm, self-inquiry, or a combination of these. Our review does not include these more classic goals of meditation, but instead focuses primarily on health benefits. We respectfully acknowledge that some experts regard this focus on specific health outcomes as a diversion from what meditation research should ideally evaluate.

Psychological Stress and Well-Being

As a mind-body method, many believe meditation uses mental processes to influence physical functioning and promote health.[1] The potential effects on function and health are postulated to occur by reducing negative emotions, cognitions, and behaviors; increasing positive emotions, cognitions, and behaviors; and altering relevant physiological processes. While some of these effects can be immediate (i.e., observed within seconds of beginning meditation), the health effects are typically postulated to occur following longer-term practice (i.e., weeks, months, or even years). For the purpose of this review, we use the phrase psychological stress and well-being to refer to a range of negative and positive emotions, cognitions, and behaviors that are known to change with exposure to acute or chronic stress. Emotions include the following: general negative affect, as well as specific emotions such as anxiety and depression; general positive affect, as well as psychological well-being; perceived stress, which generally measures a perceived loss of control; and the mental-health component of health-related quality of life. Cognitions include attention. And behaviors include a range of stress-reactive appetitive behaviors, such as eating, sleeping, smoking, and the use of alcohol or recreational drugs. Although the studies we included did not always directly link these outcomes to stress, these outcomes are generally studied in groups exposed to stress, either due to having a chronic health condition that could be construed as stressful (e.g., cancer, chronic pain, or an anxiety disorder) or due to caring for someone with a debilitating chronic medical condition (e.g., dementia).

Outcomes largely include self-reported changes in psychological stress and well-being, which range from the rare examination of well-being to the more common measurement of negative emotions and behavior, such as anxiety or sleep disturbance. During the development of this report, based on input from technical experts, we decided to include measures of pain since it was thought to be the number-one reason people meditate. We also included measurement of weight as an objective measure of eating behavior. Both pain and weight are therefore included as a fourth Key Question (KQ) based on this input. While there are many physiological/biological markers of stress, we did not include such intermediate markers in this report because we thought it was important to keep this report focused on outcomes that are clinically meaningful to patients.

Some studies investigate changes in symptoms related to the primary condition (e.g., pain in patients with low back pain, or anxiety in patients with social phobia), whereas others measure emotional symptoms in clinical groups who may or may not present with clinically significant symptoms (e.g., anxiety or depression in individuals with cancer). Because the effectiveness of meditation interventions is unclear and may vary among different subgroups, such as those with a particular clinical condition (e.g., anxiety or pain), we maintained broad inclusion criteria so as to enable subgroup analysis if possible.

Evidence to Date

Studies and reviews to date have demonstrated that both "mindfulness" and "mantra" meditation techniques reduce emotional symptoms (e.g., anxiety and depression, stress) and improve physical symptoms (e.g., pain) to a small to moderate degree.[11,15-33] The populations studied have included healthy adults as well as those with a range of clinical and psychiatric conditions.

The meditation literature has significant limitations related to inadequate control comparisons. For the most part previous reviews have included uncontrolled studies or studies that used control groups for which they did not provide any additional treatment (i.e., usual care or "waiting list"). In wait-list controlled studies, the control group receives usual care while "waiting" to receive the intervention at some time in the future, providing a usual-care control for the purposes of the study. Thus, it is unclear whether the apparently beneficial effects of meditation training are a result of the expectations for improvement that participants naturally form when obtaining this type of treatment. Additionally, many programs involve lengthy and sustained efforts on the part of both participants and trainers, possibly yielding beneficial effects from the added attention, group participation, and support participants receive as well as from the suggestion from trainers that symptoms will likely improve with these increased efforts.[34,35]

Due to the heterogeneity of control groups used in past meditation research, we chose to focus this review on only those studies that included a well-defined control group so that we could draw conclusions about the specific effects of meditation on psychological stress and well-being. An informative analogy is the use of placebos in pharmaceutical or surgical trials. Researchers typically design placebos to match to the "active intervention" in order to elicit the same expectations of benefit on the part of both provider and patient. Additionally, placebo treatment includes all components of care received by the "active" group, including office visits and patient-provider interactions in which the provider engages with the patient in the same way irrespective of which group they are randomized to. These nonspecific factors are particularly important to control when evaluation of outcome relies on patient reporting. Since double-blinding has not been feasible in the evaluation of the effects of meditation, the challenge to execute studies that are not biased by these nonspecific factors is more pressing.[13] As inquiry in this field has advanced over the last few decades, a larger number of trials have moved to a more rigorous design standard by using higher quality controls and blinded evaluators. Thus, there is a clear need to determine the specific effects of meditation based on randomized trials in which expectations for outcome and attentional support from health care professionals are controlled.

Clinical and Policy Relevance

Much uncertainty exists about the differences and similarities between the effects of various forms of meditation.[4,12] Given the increasing use of meditation across a large number of conditions, it is important for patients, clinicians, and policymakers to understand the effects of meditation, the conditions for which meditation is efficacious, and whether the type of meditation practiced influences these outcomes. While some reviews have focused on RCTs, many if not most of the included studies involved wait-list or usual-care controls. Thus, we sought to provide information on the specific incremental effects of meditation programs relative to alternative care in which expectations for outcome and attentional support from health care professionals are controlled.

Objectives

The objectives of this systematic review are to evaluate the effects of meditation programs on affect, attention, and health-related behaviors affected by stress, pain, and weight, among those with a medical or psychiatric condition in RCTs with appropriate comparators.

Scope and Key Questions

This report reviews the efficacy of meditation programs on psychological stress and well-being among those with a clinical condition. Affect refers to emotion or mood. It can be positive such as the feeling of well-being, or negative such as anxiety, depression, or stress. Studies usually measure affect through self-reported questionnaires in which the respondent describes affect over a period of time. In some studies, clinicians use structured interviews to quantify symptoms of depression. Attention refers to the ability to maintain focus on particular stimuli, and clinicians measure this directly. They measure substance use as the amount consumed or smoked over a period of time, and include alcohol consumption, cigarette smoking, or other drugs, such as cocaine. Studies measure sleep as the amount of time spent sleeping versus awake, or as overall sleep quality. They measure sleep time through either polysomnography or actigraphy, and sleep quality through self-reported questionnaires. Studies measure eating by food diaries to calculate how much energy or fat a person has consumed over a particular period of time. They measure pain similar to affect, by a self-reported questionnaire to assess how much pain an individual is experiencing. It has two dimensions, severity and interference. Studies usually measure pain severity on a numerical rating scale from 0–10 or other self-reported questionnaire. Pain interference measures how much the pain is interfering with life and studies measure it on a self-reported scale. Studies measure weight in pounds or kilograms. The KQs are as follows.

Key Question 1. What are the efficacy and harms of meditation programs on negative affect (e.g., anxiety, stress) and positive affect (e.g., well-being) among those with a clinical condition (medical or psychiatric)?

Key Question 2. What are the efficacy and harms of meditation programs on attention among those with a clinical condition (medical or psychiatric)?

Key Question 3. What are the efficacy and harms of meditation programs on health-related behaviors affected by stress, specifically substance use, sleep, and eating, among those with a clinical condition (medical or psychiatric)?

Key Question 4. What are the efficacy and harms of meditation programs on pain and weight among those with a clinical condition (medical or psychiatric)?

Analytic Framework

We present our analytic framework for the systematic review in Figure 1. The figure illustrates the populations of interest, the meditation programs, and the outcomes that we reviewed. This figure depicts the KQs within the context of the Population, Intervention, Comparator, Outcomes, Timing, and Setting (PICOTS) framework described in Table 1. Adverse events may occur at any point after the meditation program has begun.

Figure 1. Analytic framework for meditation programs conducted in clinical and psychiatric populations

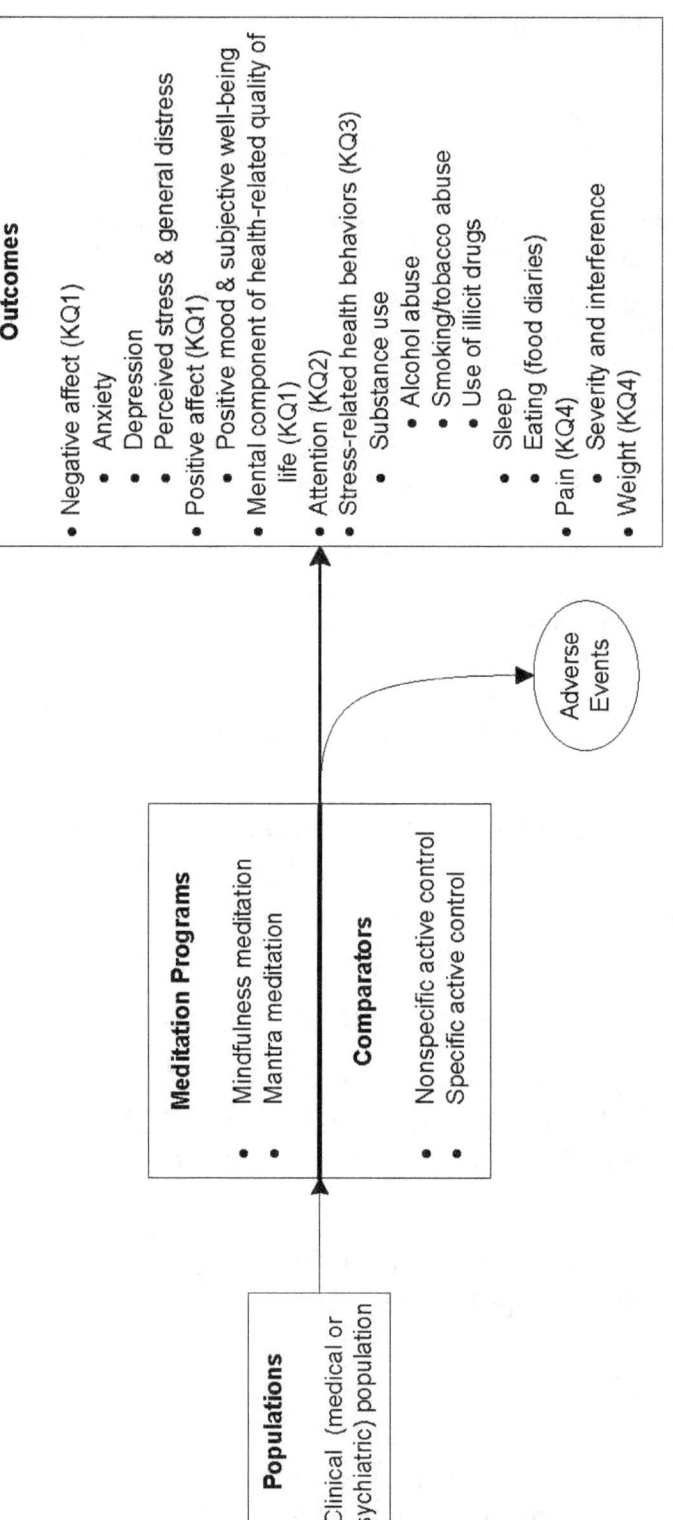

Methods

The methods for this comparative effectiveness review follow the methods suggested in the Agency for Healthcare Research and Quality (AHRQ) "Methods Guide for Effectiveness and Comparative Effectiveness Reviews" (www.effectivehealthcare.ahrq.gov/methods guide.cfm). The main sections of this chapter reflect the elements of the protocol established for comparative effectiveness reviews; certain methods map to the PRISMA checklist.[36] We carried out this systematic review according to a prespecified protocol registered at the AHRQ Web site.[37]

Topic Development

The Division of Extramural Research of the National Center for Complementary and Alternative Medicine, National Institutes of Health, nominated the topic for this report in a public process. We recruited six Key Informants to provide input on the selection and refinement of the questions for the systematic review. To develop the Key Questions (KQs), we reviewed existing systematic reviews, developed an analytic framework, and solicited input from our Key Informants through email and conference calls. We posted our draft KQs on the Effective Health Care Program Web site for public comment on October 14, 2011. We revised the KQs, as necessary, based on comments.

We drafted a protocol and recruited a multidisciplinary Technical Expert Panel (TEP), including methods experts, tai chi and qigong experts, and meditation experts. With input from the TEP and representatives from AHRQ, we finalized the protocol. Initially we planned to include physiologic outcomes and the various movement-based meditation programs. Based on expert panel input we eliminated the biological outcomes due to a need to limit the scope of this broad review, as well as a concern that a number of these outcomes, such as inflammatory markers, were felt to be more intermediate outcomes. We also eliminated the movement-based meditation programs because we felt their relevance would be greatest for the physiologic markers. We uploaded the protocol to the Effective Health Care Program Web site on February 22, 2012.

Search Strategy

We searched the following databases for primary studies: MEDLINE®, PsycINFO, Embase®, PsycArticles, SCOPUS, CINAHL, AMED, and the Cochrane Library through October 11, 2011. We developed a search strategy for MEDLINE, accessed via PubMed®, based on medical subject headings (MeSH®) terms and text words of key articles that we identified a priori (Appendix B). We reviewed the reference lists of included articles, relevant review articles, and 20 related systematic reviews to identify articles that the database searches might have missed. Our search did not have any language restrictions. We updated the search in November 2012.

We selected databases after internal deliberation and input from the TEP. We did not include meeting proceedings or abstracts of reports of unpublished studies. We searched clinicaltrials.gov. We evaluated the search strategy by examining whether it retrieved a sample of key articles. We did not limit our searches to any geographic regions. For articles written in non-English languages, we either used individuals familiar with the language or used the Google Translate Web site to assess whether an article fit our inclusion criteria.[38]

Study Selection

Two investigators independently screened title and abstracts, and excluded them if both investigators agreed that the article met one or more of the exclusion criteria. (Inclusion and exclusion criteria listed in Table 2 and the Abstract Review Form in Appendix C.) We resolved differences between investigators regarding abstract eligibility through consensus.

Citations that we promoted on the basis of title and abstract screen received a second independent screen of the full-text article (Appendix C, Article Review Form). We resolved differences regarding article inclusion through consensus. Paired investigators conducted another independent review of full-text articles to determine whether they included applicable information, and if so, included in the full-data abstraction (Appendix C, Key Question Applicability Form). We resolved disagreements about the eligibility of an article by discussion between the two reviewers or by adjudication of a third reviewer.

We required that studies reported on populations with a clinical condition, either medical or psychiatric. Although meditation programs may have an impact on healthy populations, we limited our evaluation to clinical populations. Since trials examine meditation programs in diverse populations, we defined a clinical condition broadly to include mental health/psychiatric conditions (e.g., anxiety or stress) and physical conditions (e.g., low back pain, heart disease, or advanced age). Additionally, since stress was of particular interest for meditation studies, we also included trials that studied stressed populations even though they may not have a defined medical or psychiatric diagnosis. We excluded studies among the otherwise healthy. We also excluded studies among children or adolescents because meditation instruction for non-adults is not the same as it is for adults, due to differences in maturity, understanding, and discipline. Non-adult studies would measure outcomes differently, making a synthesis difficult.

We excluded movement-based techniques that involve meditation due to the confounding effects of the exercise component of those techniques on outcomes (Table 1). To evaluate programs that are more than a brief mental exercise, yet remain broadly inclusive, we defined a meditation program as any systematic or protocolized meditation program that follows a predetermined curriculum. We defined these programs to involve, at a minimum, at least 4 hours of training with instructions to practice outside the training session.

We included both specific and nonspecific active controlled trials. We defined an active control as any control in which the control group is matched in time and attention to the intervention group. A nonspecific active control only matches time, attention and expectation similar to what a placebo pill does in a drug trial. Examples include "attention control" and "educational control." It is not a known therapy. A specific active control compares the intervention to another known therapy, such as progressive muscle relaxation.[34,35,39,40]

We defined any control group that does not match time and attention for the purposes of matching expectation as an inactive control. Examples include wait-list or usual-care controls. We excluded such trials since it would be difficult to assess whether any changes in outcomes were due to the nonspecific effects of time and attention. We excluded observational studies susceptible to confounding and selection biases.

We evaluated the effect of these meditation programs on a range of stress-related outcomes and used the framework from the Patient Reported Outcomes Measurement Information System (PROMIS) to help guide our categorization of outcomes.[41] The PROMIS framework is a National Institutes of Health-sponsored project to optimize and standardize patient reported health status tools. This framework breaks self-reported outcomes into the three broad categories of physical, mental, and social health, and then subdivides these categories further. Our outcomes included negative affect, positive affect, well-being, cognition, pain, and health-related behaviors affected by stress such as substance abuse, sleeping, and eating.[41] Based on input from technical experts, we also evaluated the effect of meditation programs on weight—an additional stress-related outcome we deemed important.

We included randomized controlled trials (RCTs) in which the control group was matched in time and attention to the intervention group. The inclusion of such trials allowed us to evaluate the specific effects of meditation programs separate from the nonspecific effects of attention and expectation. Our team thought this was the most rigorous standard for determining the efficacy of the interventions and contributing to the current literature on the effects of meditation. We did not include observational studies because they are likely to have an extremely high risk of bias due to problems such as self-selection of interventions (people who believe in the benefits of meditation or who have prior experience with meditation are more likely to enroll in a meditation program) and use of outcome measures that can be easily biased by participants' beliefs in the benefits of meditation.

Table 1. Study inclusion and exclusion criteria

PICOTS Element	Inclusion	Exclusion
Population and Condition of Interest	Adult populations (18 years or older) Clinical (medical or psychiatric) diagnosis, defined as any condition (e.g. high blood pressure, anxiety) including a stressor	Studies of children (The type and nature of meditation children receive is significantly different from adults.) Studies of otherwise healthy individuals
Interventions	Structured meditation programs (any systematic or protocolized meditation programs that follow predetermined curricula), consisting of, at a minimum, at least 4 hours of training with instructions to practice outside the training session These include: Mindfulness-based: MBSR MBCT Vipassana Zen Other mindfulness meditation Mantra-based: TM Other mantra meditation Other meditation	Meditation programs in which the meditation is not the foundation and majority of the intervention These include: DBT ACT Any of the movement-based meditations such as yoga (e.g. iyenger, hatha, shavasana), tai chi, and qi gong (chi kung) Aromatherapy Biofeedback Neurofeedback Hypnosis Autogenic training Psychotherapy Laughter therapy Therapeutic touch Eye movement desensitization reprocessing Relaxation therapy Spiritual therapy Breathing exercise, pranayama Exercise Any intervention that is given remotely, or only by video or audio to an individual without the involvement of a meditation teacher physically present

Table 1. Study inclusion and exclusion criteria (continued)

PICOTS Element	Inclusion	Exclusion
Comparisons of Interest	Active control is defined as a program that is matched in time and attention to the intervention group for the purpose of matching expectations of benefit. Some examples include "attention control," "educational control," or another therapy, such as progressive muscle relaxation, that the study compares to the intervention. A nonspecific active control only matches time and attention, and is not a known therapy. A specific active control compares the intervention to another known therapy, such as progressive muscle relaxation.	Studies that only evaluate a wait-list/usual-care control or do not include a comparison group
Outcomes	See Figure 1	All other outcomes
Study Design	RCTs with an active control	Non-RCT designs, such as observational studies
Timing and Setting	Longitudinal studies that occur in general and clinical settings	none

Note: We excluded articles with no original data (reviews, editorials, and comments), studies published in abstract form only, and dissertations.
DBT = Dialectical Behavioral Therapy; ACT = Acceptance and Commitment Therapy; KQ = Key Question; MBCT = Mindfulness-based Cognitive Therapy; RCT = Randomized Controlled Trials; MBSR = Mindfulness-based Stress Reduction; TM = Transcendental Meditation

Data Abstraction and Data Management

We used Distiller SR (Evidence Partners, 2010) to manage the screening and review process. We uploaded all citations identified by the search strategies to the system. We created standardized forms for data extraction (Appendix C). We pilot tested the forms prior to beginning the data extraction. Reviewers extracted information on general study characteristics, study participants, eligibility criteria, interventions, and the outcomes. Two investigators reviewed each article for data abstraction. For study characteristics, participant characteristics, and intervention characteristics, the second reviewer confirmed the first reviewer's data abstraction for completeness and accuracy. For outcome data and risk-of-bias scoring, we used dual and independent review. Reviewer pairs included personnel with both clinical and methodological expertise. We resolved differences between investigators regarding data through consensus.

For each meditation program we extracted information on measures of intervention fidelity including dose, training, and receipt of intervention. We measured duration and maximal hours of structured training in meditation, amount of home practice recommended, description of instructor qualifications, and description of participant adherence, if any. Many of the meditation techniques do not have clearly defined training and certification requirements for instructors. However, when available, we extracted data on whether instructors had specialized training or course certification in the particular meditative technique being assessed.

Since studies provided a variety of measures for many of our KQs, we included any RCT of a meditation program with an active control that potentially applied to any KQ. We then went through each of the papers to identify all the scales (instruments or measurement tools) that could potentially apply to a KQ. We then revised this list and organized instruments according to relevance for the KQs. We extracted data from instruments that have broad experience and that researchers commonly used to measure relevant outcomes. We prioritized instruments that were common to the numerous trials in our review, so as to allow more direct comparisons between trials (Table 2).

We entered all information from the article review process into the Distiller SR database. We used the DistillerSR database to maintain the data, which we then exported into Excel for the preparation of evidence tables.

Table 2. Organization of various scales (instruments or measurement tools) for each Key Question

Key Question 1. What are the efficacy and harms of meditation programs on negative affect (e.g. anxiety, stress) and positive affect (e.g. well-being) among those with a clinical condition (medical or psychiatric)?	
Anxiety	
General anxiety	Beck Anxiety Inventory
	Profile of Mood States, Tension
	Symptom Checklist-90 Anxiety Subscale
	State Trait Anxiety Inventory, State
	State Trait Anxiety Inventory, Trait
	Brief Symptom Inventory (18), Anxiety Subscale
	Hamilton Anxiety Rating Scale
	Institute for Personality and Ability Testing Anxiety Inventory
Worry	Penn State Worry Questionnaire
Thought emotion/ suppression	Courtauld Emotional Control, Anxiety
	White Bear Inventory (thought suppression)
Social anxiety	Liebowitz Social Anxiety, Fear
	Liebowitz Social Anxiety, Avoidance
	Liebowitz Social Anxiety, Fear and Avoidance Combined
	Social Interactions, Fear
	Social Phobia
	Fear of Negative Evaluation (brief version)
Depression	
Self-reported depression	Beck Depression Inventory
	Symptom Checklist-90 Depression Subscale
	Center for Epidemiologic Studies Depression Scale
	Profile of Mood States, Depression
	Brief Symptom Inventory (18), Depression
	Beck Depression Inventory
	Beck Depression Inventory II
	Interpersonal Sensitivity
	Self Rating Depression Scale
	Institute for Personality and Ability Testing Depression Scale
Clinician-rated depression	Structured Clinical Interview, Relapse (Y/N)
	Hamilton Psychiatric Rating Scale for Depression
Stress	
	Perceived Stress Scale (10 and 14 item)
	Life Stress Instrument
General Distress	
	Brief Symptom Inventory (18), General Symptom Severity Index
	Brief Symptom Inventory (53) Global Psychiatric Symptoms
	Positive and Negative Affect Scale—Negative mood
	Symptom Checklist-90-R Global Severity Index
	Short Form-36 Mental Health Subscale
	Profile of Mood States, Total Mood Disturbance
Negative Affect	
	Positive and Negative Affect Scale—Negative Mood

Table 2. Organization of various scales (instruments or measurement tools) for each Key Question (continued)

Well-Being	
	Sense of Coherence Scale (meaningfulness subscale)
	Quality of Well-Being Scale
Positive Mood	
	Short Form 36 Vitality Subscale
	Positive and Negative Affect Scale—Positive Mood
Positive Affect	
	Positive and Negative Affect Scale—Positive Mood
Mental Component of Health-Related Quality of Life	
	Short Form (SF) 12, SF 36, Veterans Rand 36: mental component score for all
	World Health Organization Quality of Life—Psychological
Key Question 2. What are the efficacy and harms of meditation programs on attention among those with a clinical condition (medical or psychiatric)?	
Attention	
	Attentional Network
	Stroop Color-Word Test (sustained attention)
Key Question 3. What are the efficacy and harms of meditation programs on health-related behaviors affected by stress, specifically substance use, sleep, and eating, among those with a clinical condition (medical or psychiatric)?	
Substance Use	
Alcohol	Penn Alcohol Craving Scale
	Attention (dot probe)
	Impaired Response Inhibition Scale for Alcohol
	Weekly Diary
	Daily Diary
Cocaine	Weekly Diary
Smoking	Cigarette Use
Sleep	
Summary measures	Pittsburgh Sleep Quality Index
	Insomnia Severity Index
	Epworth Sleepiness Scale
Diary	Diary (total sleep time, wake after sleep onset)
Actigraphy	Actigraphy (total sleep time, wake after sleep onset)
Eating	
Diary	7-Day Food Recall (fat/fiber/carbs)
Key Question 4. What are the efficacy and harms of meditation programs on pain and weight among those with a clinical condition (medical or psychiatric)?	
Pain	
Severity	Numeric Rating Scale 0–10 (sensation and/or unpleasantness)
	Irritable Bowel Syndrome Abdomen Pain Severity
	Pain Perception (sensory and affective)
	Short Form-36 Bodily Pain Subscale
	McGill Pain Questionnaire (current pain score)
Interference	Fibromyalgia Impact Questionnaire
	Roland Morris Disability Questionnaire
Weight (pounds or kilograms)	

All measures are direct except:
Penn Alcohol Craving Scale which is an indirect measure of alcohol consumption
Anxiety, Depression and Stress/Distress measures which are indirect measures of Negative Affect
Positive Mood and Subjective Well-being measures which are indirect measures of Positive Affect

Data Synthesis

For each KQ, we created a detailed set of evidence tables containing all information abstracted from eligible studies.

Trials used either nonspecific active controls or specific active controls (Table 1, Figure 1). Nonspecific active controls (e.g., education or attention control) control for the nonspecific effects of time, attention and expectation. Comparisons against these controls allow for assessments of the specific effectiveness of the meditation program (above and beyond the nonspecific effects of time, attention, and expectation). This is similar to a comparison against a placebo pill in a drug trial, where one is concerned with the nonspecific effects of interacting with a provider, taking a pill and expecting the pill to work. Specific active controls are therapies (e.g., exercise or progressive muscle relaxation) known or expected to change clinical outcomes. Comparisons against these controls allow for assessments of comparative effectiveness. In a drug trial, this would be similar to comparing one drug against another known drug. Since these study designs using different types of controls would yield quite different conclusions (efficacy vs. comparative effectiveness), we separated them in our analyses.

To display the outcome data, we calculated relative difference-in-change scores (i.e., the change from baseline in an outcome measure in the treatment group minus the change from baseline in the outcome measure in the control group, divided by the baseline score in the treatment group). However, many studies did not report enough information to calculate confidence intervals for the relative difference-in-change scores. When we evaluated point estimates and confidence intervals for just the post-intervention or end-of-study differences between groups, and compared these to the point estimates for the relative difference-in-change scores for those time points, some of the estimates that did not account for baseline differences appeared to favor a different group (i.e. treatment or control), when compared with the estimates that did account for baseline differences. We therefore used the relative difference-in-change scores to estimate the direction and approximate magnitude of effect for all outcomes. We used the relative difference-in-change graphs to determine consistency. They are not a statistical analysis, but a visual way to display the data. This was done by the following formula: {#(meditation T2-T1)-(control T2-T1)}/(meditation T1) where T1 is the baseline means score and T2 is the followup mean score.

For the purpose of generating an aggregate quantitative estimate of the effect of an intervention and the associated 95 percent confidence interval, we performed meta-analysis using standardized mean differences (effect sizes) calculated by Cohen's method (Cohen's d).[42] For each outcome, we displayed the resulting effect size estimate according to the type of control group and duration of followup. Some studies did not report enough information to be included in meta-analysis. For that reason, we decided to display the relative difference-in-change scores along with the effect size estimates from meta-analysis so that readers can see the full extent of the available data. We used statistical significance of the meta-analytic result to guide our reporting of precision.

We calculated point estimates for the difference-in-change scores for all outcomes. Since these studies were looking at short interventions and relatively low doses of meditation, we considered a 5 percent relative difference-in-change score to be potentially clinically significant. In synthesizing the results of these trials, we considered both statistical and clinical significance. Statistical significance is according to study-specific criteria, and we reported p-values and confidence intervals where present. We defined clinical significance as a 5 percent relative difference-in-change.

Some scales show improvement with more positive numbers, and others show more improvement with less positive numbers. After calculating the relative difference-in-change scores, we reversed the sign on the scales which showed improvement with more negative numbers so that all scales showed an improvement in the positive direction. We oriented the meta-analysis graphs similarly, so that effect sizes are shown in the direction of which treatment arm they favored rather than increases and decreases in each scale.

During data synthesis, if trials reported on more than one scale for a particular outcome, we prioritized the scale that was most common to all the trials to improve comparability between trials. To arrive at an overall strength of evidence (SOE), we used only one scale per outcome per trial in order to avoid giving extra weight to trials that reported on the same outcome with multiple scales. For this reason, although we describe the various scales reported on by the trials in the text, the graphical displays show only the scale that was compared with other studies to arrive at the SOE. Since many trials reported on the same scale at multiple time points, we provided graphs showing the effects at the end of intervention and at the end of study. Wherever meta-analysis was possible, we separated outcomes by time-point. For most, these were at 2–3 months (post intervention) and beyond 3 months (end of study). We describe relevant changes in outcomes over time in the results, but for purposes of consistency we used the first time-point only for describing the magnitude of change in the SOE tables.

Some trials specified primary and secondary outcomes, while others did not. Since the direction and magnitude may differ based on whether it is a primary or secondary outcome, we categorized and labeled each outcome as primary or secondary on the difference-in-change graphs. For trials that did not specify a primary or secondary outcome, two reviewers independently assessed whether an outcome was identified as a primary focus of the study or if it was the outcome that the population was selected on, and these were classified as primary outcomes. We resolved any conflicts by consensus.

Although some trials had more than two arms, we report the sample sizes only for the two arms we examined. The numbers reported are the numbers that the trials used to calculate their effects. If a trial had some attrition but imputed data for the missing participants, then we reported those intent-to-treat (ITT) numbers. If a trial did not impute data for the missing participants, we reported the numbers they used to calculate effects. For this reason, our report of the number of participants randomized in each trial may differ from the number of participants the trials reported as randomized.

We combined stress and distress into a single outcome due to the paucity of studies and similarities between these outcomes. For studies that reported on both a stress and a distress scale, we prioritized using the scale that was most common in the group of studies. For the same reasons, we also combined well-being and positive mood into the single outcome of positive affect.[43]

To analyze the effects of meditation programs on negative affect, we combined one negative affect scale per trial with the others. Since some trials reported on more than one negative affect scale, we prioritized anxiety, then depression, then stress/distress. Anxiety is a primary dimension of negative affect and a common symptom of stress. Anxiety is highly correlated with depressive symptoms, and thus, when more than one measure of negative affect is available we consider anxiety a good primary marker of negative affect.[44] We also conducted a sensitivity analysis by reversing the prioritization order, prioritizing stress/distress over depression, and depression over anxiety. For the large bulk of outcomes, we rated measures as direct measures of that outcome. However, since anxiety, depression, stress, and distress are components of negative affect, we rated them as indirect measures of negative affect. If a direct measure of negative affect was available (e.g. positive and negative affect schedule), we used that measure instead of any indirect measures.

Assessment of Methodological Quality of Individual Studies

We assessed the risk of bias in studies independently and in duplicate based on the recommendations in the Guide for Conducting Comparative Effectiveness Reviews.[45] We supplemented these tools with additional assessment questions based on the Cochrane Collaboration's Risk of Bias Tool.[46,47] While many of the tools to evaluate risk of bias are common to behavioral as well as pharmacologic interventions, some items are more specific to behavioral interventions. After discussion with experts in meditation programs and clinical trials, we emphasized four major and four minor criteria in assessing bias of meditation programs. The four major criteria were: matching control for time and attention; description of withdrawals and dropouts; attrition; and blinding of outcome assessors. We considered as minor criteria the description of randomization, allocation concealment, ITT analysis, and credibility evaluation (Table 3).

Matching controls for time and attention is prerequisite to matching expectations of benefit. We extracted data on time and attention for both groups. If the control gave at least 75 percent of the time and attention given the intervention arm, we gave it credit for matching. Evaluating credibility is also an important, albeit followup step. Clearly identifying the number of withdrawals and dropouts is necessary for estimating the role that it may play in biasing the results. If attrition was very large, greater than 20 percent, we felt it reflected a potentially large bias and lower quality of trial. Finally, although double blinding is not possible, single blinding of the data collectors is possible and important in reducing risk of bias. While all studies should clearly describe the randomization procedure rather than just stating that "participants were randomized," we felt that some studies, especially older ones, may have conducted appropriate randomization but just not reported the procedures in detail. We therefore listed this as a minor criterion. The same applied for ITT analysis. However, if a study stated they conducted an ITT analysis but did not impute missing data, we did not give those studies points for an ITT analysis. Credibility is evaluated by administration of a scale that measures a participant's expectations of benefit before or during the trial. If credibility scores are similar in both arms of a trial, it suggests that those in the control group had similar beliefs and expectations of benefit as the treatment arm. We only gave 1 point for this if the trial specified administration of a measure of credibility.

We assigned 2 points each to the major criteria, weighting them more in assessing risk of bias (Table 3). We assigned 1 point each to the minor criteria. Studies could therefore receive a total of 12 points. If studies met a minimum of three major criteria and three minor criteria (9–12 points), we classified it as having "low risk of bias." Studies receiving 6–8 points were classified as having "medium risk of bias," and studies receiving 5 or less points were classified as having "high risk of bias." Using this scoring system, we would still consider a study that did not meet one major criterion low risk of bias if it met other minor criteria. We could only grade a study that did not meet two major criterions as medium risk of bias or high risk of bias.

Low risk-of-bias studies had the least bias and we considered the results valid. Medium risk-of-bias studies were susceptible to some bias, but not enough to invalidate the results. High risk-of-bias studies had significant flaws that might have invalidated the results. In addition, if there were other issues with the studies that were not captured by the above criteria, such as significantly greater than 20 percent attrition (e.g. 40 or 50 percent attrition) or significant errors in reporting, we categorized such studies as high risk of bias on a study-by-study basis.

Table 3. List of major and minor criteria in assessing risk of bias

Major Criteria*	Minor Criteria*
<ul><li>Was the control matched for time and attention by the instructors?</li><li>Was there a description of withdrawals and dropouts?</li><li>Was attrition < 20% at the end of treatment? As several studies did not calculate attrition starting from the original number randomized, we recalculated the attrition from the original number randomized.</li><li>Were those who collected data on the participants blind to the allocation?</li></ul>	<ul><li>Was the method of randomization described in the paper? To answer "yes" for this question, the papers had to give some description of the randomization procedure.</li><li>Was allocation concealed?</li><li>Was intent-to-treat analysis used? To answer "yes" for this question, the paper must impute non-completer or other missing data, and do this from the original number randomized.</li><li>Was the credibility evaluated, and if so, was it comparable? If credibility was not evaluated, or if it was evaluated but not comparable, then it did not receive a point.</li></ul>

*We assigned 2 points each to the major criteria, weighting them more in assessing risk of bias. We assigned 1 point each to the minor criteria. Studies could therefore receive a total of 12 points. If studies met a minimum of three questions from major and three from minor (9–12 points), we assigned it a grade of "low risk of bias." For studies ranging 6–8 points, we assigned a "medium risk of bias," and for studies scoring 5 or less points, we assigned a "high risk of bias."

Assessment of Potential Publication Bias

Sometimes studies with positive results for a particular outcome get published while studies with negative results do not, erroneously leading readers to conclude that an intervention has positive effects on a given outcome when it may not. Even when an intervention does have an effect on an outcome, we expect that the distribution of results (by chance) will include null results. When conducting a meta-analysis, a funnel plot allows us to see if the results of the studies were spread in a distribution reflecting what we might expect by chance. It assumes that the largest studies will be near the average, and small studies will be spread on both sides of the average. However, this requires that we have the data to represent the results of each study in a meta-analysis. Anticipating that we might not find enough studies to support a quantitative assessment of publication bias, we conducted a qualitative assessment of publication bias by reviewing all the RCTs of meditation listed in the clinicaltrials.gov registry. We searched for any trials that completed recruitment 3 or more years ago that did not publish results, or that listed outcomes for which they did not report results.[48] To assess for selective outcomes reporting, we examined the methods section for all the scales used to measure outcomes and assessed whether the studies had reported results for all of them.

Strength of the Body of Evidence

After synthesizing the evidence, two reviewers graded the quantity and quality of the best available evidence addressing KQs1–4 by adapting an evidence grading scheme recommended in the "Methods Guide for Effectiveness and Comparative Effectiveness Reviews."[45] In assigning evidence grades, we considered the four recommended domains, including risk of bias in the included studies, consistency across studies, precision of the pooled estimate or the individual study estimates, and directness of the evidence.

We derived the risk of bias for an individual study from the algorithm described above. We assessed the aggregate risk of bias of studies and integrated these assessments into a qualitative assessment of the summary risk-of-bias score. Since the studies in our evidence base were at varying risk of bias, we based most aggregate scores on a combination of high, moderate, or low risk-of-bias ratings. Where there was heterogeneity, we prioritized the lowest risk-of-bias studies.

We used the direction of effect of outcomes falling in the same category, irrespective of statistical significance, to evaluate consistency. In evaluating consistency, due to the heterogeneity of studies, we qualitatively considered giving greater weight to low risk-of-bias studies and/or those with large sample sizes if they were accompanied by one to two other conflicting studies that were of high risk of bias. If all the studies in an evidence base showed a similar direction of effect, we rated the evidence base as consistent. We rated single studies as consistency unknown.

We assessed the precision of individual studies by evaluating the statistical significance of a comparison through meta-analysis. To evaluate precision, we used confidence intervals or p-values. When we did not have a meta-analysis, we prioritized difference-in-change or "group-by-time interaction" confidence intervals or p-values where available. We found that few of the studies reported effect sizes and 95 percent confidence intervals. We estimated the confidence intervals for some of the outcomes. If all studies in an evidence base were precise, we rated the evidence base to be precise. We designated as imprecise studies whose effect size overlapped with the line of no difference. When studies did not report measures of dispersion or variability, we rated the precision as unknown.

We rated the evidence as being direct if the intervention was directly linked to the patient oriented outcomes of interest. We rated the evidence as indirect when studies measured the outcome using scales such as Penn alcohol craving scale, impaired response inhibition scale for alcohol use, and attention dot scales, as these were indirect measures of substance use behavior. We conducted internal deliberations to arrive at a consensus of what was direct or indirect. For the large bulk of outcomes, we rated measures as direct measures of that outcome. However, since anxiety, depression, and stress/distress are components of negative affect, we rated them as indirect measures of negative affect. If direct measures of negative affect such as the positive and negative affect schedule were available, we used that measure instead of any indirect measures. Similarly, we rated well-being and positive mood as indirect measures of positive affect.

To incorporate multiple domains into an overall grade of the SOE, we used the estimate of the summary risk-of-bias score, directness, consistency, and precision to evaluate an intervention. We used a qualitative approach to incorporating these multiple domains into an overall grade. We initially assigned SOE for all outcomes based on their risk-of-bias ratings. We assigned low risk-of-bias studies a high SOE and vice versa. We rated consistent, precise, and direct evidence from such low risk-of-bias studies as high-grade SOE. We downgraded the SOE when we could not determine consistency (i.e., single study) or when we deemed results inconsistent. We downgraded the SOE when evidence was indirect. Imprecision or unknown precision also led to a downgrade in the SOE (Figure 2).

We classified evidence pertaining to KQs1–4 into four categories: (1) "High" grade, indicating high confidence that the evidence reflects the true effect, and further research is very unlikely to change our confidence in the estimate of the effect; (2) "Moderate" grade, indicating moderate confidence that the evidence reflects the true effect, and further research may change our confidence in the estimate of the effect and may change the estimate; (3) "Low" grade, indicating low confidence that the evidence reflects the true effect, and further research is likely to change our confidence in the estimate of the effect and is likely to change the estimate; and (4) "Insufficient" grade, indicating evidence is either unavailable or inadequate to draw a conclusion.

We did not incorporate the optional domain of publication bias in the evidence grade. However, if we found qualitative evidence of publication bias, the ultimate conclusions took that into consideration. Thus, low SOE with probable publication bias translated into a very weak conclusion.

Figure 2. Algorithm for rating the strength of evidence

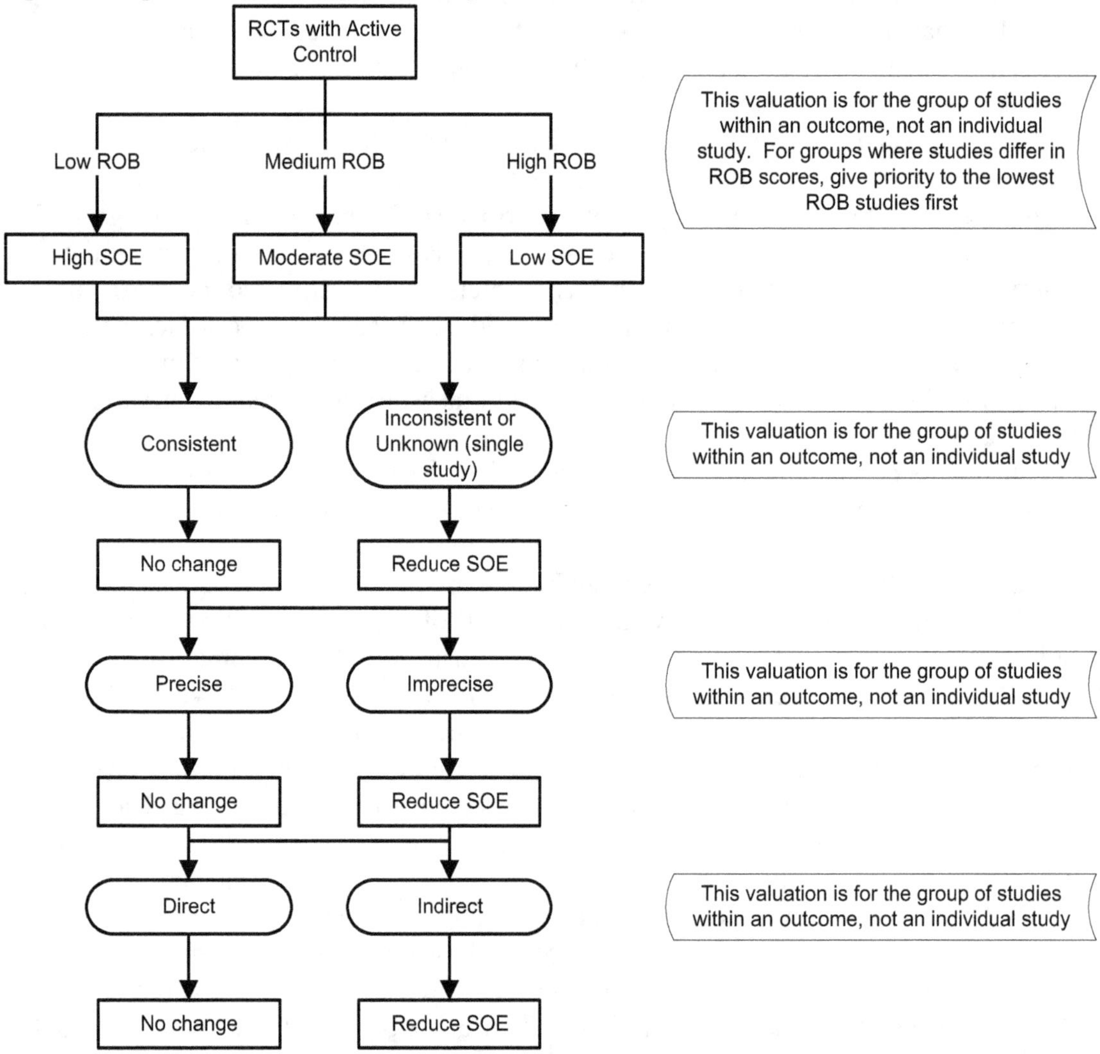
RCTs with Active Control
Low ROB
Medium ROB
High ROB
High SOE
Moderate SOE
Low SOE
This valuation is for the group of studies within an outcome, not an individual study. For groups where studies differ in ROB scores, give priority to the lowest ROB studies first
Consistent
Inconsistent or Unknown (single study)
This valuation is for the group of studies within an outcome, not an individual study
No change
Reduce SOE
Precise
Imprecise
This valuation is for the group of studies within an outcome, not an individual study
No change
Reduce SOE
Direct
Indirect
This valuation is for the group of studies within an outcome, not an individual study
No change
Reduce SOE

Definitions

Risk of Bias (ROB):	Low, Medium, or High based on 4 major and 4 minor criteria
Consistency:	The direction of effect, irrespective of statistical significance
Precision:	Confidence interval or p-values, prioritizing difference-in-change values or "group x time interaction" values
Directness:	If not a direct measure of an outcome, categorized as indirect

Assumptions

- All outcomes have at least 1 study
- Studies start out with a SOE grading based on ROB
- Then based on other criteria, they either maintain that SOE grade or are downgraded one notch. They do not upgrade.

Abbreviations: RCTs = Randomized controlled trials; ROB = Risk of bias; SOE= Strength of evidence

Applicability

We assessed applicability separately for the different outcomes for the entire body of evidence guided by the PICOTS framework as recommended in the "Methods Guide for Effectiveness and Comparative Effectiveness Reviews."[45] One of the potential factors we assessed was intervention fidelity (e.g., duration of structured meditation training, total amount of meditation practice (dose of meditation), subject adherence with meditation, subject proficiency with meditation, instructor qualifications, and study selection criteria for participants). We also assessed the selection process of these studies to evaluate the concern that participants in meditation studies are highly-selected, such as trained meditators. In addition, we assessed whether findings were applicable to various ethnic groups or whether the applicability of evidence was limited by race, ethnicity, or education.

Peer Review and Public Commentary

We invited experts in mind/body medicine and TM, as well as individuals representing stakeholder and user communities to provide external peer review of this comparative effectiveness review; AHRQ and an associate editor also provided comments. The draft report was posted on the AHRQ Web site for 4 weeks to elicit public comment. We addressed all reviewer comments, revising the text as appropriate, and documented everything in a disposition of comments report that we will make available 3 months after AHRQ posts the final comparative effectiveness review on its Web site.

Results

Results of the Search

Figure 3 summarizes the search results. The literature search identified 17,801 unique citations. During the title and abstract screening, we excluded 16,177 citations, during the article screening, we excluded 1,447 citations, and during Key Question (KQ) applicability screening we excluded an additional 136 articles (Appendix D). In total 41 articles met our inclusion criteria and were included in our review.

Figure 3. Summary of the literature search

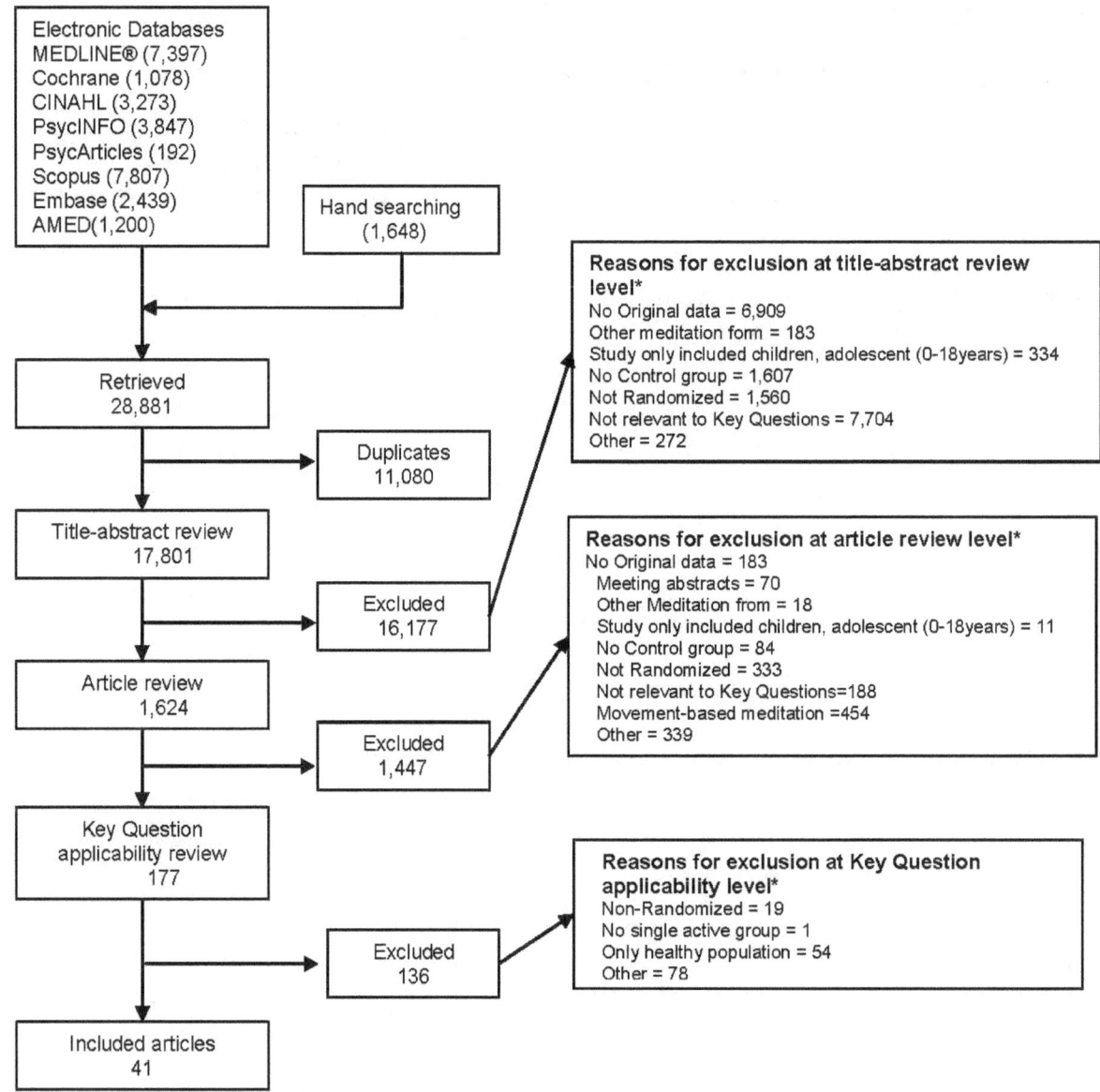

*Total exceeds the number in the exclusion box because reviewers were allowed to mark more than 1 reason for exclusion

Description of Types of Trials Retrieved

Of the included trials, 32 addressed KQ1 (negative and positive affect), one trial addressed KQ2 (attention), 13 trials addressed KQ3 (health-related behaviors affected by stress), and 14 addressed KQ4 (pain and weight). The majority of trials targeted patient populations with mental health or substance abuse problems (n=20). Other population groups under investigation included individuals with breast cancer (n=2), cardiovascular disease (hypertension and congestive heart failure (CHF) (n=4), chronic pain (n=5), human immunodeficiency virus (HIV) (n=2), diabetes and other metabolic disorders (n=3), respiratory diseases such as chronic obstructive pulmonary disorder (COPD), asthma or history of colds (n=3), tinnitus (n=1), and organ transplant recipients (n=1) (Table 4).

The interventions included mindfulness-based stress reduction (MBSR) (n=16), mindfulness-based cognitive therapy (MBCT) (n=4), modified MBSR or similar mindfulness training (n=11), transcendental meditation (TM) (n=7), and other mantra meditation (n=3) (Table 4). The trials took place in various countries: U.S. trials (n=28), Non-U.S. trials (n=13) (Table 4).

Since the amount of training and practice in any meditation program may affect its results, we collected this information and found a fair range in the quality of information reported. Not all trials reported on amount of training and home practice recommended. In general, MBSR programs provided 20–27.5 hours of training over 8 weeks. The modified mindfulness trials generally provided about half this level of training (8–13.5 hours of training over 4–8 weeks) as did other mantra programs (7.5–8 hours of training over 5–8 weeks). TM trials generally provided more training (16–39 hours) over longer periods of time (3–12 months) (Tables 5 and 6).

Most trials did not describe the specific expertise of the trainers. Only five of the trials reported the trainers' actual meditation experience (ranging between 4 months to 25 years) and six reported the trainers' actual teaching experience (ranging between 0–15.7 years).

We rated 10 trials as low risk of bias, 20 as medium risk of bias, and 11 as high risk of bias (Table 7).

Table 4. Characteristics of included trials

Author, Year	Study Objective	Sample Size (N)	Study Location	Medical or Psychiatric Condition of the Study Population	Intervention and Comparator	Outcome(s) (KQs)
Mindfulness Meditation						
Barrett, 2012[49]	Evaluated potential preventive effects of meditation compared with exercise on incidence, duration, and severity of acute respiratory infection illness	154	United States	Community dwelling older adults with cold in preceding years	MBSR vs. specific active control (exercise)	Anxiety (KQ 1) Stress (KQ1) Subjective well-being (KQ 1) QOL (KQ 1) Sleep (KQ 3)
Brewer, 2009[49]	Assessed group MT compared with CBT in substance use and treatment acceptability, and specificity of MT compared with CBT in targeting stress reactivity	36	United States	Patients with alcohol and/or cocaine use disorders	Group MT vs. specific active control (CBT)	Substance use—alcohol and/or cocaine (KQ 3) Adverse Events
Brewer, 2011[50]	Evaluated the effect of mindfulness training on smoking cessation through randomized clinical trials	88	United States	Nicotine-dependent adults with interest in smoking cessation	MT vs. specific active control (American Lung Association's (FFS) treatment)	Substance use (KQ 3) Adverse Events
Chiesa A, 2012[51]	Compared MBCT with a psycho-education for the treatment of patients with major depression	18	Italy	Patients with major depression	MBCT vs. NSAC (education)	Anxiety (KQ 1) Depression (KQ 1) Subjective well-being (KQ 1)
Delgado LC, 2010[51]	Examined psychological and physiological indices of emotional regulation in non-clinical high worriers after a mindfulness-based training program aimed at reducing worry	36	Spain	Patients with chronic worry	MBCT/modified MBCT vs. specific active control (progressive muscle relaxation)	Worry (KQ 1) General distress (KQ1) Positive mood (KQ 1)
Garland EL, 2010[52]	Assessed the effect of MT to disrupt the risk chain of stress-precipitated alcohol relapses	53	United States	Alcohol-dependent adults	Mindfulness-based interventions vs. NSAC (alcohol abstinence support group)	Stress (KQ 1) General Distress (KQ 1) Substance use (KQ 3)

Table 4. Characteristics of included trials (continued)

Author, Year	Study Objective	Sample Size (N)	Study Location	Medical or Psychiatric Condition of the Study Population	Intervention and Comparator	Outcome(s) (KQs)
Gaylord SA, 2011[53]	Assessed the feasibility and efficacy of a group program of mindfulness training, a cognitive behavioral technique, for women with IBS	97–22 dropped before intervention started. (75)	United States	Women with Irritable Bowel Syndrome	MBSR vs. specific active control (IBS support group)	Depression (KQ 1) General distress (KQ 1) Pain severity (KQ 4) Adverse Events
Gross CR, 2010[54]	Assessed the efficacy of MBSR in reducing symptoms of anxiety, depression, and poor sleep in transplant patients	150	United States	Solid organ transplant recipients	MBSR vs. NSAC (peer-led health education)	Anxiety (KQ 1) Depression (KQ 1) Positive mood (KQ 1) QOL (KQ 1) Sleep (KQ 3) Pain severity (KQ 4) Adverse Events
Gross CR, 2011[55]	Investigated the potential of MBSR as a treatment for chronic primary insomnia.	30	United States	Adults with primary chronic insomnia	MBSR vs. specific active control (PCT with eszopiclone)	Anxiety (KQ 1) Depression (KQ 1) QOL (KQ 1) Sleep (KQ 3) Adverse Events
Hebert JR, 2001[56]	Assessed the effectiveness of an intensive dietary intervention on diet and body mass in women with breast cancer	172	United States	Patients with breast cancer	MBSR-based clinic program vs. NSAC (NEP)	Eating (KQ 3) Weight (KQ 4)
Henderson VP, 2011[57]	Assessed the effectiveness of a MBSR program on QOL and psychosocial outcomes in women with early-stage breast cancer, using a three-armed randomized controlled clinical trial	172	United States	Women with early stage breast cancer	MBSR vs. NSAC (NEP)	Anxiety (KQ 1) Thoughts/emotion suppression (KQ 1) Depression (KQ 1) Subjective well-being (KQ 1)
Jazaieri, 2012[58]	Assessed the efficacy of MBSR in the treatment of SAD	56	United States	Patients with Social anxiety disorder	MBSR vs. specific active control (aerobic exercise)	Social anxiety (KQ 1) Depression (KQ 1) Stress (KQ1) Subjective well-being (KQ 1)

Table 4. Characteristics of included trials (continued)

Author, Year	Study Objective	Sample Size (N)	Study Location	Medical or Psychiatric Condition of the Study Population	Intervention and Comparator	Outcome(s) (KQs)
Koszycki D, 2007[58]	Evaluated how well MBSR compared with a first-line psychological intervention works for the treatment of SAD	53	Canada	Patients with generalized social anxiety disorder	MBSR vs. specific active control (CBT)	Social anxiety (KQ 1) Depression (KQ 1)
Kuyken W, 2008[59]	Assessed whether, among patients with recurrent depression who are treated with antidepressant medication, MBCT is comparable to treatment with m-ADM in (a) depressive relapse prevention, (b) key secondary outcomes, and (c) cost effectiveness	123	U.K.	Patients with depression	MBCT vs. specific active controls (antidepressant tapering or M-ADM)	Depression (KQ 1) QOL (KQ 1) Adverse Events
Lee SH, 2006[60]	Examined the effectiveness of a MBSR program in patients with anxiety disorder	46	South Korea	Patients with generalized anxiety disorder or panic disorder	MBSR vs. NSAC (anxiety disorder education program)	Anxiety (KQ 1)
Malarkey, 2012[61]	Evaluated if MBI-ld could produce a greater decrease in CRP, IL-6 and cortisol compared with an active control group receiving a lifestyle education program	186	United States	University faculty and staff with risk of cardiovascular disease and CRP>3.0	MBI-ld vs. NSAC (lifestyle education)	Depression (KQ 1) Stress (KQ 1) Sleep (KQ 3)
Miller, 2012[62]	Compared mindful eating with diabetes self-management education for weight management and glycemic control in adults with type 2 diabetes mellitus	68	United States	Overweight DM patients	MB-EAT vs. specific active controls (smart choices program)	Weight (KQ 4)

Table 4. Characteristics of included trials (continued)

Author, Year	Study Objective	Sample Size (N)	Study Location	Medical or Psychiatric Condition of the Study Population	Intervention and Comparator	Outcome(s) (KQs)
Moritz S, 2006[63]	Evaluated the efficacy of a home study-based spirituality program on mood disturbance in emotionally distressed patients	165	Canada	Patients with psychological distress	MBSR vs. specific active controls (spirituality)	Anxiety (KQ 1) Depression (KQ1) General distress (KQ 1) Positive mood (KQ 1) QOL (KQ 1) Pain severity (KQ 4)
Morone N E, 2009[64]	Assessed the impact of an 8-week mindfulness meditation program on disability, psychological function, and pain severity in community-dwelling older adults with chronic low back pain, and to test the education control program for feasibility	40	United States	Community dwelling older adults with chronic low back pain	MBSR vs. NSAC (health education program)	Pain severity (KQ 4) Pain interference (KQ 4) Adverse Events
Mularski RA, 2009[65]	Tested the efficacy of MBBT (a hybrid of the Relaxation Response training and MBSR training) on improving symptoms and health-related QOL in those with COPD	86	United States	Patients with COPD	MBBT vs. NSAC (support group)	Stress (KQ 1) QOL (KQ 1)
Oken BS, 2010[66]	Evaluated whether a mindfulness meditation intervention may be effective in caregivers of close relatives with dementia and to help refine the protocol for future larger trials	31	United States	Caregivers of close relatives with dementia	MBCT vs. NSAC (education or respite care)	Depression (KQ 1) Stress (KQ 1) Attention (KQ 2)
Pbert L, 2012[67]	Evaluated the efficacy of MBSR in improving QOL and lung function in patients with asthma	83	United States	Patients with persistent asthma	MBSR vs. NSAC (healthy living course)	Stress (KQ 1) QOL (KQ 1)

Table 4. Characteristics of included trials (continued)

Author, Year	Study Objective	Sample Size (N)	Study Location	Medical or Psychiatric Condition of the Study Population	Intervention and Comparator	Outcome(s) (KQs)
Philippot P, 2011[67]	Examined the relative effectiveness of two psychological interventions for treating tinnitus	30	Belgium	Patients with tinnitus	MBCT/ modified MBCT vs. specific active controls (relaxation training or CBT)	Anxiety (KQ 1) Depression (KQ1) Attention (KQ 2)
Piet J, 2010[68]	Pilot tested MBCT alone and in combination with CBGT for young adults with social phobia	26	Denmark	Adults with social phobia	MBCT/modified MBCT vs. relaxation training specific active control (CBT)	Social anxiety (KQ 1) Depression (KQ 1) General distress (KQ 1)
Plews-Ogan M, 2005[69]	Assessed the feasibility of studying MBSR and massage for the management of chronic pain and to estimate their effects on pain and mood.	30	United States	Patients with chronic musculoskeletal pain	MBSR vs. specific active control (weekly massage)	Subjective well-being (KQ 1) Pain severity (KQ 4)
Schmidt S, 2010[70]	Studied the efficacy of MBSR for enhanced well-being of fibromyalgia patients investigated in a three-armed trial	177	Germany	Women with fibromyalgia	MBSR vs. specific active controls (progressive muscle relaxation and stretching)	Anxiety (KQ 1) Depression (KQ 1) Sleep (KQ 3) Pain severity (KQ 4)
Segal ZV, 2010[71]	Compared rates of relapse in depressed patients in remission receiving MBCT against maintenance antidepressant pharmacotherapy, the current standard of care	84	Canada	Patients with recurrent depression	MBCT vs. specific active control (maintenance antidepressant therapy)	Depression (KQ 1)
Seyedalinaghi, 2012[71]	Evaluated the immediate and long-term effectiveness of MBSR on markers of health among HIV patients, using a randomized controlled trial	245	Iran	Adults with HIV infection	MBSR vs. NSAC (education and support)	Distress and negative affect (KQ 1)

Table 4. Characteristics of included trials (continued)

Author, Year	Study Objective	Sample Size (N)	Study Location	Medical or Psychiatric Condition of the Study Population	Intervention and Comparator	Outcome(s) (KQs)
Whitebird, 2012[72]	Compared the effectiveness of MBSR intervention with a community caregiver education and support intervention for family caregivers of people with dementia	7	United States	Caregivers of close relatives with dementia	MBSR vs. NSAC (education and support)	Anxiety (KQ 1) Depression (KQ 1) Stress (KQ 1) QOL (KQ 1)
Wolever, 2012[73]	Evaluated the viability and proof of concept for mindfulness based compared with yoga-based intervention, setting the stage for a larger cost-effectiveness trial and also to evaluate online and in-person delivery of the mindfulness-based intervention	239	United States	Employees working in a high stress environment inside a national health insurance agency	Mindfulness based intervention vs. specific active control (vinyana yoga)	Depression (KQ 1) Stress (KQ 1) Sleep (KQ 3) Pain severity (KQ 4)
Wong SY-S, 2011[74]	Compared the clinical effectiveness of the MBSR program with an MPI program in terms of pain intensity, pain-related distress, QOL, and mood in patients with chronic pain	99	Hong Kong	Patients with chronic pain	MBSR vs. specific active control (MPI)	Anxiety (KQ 1) Depression (KQ 1) QOL (KQ 1) Pain severity (KQ 4)

Table 4. Characteristics of included trials (continued)

Author, Year	Study Objective	Sample Size (N)	Study Location	Medical or Psychiatric Condition of the Study Population	Intervention and Comparator	Outcome(s) (KQs)
Mantra Meditation						
Bormann JE, 2006[75]	Examined the efficacy of a psycho-spiritual intervention of mantra repetition—a word or phrase with spiritual associations repeated silently throughout the day—on psychological distress (intrusive thoughts, stress, anxiety, anger, and depression), QOL enjoyment, satisfaction, and existential spiritual well-being in HIV-infected adults	93	United States	Adults with HIV infection	Mantra Meditation vs. NSAC (education)	Anxiety (KQ 1) Stress (KQ 1) Depression (KQ 1)
Castillo-Richmond, 2000[76]	Assessed if stress reduction with the TM program can decrease CHD risk factors and cardiovascular mortality in African Americans	138	United States	Hypertension (high normal blood pressure, stage I, or stage II hypertension	TM vs. NSAC (health education)	Substance use—smoking (KQ 3) Weight (KQ 4)
Elder, 2006[77]	Assessed the feasibility and clinical impact of a whole-system, Ayurvedic intervention for newly diagnosed people with type 2 diabetes	60	United States	Diabetic patients in primary care setting	TM vs. NSAC (diabetes education classes)	Weight (KQ 4) Adverse Events
Jayadevappa R, 2007[78]	Evaluated the effectiveness of a TM stress reduction program for African Americans with CHF	23	United States	African American patients with CHF	TM vs. NSAC (health education)	Stress (KQ 1) Depression (KQ 1) Subjective well-being (KQ 1) Positive mood (KQ 1) Pain severity (KQ 4)

Table 4. Characteristics of included trials (continued)

Author, Year	Study Objective	Sample Size (N)	Study Location	Medical or Psychiatric Condition of the Study Population	Intervention and Comparator	Outcome(s) (KQs)
Lehrer PM, 1983[79]	Compared mantra meditation and progressive relaxation treatments and their effect on anxiety among anxious participants	61	United States	Adults with anxiety	Mantra meditation vs. specific active control (relaxation program)	Anxiety (KQ 1) Depression (KQ 1)
Murphy TJ, 1986[80]	Assessed the effects of exercise and meditation on alcohol consumption in social drinkers	60	United States	High-volume drinkers	Mantra meditation vs. specific active control (running exercise)	Substance use—alcohol (KQ 3)
Paul-Labrador M, 2006[81]	Evaluated the efficacy of TM on components of the metabolic syndrome and CHD	103	United States	Patients with stable CHD	Mantra Meditation vs. NSAC (health education)	Anxiety (KQ 1) Depression (KQ 1) Stress (KQ 1) Adverse Events
Schneider, 2012[82]	Evaluated the effectiveness of TM stress reduction for African American with coronary artery disease	201	United States	African American patients with CAD	TM vs. NSAC (cardiovascular health education)	Depression (KQ 1) Substance abuse (KQ 2) Eating (KQ 3) Weight (KQ 4)
Smith JC, 1976[83]	The objective was to Assessed whether the crucial therapeutic component of TM is or is not the TM exercise	139	United States	Anxious college students	Mantra meditation vs. NSAC (relaxation program)	Anxiety (KQ 1)
Taub E, 1994[84]	Assessed whether TM has an effect on prelapse prevention in alcoholics.	125	United States	Alcoholics in recovery program	TM vs. SAC Biofeedback	Substance Use (KQ3)

Note: CBT = Cognitive Behavioral Therapy; CBGT = Cognitive Behavioral Group Therapy; FFS = Freedom from Smoking; M-ADM = Maintenance Antidepressant Monotherapy; MBBT = Mindfulness-based Breathing Therapy; MBCT = Mindfulness-based Cognitive Therapy; MBSR = Mindfulness-based Stress Reduction; MPI = Multidisciplinary Pain Intervention; MT = Mindfulness Training; NEP = Nutrition Education Program; PCT = Pharmacotherapy; TM = Transcendental Meditation; CHF = Congestive Heart Failure; IBS = Irritable Bowel Syndrome; MPI = Meditation Practice Institute; SAD = Social Anxiety Disorder; QOL = Quality of Life; COPD = Chronic Obstructive Pulmonary Disorder; CHD = Chronic Heart Disease; HIV = Human Immunodeficiency Virus; KQ = Key Question; NSAC = Nonspecific Active Control; SAC = Specific Active Control; CSM = Clinically Standardized Meditation; CAD = Coronary Artery Disease

Table 5. Training dose for included trials over duration of training period (numbers are calculated from information provided in trials)

Author, Year	Intervention	Training Duration (weeks)	Total Training Dose (hours)	Recommended Home Practice over Training Period (hours)
Mindfulness Meditation				
Barrett, 2012[85]	MBSR	8	20	42
Brewer, 2009[49]	MB Relapse Prevention	9	9	NP
Brewer, 2011[50]	MM	4	12	NP
Chiesa, 2012[86]	MBCT	8	16	NP
Delgado LC, 2010[51]	MM	5	10	NP
Garland EL, 2010[52]**	MBCT	10	NP	NP
Gaylord SA, 2011[53]*	MM	8	23	NP
Gross CR, 2010[54]*	MBSR	8	27	NP
Gross CR, 2011[55]	MBSR	8	26	36
Hebert JR, 2001[56]*	MM	15	45	NP
Henderson VP, 2011[57]	MBSR	8	25	NP
Jazaieri, 2012[87]	MBSR	8	25	28.3 (actual mean hrs.)
Koszycki D, 2007[58]	MBSR	8	27.5	28
Kuyken W, 2008[59]*	MBCT	8	24	37.5
Lee SH, 2006[60]	MM	8	8	NP
Malarkey, 2012[61]	MBI	8	9	18.5
Miller, 2012[62]	MB	12	25	NP
Moritz S, 2006[63]*	MBSR	8	12	NP
Morone N E, 2009[64]	MM	8	12	42
Mularski R A, 2009[65]	MBBT	8	8	NP
Oken BS, 2010[66]	MBSR/MBCT	7	9	NP
Pbert L, 2012[88]	MBSR	8	26	24
Philippot P, 2011[67]	MM	6	13.5	NP
Piet J, 2010[68]	MBCT	8	16	28
Plews-Ogan M, 2005[69]	MBSR	8	20	NP
Schmidt S, 2010[70]	MBSR	8	27	42
Segal ZV, 2010[71]*	MBCT	8	23	NP
Seyedalinaghi, 2012[89]*	MBSR	8	25	NP
Whitebird, 2012[72]	MBSR	8	25	26.7 (actual mean hrs.)
Wolever, 2012[73]	MM	12	14	NP
Wong SY-S, 2011[74]	MBSR	8	27	NP
Mantra Meditation				
Bormann JE, 2006[75]	Mantra	5	7.5	NP
Castillo-Richmond, 2000[76]**	TM	1	NP	120.6
Elder, 2006[77]**	TM	NP	NP	90
Jayadevappa R, 2007[78]*	TM	24	22.5	90
Lehrer PM, 1983[79]	Mantra	5	7.5	NP
Murphy, 1986[80]	Mantra	8	8	37.52
Paul-Labrador M, 2006[81]	TM	16	39	NP
Schneider, 2012[90]*	TM	5.4 yrs.	78	1310
Smith JC, 1976[83]**	TM	25	NP	87.5
Taub E, 1994[84]	TM	4	19	NP

* These studies did not explicitly describe training amounts. Numbers were estimated from available information.
** These studies did not give enough information to estimate or calculate training dose.
Note: NP=Not Provided; MBSR = Mindfulness-based Stress Reduction; MBCT = Mindfulness-based Cognitive Therapy; MBRP = Mindfulness-based Relapse Prevention; MBBT = Mindfulness=based Breathing Therapy; MM = Mindfulness Meditation, typically a variant of MBSR; TM = Transcendental Meditation

Table 6. Teacher qualifications for included trials

Author, Year	Intervention	Teacher Trained in Meditation Technique?	Certified?	Years of Meditation Experience?	Years of Teaching Experience in Meditation?
Mindfulness Meditation					
Barrett, 2012[85]	MBSR	Y	NP	NP	NP
Brewer, 2009[49]	MBRP	Y	NP	12	Several
Brewer, 2011[50]	MM	Y	NP	>13	NP
Chiesa, 2012[86]	MBCT	Y	Y	NP	NP
Delgado, 2010[51]	MM	NP	NP	NP	NP
Garland, 2010[52]	MBCT	NP	NP	NP	NP
Gaylord, 2011[53]	MM	Y	NP	NP	NP
Gross, 2010[54]	MBSR	Y	NP	NP	NP
Gross, 2011[55]	MBSR	Y	Y	NP	NP
Herbert, 2001[56]	MM	NP	NP	NP	NP
Henderson VP, 2011[57]	MBSR	Y	NP	NP	NP
Jazaieri, 2012[87]	MBSR	Y	NP	NP	15.7
Koszycki D, 2007[58]	MBSR	Y	NP	NP	NP
Kuyken, 2008[59]	MBCT	Y	Y	NP	NP
Lee, 2006[60]	MM	Y	NP	NP	5
Malarkey, 2012[61]	MBI	Y	NP	15	Y
Miller, 2012[62]	MB	NP	NP	NP	NP
Moritz, 2006[63]	MBSR	NP	NP	NP	NP
Morone, 2009[64]	MM	Y	Y	25	Y
Mularski, 2009[65]	MBBT	Y	Y	Several	Several
Oken, 2010[66]	MBSR/MBCT	Y	NP	NP	NP
Pbert L, 2012[88]	MBSR	NP	NP	NP	NP
Philippot, 2011[67]	MM	Y	NP	3	NP
Piet, 2010[68]	MBCT	Y	NP	NP	NP
Plews-Ogan, 2005[69]	MBSR	NP	NP	NP	NP
Schmidt S, 2010[70]	MBSR	Y	Y	NP	7
Segal, 2010[71]	MBCT	Y	Y	NP	NP
Seyedalinaghi, 2012[89]	MBSR	Y	NP	NP	NP
Whitebird ,2012[72]	MBSR	Y	NP	NP	NP
Wolever, 2012[73]	MM	Y	Y	NP	NP
Wong, 2011[74]	MBSR	Y	NP	NP	NP
Mantra Meditation					
Borman, 2006[75]	Mantra	Y	NP	NP	NP
Castillo-Richmond, 2000[76]	TM	NP	Y	NP	NP
Elder, 2006[77]	TM	Y	NP	NP	NP
Jayadevappa, 2007[78]	TM	Y	Y	NP	NP
Lehrer, 1983[79]	Mantra	Y	NP	0.33	0
Murphy, 1986[80]	Mantra	NP	NP	Y	NP
Paul-Labrador, 2006[81]	TM	Y	NP	NP	NP
Schneider, 2012[90]	TM	Y	Y	NP	NP
Smith, 1976[83]	TM	Y	Y	NP	NP
Taub, 1994[84]	TM	Y	Y	NP	NP

Note: NP=Not Provided; MBSR = Mindfulness-based Stress Reduction; MBCT = Mindfulness-based Cognitive Therapy; MBRP = Mindfulness-based Relapse Prevention; MBBT = Mindfulness-based Breathing Therapy; MM = Mindfulness Meditation, typically a variant of MBSR; TM = Transcendental Meditation

Table 7. Risk of bias for included trials

Author, Year	Major Criteria				Minor Criteria				Score	ROB
	Q1: Matched for time/ attention	Q2: Withdrawals & Dropouts described	Q3 Attrition less than 20%	Q4: Single Blinding	Q5: randomization method	Q6: AC	Q7: ITT	Q8: credibility comparable		
Mindfulness										
Barrett, 2012[85]	1	1	1	0	1	1	0	0	8	Medium
Brewer, 2009[49]	1	1	0	0	1	0	0	1	6**	High
Brewer, 2011[50]	1	1	0	0	1	0	0	0	5	High
Chiesa, 2012[86]	1	1	0	0	1	0	0	1	6	Medium
Delgado LC, 2010[51]	1	1	1	0	0	0	0	0	6	Medium
Garland E L, 2010[52]	1	1	0	1	0	0	0	1	7	Medium
Gaylord SA, 2011[53]	1	1	0	1	1	0	0	1	8	Medium
Gross CR, 2010[54]	1	1	1	0	1	0	0	0	7	Medium
Gross CR, 2011[55]	1	1	1	0	1	1	0	0	8	Medium
Hebert JR, 2001[56]	1	1	1	0	0	0	0	0	6	Medium
Henderson VP, 2011[57]	1	1	1	0	1	0	0	0	7	Medium
Jazaieri, 2012[87]	1	1	0	0	1	0	0	0	5	High
Koszycki D, 2007[58]	1	1	0	0	0	0	1	0	5	High
Kuyken W, 2008[59]	1	1	1	1	1	0	1	0	10	Low
Lee SH, 2006[60]	1	1	1	0	0	0	1	0	7	Medium
Moritz S, 2006[63]	1	1	1	0	1	1	1	0	9	Low
Morone NE, 2009[64]	1	1	1	1	1	1	0	1	11	Low
Mularski RA, 2009[65]	1	1	0	0	1	1	0	1	7**	High
Oken BS, 2010[66]	1	1	0	1	1	0	0	1	8	Medium
Pbert, 2013[88]	1	1	1	1	1	0	0	0	9	Low
Philippot P, 2011[67]	1	1	1	0	1	0	0	0	7	Medium
Piet J, 2010[68]	1	1	1	0	1	0	1	0	8	Medium

Table 7. Risk of bias for included trials (continued)

Author, Year	Major Criteria				Minor Criteria				Score	ROB
	Q1: Matched for time/ attention	Q2: Withdrawals & Dropouts described	Q3 Attrition less than 20%	Q4: Single Blinding	Q5: random-ization method	Q6: AC	Q7: ITT	Q8: credibility comparable		
Plews-Ogan M, 2005[69]	1	1	0	0	1	0	0	0	5	High
Schmidt S, 2010[70]	1	1	1	0	1	1	0	0	8	Medium
Segal ZV, 2010[71]	1	1	0	1	1	1	1	0	9	Low
Seyedalinaghi, 2012[89]	0	1	0	0	1	1	0	0	4	High
Whitebird, 2012[72]	1	1	1	0	1	0	1	0	8	Medium
Wong SY-S, 2011[74]	1	1	1	1	1	1	1	0	11	Low
Wolever, 2012[73]	1	1	1	0	0	0	1	0	7	Medium
Mantra										
Bormann JE, 2006[75]	1	1	0	0	1	0	1	0	6	Medium
Castillo-Richmond, 2000[76]	1	1	0	1	1	0	0	0	7*	High
Elder, 2006[77]	0	1	1	0	1	1	0	0	6	Medium
Jayadevappa R, 2007[78]	1	1	1	1	1	0	1	0	10	Low
Lehrer PM, 1983[79]	1	1	1	0	0	0	0	1	7	Medium
Murphy TJ, 1986[80]	1	1	0	0	1	0	0	0	5	High
Paul-Labrador M, 2006[81]	1	1	1	1	1	0	0	0	9	Low
Schneider, 2012[90]	1	1	1	1	1	1	1	0	11	Low
Smith JC, 1976[83]	1	1	0	0	1	0	0	0	5	High
Taub E, 1994[84]	1	1	1	0	1	0	0	0	7	Medium

Major Criteria: Q 1: Was the Control Matched for Time and Attention by the Instructors? Q2: Was There a Description of Withdrawals and Dropouts? Q3: Was Attrition <20% at the End of Treatment? Q4: Single blinding employed?
Minor Criteria: Q5: Was the Method of Randomization Described in the Paper? Q6: Was Allocation Concealed? Q7: Was ITT Used? Q8: Was the Credibility Comparable? ROB = Risk of Bias.

Score calculated by multiplying each major criteria by two and then adding across all eight questions. <6= high ROB, 6–8 = medium ROB, 9–12 = low ROB.
* Scored as high due to uncertain sampling method
** Scored as high due to very high attrition, 42% for Mularski and 61% for Brewer

Key Question Results

Since there were numerous scales for the different measures of affect, as well as subgroups within each affect, we organized the scales to best represent the clinically relevant aspects of each affect. For this review, the comparisons with nonspecific active controls were the most meaningful as they allowed a consistent comparison with a similar control group across all outcomes (efficacy). Comparisons with specific active controls were more difficult to draw conclusions from due to the large heterogeneity of type and strength of control groups (comparative effectiveness). Therefore, our results are presented first for all the comparisons with nonspecific active controls, and then for the specific active controls. We present summary results for all outcomes in Figure 4a (comparisons with nonspecific active controls) and 4b (comparisons with specific active controls) prior to describing each of the sections in detail. Tables 8–16 give synthesis summaries of all the trials by outcome.

Figure 4a. Summary across measurement domains of comparisons of meditation with nonspecific active controls
[See combined legend for Figures 4a and 4b following the figures for further information, including explanations of symbols and definitions of lettered footnotes]

Outcome	Meditation Program	Population	Direction[1] (Magnitude[2]) of Effect	Number of Trials Total [PO]: PA (MA)[3], total N	SOE[4]
Anxiety (KQ1)	Mindfulness	Various	↑ (0% to +44%)	7 [3]: 6 (6), N=558	Moderate for ↑
	Mantra	Various	∅ (−3% to +6%)	3 [2]: 3 (3), N=237	Low for ∅
Depression (KQ1)	Mindfulness	Various	↑ (0% to +52%)	9 [4]: 8 (8), N=768	Moderate for ↑
	Mantra	Various	↑↓ (−19% to +46%)	4 [1]: 4 (2), N=420	Insufficient
Stress/Distress (KQ1)	Mindfulness	Various	↑ (+1% to +21%)	8 [3]: 6 (6), N=697 *	Low for ↑
	Mantra	Select	∅ (−6% to +1%)	3 [1]: 3 (2), N=219	Low for ∅
Negative Affect (KQ1)	Mindfulness	Various	↑ (0% to +44%)	13 [5]:11 (11), N=1102+	Low for ↑
	Mantra	Various	↑↓ (−3% to +46%)	5 [2]: 5 (0), N=438 **	Insufficient
Positive Affect (KQ1)	Mindfulness	Various	↑ (+1% to +55%)	3 [0]: 3 (3), N=255	Insufficient
	TM (Mantra)	CHF	∅ (+2%)	1 [0]: 1 (0), N=23	Insufficient
Quality of Life (KQ1)	Mindfulness	Various	↑ (+5% to +28%)	4 [2]: 4 (3), N=346	Low for ↑
Attention (KQ2)	Mindfulness	Caregivers	↑ (+15% to +81%)	1 [0]: 1 (0), N=21	Insufficient
Sleep (KQ3)	Mindfulness	Various	↑↓ (−3% to +24%)	4 [1]: 3 (3), N=451	Insufficient
Substance Use (KQ3)	TM	CAD	∅	1 [2]: 0 (0), N=201	Insufficient
Pain (KQ4)	Mindfulness	Select	↑ (+5% to +31%)	4 [2]: 4 (4), N=341	Moderate for ↑
	TM (Mantra)	CHF	∅ (−2%)	1 [2]: 1 (0), N=23	Low for ∅
Weight (KQ4)	TM (Mantra)	Select	∅ (−1% to +2%)	3 [0]: 2 (0), N=297	Low for ∅

−1 Favors Meditation   0 Favors Control   1

35

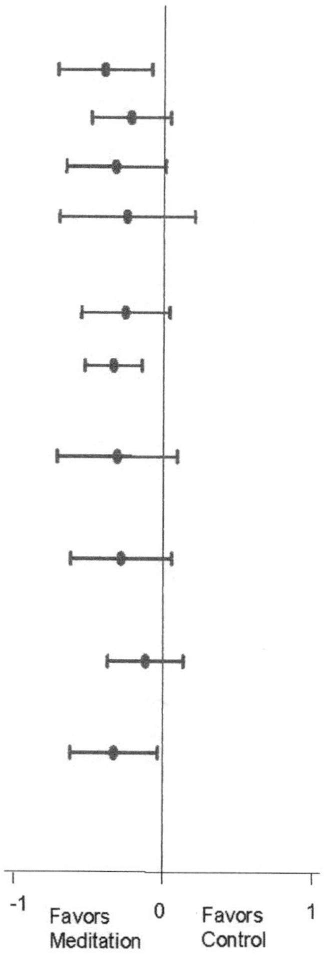

Figure 4b. Summary across measurement domains of comparisons of meditation with specific active controls
[See combined legend for Figures 4a and 4b following the figures for further information, including explanations of symbols and definitions of lettered footnotes]

Outcome	Meditation Program	Population	Direction[1] (Magnitude[2]) of Effect	Number of Trials Total [PO]: PA (MA)[3], total N	SOE[4]
Anxiety (KQ1)	Mindfulness	Various	↑↓ (−39% to +8%)	9 [5]: 9 (8), N=526	Insufficient
	CSM (mantra)	Anxiety	↓ (−6%)	1 [1]: 1 (0), N=42	Insufficient
Depression (KQ1)	Mindfulness	Various	↑↓ (−32% to +23%)	11 [5]:11 (9), N=821	Insufficient
	CSM (mantra)	Anxiety	↓ (−28%)	1 [1]: 1 (0), N=42	Insufficient
Stress/Distress (KQ1)	Mindfulness	Various	↑↓ (−24% to +18%)	6 [4]: 6 (6), N=508	Insufficient
Positive Affect (KQ1)	Mindfulness	Various	↑↓ (−45% to +10%)	4 [2]: 4 (4), N=297	Insufficient
Quality of Life (KQ1)	Mindfulness	Various	↑↓ (−23% to +9%)	6 [1]: 6 (5), N=472	Insufficient
KQ3: Sleep	Mindfulness	Various	↑↓ (−2% to +15%)	3 [1]: 3 (2), N=311	Insufficient
KQ3: Eating	Mindfulness	Select	↓ (−6% to −15%)	2 [1]: 2 (0), N=158	Insufficient
KQ3: Smoking/Alcohol	Mindfulness	Substance abuse	↑ (Ø to +21%)	2 [2]: 1 (0), N=95	Insufficient
KQ3: Alcohol Only	Mantra	Alcoholic	Ø (−5% to −36%)	2 [2]: 2 (0), N=145	Low for Ø
Pain (KQ4)	Mindfulness	Select	Ø (−1% to −32%)	4 [2]: 4 (4), N=410	Low for Ø
Weight (KQ4)	Mindfulness	Select	Ø (−2% to +1%)	2 [2]: 2 (0), N=151	Low for Ø

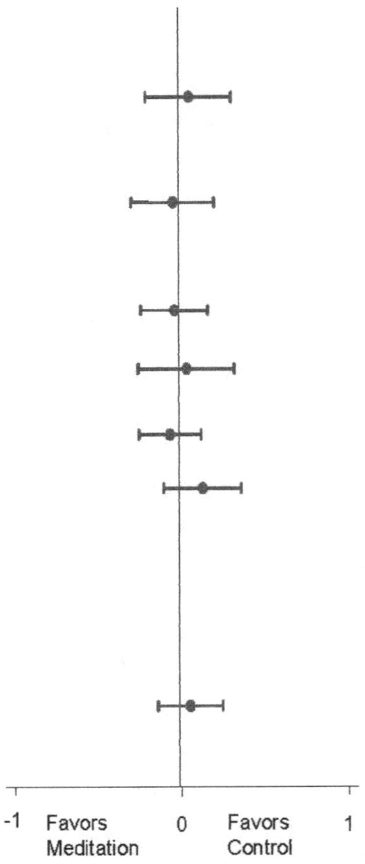

Notes: SOE = Strength of Evidence; PO = Number of trials in which this was a primary outcome for the trial; PA = Primary Analysis; MA = Meta-analysis; CSM = Clinically Standardized Meditation, a mantra meditation program; CHF = Congestive Heart Failure; CA = Cancer
Meta-analysis figure shows Cohen's d with the 95% CI

Legend for Figure 4a and Figure 4b
The figure on the far right shows the effect size estimates using Cohen's d (in standard deviation units with the associated 95% confidence interval) whenever sufficient data were available to perform a meta-analysis. For comparisons with nonspecific active control (NSAC), all eligible studies were included in the analysis for the outcomes of pain and positive affect for mindfulness trials, and for the outcome of anxiety for mantra. For comparisons with specific active control (SAC), all eligible studies were included in the analysis for the outcome of stress/distress, positive affect and pain for mindfulness trials. For all other meta-analyses, only a subset of eligible studies was included because data was missing in some studies. The meta-analysis results should be interpreted with caution because the inconsistent reporting of data suggests possible reporting bias.

Direction: direction of change in the outcome across trials, based on the relative difference between groups in how the outcome measure changed from baseline in each trial. This is calculated as the difference between the change over time in the meditation group and the change over time in the control group, divided by the baseline mean for the meditation group.
↑ indicates that the meditation group improved relative to the control group (with a relative difference generally greater than or equal to 5% across trials).
↓ indicates the meditation group worsened relative to the control group (with a relative difference generally greater than or equal to 5% across trials).
Ø indicates a null effect (with a relative difference generally less than 5% across trials).
↑↓ inconsistent findings (some trials reported improvement with meditation (relative to control) while others showed no improvement or improvement in the control group (relative to meditation).

Magnitude: range of estimates across all trials in a particular domain based on the relative difference between groups in how the outcome measure changed from baseline in each trial. This is a relative percentage difference calculated as: {# (Meditation T2 - Meditation T1) - (Control T2 - Control T1)}/ (Meditation T1) where T1 = baseline mean and T2 = follow up mean (after intervention or at the end of the study). This is a simple range of estimates, not a meta-analysis.

Total number: the number of trials that measured this outcome; PO - the number of trials for which this outcome was a primary outcome; PA – the primary analysis (PA) - refers to the number of trials which reported information allowing calculation of the relative difference between groups in the change score; MA – refers to the number of trials reporting sufficient information to be included in a meta-analysis. N refers to the total sample size.

Strength of evidence (SOE): based on aggregate risk of bias, consistency across studies, directness of measures, and precision of estimates. SOE rating is given for the direction of effect in most cases. In some cases, such as mantra meditation programs for anxiety, although the relative differences between groups in the change scores showed inconsistency in findings, the meta-analysis gave a precise estimate favoring one direction.

Table 8. Synthesis summary for anxiety

Author, year	Meditation Program	Type of Active Control	Risk of Bias	Program Training (hrs)	Home-work (hrs)	Program Duration (wks)	Scale	Outcome at End of Treatment	Outcome at End of Study	Population	N
Henderson, 2011[57]	MBSR	NSAC	7	25	?	8	BAI	ns	ns	breast cancer	100
Gaylord, 2011[53]	MBSR	NSAC	8	23*	Y	8	BSI-18	Ø/↑	+	IBS	75
Schmidt, 2010[70]	MBSR	NSAC	8	27	42	8	STAI trait	Ø/↑	+/Ø	fibromyalgia	109
Gross, 2010[54]	MBSR	NSAC	7	27	Y	8	STAI	↑	↑	organ transplant	137
Whitebird, 2012[72]	MBSR	NSAC	8	25	26.7	8	STAI state	Ø	Ø	dementia caregivers	78
Lee, 2006[60]	MM	NSAC	7	8	Y	8	STAI trait	+		anxiety	41
Chiesa, 2012[86]	MBCT	NSAC	6	16	?	8	BAI	↑		depression	18
Wong, 2011[74]	MBSR	Pain AC	11	27	Y	8	STAI Trait	Ø	Ø	chronic pain	99
Gross, 2011[55]	MBSR	Drug	8	26	36	8	STAI state	Ø	Ø/↑	insomnia	27
Koszycki, 2007[58]	MBSR	CBGT	5	27.5	28	8	SIAS	↓		anxiety	53
Barrett, 2012[85]	MBSR	Exercise	8	20	42	8	STAI state	Ø	Ø	cold/URI	98
Jazaieri, 2012[87]	MBSR	Exercise	5	25	28.3	8	Liebowitz SAS	↑	Ø	Social anxiety disorder	56
Moritz, 2006[63]	MBSR	Spirituality	9	12*	Y	8	POMS Tension	⊖		mood disturbance (POMS)	110
Philippot, 2011[67]	MBCT	Relaxation	7	13.5	Y	6	STAI	↑	↑	Tinnitus	25
Delgado, 2010[51]	MM	PMR	6	10	Y	5	STAI Trait	Ø		worriers	32
Piet, 2010[68]	MBCT	CBGT	8	16	28	8	BAI	↓		social phobia	26
Bormann, 2006[75]	Mantra	NSAC	6	7.5	Y	5	STAI Trait	Ø/↑	Ø	HIV	93
Paul-Labrador, 2006[81]	TM	NSAC	9	39	Y	16	STAI Trait	Ø	Ø	CAD	103
Smith, 1976[83]	TM	NSAC	5	?	87.5	25	STAI Trait	Ø		anxious people	41
Lehrer, 1983[79]	CSM	PMR	7	7.5	y	5	STAI Trait	Ø/↓		anxiety	42

Notes: *=estimated; Ø=no effect (within + or − 5%); +=improved and statistically significant; ++=improved & statistically significant; Ø/↓= borderline worsened; Ø/↑= borderline improved; +/Ø = less than or equal to 5% improvement, but statistically significant; ↑/+= improved with borderline statistical significance; ?= unclear; Y= yes, homework was prescribed but amount not reported; ns= not significant, not reported; NSAC = Nonspecific active control; MBSR = mindfulness-based stress reduction; MM = mindfulness meditation; MBCT = mindfulness based cognitive therapy; TM = transcendental meditation; CSM = clinically standardized meditation; PMR = progressive muscle relaxation; CBGT = cognitive behavioral group therapy; Pain AC = pain active control; BAI = beck anxiety inventory; BSI-18 = brief symptom inventory 18; STAI = state trait anxiety inventory; SIAS = social interaction anxiety scale; POMS = profile of mood states; SAS = social anxiety scale

Table 9. Synthesis summary for depression

Author, year	Meditation Program	Type of Active Control	Risk of Bias	Program Training (hrs)	Home-work (hrs)	Program Duration (wks)	Scale	Outcome at End of Treatment	Outcome at End of Study	Population	N
Henderson, 2011[57]	MBSR	NSAC	7	25	?	8	SCL90 Dep	+	↑	breast cancer	105
Gaylord, 2011[53]	MBSR	NSAC	8	23*	Y	8	BSI18 Dep	Ø	Ø	IBS	75
Schmidt, 2010[70]	MBSR	NSAC	8	27	42	8	CESD	Ø	↑	fibromyalgia	109
Gross, 2010[54]	MBSR	NSAC	7	27	Y	8	CESD	↑	↑	organ transplant	137
Whitebird, 2012[72]	MBSR	NSAC	8	25	26.7	8	CESD	+	↑	dementia caregivers	78
Oken,2010[66]	MM	NSAC	8	9	Y	7	CESD	↑		dementia caregivers	19
Lee, 2006[60]	MM	NSAC	7	8	Y	8	SCL90 Dep	↑		anxiety	41
Malarkey,2012[61]	MM	NSAC	9	9	18.5	8	CESD	ns		CRP>3.0	186
Chiesa, 2012[86]	MBCT	NSAC	6	16	?	8	HAMD	+		depression	18
Wong, 2011[74]	MBSR	Pain AC	11	27	Y	8	CESD	Ø	Ø	chronic pain	99
Gross, 2011[55]	MBSR	drug	8	26	36	8	CESD	↑	↓	insomnia	27
Koszycki, 2007[58]	MBSR	CBGT	5	27.5	28	8	BDI	Ø		anxiety	53
Moritz, 2006[63]	MBSR	Spirituality	9	12*	Y	8	POMS dep	↓		mood disturbance (POMS)	110
Jazaieri,2012[87]	MBSR	exercise	5	25	28.3	8	BDI II	↑	↑	Social anxiety disorder	56
Philippot, 2011[67]	MBCT	relaxation	7	13.5	Y	6	BDI	↑	Ø	Tinnitus	25
Delgado, 2010[51]	MM	PMR	6	10	Y	5	BDI	↑		worriers	32
Wolever, 2012[73]	MM	Viniyoga	7	14	?	12	CESD	↑		stressed employees	186
Piet, 2010[68]	MBCT	CBGT	8	16	28	8	BDI	↓		social phobia	26
Segal, 2010[71]	MBCT	drug	9	23*	Y	8	SCID		↑	depression	84
Kuyken, 2008[59]	MBCT	drug	10	24*	37.5	8	BDI	↑	↑	depression	123
Paul-Labrador, 2006[81]	TM	NSAC	9	39	Y	16	CESD		↑	CAD	103
Jayadevappa, 2007[78]	TM	NSAC	10	22.5*	90	25	CESD		↑	CHF	23
Schneider, 2012[90]	TM	NSAC	11	~78*	1310	5.4 yrs	CESD		↑	CAD	201
Bormann, 2006[75]	Mantra	NSAC	6	7.5	Y	5	CESD	Ø	↓	HIV	93
Lehrer, 1983[79]	CSM	PMR	7	7.5	y	5	SCL90 Dep	↓		anxiety	42

*=estimated; Ø=no effect (within + or − 5%); +=borderline improved; ↑= improved and statistically significant; ↑= favors meditation > 5% but non significant; ↓=favors control > 5% but non significant; ⊖ = worsened & statistically significant; Ø/↑= borderline worsened; ?= unclear; Y= yes, homework was prescribed but amount not specified; ns= not significant, not reported; NSAC = Nonspecific active control; MBSR = mindfulness-based stress reduction; MM = mindfulness meditation; MBCT = mindfulness based cognitive therapy; TM = transcendental meditation; CSM = clinically standardized meditation; PMR = progressive muscle relaxation; CBGT = cognitive behavioral group therapy; Pain AC = pain active control; BSI-18 = brief symptom inventory 18; POMS = profile of mood states; BDI=Becks Depression Inventory; CESD=Center for Epidemiologic Studies Depression Scale; IBS=Irritable Bowel Syndrome; SCID= Structured Clinical Interview ; HAM-D= Hamilton Psychiatric Rating Scale for Depression; CAD=Coronary Artery Disease;CHF=;Congestive Heart Failure; CRP=C-reactive protein

Table 10. Synthesis summary for stress/distress

Author, year	Meditation Program	Type of Active Control	Risk of Bias	Program Training (hrs)	Home-work (hrs)	Program Duration (wks)	Scale	Outcome at End of Treatment	Outcome at End of Study	Population	N
Gaylord, 2011[53]	MBSR	NSAC	8	23*	Y	8	BSI Gen Sx	Ø/↑	Ø/+	IBS	75
Whitebird, 2012[72]	MBSR	NSAC	8	25	26.7	8	PSS	+	+	dementia caregivers	78
SeyedAlinaghi, 2012[89]	MBSR	NSAC	4	25*	y	8	SCL90R	↑	↓	HIV	171
Pbert L, 2012[88]	MBSR	NSAC	9	26	24	8	PSS	↑/+	+	Asthmatics	82
Oken, 2010[66]	MM	NSAC	8	9	Y	7	PSS	↑		dementia caregivers	19
Garland, 2010[52]	MORE	NSAC	7	?	17.5	10	PSS	+		alcohol	37
Mularski, 2009[65]	MBBT	NSAC	High	8	Y	8	PSS	Ø		COPD	49
Malarkey, 2012[61]	MM	NSAC	9	9	18.5	8	PSS	ns		CRP>3.0	186
Jazaieri, 2012[87]	MBSR	exercise	5	25	28.3	8	PSS	↑		Anxiety	56
Barrett, 2012[85]	MBSR	exercise	8	20	42	8	PSS	Ø	Ø	colds in past yr	98
Moritz, 2006[63]	MBSR	Spirituality	9	12*	Y	8	POMS total mood disturbance	⊖	↓	mood disturbance (POMS)	110
Delgado, 2010[51]	MM	PMR	6	10	Y	5	PANAS-N	Ø/↓		worriers	32
Wolever, 2012[73]	MM	Viniyoga	7	14	?	12	PSS	Ø		stressed employees	186
Piet, 2010[68]	MBCT	CBGT	8	16	28	8	SCL90 GSI	↓		social phobia	26
Paul-Labrador, 2006[81]	TM	NSAC	9	39	Y	16	Life Stress Instrument	Ø/↓	Ø	CAD	103
Jayadevappa, 2007[78]	TM	NSAC	10	22.5*	90	25	PSS	Ø	Ø	CHF	23
Bormann, 2006[75]	Mantra	NSAC	6	7.5	Y	5	PSS	Ø	Ø	HIV	93

Notes: *=estimated; Ø=no effect (within + or − 5%); +=improved and statistically significant; ↑=improved meditation > 5% but non significant; ⊖ = worsened & statistically significant; Ø/↑ = borderline improved; Ø/↓= borderline worsened; ↑/+= improved with borderline statistical significance; ?= unclear; Y= yes, homework was prescribed but amount not specified; ns= not significant, not reported ;NSAC = Nonspecific active control; MBSR = mindfulness-based stress reduction; MM = mindfulness meditation; MBCT = mindfulness based cognitive therapy; TM = transcendental meditation; PMR = progressive muscle relaxation; MORE=Mindfulness oriented Recovery Enhancement; BSI Gen SX=Brief Symptom Inventory ;PSS=Perceived Stress Scale; SCL90R=Symptom Checklist-90; PANAS-N=Positive and Negative Affect Scale-negative mood; SCL90 GSI=Symptom Checklist 90- Global Severity Index; IBS=Irritable Bowel Syndrome ; HIV=Human Immunodeficiency Virus; COPD=Chronic Obstructive Pulmonary Disease; CAD=Coronary Artery Disease, CHF=Congestive Heart Failure

Table 11. Synthesis summary for negative affect

Author, year	Meditation Program	Type of Active Control	Risk of Bias	Program Training (hrs)	Home-work (hrs)	Program Duration (wks)	Scale	Outcome at End of Treatment	Outcome at End of Study	Population	N
Henderson, 2011[57]	MBSR	NSAC	7	BAI	ns	ns	SCL90 Dep	+	↑	breast cancer	100
Gaylord, 2011[53]	MBSR	NSAC	8	BSI-18 Anxiety	Ø/↑	+	BSI Gen Sx	Ø/↑	Ø/+	IBS	75
Schmidt, 2010[70]	MBSR	NSAC	8	STAI trait	Ø/↑	+/Ø	CESD	Ø	↑	fibromyalgia	109
Oken, 2010[66]	MM	NSAC	8	CESD	↑		PSS	↑		dementia caregivers	19
Gross, 2010[54]	MBSR	NSAC	7	STAI	↑	↑	CESD	↑	↑	organ transplant	137
Garland, 2010[52]	MT	NSAC	7	PSS	+		PSS	+		alcohol	37
Mularski, 2009[65]	MBBT	NSAC	High	PSS	Ø		PSS	Ø		COPD	49
Lee, 2006[60]	MM	NSAC	7	STAI trait	+		SCL90 Dep	↑		anxiety	41
Malarkey, 2012[61]	MM	NSAC	9	CESD	ns		PSS	ns		CRP > 3.0	186
Whitebird, 2012[72]	MBSR	NSAC	8	STAI state	Ø	Ø	PSS	+	+	dementia caregivers	78
Chiesa, 2012[86]	MBCT	NSAC	6	BAI	↑		HAMD	+		depression	18
Seyedalinaghi, 2012[89]	MBSR	NSAC	4	SCL90R	↑	↓	SCL90R	↑	↓	HIV in Iran	171
Pbert L, 2012[88]	MBSR	NSAC	9	PSS	↑/+	+	PSS	↑/+	+	Asthmatics	82
Bormann, 2006[75]	Mantra	NSAC	6	STAI Trait	Ø/↑	Ø	PSS	Ø	Ø	HIV	93
Paul-Labrador, 2006[81]	TM	NSAC	9	STAI Trait	Ø		Life Stress Instrument	Ø/↓		CAD	103
Smith, 1976[83]	TM	NSAC	5	STAI Trait	Ø		STAI Trait	Ø		anxious people	41
Jayadevappa, 2007[78]	TM	NSAC	10	CESD	↑	↑	PSS	Ø	Ø	CHF	23
Schneider, 2012[90]	TM	NSAC	11	CESD		↑	CESD		↑/Ø	CAD	178

Notes: *=estimated; Ø=no effect (within + or − 5%); +=improved and statistically significant; ↑= favors meditation > 5% but non significant; ↓=favors control > 5% but non significant; ⊖ = worsened & statistically significant; Ø/↓= borderline worsened; Ø/↑= borderline improved; ?= unclear; Y= yes, homework was prescribed but amount not specified; ns= not significant, not reported; CESD=;NSAC = Nonspecific active control; MBSR = mindfulness-based stress reduction; MM = mindfulness meditation; TM = transcendental meditation; MT=Mindfulness Training; BAI = Beck anxiety inventory; BSI-18 = brief symptom inventory 18; STAI = state trait anxiety inventory; PSS=Perceived Stress Scale; SCL90 Dep= Symptom checklist 90 depression; IBS= Irritable bowel Syndrome; CRP=c-reactive protein; CHF=Congestive heart failure; CAD=Coronary Artery Disease; COPD=Chronic obstructive Pulmonary Disease

Table 12. Synthesis summary for positive affect (well being and positive mood)

Author, year	Meditation Program	Type of Active Control	Risk of Bias	Program Training (hrs)	Home-work (hrs)	Program Duration (wks)	Scale	Outcome at End of Treatment	Outcome at End of Study	Population	N
Henderson, 2011[57]	MBSR	NSAC	7	25	?	8	SOC:MS	+/Ø	Ø	breast cancer	100
Gross, 2010[54]	MBSR	NSAC	7	27	Y	8	SF36 V	Ø	↑	organ tx	137
Chiesa, 2012[86]	MBCT	NSAC	6	16	?	8	PGWBI	+		depression	18
Moritz, 2006[63]	MBSR	Spirituality	9	12*	Y	8	SF36 V	⊖		mood disturbance (POMS)	110
Barrett, 2012[85]	MBSR	exercise	8	20	42	8	PANAS-p	Ø	Ø	cold in past year	98
Jazaieri, 2012[87]	MBSR	exercise	5	25	28.3#	8	SWLS	↑		Anxiety	56
Delgado, 2010[51]	MM	PMR	6	10	Y	5	PANAS-p	Ø		worriers	33
Jayadevappa, 2007[78]	TM	NSAC	10	22.5*	90	25	SF36 V	Ø	Ø	CHF	23

Notes: *=estimated; Ø=no effect (within + or − 5%); +=improved and statistically significant; ↑= favors meditation > 5% but non significant; ⊖ = worsened & statistically significant; ?= unclear; Y= yes, homework was prescribed but amount not specified; ns= not significant, not reported; ; NSAC = Nonspecific active control; MBSR = mindfulness-based stress reduction; MM = mindfulness meditation; MBCT = mindfulness based cognitive therapy; TM = transcendental meditation; PMR = progressive muscle relaxation; SF 36V=Short Form 36 Veteran Rand; PGWBI=Psychological General Well-Being Index ; PANAS-p=Positive and Negative Affect Scale-positive mood ; SWLS= Satisfaction with Life Scale; CHF= Congestive Heart Failure; POMS=Profile of Mood States

Table 13. Synthesis summary for quality of life/mental component of health-related quality of life

Author, year	Meditation Program	Type of Active Control	Risk of Bias	Program Training (hrs)	Homework (hrs)	Program Duration (wks)	Scale	Outcome at End of Treatment	Outcome at End of Study	Population	N
Gross, 2010[54]	MBSR	NSAC	7	27	Y	8	SF12:MC	Ø/↑	Ø/↑	organ transplant	137
Whitebird, 2012[72]	MBSR	NSAC	8	25	26.7#	8	SF12:MC	+	+	dementia caregivers	78
Pbert L, 2012[88]	MBSR	NSAC	9	26	24	8	Asthma QoL:Emotion	↑	+	Asthmatics	82
Mularski, 2009[65]	MBBT	NSAC	poor	8	Y	8	VR36: MC	↑		COPD	49
Wong, 2011[74]	MBSR	Pain AC	11	27	Y	8	SF12:MC	Ø	Ø	chronic pain	99
Gross, 2011[55]	MBSR	drug	8	26	36	8	SF12:MC	Ø		insomnia	27
Moritz, 2006[63]	MBSR	Spirituality	9	12*	Y	8	SF36:MC	⊖	→	mood disturbance (POMS)	110
Plews-Ogan, 2005[69]	MBSR	Massage	5	20	Y	8	SF12:MC	→	↑	chronic pain	15
Barrett, 2012[85]	MBSR	exercise	8	20	42	8	SF12:MC	Ø	Ø	cold in past year	98
Kuyken, 2008[59]	MBCT	drug	10	24*	37.5	8	WHOQL	+	+	depression	123

Notes: *=estimated; Ø=no effect (within + or − 5%); +=improved (within + or − 5%); += improved and statistically significant; ↑= favors meditation > 5% but non significant; ⊖ = worsened & statistically significant; Ø/↑= borderline improved; ?= unclear; Y= yes, homework was prescribed but amount not specified; ns= not significant, not reported; ; MBSR = mindfulness-based stress reduction; MBCT = mindfulness based cognitive therapy; Pain AC = pain active control; POMS = profile of mood states; SF12: MC= Short Form-12: Mental Component Score of Health-related Quality of Life; QoL=Quality of Life; SF36=MC= Short Form-36: Mental Component Score of Health-related Quality of Life; WHOQL= World Health Organization Quality of Life Assessment; COPD=Chronic obstructive pulmonary Disease

Table 14. Synthesis summary for substance use, eating, sleep

Author, year	Meditation Program	Type of Active Control	Risk of Bias	Program Training (hrs)	Home-work (hrs)?	Program Duration	Domain	Scale	Outcome at End of Treatment	Outcome at End of Study	Population	N
Mindfulness												
Schmidt, 2010[70]	MBSR	NSAC	8	27	42	8	Sleep	PSQI	Ø	Ø	fibromyalgia	109
Oken, 2010[66]	MM	NSAC	8	9	Y	7	Sleep	PSQI	Ø		dementia caregivers	19
Gross, 2010[54]	MBSR	NSAC	7	27	Y	8	Sleep	PSQI	↑/+	+	organ transplant	137
Malarkey, 2012[61]	MM	NSAC	9	9	18.5	8	Sleep	PSQI	ns		CRP>3.0	186
Wolever, 2012[73]	MM	exercise	7	14	?	12	Sleep	PSQI	Ø		stressed employees	186
Gross, 2011[55]	MBSR	drug	8	26	36	8	Sleep	PSQI	↑	Ø	insomnia	27
Barrett, 2012[85]	MBSR	exercise	8	20	42	8	Sleep	PSQI	Ø	Ø	cold/URI	98
Mindfulness												
Hebert, 2001[56]	MBSR	Nutrition Education	6	45*	?	15	Eating	Kcals/day	Ø	Ø	breast cancer	106
Miller, 2012[62]	MB-EAT	Smart Choices	5	25	Y	12	Eating	kcal/day	↓	↓	diabetes	52
Brewer, 2011[50]	MT	Lung Assoc FFS	5	12	Y	4	Smoking	cigs/day	↑/+	+	smokers	71
Mantra												
Brewer, 2009[49]	MT	CBT	poor	9	?	9	ETOH	drinks/day	ns		substance abuse	24
Murphy, 1986[80]	CSM	running	5	8	37.5	8	ETOH	drinks/week	⊖		alcohol	27
Taub, 1994[84]	TM	BF	7	19	?	4	ETOH	% days abstinent	Ø / ↓		alcohol	118

Notes: *=estimated; Ø=no effect (within + or − 5%); +=improved and statistically significant (within + or − 5%); +=improved and statistically significant; ↑= favors meditation > 5% but non significant; ⊖ = worsened & statistically significant; Ø/↓= borderline worsened; Ø/↑= borderline improved; ?= unclear; Y= yes, homework was prescribed but amount not specified; ns= not significant, not reported ; NSAC = Nonspecific active control; MBSR = mindfulness-based stress reduction; MM = mindfulness meditation; MB-EAT= Mindfulness Based Eating Training Program; MT=Mindfulness Training; BF=Biofeedback; CBT=Cognitive Behavioral Therapy ;CSM= clinically standardized meditation; ETOH=Ethanol; FFS=Freedom from Smoking; TM = transcendental meditation; PSQI=Pittsburgh Sleep Quality Index; ETOH=ethanol; cigs/day=cigarettes/day; CPR=c-reactive protein; URI=Upper Respiratory Infection

Table 15. Synthesis summary for pain

Author, year	Meditation Program	Type of Active Control	Risk of Bias	Program Training (hrs)	Home-work (hrs)	Program Duration (wks)	Scale	Outcome at End of Treatment	Outcome at End of Study	Population	N
Gaylord, 2011[53]	MBSR	NSAC	8	23*	Y	8	IBS Pain	+	+	IBS	75
Schmidt, 2010[70]	MBSR	NSAC	8	27	42	8	PPS Sens	↑/Ø	Ø	fibromyalgia	109
Gross, 2010[54]	MBSR	NSAC	7	27	Y	8	SF36BP	↑/Ø	↑/Ø	organ transplant	122
Morone, 2009[64]	MBSR	NSAC	11	12	42	8	SF36BP	↑	Ø	Low back pain	35
Wong, 2011[74]	MBSR	Pain AC	11	27	Y	8	NRS	Ø	Ø	chronic pain	99
Moritz, 2006[63]	MBSR	Spirituality	9	12*	Y	8	SF36BP	↓/Ø		mood disturbance (POMS)	110
Plews-Ogan, 2005[69]	MBSR	Massage	5	20	Y	8	NRS	→	→	chronic pain	15
Wolever, 2012[73]	MM	Viniyoga	7	14	?	12	NRS	→		stressed employees	186
Jayadevappa, 2007[78]	TM	NSAC	10	22.5*	90	25	SF36BP	Ø	↑/Ø	CHF	23

Notes: *=estimated; Ø=no effect (within + or − 5%); +=improved and statistically significant; ↑= favors meditation > 5% but non significant; ↓= favors control > 5% but non significant; Ø/↓= borderline worsened; Ø/↑= borderline improved; ?= unclear; Y= yes, homework was prescribed but amount not specified; ns= not significant, not reported; NSAC = Nonspecific active control; MBSR = mindfulness-based stress reduction; MM = mindfulness meditation; TM = transcendental meditation; POMS = profile of mood states; PPS Sens= Pain perception sensory; SF 36 BP=Short Form 36 Bodily Pain; NRS=Numeric Rating Scale; IBS= Irritable Bowel Syndrome; CHF=Congestive heart Failure

Table 16. Synthesis summary for weight

Author, year	Meditation Program	Type of Active Control	Risk of Bias	Program Training (hrs)	Homework (hrs)	Program Duration (wks)	Scale	Outcome at End of Treatment	Outcome at End of Study	Population	N
Hebert, 2001[56]	MBSR	Nutrition Education	6	45*	?	15	kg	Ø	Ø	breast cancer	99
Miller, 2012[62]	MBSR	Smart Choices	5	25	Y	12	kg	Ø	Ø	diabetes	52
Elder, 2006[77]	TM	NSAC	6	?	90	?	kg	Ø		diabetes	54
Castillo-Richmond, 2000[76]	TM	NSAC	poor	?	120.6	12	kg	Ø		hypertensive AA	**60/170**
Schneider, 2012[90]	TM	NSAC	11	~78*	1310	5.4 yrs	BMI		ns	CAD	183

Notes: *=estimated; Ø=no effect (within + or – 5%); ?= unclear; Y= yes, homework was prescribed but amount not specified; ns= not significant, not reported; NSAC = Nonspecific active control; MBSR = mindfulness-based stress reduction; TM = transcendental meditation; CAD=Coronary Artery Disease; BMI=Body Mass Index

Key Question 1. What are the efficacy and harms of meditation programs on negative affect (e.g., anxiety, stress) and positive affect (e.g., well-being) among those with a clinical condition (medical or psychiatric)?

Key Points and Evidence Grades

Comparisons With <u>Nonspecific</u> Active Controls

Anxiety
- The strength of evidence is moderate that mindfulness meditation programs result in a small improvement in anxiety among various clinical populations when compared with a nonspecific active control. We based this rating on overall medium risk of bias, consistent findings for a small positive effect, directness of measures, and precise estimates.
- The strength of evidence is low that mantra meditation programs do not have an effect on anxiety among various clinical populations when compared with a nonspecific active control. We based this rating on overall medium risk of bias, consistent findings, directness of measures, and imprecise estimates.

Depression
- The strength of evidence is moderate that mindfulness meditation programs improve symptoms of depression among various clinical populations when compared with a nonspecific active control. We based this rating on overall medium risk of bias, consistent findings for a positive effect, directness of measures, and precise estimates. However, since one trial is missing from the meta-analysis and the post-intervention I^2 is high, this strength of evidence warrants a cautious interpretation.
- The strength of evidence is insufficient that mantra meditations have an effect on symptoms of depression among cardiac and HIV populations when compared with a nonspecific active control. We based this rating on overall medium risk of bias, inconsistent findings, directness of measures, and imprecise estimates.

Stress/Distress
- The strength of evidence is low that mindfulness meditation programs result in a small improvement in stress and distress among various clinical populations when compared with a nonspecific active control. We based this rating on overall medium risk of bias, inconsistent findings, directness of measures, and precise estimates.
- The strength of evidence is low that mantra meditation programs have no effect on stress when compared with a nonspecific active control. We based this rating on overall medium risk of bias, consistent findings of a null effect, directness of measures, and imprecise estimates.

Negative Affect
- The strength of evidence is low that mindfulness meditation programs improve negative affect among various clinical populations when compared with a nonspecific active

control. We based this rating on overall medium risk of bias, consistent results, indirect measures of negative affect, and precise estimates.
- The strength of evidence is insufficient that mantra programs have an effect on negative affect among various clinical populations when compared with a nonspecific active control. We based this rating on overall medium risk of bias, inconsistent results, indirect measures of negative affect, and imprecise estimates.

Positive Affect
- The strength of evidence is insufficient that mindfulness meditation programs have an effect on positive affect when compared with a nonspecific active control. We based this rating on medium risk of bias, consistent findings, indirect measures, and imprecise estimates.
- The strength of evidence is insufficient about the effects of TM on positive affect when compared with a nonspecific active control. We based this rating on a single low risk-of-bias study, unknown consistency, indirect measures, and imprecise estimates.

Mental Component of Health-Related Quality of Life
- The strength of evidence is low that mindfulness meditation programs improve the mental component of health-related quality of life (QOL) in various patients as compared with a nonspecific active control. We based this rating on overall medium risk of bias, consistent findings, direct measures, and imprecise estimates.

Comparisons With <u>Specific</u> Active Controls

Anxiety
- The strength of evidence is insufficient that mindfulness meditation programs have an effect on anxiety among various clinical populations when compared with a variety of specific active controls. We based this rating on overall medium risk of bias, inconsistent findings, directness of measures, and imprecise estimates.
- The strength of evidence is insufficient about the effects of clinically standardized meditation on anxiety in an anxious population when compared with progressive muscle relaxation. We based this rating on a single study with medium risk of bias, unknown consistency, directness of measures, and imprecise estimates.

Depression
- The strength of evidence is insufficient that mindfulness meditation programs have an effect on depressive symptoms among various clinical populations compared with a variety of specific active controls. We based this rating on overall medium risk of bias, inconsistent results, direct measures, and imprecise estimates.
- The strength of evidence is insufficient that clinically standardized meditation has an effect on depressive symptoms in an anxious population compared with progressive muscle relaxation. We based this rating on a single study with medium risk of bias, unknown consistency, direct measures, and imprecise estimates.

Stress/Distress
- The strength of evidence is insufficient that mindfulness meditation programs affect distress among those with mood disturbance or symptoms of anxiety compared with a variety of specific active controls. We based this rating on overall medium risk of bias, inconsistent results, direct measures, and imprecise estimates.

Positive Affect
- The strength of evidence is insufficient that mindfulness meditation programs have an effect on positive affect among those with a mood disturbance or symptoms of anxiety when compared with a variety of specific active controls. We based this rating on overall medium risk of bias, inconsistent findings, indirect measures, and imprecise estimates.

Mental Component of Health-Related Quality of Life
- The strength of evidence is insufficient that mindfulness meditation programs have an effect on the mental component of health-related QOL among various clinical populations when compared with a variety of specific active controls. We based this rating on overall medium risk of bias, inconsistent findings, direct measures, and imprecise estimates.

Harms
- Four studies reported on adverse events, but participants experienced no adverse events and 28 studies did not report on adverse events.

Trial Characteristics

We included 32 trials for this KQ, of which 19 took place in the United States. Three trials took place in Canada. Seven trials took place in Europe, including Belgium, the United Kingdom (two trials), Spain, Denmark, Italy, and Germany. The remaining three trials were done in Hong Kong, South Korea, and Iran. Twenty-two of the trials took place in an outpatient setting, two in a university setting, and one in multiple settings; the remaining trials did not report the setting or it was unclear.

Nine trials explicitly reported the time period of recruitment. The year when recruitment started ranged from 1998 to 2010 in these trials. Twenty-five trials reported the trial duration, which ranged from 5 weeks to 9.3 years. All trials reported the length of treatment. The length of additional followup after treatment ranged from none (i.e. treatment assessed at its end) to over 9 years.

Eleven trials excluded patients with past or present substance abuse, 20 trials had exclusion criteria related to psychiatric conditions or treatment, and 20 trials excluded patients according to some medical diagnostic criteria (Appendix E, Evidence Table E2). Most trials (N=18) were of medium risk of bias, five were of high risk of bias, and nine were of low risk of bias.

Population Characteristics

The majority of trials recruited populations with chronic medical conditions, anxiety, or depression. Information was not available for the majority of trials on racial, ethnic, education, or gender composition.

The sample size of the trials ranged from 23–201, with a median sample size of 83. In eight trials the participants were from populations with psychiatric disorders, and in 16 trials the participants were from medical populations, including substance abuse, chronic pain, and fibromyalgia. Of the trials in medical populations, three trials were of subjects with acute or chronic pain or fibromyalgia;[69,70,74] seven trials were of subjects with anxiety disorders, anxiety trait, or worry;[51,58,60,68,79,83,88] three trials were of subjects with depression;[59,71,86] and 13 trials were of subjects with chronic medical conditions, including metabolic syndrome, COPD, HIV, asthma, and CHF.[53-55,57,65-67,75,78,81,88-90]. Twenty-eight trials provided information on the gender characteristics of the participants. In five trials, the population was 100 percent female.[51,53,57,66,70] The mean percentage of female participants in the remaining trials was 56 percent.

Thirty trials provided information on the age distribution of the trial population. The mean age in these trials ranged from 21.8–67.4 years (median=47). Only 16 trials provided information on racial or ethnic characteristics of their trial population. The proportion of white subjects among these populations ranged from 0 percent (in trials of African Americans with CHF) to 99 percent.[78] Twenty trials provided information on the level of completed education among trial participants (Appendix E, Evidence Table E3).

Intervention Characteristics

In the intervention arms, 14 trials administered MBSR, four administered MBCT, eight administered a mindfulness variant, four administered TM, and two administered other mantra meditations.

Mindfulness Trials

The mindfulness trials conducted a weekly training session that typically ran for 6–8 weeks. Exceptions include one mindfulness meditation trial that ran for 5 weeks on high worriers,[51], another that ran for 12 weeks with stressed employees [73], and one that ran for 10 weeks on alcohol-dependent people.[52]

Twelve of the 14 MBSR trials provided training that generally ranged from 20–27.5 hours; two trials did not clearly specify training time. Of those two, one used MBSR as a control group for a spirituality intervention; we estimated the maximal training time for that trial at 12 hours.[63] All MBSR trials, except two,[56,57] noted that they provided homework. Seven MBSR trials specified the amount of homework, which ranged from 24–42 hours over an 8-week period. Eleven of 14 MBSR trials noted that the teachers were trained, two noted they were certified, and three trials noted that their teachers had between 5–15.7 years of teaching experience. Three trials did not report on teacher qualifications. Seven of the MBSR trials used a nonspecific active control and seven used a specific active control.

For the four MBCT trials, the amount of meditation training ranged from 16–24 hours over an 8-week period. All but one of the trials[86] recommended home practice, and only two specified the amount, which ranged from 28–37.5 hours over the 8-week period. One reported the teacher was trained, and three reported the teachers were trained and certified. None gave details on amount of meditation or teaching experience. One used a nonspecific active control and three used a specific active control (Table 5).

Among the remaining eight mindfulness-variant trials, the amount of training ranged from 8–13.5 hours over 5–12 weeks. All except one recommended home practice and two trials specified the amount of home practice, which ranged from 17.5–18.5 hours over the training period. Seven of eight trials reported that their teachers were trained, and two noted that the amount of teaching experience ranged from 3–5 years. One trial did not report anything regarding teacher qualifications. Five used a nonspecific active control and three used a specific active control (Table 6).

Mantra Trials

The four TM trials generally had a format generally consistent with TM training.[78,81,83,90] There was an initial period of daily training for 1–1.5 hours for about 1 week, followed by periodic checks lasting 30–60 minutes over the followup period. One TM trial did not give enough information to calculate a training amount. All trials recommended daily homework, with the two 6-month trials recommending approximately 90 hours. The TM trials all use trained and certified teachers, although none specified the amount of meditation or teaching experience these teachers had. All four trials used a nonspecific active control.

Two trials used a mantra and were not of the TM tradition. Bormann et al. used mantras representing various spiritual traditions, based on the Easwaran approach.[75,90] Lehrer et al. used a clinically standardized meditation program.[79] Both trials consisted of no more than 7.5 hours of training over a 5-week period, with instructions to practice at home. Both studies reported that teachers were trained. The teachers for clinically standardized meditation were undergraduate and graduate students who had 4 months of training and had no prior meditation teaching experience.

Outcomes

Comparisons With Nonspecific Active Controls

Anxiety

Seven mindfulness meditation programs and three mantra meditation programs trials examined the effect of the meditation program on anxiety as compared with a nonspecific active control.[53,54,57,60,70,72,75,81,83,86,91] The trials included in this analysis used three measures of anxiety. We selected measures that are widely used in trials of anxiety, giving preference to those that most of the other trials in their comparison group used. This was to maintain as much homogeneity in the outcome scale as possible (Appendix E).

One mindfulness meditation program trial found nonsignificant results for its anxiety measure and did not report the data.[57]

Mindfulness Meditation Programs Versus Nonspecific Active Controls

Seven trials compared mindfulness meditation programs to nonspecific active controls for this outcome, and tended to show a small effect (Table 8, Figure 5). Five were MBSR trials, one was MBCT, and one was a modified version of MBSR. Four trials used the state trait anxiety inventory (STAI), while others used the brief symptom inventory anxiety subscale 18 or Beck anxiety inventory (BAI) scale. The five MBSR trials gave an equivalent amount of training, ranging from 23–27 hours, while the modified mindfulness trial gave 8 hours of training. The trials did not give enough information on the amount of home practice recommended or completed.

Among the trials that reported scores, a difference-in-change calculation shows that all had a 0.3–44 percent improvement post intervention (8 weeks), and a −2.3 to +6.8 percent improvement at the end of the trial (3–6 months). The trial conducted in Korea showed statistically significant results by the end of treatment, and the results reached statistical significance at the end of the study period for two other trials.

Gross et al. randomized patients with an organ transplant (n=138) to 8 weeks of MBSR or health education arms.[54] Anxiety was a primary outcome measure and it saw nonsignificant changes at 8 weeks and 6 months. Schmidt et al. randomized women with fibromyalgia (n=177) to one of three arms: (1) MBSR, (2) a nonspecific active control, or (3) a wait list.[70] The anxiety scale was a secondary outcome. The MBSR group showed a statistically significant 4.6 percent decrease in STAI trait score at 4 months (p=0.02) compared with the nonspecific active control. Gaylord et al. randomized women to an MBSR program adapted for individuals with irritable bowel syndrome (IBS) or a nonspecific active control (n=97).[53] The MBSR group showed a 6.8 percent change over baseline at 3 months (p=0.02). In a three-arm randomized clinical trial of women with early stage breast cancer, Henderson et al.[57] examined the effect of MBSR (n=100). They found no differences in scores of the BAI or the symptom checklist 90 (SCL-90) phobic anxiety scores, and did not report either set of scores.

Lee et al. randomized patients with anxiety disorders (n=46) recruited from a psychiatric hospital or its clinics in South Korea, to either an 8-week mindfulness-based stress management program or nonspecific active control (anxiety disorder-based education).[60] It was the only trial to use anxiety patients. The Korean meditation program did not appear to be a direct derivative of MBSR as most other trials in this review are, but shared overlapping features of mindfulness meditation. Outcome measures included both self-report measures (State-Trait Anxiety Inventory, State and Trait subscales; SCL-90 anxiety subscale; and a clinician-rated measure Hamilton psychiatric rating scale for anxiety. The trial standardized all of the self-report measures in Korean. The program provided 8 hours of training targeted towards anxiety reduction, with unspecified amount of home practice. At the end of 8 weeks of treatment, the meditation group showed a significantly greater improvement (p <.05) in all outcome measures compared with the education group, with relatively large effects (15–43 percent overall reduction on the measures compared with the education group). Of note, the trial saw the largest reduction (43 percent) on the clinician-rated Hamilton anxiety rating scale. This trial had a medium risk of bias.

Whitebird et al. randomized patients who were caregivers of family members with dementia (n=78) to either MBSR or education support group. This trial did not specify primary or secondary outcomes, but categorized anxiety as a primary focus of the study. The MBSR group showed no difference in the STAI state scores as compared with the education support group. We rated this trial as medium risk of bias. It provided 25 hours of training over 8 weeks by a trained teacher, with an average of 26.7 hours of homework completed by the participants.

Chiesa et al. randomized patients with major depression (n=18) who failed to achieve remission after at least 8 weeks of antidepressant therapy, to either MBCT or nonspecific active control. The trial found a nonsignificant 44 percent reduction in the BAI, which was a secondary outcome. We rated this trial as medium risk of bias. It provided 16 hours of training over 8 weeks by a trained and certified teacher, with unspecified home practice.

We conducted two meta-analyses, one of post-intervention outcomes at 8 weeks and one of end of study outcomes at 3–6 months (Figures 6–7). Both showed small and significant effect sizes favoring meditation, generally consistent with the difference-in-change analysis (Figure 5). Since the I^2 on the post-intervention meta-analysis was large and significant, we conducted a sensitivity analysis by removing the outlier trial by Lee et al. The effect size dropped to −0.24 (−0.44, −.04) with an I^2 of 0 percent (p=.49), and did not change our conclusions. Of note, these effect sizes do not account for the baseline differences and therefore may not be entirely consistent with the difference-in-change graphs.

In summary, the Korean meditation trial used an anxious population and showed large effect sizes on all measures of anxiety. The remaining trials used diverse clinical populations; among these, two trials showed small significant effects at 3–4 months. There was general consistency among all three measures of anxiety. All seven trials had a medium risk of bias.

The strength of evidence is moderate that mindfulness meditation programs result in a small improvement in anxiety among various clinical populations when compared with a nonspecific active control. We based this rating on overall medium risk of bias, consistent findings for a small positive effect, directness of measures, and precise estimates (Table 17).

Table 17. Grade of trials addressing the efficacy of mindfulness meditation program on anxiety compared with nonspecific active controls among various populations

Number of Trials; Subjects	Domains Pertaining to Strength of Evidence				Magnitude of Effect and Strength of Evidence
	Risk of Bias	Consistency	Directness	Precision	
Anxiety					Moderate SOE of an improvement
7; 558	Medium	Consistent	Direct	Precise	0.3% to 44% improvement favoring meditation

Note: SOE = Strength of Evidence

Figure 5. Relative difference between groups in the changes in measures of general anxiety, in the mindfulness versus nonspecific active control studies

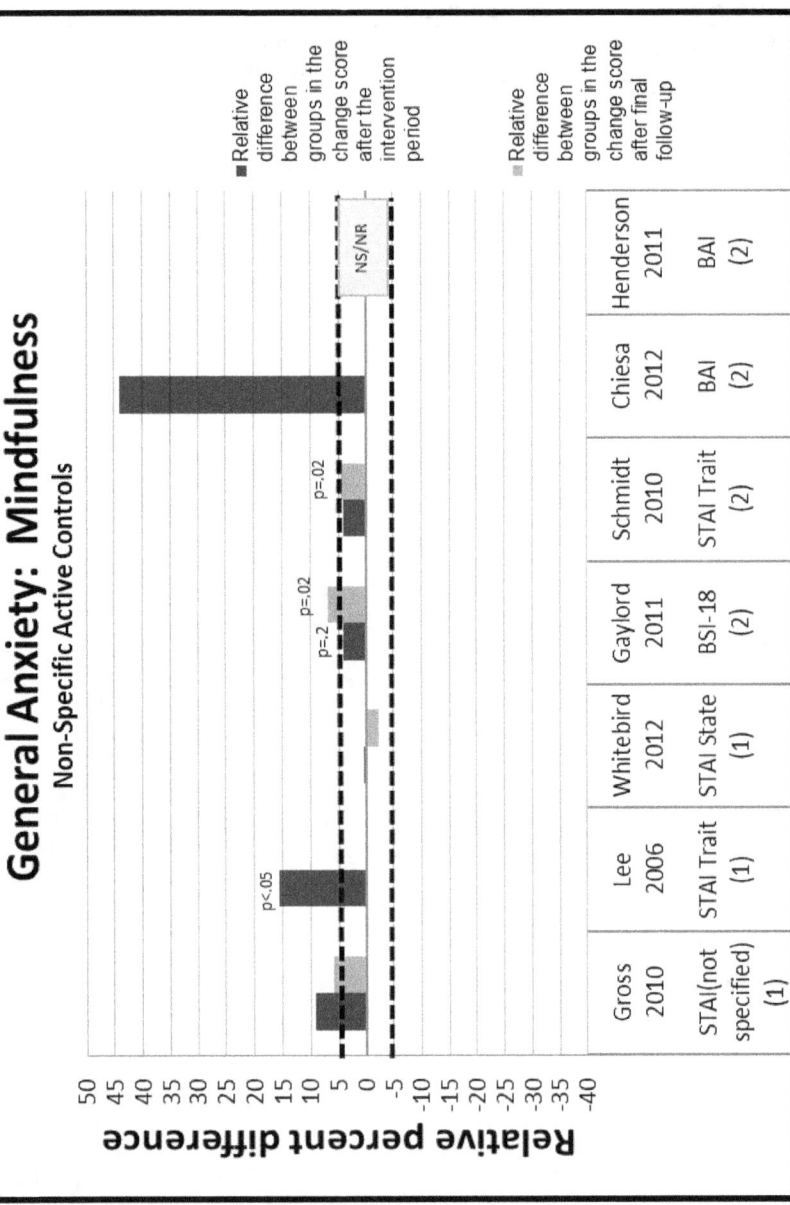

1. **Relative difference between groups in the change score.** This is a relative percent difference, using the baseline mean in the meditation group as the denominator. For example, if the meditation group improves from a 10 to 19 on a mental health scale and the control group improves from 11 to 16 on the same scale, the relative difference between groups in the change score is: $(((19-10)-(16-11))/10) \times 100 = 40\%$. The interpretation is that there is a 40% relative improvement on the mental health scale in the meditation group compared with the control group. See appendix E for absolute difference-in-change score values. Improvement in all scales is indicated in the positive direction. A positive relative percent difference means that the score improved more in the intervention group than in the control group
2. (1): Primary outcome. If the trial did not specify primary or secondary outcomes, this is either the outcome that the population was selected on or identified as a primary focus of the study. (2): Secondary outcome. If the trial did not specify primary or secondary outcomes, then this is not the outcome that the population was selected nor identified as a primary focus of the study.
3. NR / NS = Not Reported/Not significant. The trial measured this outcome and stated they were nonsignificant, and did not report actual results.
4. Black dotted lines from −5% to +5% indicate our criteria for no effect. It does not indicate statistical significance.
5. A p value above or below a bar indicates statistical significance reported in the original study publication. If there is no p value, the outcome was not significant in the original publication.
6. BSI-18=Brief Symptom Inventory 18, Anxiety subscale; STAI = State Trait Anxiety Inventory; BAI = Beck Anxiety Inventory; SCL90 = Symptom Checklist 90, anxiety subscale

Figure 6. Meta-analysis of the effects of meditation programs on anxiety with up to 12 weeks of followup

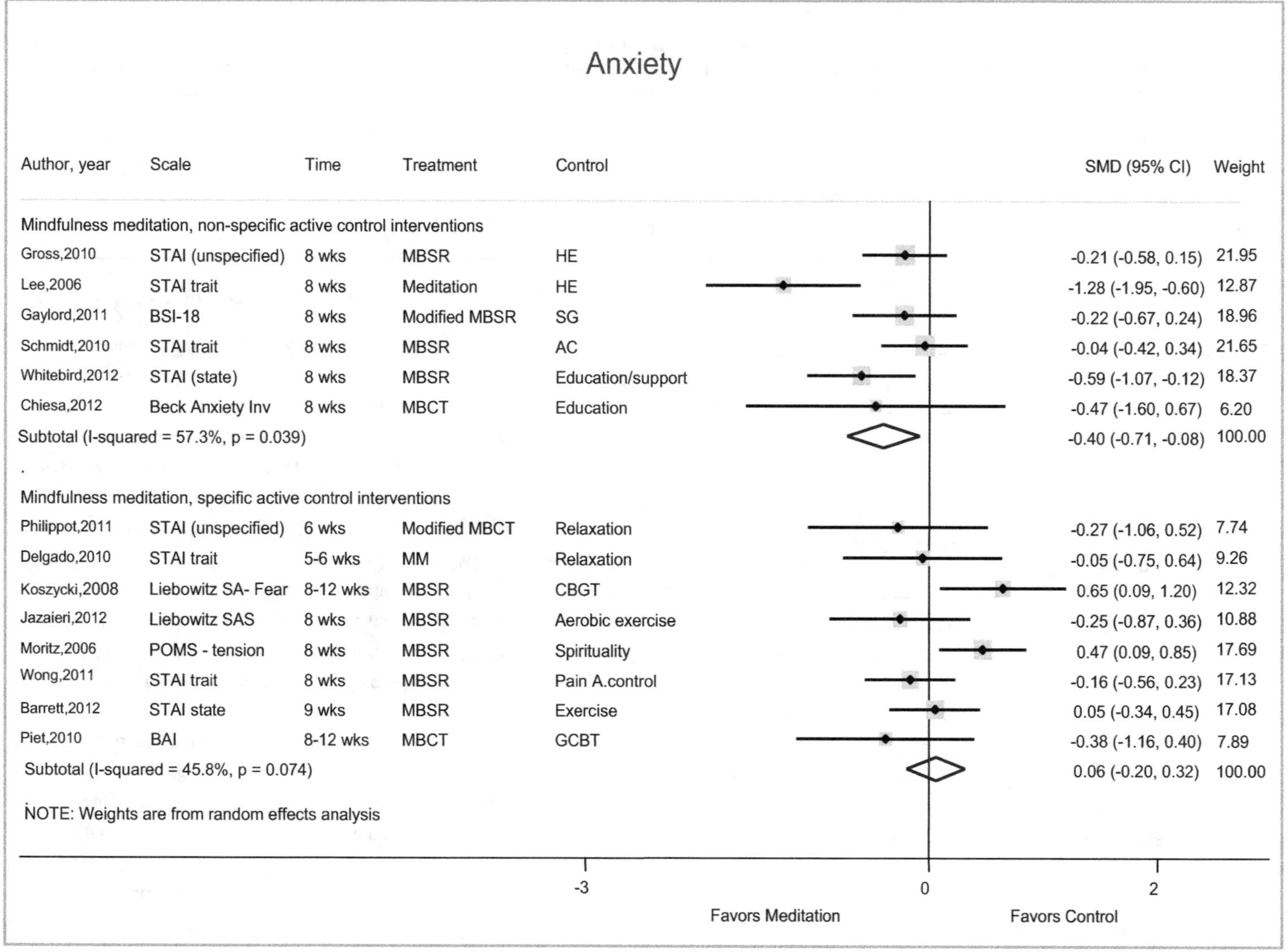

Author, year	Scale	Time	Treatment	Control	SMD (95% CI)	Weight
Mindfulness meditation, non-specific active control interventions						
Gross, 2010	STAI (unspecified)	8 wks	MBSR	HE	-0.21 (-0.58, 0.15)	21.95
Lee, 2006	STAI trait	8 wks	Meditation	HE	-1.28 (-1.95, -0.60)	12.87
Gaylord, 2011	BSI-18	8 wks	Modified MBSR	SG	-0.22 (-0.67, 0.24)	18.96
Schmidt, 2010	STAI trait	8 wks	MBSR	AC	-0.04 (-0.42, 0.34)	21.65
Whitebird, 2012	STAI (state)	8 wks	MBSR	Education/support	-0.59 (-1.07, -0.12)	18.37
Chiesa, 2012	Beck Anxiety Inv	8 wks	MBCT	Education	-0.47 (-1.60, 0.67)	6.20
Subtotal (I-squared = 57.3%, p = 0.039)					-0.40 (-0.71, -0.08)	100.00
Mindfulness meditation, specific active control interventions						
Philippot, 2011	STAI (unspecified)	6 wks	Modified MBCT	Relaxation	-0.27 (-1.06, 0.52)	7.74
Delgado, 2010	STAI trait	5-6 wks	MM	Relaxation	-0.05 (-0.75, 0.64)	9.26
Koszycki, 2008	Liebowitz SA- Fear	8-12 wks	MBSR	CBGT	0.65 (0.09, 1.20)	12.32
Jazaieri, 2012	Liebowitz SAS	8 wks	MBSR	Aerobic exercise	-0.25 (-0.87, 0.36)	10.88
Moritz, 2006	POMS - tension	8 wks	MBSR	Spirituality	0.47 (0.09, 0.85)	17.69
Wong, 2011	STAI trait	8 wks	MBSR	Pain A.control	-0.16 (-0.56, 0.23)	17.13
Barrett, 2012	STAI state	9 wks	MBSR	Exercise	0.05 (-0.34, 0.45)	17.08
Piet, 2010	BAI	8-12 wks	MBCT	GCBT	-0.38 (-1.16, 0.40)	7.89
Subtotal (I-squared = 45.8%, p = 0.074)					0.06 (-0.20, 0.32)	100.00

NOTE: Weights are from random effects analysis

Favors Meditation | Favors Control

Notes: AC = Active Control; BAI = Beck Anxiety Inventory; BSI = Brief Symptom Inventory; CBGT = Cognitive Behavioral Group Therapy; HE=Health Education; MM = Mindfulness Meditation; MBSR = Mindfulness Based Stress Reduction; MBCT = Mindfulness-based Cognitive Therapy; POMS = Profile of Mood States; SCL = Symptom Checklist; SG = Support Group; STAI = State Trait Anxiety Inventory; wks = weeks
Text describing results for comparisons with specific active controls for anxiety starts on page 86

Figure 7. Meta-analysis of the effects of meditation programs on anxiety after 3–6 months of followup

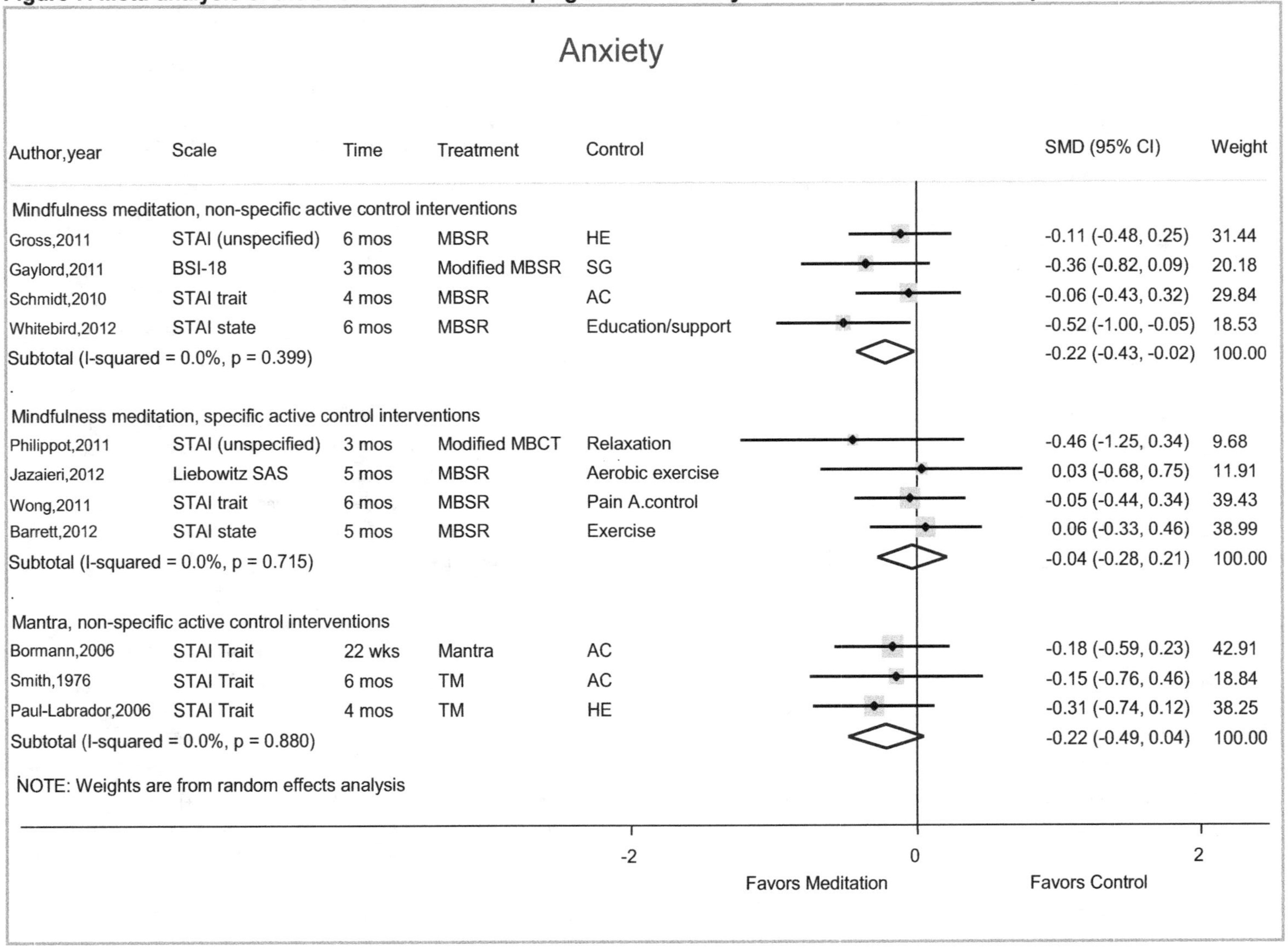

Anxiety

Author, year	Scale	Time	Treatment	Control	SMD (95% CI)	Weight
Mindfulness meditation, non-specific active control interventions						
Gross, 2011	STAI (unspecified)	6 mos	MBSR	HE	-0.11 (-0.48, 0.25)	31.44
Gaylord, 2011	BSI-18	3 mos	Modified MBSR	SG	-0.36 (-0.82, 0.09)	20.18
Schmidt, 2010	STAI trait	4 mos	MBSR	AC	-0.06 (-0.43, 0.32)	29.84
Whitebird, 2012	STAI state	6 mos	MBSR	Education/support	-0.52 (-1.00, -0.05)	18.53
Subtotal (I-squared = 0.0%, p = 0.399)					-0.22 (-0.43, -0.02)	100.00
Mindfulness meditation, specific active control interventions						
Philippot, 2011	STAI (unspecified)	3 mos	Modified MBCT	Relaxation	-0.46 (-1.25, 0.34)	9.68
Jazaieri, 2012	Liebowitz SAS	5 mos	MBSR	Aerobic exercise	0.03 (-0.68, 0.75)	11.91
Wong, 2011	STAI trait	6 mos	MBSR	Pain A.control	-0.05 (-0.44, 0.34)	39.43
Barrett, 2012	STAI state	5 mos	MBSR	Exercise	0.06 (-0.33, 0.46)	38.99
Subtotal (I-squared = 0.0%, p = 0.715)					-0.04 (-0.28, 0.21)	100.00
Mantra, non-specific active control interventions						
Bormann, 2006	STAI Trait	22 wks	Mantra	AC	-0.18 (-0.59, 0.23)	42.91
Smith, 1976	STAI Trait	6 mos	TM	AC	-0.15 (-0.76, 0.46)	18.84
Paul-Labrador, 2006	STAI Trait	4 mos	TM	HE	-0.31 (-0.74, 0.12)	38.25
Subtotal (I-squared = 0.0%, p = 0.880)					-0.22 (-0.49, 0.04)	100.00

NOTE: Weights are from random effects analysis

-2 Favors Meditation 0 Favors Control 2

Notes: AC = Active Control; BSI = Brief Symptom Inventory; CSM = Clinically Standardized; HE = Health Education; MBCT=Mindfulness-based Cognitive Therapy; MBSR = Mindfulness Based Stress Reduction; mos = months; SG = Support Group; STAI = State Trait Anxiety Inventory; TM = Transcendental Meditation; wks = weeks
Text describing results for comparisons with **specific** active controls for anxiety starts on page 86

Mantra Mindfulness Programs Versus <u>Nonspecific</u> Active Controls

Two trials of TM and one trial of another mantra meditation programs evaluated an anxiety outcome (Table 8).

Bormann et al. randomized HIV-infected adults (n=93) to a mantra meditation or an education group. The intervention was 10 weeks with a 22-week followup, and provided 7.5 hours of training and unspecified amount of home practice over 10 weeks.[75] At 10 weeks, the difference-in-change score on the STAI trait scale was 6.1 percent favoring the mantra group; however, this was not statistically significant. This difference reduced to 2.1 percent at 22 weeks. This trial had a medium risk of bias. It listed anxiety as one of seven primary outcomes.

Smith et al. randomized university students (n=100) interested in an anxiety reducing technique to either TM or a sham meditation program to match expectations, time, and attention.[83] This trial had 59 percent attrition and was also categorized as high risk of bias. The trial did not report on amount of meditation training given but it estimated a maximum home practice of 87.5 hours over 6 months. STAI trait score was a primary outcome, and at 6 months, the difference-in-change scores were not different between the two groups.

Paul-Labrador et al. randomized participants with stable coronary heart disease (n=103) to 16 weeks of either TM or health education.[81] The STAI measured anxiety as a secondary outcome. The program provided up to 39 hours of training over 16 weeks with an unspecified amount of home practice. At 16 weeks of followup, the difference-in-change between the two groups was only 2.8 percent favoring the control, and was nonsignificant. This was a well-designed trial with a low risk of bias and relatively large sample size.

Overall, two TM trials had point estimates favoring the null, including one for which anxiety was a primary outcome. The largest and highest quality trial using cardiac patients showed no effect of TM compared with a nonspecific control trial.[81] The other mantra trial among HIV patients had similarly null effects on anxiety. The difference-in-change graphs showed consistent results favoring a null effect (Figure 8). The meta-analysis of mantra meditation programs on anxiety was also nonsignificant (Figure 7).

The strength of evidence is low that mantra meditation programs do not have an effect on anxiety among various clinical populations when compared with a nonspecific active control. We based this rating on overall medium risk of bias, consistent findings, directness of measures, and imprecise estimates (Table 18). An evaluation of TM programs only does not change this conclusion.

Table 18. Grade of trials addressing the efficacy of mantra meditation programs on anxiety compared with nonspecific active controls among various populations

Number of Trials; Subjects	Domains Pertaining to Strength of Evidence				Magnitude of Effect and Strength of Evidence
	Risk of Bias	Consistency	Directness	Precision	
Anxiety					Low SOE of no effect on measures of anxiety
3; 237	Medium	Consistent	Direct	Imprecise	−2.8% to +6.1%

Note: SOE = Strength of Evidence

Figure 8. Relative difference between groups in the changes in measures of general anxiety, in the mantra versus nonspecific active control/specific active control studies

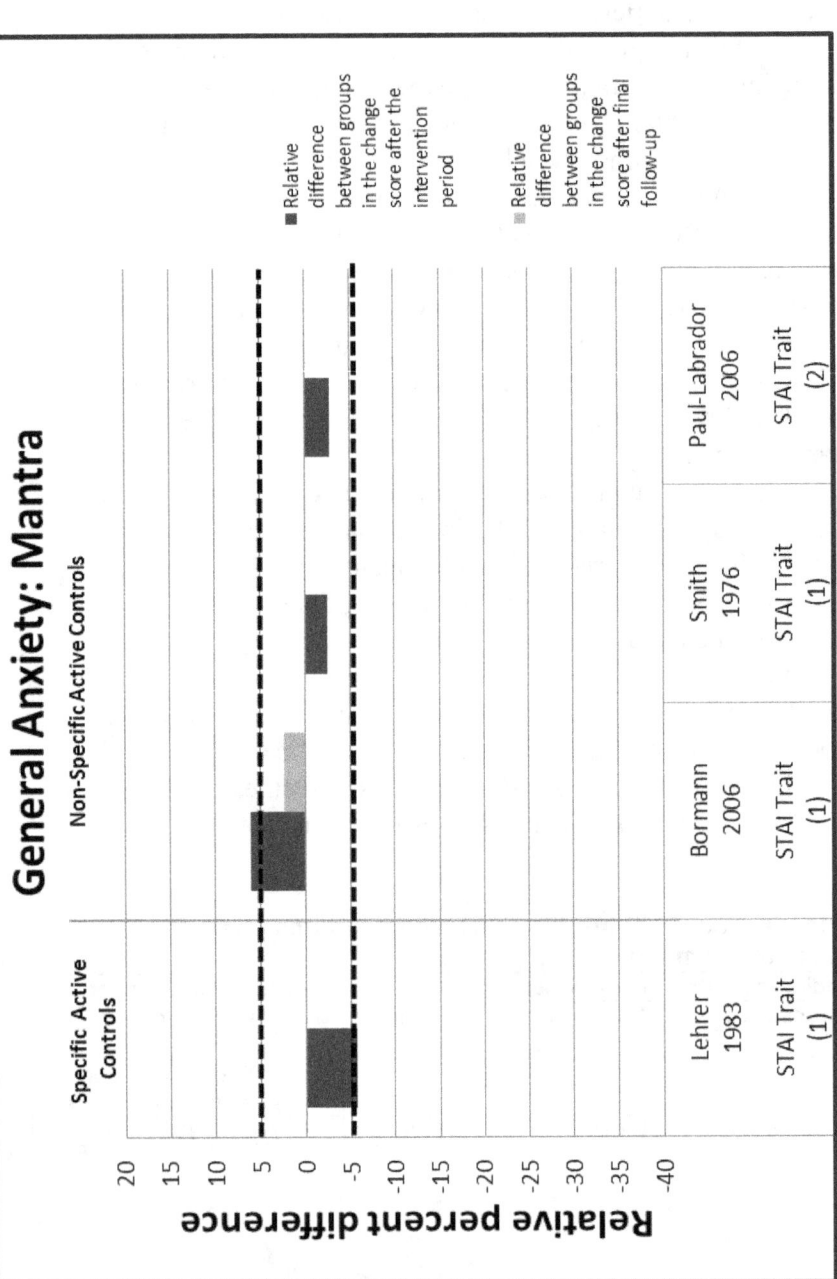

1. **Relative difference between groups in the change score.** This is a relative percent difference, using the baseline mean in the meditation group as the denominator. For example, if the meditation group improves from a 10 to 19 on a mental health scale and the control group improves from 11 to 16 on the same scale, the relative difference between groups in the change score is: $(((19-10)-(16-11))/10) \times 100 = 40\%$. The interpretation is that there is a 40% relative improvement on the mental health scale in the meditation group compared with the control group. See appendix E for absolute difference-in-change score values. Improvement in all scales is indicated in the positive direction. A positive relative percent difference means that the score improved more in the intervention group than in the control group
2. (1): Primary outcome. If the trial did not specify primary or secondary outcomes, this is either the outcome that the population was selected on or identified as a primary focus of the study. (2): Secondary outcome. If the trial did not specify primary or secondary outcomes, then this is not the outcome that the population was selected nor identified as a primary focus of the study.
3. NR / NS = Not Reported/Not significant. The trial measured this outcome and stated they were nonsignificant, and did not report actual results.
4. Black dotted lines from −5% to +5% indicate our criteria for no effect. It does not indicate statistical significance.
5. A p value above or below a bar indicates statistical significance reported in the original study publication. If there is no p value, the outcome was not significant in the original publication.
6. STAI = State Trait Anxiety Inventory.

Depression

Mindfulness Meditation Programs Versus <u>Nonspecific</u> Active Control

Five trials compared MBSR with a nonspecific active control (Table 9).[53,54,57,70,72] All were rated as medium risk of bias and had sample sizes ranging from 75–137. These five trials provided between 23–27 hours of training with unclear amounts of home practice. In addition, three trials compared a modified MBSR program with a nonspecific active control.[60,61,66] These three were at medium to low risk of bias, provided 8–9 hours of training with unclear amounts of home practice, and had sample sizes ranging from 19–186. One trial compared MBCT with a nonspecific active control.[86] This trial had medium risk of bias, provided 16 hours of training with unclear amounts of home practice. These nine trials included diverse populations. Five trials used the Center for Epidemiologic Studies Depression Scale (CES-D), two used the Symptom Checklist 90 (SCL90) Depression subscale, and one used the Brief Symptom Inventory 18 depression subscale.

Henderson et al. randomized patients with early-stage breast cancer (n=100) to MBSR or a nutrition education program. They used two scales to measure depression. They found nonsignificant results on their main measure of depression, the Beck Depression Inventory (BDI), and did not report values. However, this trial measured numerous outcomes and did not correct for multiple comparisons. A difference-in-change estimate revealed a 49 percent improvement on the SCL-90 depression subscale (p<.05). Gaylord et al. randomized women with IBS (n=75) to MBSR versus a support program for women with IBS and showed no significant difference between trial arms at 2 or 3 months.[53] Schmidt et al. randomized women with fibromyalgia (n=109) to MBSR or nonspecific active control. The MBSR arm showed no changes at 8 weeks but showed a 12.4 percent nonsignificant improvement in the CES-D at 4 months compared with the control arm.[70] Gross et al. randomized solid organ transplant patients, post-surgery, (n=137) to MBSR versus health education. A difference-in-change calculation showed that MBSR participants had 25.8–31.8 percent reductions in the CES-D that were consistently maintained between 2–12 months. However, these changes did not reach significance (p=0.10).[54] Whitebird et al. randomized patients who were caregivers of family members with dementia (n=78) to either MBSR or education support group. This trial did not specify primary or secondary outcomes, but categorized depression as a primary focus of the study. The MBSR group showed a 29.1 and 10.6 percent reduction in CES-D scores at post intervention and 6 months, respectively, (p=.07 for overall reductions) as compared with the education support group. We rated this trial as medium risk of bias. It provided 25 hours of training over 8 weeks by a trained teacher, with an average of 26.7 hours of homework completed by the participants.

Chiesa et al. randomized patients with major depression (n=18) who failed to achieve remission after at least 8 weeks of antidepressant therapy, to either MBCT or nonspecific active control. The trial found a 51.6 percent reduction (p=.04) in the Hamilton rating scale for depression. We rated this trial as medium risk of bias. It provided 16 hours of training over 8 weeks by a trained and certified teacher, with unspecified home practice.

Three trials evaluated other mindfulness programs against a nonspecific active control. Oken et al. randomized people who take care of elderly relatives with dementia (n=19) to mindfulness meditation program or a nonspecific active control.[66] This trial found a nonsignificant 10.1 percent improvement on CES-D favoring the mindfulness group. This trial had a medium risk of bias, provided 9 hours of training over 7 weeks by a trained teacher and an unspecified amount of home practice.

Malarkey et al. randomized people, who either had or were at risk for cardiovascular disease due to elevated C-Reactive protein levels (n=186), to mindfulness meditation or nonspecific active control.[61] It provided 9 hours of abbreviated MBSR training at work with approximately 18.5 hours of homework over 8 weeks. At 8 weeks, the trial found no differences between the groups, but did not provide data for comparisons of the size of effect. This trial had a low risk of bias.

Lee et al. randomized 46 patients with anxiety disorders recruited from a psychiatric hospital or its clinics in South Korea, to either an 8-week mindfulness-based stress management program or nonspecific active control group (anxiety disorder-based education).[60] The Korean meditation program did not appear to be a derivative of MBSR or MBCT as most other trials in this review are, but shared some overlapping features of mindfulness meditation. It found nonsignificant 30.3 percent reduction in the BDI and 17.4 percent reduction in SCL-90 depression scores. The trial standardized all of the self-report measures in Korean. The program provided 8 hours of training targeted towards anxiety reduction, with unspecified amount of home practice. This trial had a medium risk of bias.

In summary, these nine trials used diverse populations of patients, with only one of them overtly depressed. The difference-in-change graphs showed generally consistent findings favoring an improvement in depressive symptoms across studies. Two of the four trials in which depression was a primary outcome showed statistically significant results (Figure 9). The study by Malarkey had nonsignificant results, but also started out with much lower CES-D scores as compared with the other trials. We performed two meta-analyses, one of 2-month outcomes and the other of 3–6 month outcomes. The meta-analyses at 2 months found small and marginally nonsignificant effects of mindfulness meditation programs on depressive symptoms, while the meta-analysis at 3–6 months found small but significant effects (Figures 10 and 11). The 2-month meta-analysis also had a high I^2 (p=.012). These meta-analysis do not take into account the baseline differences, while the difference-in-change analysis do take the baseline differences into account.

The strength of evidence is moderate that mindfulness meditation programs improve symptoms of depression among various clinical populations when compared with a nonspecific active control. We based this rating on overall medium risk of bias, consistent findings for a positive effect, directness of measures, and precise estimates (Table 19). However, since one trial is missing from the meta-analysis and the post-intervention I^2 is high, this strength of evidence warrants a cautious interpretation.

Table 19. Grade of trials addressing the efficacy of mindfulness meditation programs on symptoms of depression compared with nonspecific active controls among clinical populations

Number of Trials; Subjects	Domains Pertaining to Strength of Evidence				Magnitude of Effect and Strength of Evidence
	Risk of Bias	Consistency	Directness	Precision	
Depressive symptoms					Moderate SOE of an improvement in depressive symptoms
9; 768	Medium	Consistent	Direct	Precise	−0.1% (favoring null) to +51.6% (favoring mindfulness meditation program)

Note: SOE = Strength of Evidence

Figure 9. Relative difference between groups in the changes in measures of depression, in the mindfulness versus nonspecific active control studies

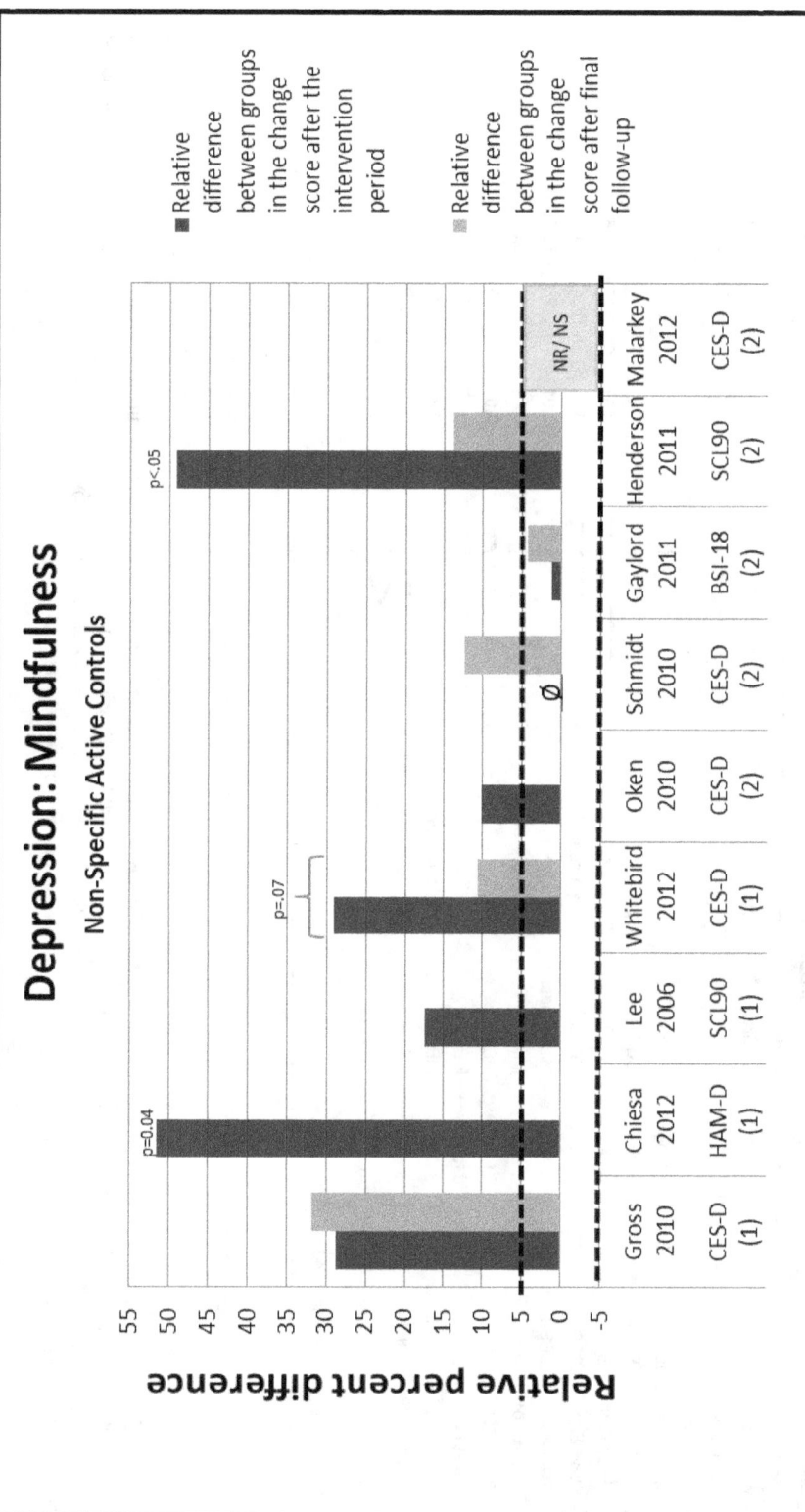

1. **Relative difference between groups in the change score.** This is a relative percent difference, using the baseline mean in the meditation group as the denominator. For example, if the meditation group improves from a 10 to 19 on a mental health scale and the control group improves from 11 to 16 on the same scale, the relative difference between groups in the change score is: (((19-10)-(16-11))/10)x100=40%. The interpretation is that there is a 40% relative improvement on the mental health scale in the meditation group compared with the control group. See appendix E for absolute difference-in-change score values. Improvement in all scales is indicated in the positive direction. A positive relative percent difference means that the score improved more in the intervention group than in the control group
2. (1): Primary outcome. If the trial did not specify primary or secondary outcomes, this is either the outcome that the population was selected on or identified as a primary focus of the study. (2): Secondary outcome. If the trial did not specify primary or secondary outcomes, then this is not the outcome that the population was selected nor identified as a primary focus of the study.
3. NR/NS = Not Reported/Not significant. The trial measured this outcome and stated they were nonsignificant, and did not report actual results.
4. Black dotted lines from −5% to +5% indicate our criteria for no effect. It does not indicate statistical significance.
5. A p value above or below a bar indicates statistical significance reported in the original study publication. If there is no p value, the outcome was not significant in the original publication.
6. BSI-18=Brief Symptom Inventory 18, Anxiety subscale; CES-D=Center for Epidemilogic Studies Depression Scale; HAM-D=Hamilton Psychiatric Rating Scale for depression; SCL90 = Symptom Checklist 90, anxiety subscale

Figure 10. Meta-analysis of the effects of meditation programs on depression with up to 3 months of followup

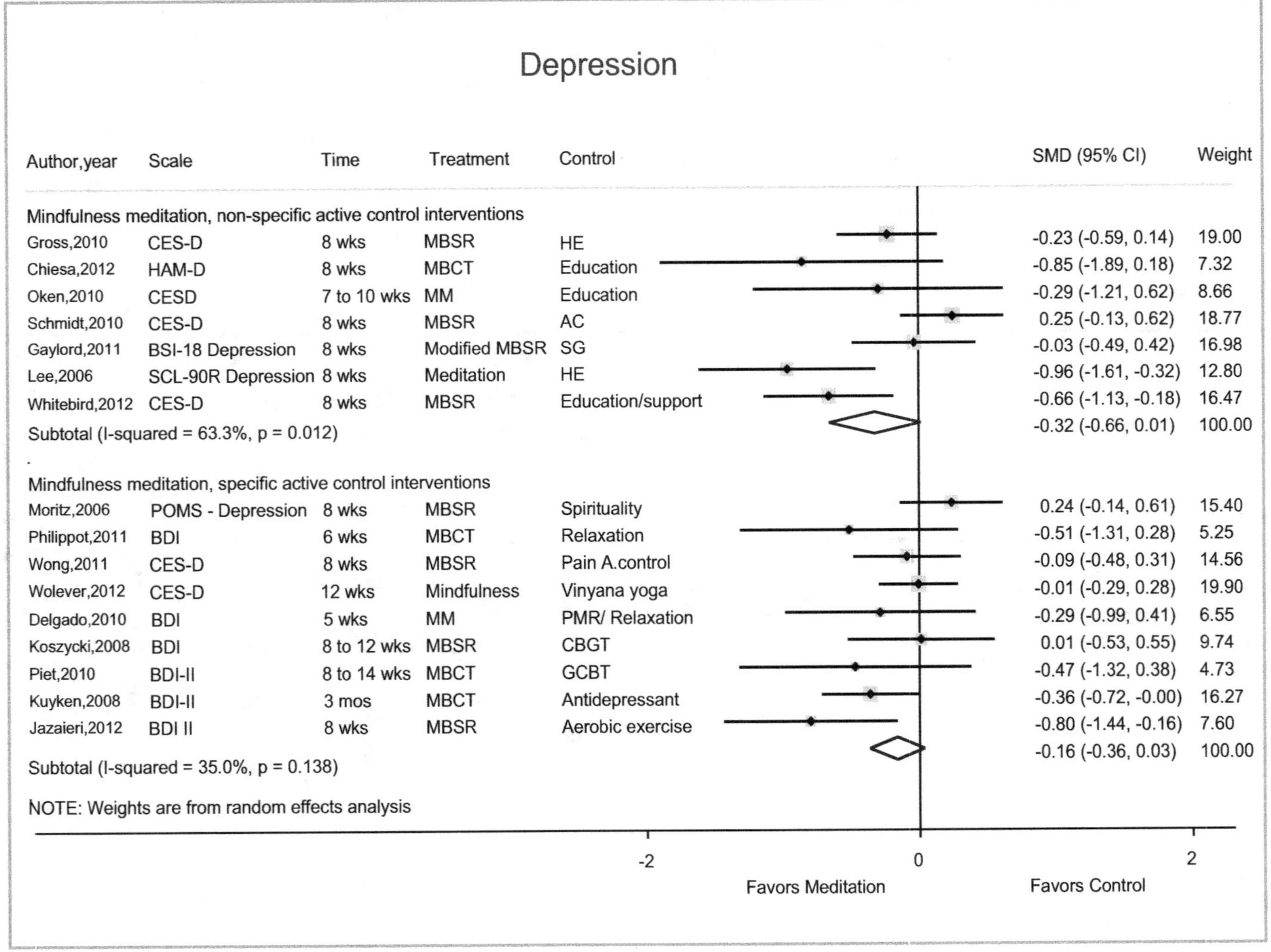

Depression

Author, year	Scale	Time	Treatment	Control	SMD (95% CI)	Weight
Mindfulness meditation, non-specific active control interventions						
Gross, 2010	CES-D	8 wks	MBSR	HE	-0.23 (-0.59, 0.14)	19.00
Chiesa, 2012	HAM-D	8 wks	MBCT	Education	-0.85 (-1.89, 0.18)	7.32
Oken, 2010	CESD	7 to 10 wks	MM	Education	-0.29 (-1.21, 0.62)	8.66
Schmidt, 2010	CES-D	8 wks	MBSR	AC	0.25 (-0.13, 0.62)	18.77
Gaylord, 2011	BSI-18 Depression	8 wks	Modified MBSR	SG	-0.03 (-0.49, 0.42)	16.98
Lee, 2006	SCL-90R Depression	8 wks	Meditation	HE	-0.96 (-1.61, -0.32)	12.80
Whitebird, 2012	CES-D	8 wks	MBSR	Education/support	-0.66 (-1.13, -0.18)	16.47
Subtotal (I-squared = 63.3%, p = 0.012)					-0.32 (-0.66, 0.01)	100.00
Mindfulness meditation, specific active control interventions						
Moritz, 2006	POMS - Depression	8 wks	MBSR	Spirituality	0.24 (-0.14, 0.61)	15.40
Philippot, 2011	BDI	6 wks	MBCT	Relaxation	-0.51 (-1.31, 0.28)	5.25
Wong, 2011	CES-D	8 wks	MBSR	Pain A.control	-0.09 (-0.48, 0.31)	14.56
Wolever, 2012	CES-D	12 wks	Mindfulness	Vinyana yoga	-0.01 (-0.29, 0.28)	19.90
Delgado, 2010	BDI	5 wks	MM	PMR/ Relaxation	-0.29 (-0.99, 0.41)	6.55
Koszycki, 2008	BDI	8 to 12 wks	MBSR	CBGT	0.01 (-0.53, 0.55)	9.74
Piet, 2010	BDI-II	8 to 14 wks	MBCT	GCBT	-0.47 (-1.32, 0.38)	4.73
Kuyken, 2008	BDI-II	3 mos	MBCT	Antidepressant	-0.36 (-0.72, -0.00)	16.27
Jazaieri, 2012	BDI II	8 wks	MBSR	Aerobic exercise	-0.80 (-1.44, -0.16)	7.60
Subtotal (I-squared = 35.0%, p = 0.138)					-0.16 (-0.36, 0.03)	100.00

NOTE: Weights are from random effects analysis

Favors Meditation Favors Control

Notes: AC = Active Control; BDI = Beck Depression Inventory; BSI = Beck Stress Inventory; CES-D = Center for Epidemiological Studies Depression Scale; CBGT = Cognitive Behavioral Group Therapy; HE = Health Education; MBCT=Mindfulness-based Cognitive Therapy; MBSR = Mindfulness Based Stress Reduction; mos = Months; POMS = Profile of Mood States; SG = Support Group; SCL= Symptom Checklist; STAI = State Trait Anxiety Inventory; TM = Transcendental Meditation; wks = weeks
Text describing results for comparisons with **specific** active controls for depression starts on page 99

Figure 11. Meta-analysis of the effects of meditation programs on depression after 3–6 months of followup

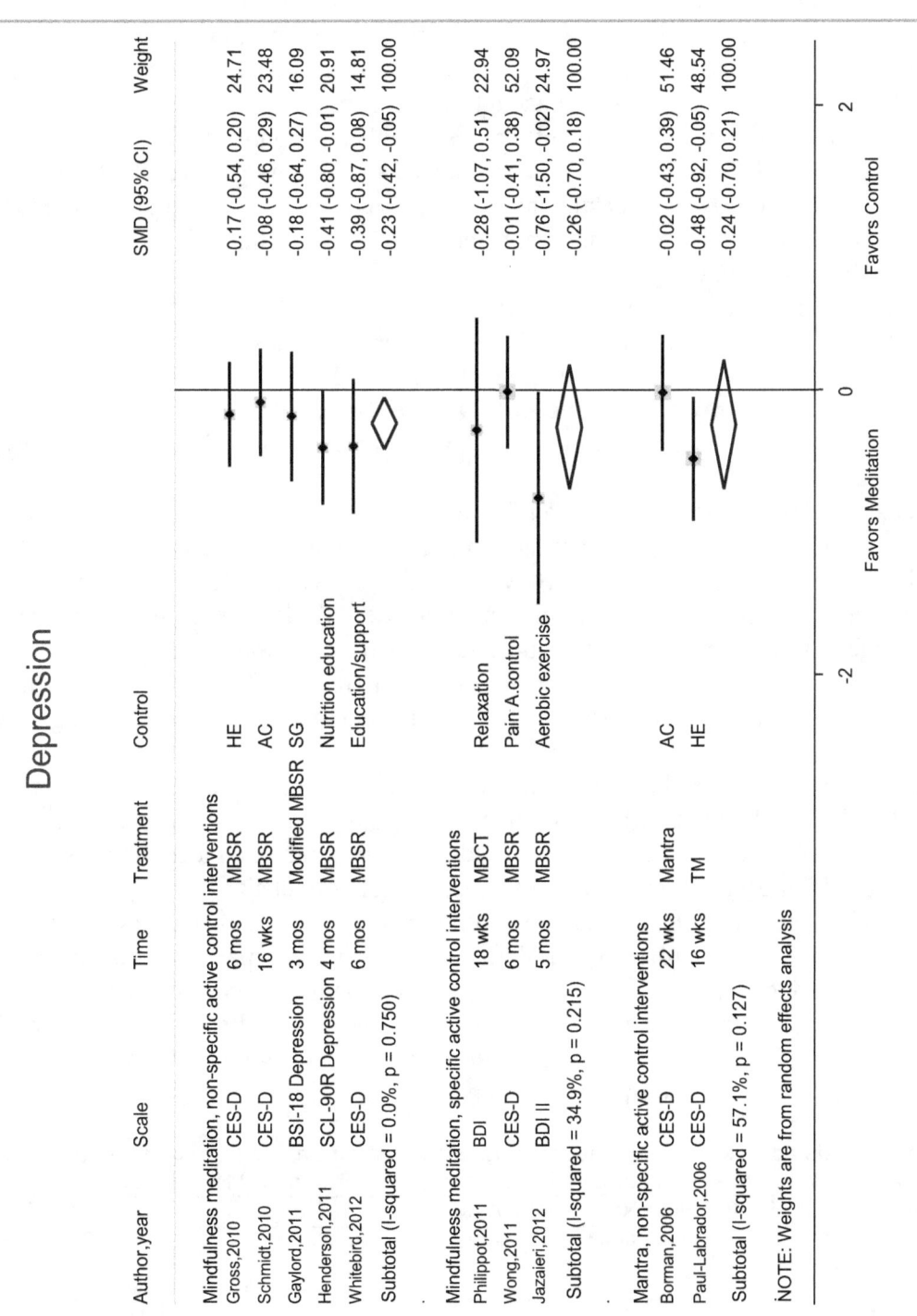

Notes: AC = Active Control; BDI = Beck Depression Inventory; BSI = Beck Stress Inventory; CES-D = Center for Epidemiological Studies Depression Scale; HE = Health Education; MBSR = Mindfulness Based Stress Reduction; mos = months; POMS = Profile of Mood States; SCL= Symptom Checklist; SG = Support Group; TM = Transcendental Meditation; wks = weeks

Text describing results for comparisons with **specific** active controls for depression starts on page 99

Mantra Meditation Programs Versus Nonspecific Active Control

Three trials of TM assessed a depression outcome among cardiac patients. One trial of other mantra assessed depression as an outcome among HIV patients. We rated all three TM trials as low risk of bias and the other mantra trial as medium risk of bias. The TM studies ranged from 22–39 hours of training over 16–25 weeks, although one trial lasted on average 5.4 years with an estimated training time of 78 hours and 1,310 homework hours. The other mantra trial in HIV patients provided 7.5 hours of training over 5 weeks (Table 9).

Paul-Labrador et al. randomized 103 participants with stable coronary heart disease to 16 weeks of either TM or health education.[81] The team measured depression as a secondary outcome using the Center for Epidemiologic Studies depression scale (CES-D). They provided up to 39 hours of training over 16 weeks with an unspecified amount of home practice. At 16 weeks of followup, the difference-in-change between the two groups was 19.1 percent favoring the control, and was nonsignificant. This trial had a low risk of bias.

Jayadevappa et al. randomized CHF patients (n=23) to either 3 months of TM or health education and used the CES-D scale to assess depression as a secondary outcome.[78] Post-intervention, difference-in-change point estimates were 46.1 and 49 percent at 3 and 6 months respectively. The trial reported these results as nonsignificant. This trial had a low risk of bias, and provided 22.5 hours of training over 6 months by trained and certified teachers. It recommended up to 90 hours of home practice during this time.

Schneider et al. randomized 201 patients with coronary artery disease to either TM or nonspecific active control. The study followed patients on average for 5.4 years. It found a nonsignificant 6.8 percent improvement in the CES-D score compared with control. This trial had a low risk of bias, and provided an estimated 78 hours of training over the study period by trained and certified teachers.

Bormann et al. randomized HIV-infected adults (n=93) to mantra meditation or an education group with primary outcomes related to the reduction of intrusive thoughts and improvement in QOL and well-being.[75] The intervention was 10 weeks with a 22-week followup, and provided 7.5 hours of training and unspecified amount of home practice.[75] At 10 weeks, the difference-in-change score on the center for epidemiologic studies depression scale was 1.6 percent and was not statistically significant. This difference increased to 20.1 percent at 22 weeks favoring the control (p=.07). This trial had a medium risk of bias. It listed depression as one of seven primary outcomes.

In summary, the difference-in-change graphs showed inconsistent results (Figure 12). All three of the TM trials were low risk of bias, conducted in cardiac patients, and depression was a secondary outcome. Only two of the four trials provided data to conduct a meta-analyses at 4–6 months of followup (Figure 11), showing a small nonsignificant effect size.

The strength of evidence is insufficient that mantra meditation programs have an effect on symptoms of depression among cardiac and HIV populations when compared with a nonspecific active control. While two of the TM trials did not have data to be included in the meta-analysis, due to conflicting results in the difference-in-change analysis, we do not believe that data would change our conclusions. We based this rating on overall medium risk of bias, inconsistent findings, directness of measures, and imprecise estimates (Table 20).

Table 20. Grade of trials addressing the efficacy of mantra meditation program on symptoms of depression compared with nonspecific active controls among cardiac and HIV populations

Number of Trials; Subjects	Domains Pertaining to Strength of Evidence				Magnitude of Effect and Strength of Evidence
	Risk of Bias	Consistency	Directness	Precision	
Depressive symptoms					Insufficient SOE of an effect
4;420	Medium	Inconsistent	Direct	Imprecise	−19.1% to +46.1%

Note: SOE = Strength of Evidence

Figure 12. Relative difference between groups in the changes in measures of depression, in the mantra versus nonspecific active control/specific active control studies

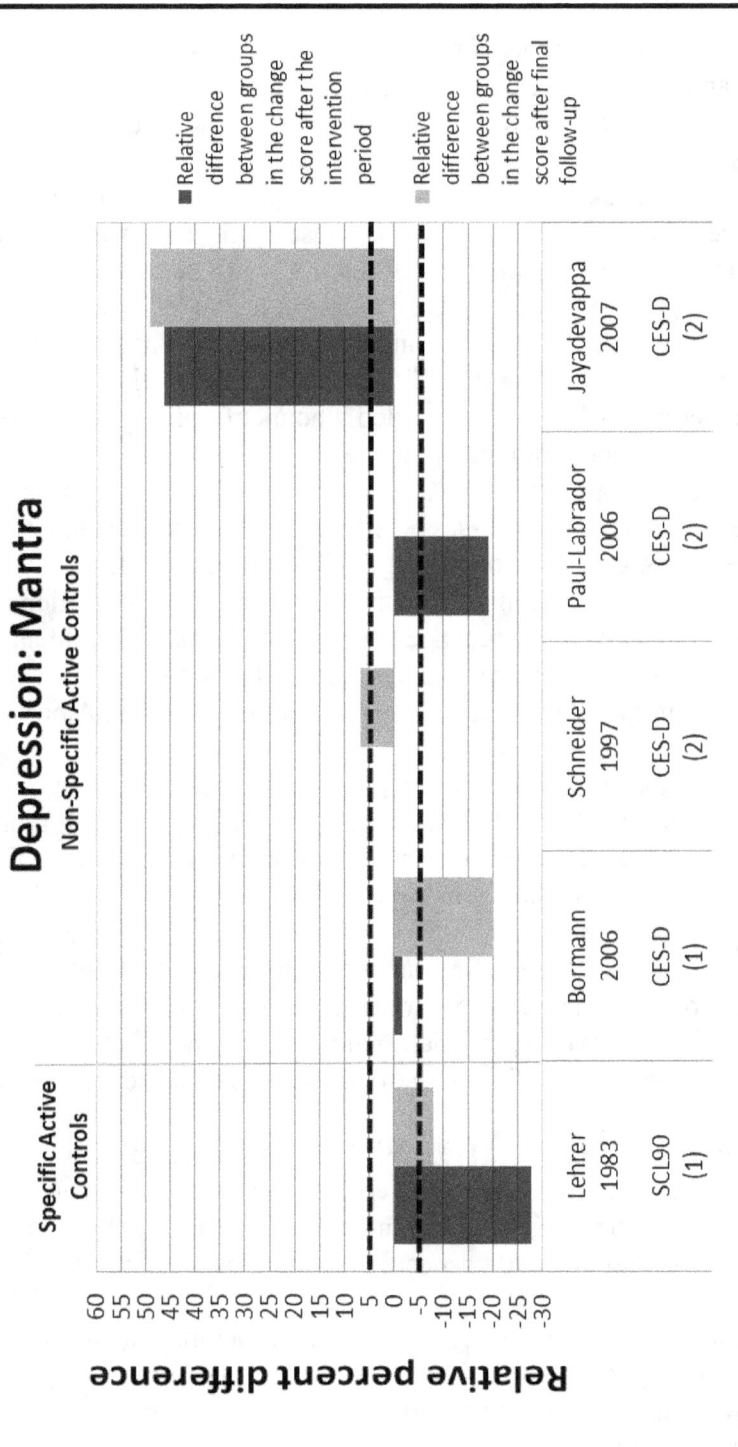

1. **Relative difference between groups in the change score.** This is a relative percent difference, using the baseline mean in the meditation group as the denominator. For example, if the meditation group improves from a 10 to 19 on a mental health scale and the control group improves from 11 to 16 on the same scale, the relative difference between groups in the change score is: $(((19-10)-(16-11))/10) \times 100 = 40\%$. The interpretation is that there is a 40% relative improvement on the mental health scale in the meditation group compared with the control group. See appendix E for absolute difference-in-change score values. Improvement in all scales is indicated in the positive direction. A positive relative percent difference means that the score improved more in the intervention group than in the control group.
2. (1): Primary outcome. If the trial did not specify primary or secondary outcomes, this is either the outcome that the population was selected on or identified as a primary focus of the study. (2): Secondary outcome. If the trial did not specify primary or secondary outcomes, then this is not the outcome that the population was selected nor identified as a primary focus of the study.
3. NR / NS = Not Reported/Not significant. The trial measured this outcome and stated they were nonsignificant, and did not report actual results.
4. Black dotted lines from −5% to +5% indicate our criteria for no effect. It does not indicate statistical significance.
5. A p value above or below a bar indicates statistical significance reported in the original study publication. If there is no p value, the outcome was not significant in the original publication.
6. CES-D=Center for Epidemilogic Studies Depression Scale; SCL90 = Symptom Checklist 90, anxiety subscale

Stress and Distress

Mindfulness Meditation Programs Versus <u>Nonspecific</u> Active Control

Eight trials compared mindfulness meditation programs with nonspecific active controls, and evaluated stress or distress as an outcome (Table 10).[52,53,61,65,66,72,88,89] Four used MBSR and four used an abbreviated version of MBSR. We rated two as low risk of bias, four as medium risk of bias, and two as high risk of bias. These trials involved diverse patient groups including patients suffering from IBS, lung disease, and HIV, as well as alcoholics and caregivers of family members with dementia. The trial sizes ranged from 19–186. Six trials used a measure of stress and two used a measure of distress.

Oken et al. randomized people who take care of elderly relatives with dementia (n=19) to mindfulness meditation or a nonspecific active control.[66] The purpose of this trial was to see if mindfulness meditation would decrease stress in caregivers of relatives with dementia. For inclusion, participants had to endorse greater than 9 points on the perceived stress scale (PSS). Although stress was a primary outcome, the PSS was a secondary measure for this trial. This trial found a nonsignificant 14.1 percent improvement on the PSS favoring the mindfulness meditation group. This trial had a medium risk of bias, provided 9 hours of training over 7 weeks by a trained teacher, and an unspecified amount of home practice.

Garland et al.[52] assessed the effects of a modified MBCT for alcoholics versus a nonspecific active control on alcohol dependent adults (n=37) to assess whether mindfulness meditation could disrupt the risk chain of stress-precipitated alcohol relapse. The intervention lasted 10 weeks and did not specify information on the amount of training provided, although participants could have done a maximum of 17.5 hours of home practice over the 10 weeks. This trial had a medium risk of bias and found a statistically significant 21.2 percent reduction in the PSS favoring the mindfulness meditation group (p=.03). This trial studied mostly African American males.

Mularski et al. randomized elderly patients, predominantly men, with moderate to severe chronic obstructive pulmonary disorder (n=49) to MBBT or an active support group.[65] It found no difference in perceived stress scores between the two arms of the trial after 2 months. This trial suffered from a 42 percent attrition rate and had a high risk of bias.

Malarkey et al. randomized people, who either had or were at risk for cardiovascular disease due to elevated C-reactive protein levels (n=186), to mindfulness meditation or nonspecific active control.[61] It provided 9 hours of abbreviated MBSR training at work with approximately 18.5 hours of homework over 8 weeks. At 8 weeks, the trial found no differences between the groups, but did not provide data for comparisons of the size of effect. This trial had a low risk of bias.

Gaylord et al. randomized women with IBS (n=75) to MBSR versus support program for women with IBS, and showed no significant difference (3.6 percent favoring MBSR) between trial arms at 2 months on the BSI 18.[53] At 6 months this had increased slightly to 5.2 percent (p=.049). The trial provided 23 hours of training and unspecified amount of home practice. It had a medium risk-of-bias.

Whitebird et al. randomized patients who were caregivers of family members with dementia (n=78) to either MBSR or education support group. This trial did not specify primary or secondary outcomes, but categorized stress/distress as a primary focus of the study. The MBSR group showed a 19.3 and 12.7 percent reduction in perceived stress scores at post intervention and 6 months respectively (p=.01 for overall reductions), as compared with the education support group. This trial provided 25 hours of training over 8 weeks by a trained teacher, with an average of 26.7 hours of homework completed by the participants. It had a medium risk of bias.

Seyedalinaghi et al. randomized HIV positive patients in Iran to MBSR or nonspecific active control (n=171). The trial did not specify primary or secondary outcomes, but stress/distress was a primary focus of the study. This trial provided approximately 25 hours of training over 8 weeks by trained teaches, and unspecified amount of homework, and had a high risk of bias. The trial found a 11 percent improvement in the SCL-90 revised at the end of the intervention, and a 4.9 percent worsening at 12 months compared with control. The overall effect was significant at p<.001.

Pbert et al. randomized asthmatics to MBSR or education control (n=82), and found 16.2 percent (p=.055) and 26 percent (p=.001) improvement at 10 weeks and 12 months, respectively. The trial provided 26 hours of training over 8 weeks with approximately 24 hours of recommended home practice, and did not provide information about the teachers. It had a low risk of bias.

The difference-in-change graphs generally showed consistent effects on measures of stress and distress favoring a reduction in the mindfulness groups (Figure 13). The effect size calculations included six trials and excluded two (Figure 14). However, we felt an overall meta-analysis of this data would be biased since the largest included trial[89] had a high risk of bias and carried nearly 40 percent of the statistical weight, while an even larger trial with null results that had a low risk of bias was excluded.[61] Therefore, we did not present an overall effect size. Because the largest (and lowest risk-of-bias) trial by Malarkey et al.[61] was inconsistent with the others trials on stress/distress, we rate the overall evidence as inconsistent. In the absence of an overall effect size, we rate the precision of the group of studies as precise due to the majority of trials (5 of 8) finding statistically significant results.

The strength of evidence is low that mindfulness meditation programs result in a small improvement in stress and distress among various clinical populations when compared with a nonspecific active control. We based this rating on overall medium risk of bias, inconsistent findings, directness of measures, and precise estimates (Table 21).

Table 21. Grade of trials assessing the efficacy of mindfulness programs on stress and distress compared with nonspecific active controls among various populations

Number of Trials; Subjects	Domains Pertaining to Strength of Evidence				Magnitude of Effect and Strength of Evidence
	Risk of Bias	Consistency	Directness	Precision	
Stress & Distress					Low SOE of an effect
8; 697	Medium	Inconsistent	Direct	Precise	1.4% to 21.2% improvement in stress & distress

Note: SOE = Strength of Evidence

Figure 13. Relative difference between groups in the changes in measures of stress/distress, in the mindfulness versus nonspecific active control studies

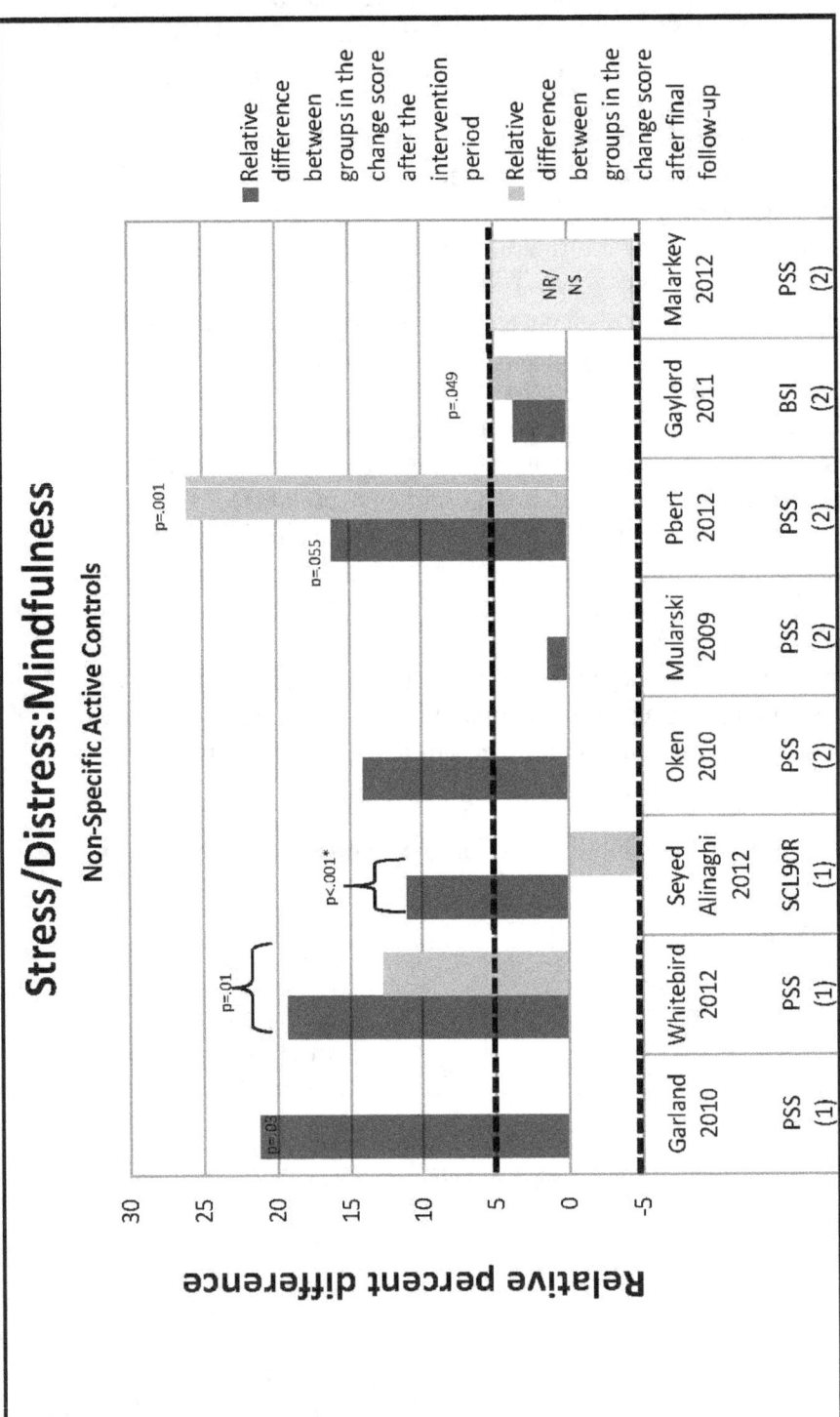

1. **Relative difference between groups in the change score.** This is a relative percent difference, using the baseline mean in the meditation group as the denominator. For example, if the meditation group improves from a 10 to 19 on a mental health scale and the control group improves from 11 to 16 on the same scale, the relative difference between groups in the change score is: $(((19-10)-(16-11))/10) \times 100 = 40\%$. The interpretation is that there is a 40% relative improvement on the mental health scale in the meditation group compared with the control group. See appendix E for absolute difference-in-change score values. Improvement in all scales is indicated in the positive direction. A positive relative percent difference means that the score improved more in the intervention group than in the control group
2. (1): Primary outcome. If the trial did not specify primary or secondary outcomes, this is either the outcome that the population was selected on or identified as a primary focus of the study. (2): Secondary outcome. If the trial did not specify primary or secondary outcomes, then this is not the outcome that the population was selected nor identified as a primary focus of the study.
3. NR / NS = Not Reported/Not significant. The trial measured this outcome and stated they were nonsignificant, and did not report actual results.
4. Black dotted lines from −5% to +5% indicate our criteria for no effect. It does not indicate statistical significance.
5. A p value above or below a bar indicates statistical significance reported in the original study publication. If there is no p value, the outcome was not significant in the original publication.
6. BSI = Beck Stress Inventory; PSS = Perceived Stress Scale; SCL = Symptom Checklist-90 Depression Subscale.

Figure 14. Meta-analysis of the effects of meditation programs on stress/distress with up to 16 weeks of followup

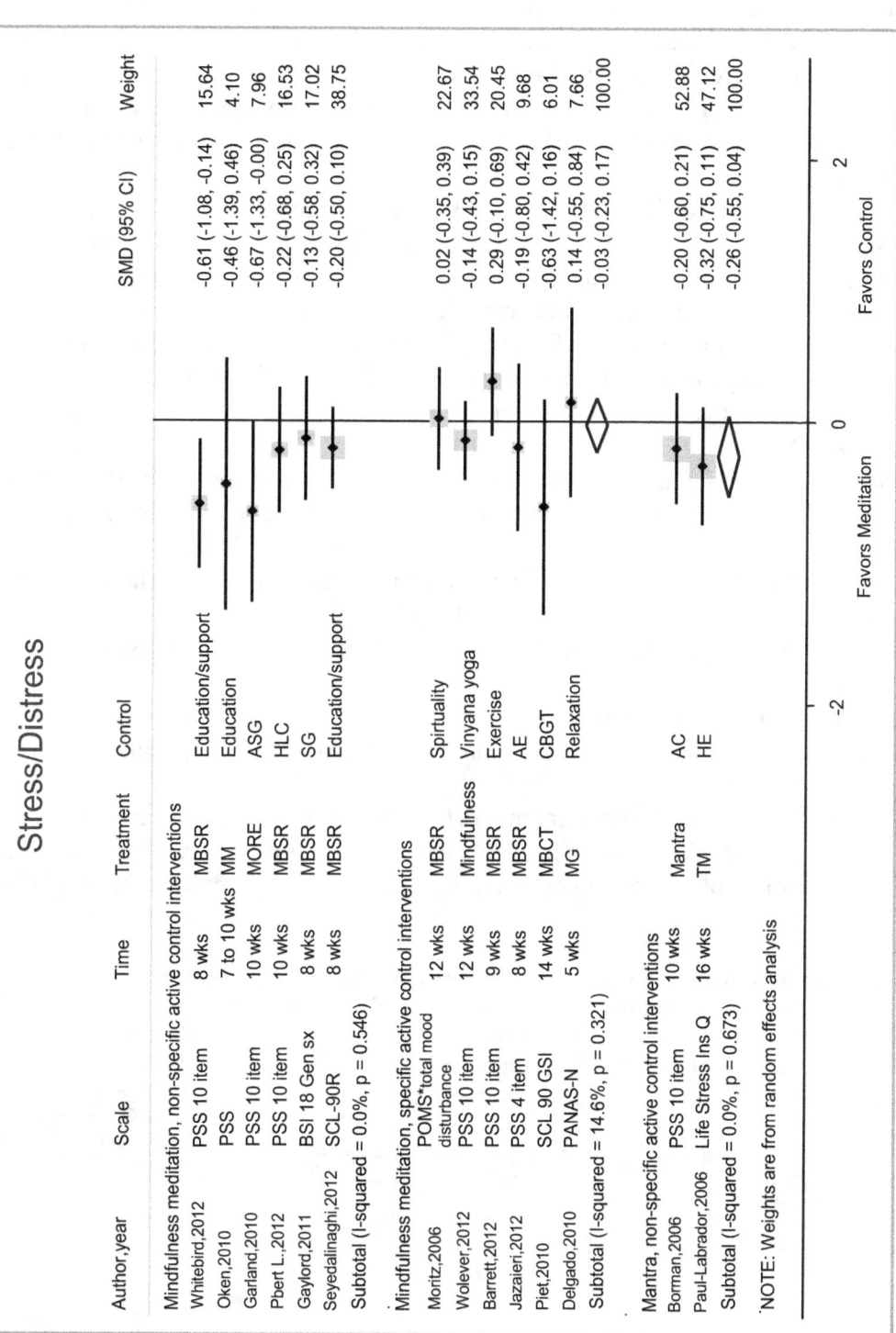

Notes: AC = Active Control; AE = Aerobic Exercise; ASG = Alcohol Dependence Support Group; BSI = Beck Stress Inventory; CBGT = Cognitive Behavioral Group Therapy; HE = Health Education; HLC = Healthy Living Course; MBSR = Mindfulness-based Stress Reduction; MBCT = Mindfulness-based Cognitive Therapy; MM = Mindfulness Meditation; MORE = Mindfulness-oriented Recovery Enhancement; PANAS-N = Positive and Negative Affect Scale - Negative mood; POMS = Profile of Mood States; PSS = Perceived Stress Scale; SCL = Symptom Checklist; SG = Support Group; TM = Transcendental Meditation.
Text describing results for comparisons with **specific** active controls for stress/distress starts on page 103

Mantra Meditation Programs Versus <u>Nonspecific</u> Active Control

Three trials of mantra meditation programs evaluated stress as an outcome for cardiac patients (Table 10). Two were TM and one used another mantra meditation program. Both TM trials studied cardiac patients and both had a low risk of bias. One used the Life Stress Instrument Questionnaire and the other used the PSS. The other mantra meditation trial studied HIV patients and used the PSS.

Paul-Labrador et al. randomized patients with stable coronary heart disease (n=103) to 16 weeks of either TM or health education.[81] Stress was a secondary outcome measured by the Life Stress Instrument Questionnaire. The program provided up to 39 hours of training over 16 weeks with an unspecified amount of home practice. At 16 weeks of followup, the difference-in-change between the two groups was 5.9 percent favoring the control, and was nonsignificant. This trial had a low risk of bias.

Jayadevappa et al. randomized CHF patients (n=23) to either 3 months of TM or health education, assessing stress as a secondary outcome using the PSS scale.[78] With 100 percent trial completion and a 95 percent compliance rate among the originally randomized subjects, there was no difference in perceived stress scores between the two groups at 3 or 6 months. Difference-in-change point estimates were 0.9 and 1.3 percent at 3 and 6 months, respectively. These were reported as nonsignificant. This trial provided 22.5 hours of training over 6 months by trained and certified teachers and recommended up to 90 hours of home practice during this time. It had a low risk of bias.

Bormann et al. randomized adults with HIV (n=93) to mantra meditation or an education group with primary outcomes related to the reduction of intrusive thoughts and improvement in QOL and well-being.[75] The intervention was 10 weeks with a 22-week followup, and provided 7.5 hours of training and unspecified amount of home practice over 10 weeks.[75] The difference-in-change score on the PSS was 1.2 and 3 percent at 10 and 22 weeks, respectively, favoring the null, and was not statistically significant. This trial had a medium risk of bias. Stress was one of seven primary outcomes.

The difference-in-change graphs showed consistent findings of a null effect of mantra meditation programs on stress (Figure 15). A meta-analysis of two of the trials suggested a small nonsignificant effect (Figure 14).

The strength of evidence is low that mantra meditation programs have no effect on stress when compared with a nonspecific active control. We based this rating on overall medium risk of bias, consistent findings of a null effect, directness of measures, and imprecise estimates (Table 22).

Table 22. Grade of trials addressing the efficacy of mantra meditation programs on stress compared with nonspecific active controls among cardiac and HIV patients

Number of Trials; Subjects	Domains Pertaining to Strength of Evidence				Magnitude of Effect and Strength of Evidence
	Risk of Bias	Consistency	Directness	Precision	
Stress					Low SOE of no effect on measures of stress
3; 219	Medium	Consistent	Direct	Imprecise	−5.9% to +1.2%

Note: SOE = Strength of Evidence

Figure 15. Relative difference between groups in the changes in measures of stress, in the mantra versus nonspecific active control studies

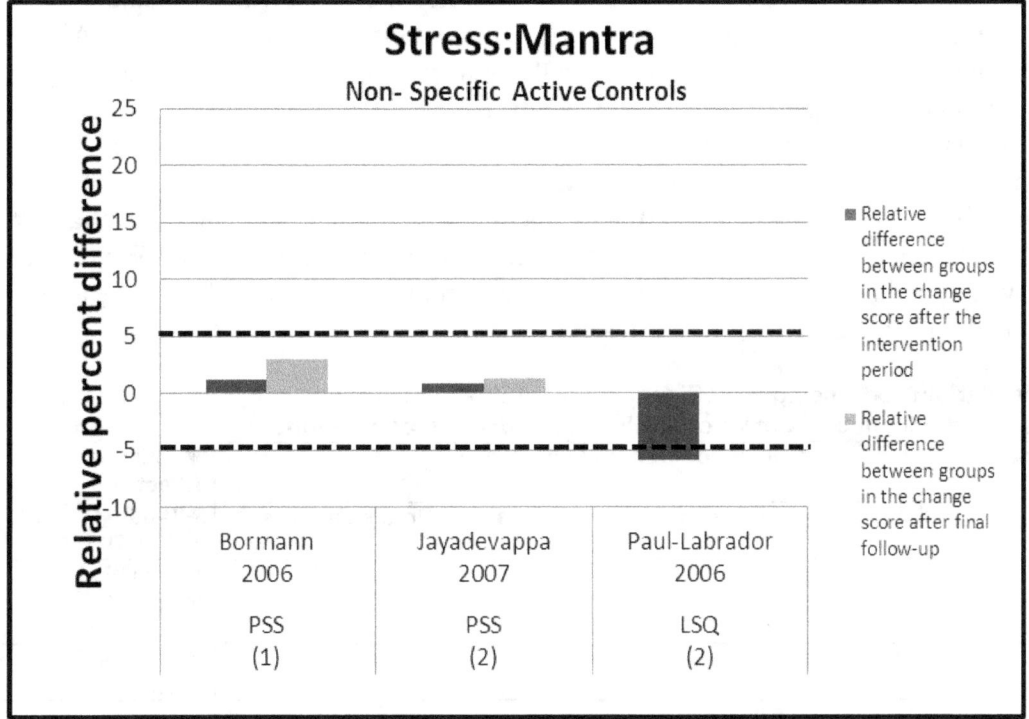

1. **Relative difference between groups in the change score**. This is a relative percent difference, using the baseline mean in the meditation group as the denominator. For example, if the meditation group improves from a 10 to 19 on a mental health scale and the control group improves from 11 to 16 on the same scale, the relative difference between groups in the change score is: (((19-10)-(16-11))/10)x100=40%. The interpretation is that there is a 40% relative improvement on the mental health scale in the meditation group compared with the control group. See appendix E for absolute difference-in-change score values. Improvement in all scales is indicated in the positive direction. A positive relative percent difference means that the score improved more in the intervention group than in the control group
2. (1): Primary outcome. If the trial did not specify primary or secondary outcomes, this is either the outcome that the population was selected on or identified as a primary focus of the study. (2): Secondary outcome. If the trial did not specify primary or secondary outcomes, then this is not the outcome that the population was selected nor identified as a primary focus of the study.
3. NR / NS = Not Reported/Not significant. The trial measured this outcome and stated they were nonsignificant, and did not report actual results.
4. Black dotted lines from −5% to +5% indicate our criteria for no effect. It does not indicate statistical significance.
5. A p value above or below a bar indicates statistical significance reported in the original study publication. If there is no p value, the outcome was not significant in the original publication.
6. PSS = Perceived Stress Scale (PSS); LSQ = Life Stress Ins Q

Negative Affect

Mindfulness Meditation Programs Versus <u>Nonspecific</u> Active Control

Thirteen trials compared mindfulness meditation programs with nonspecific active controls, and evaluated a negative affect outcome (Table 11). Since some trials reported on more than one outcome, for these trials we prioritized anxiety over depression and depression over stress/distress as indirect measures of negative affect. None of the trials used a direct measure of negative affect. Seven trials reported on anxiety, two on depression, and four on stress/distress. The trials included diverse populations, ranging in sample size from 18–186. Two trials had a low risk of bias, nine had a medium risk of bias, and two had a high risk of bias. For five of the trials the outcome was a primary outcome. We previously described these trials, and displayed them in graphical form in Figure 16. The difference-in-change graphs showed a consistent improvement in negative affect when we compared mindfulness meditation programs to a nonspecific active control. Two trials showed small nonsignificant effects, which became significant at the end of study, and four trials showed significant effects post-intervention. A meta-analysis of these trials showed a small statistically significant effect size of 0.34 favoring meditation (Figure 17). We conducted a sensitivity analysis reversing our prioritization order, prioritizing stress/distress over depression and depression over anxiety, to see if this would change our conclusions (Figures 18–19). Both analyses gave similar results.

The strength of evidence is low that mindfulness meditation program improve negative affect among various clinical populations when compared with a nonspecific active control. We based this rating on overall medium risk of bias, consistent results, indirect measures of negative affect, and precise estimates (Table 23).

Table 23. Grade of trials addressing the efficacy of mindfulness meditation programs on negative affect compared with nonspecific active controls among diverse populations

Number of Trials; Subjects	Domains Pertaining to Strength of Evidence				Magnitude of Effect and Strength of Evidence
	Risk of Bias	Consistency	Directness	Precision	
Negative Affect					Low SOE of an improvement in negative affect
13; 1102	Medium	Consistent	Indirect	Precise	0.3% to 44% improvement

Note: SOE = Strength of Evidence

Figure 16. Relative difference between groups in the changes in negative affect, in the mindfulness versus nonspecific active control studies

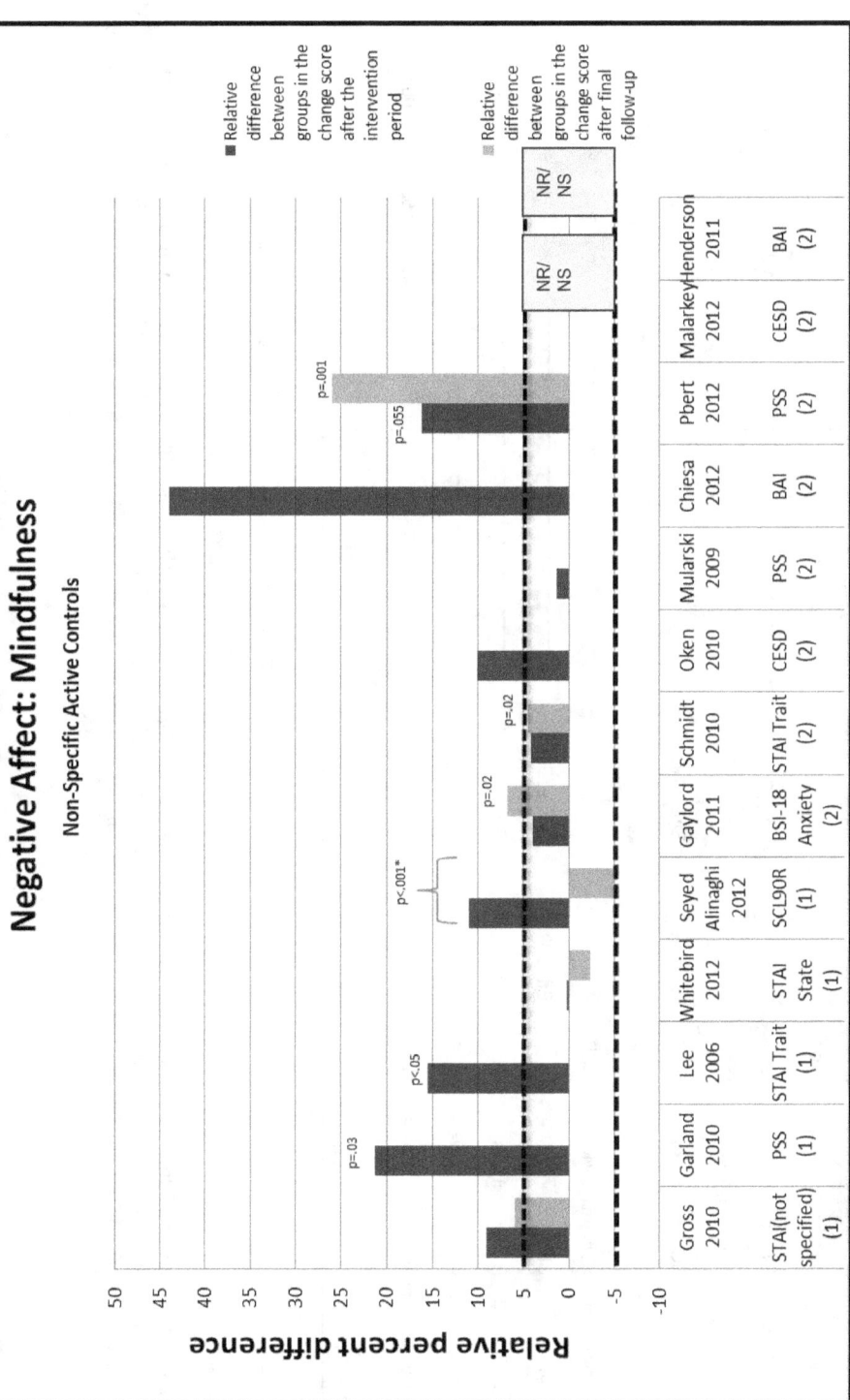

1. **Relative difference between groups in the change score.** This is a relative percent difference, using the baseline mean in the meditation group as the denominator. For example, if the meditation group improves from a 10 to 19 on a mental health scale and the control group improves from 11 to 16 on the same scale, the relative difference between groups in the change score is: (((19-10)-(16-11))/10)x100=40%. The interpretation is that there is a 40% relative improvement on the mental health scale in the meditation group compared with the control group. See appendix E for absolute difference-in-change score values. Improvement in all scales is indicated in the positive direction. A positive relative percent difference means that the score improved more in the intervention group than in the control group
2. (1): Primary outcome. If the trial did not specify primary or secondary outcomes, this is either the outcome that the population was selected on or identified as a primary focus of the study. (2): Secondary outcome. If the trial did not specify primary or secondary outcomes, then this is not the outcome that the population was selected nor identified as a primary focus of the study.
3. NR/NS = Not Reported/Not significant. The trial measured this outcome and stated they were nonsignificant, and did not report actual results.
4. Black dotted lines from −5% to +5% indicate our criteria for no effect. It does not indicate statistical significance.
5. A p value above or below a bar indicates statistical significance reported in the original study publication. If there is no p value, the outcome was not significant in the original publication.
6. BAI=Beck Anxiety inventory; BSI-18: Brief Symptom Inventory; CESD = Center for Epidemiologic Studies Depression Scale; STAI = State Trait Anxiety Inventory; PSS = Perceived Stress Scale; SCL90: Symptom Checklist-90.

Figure 17. Meta-analysis of the effects of meditation programs on negative affect—main analysis (mindfulness meditation versus nonspecific active control interventions)

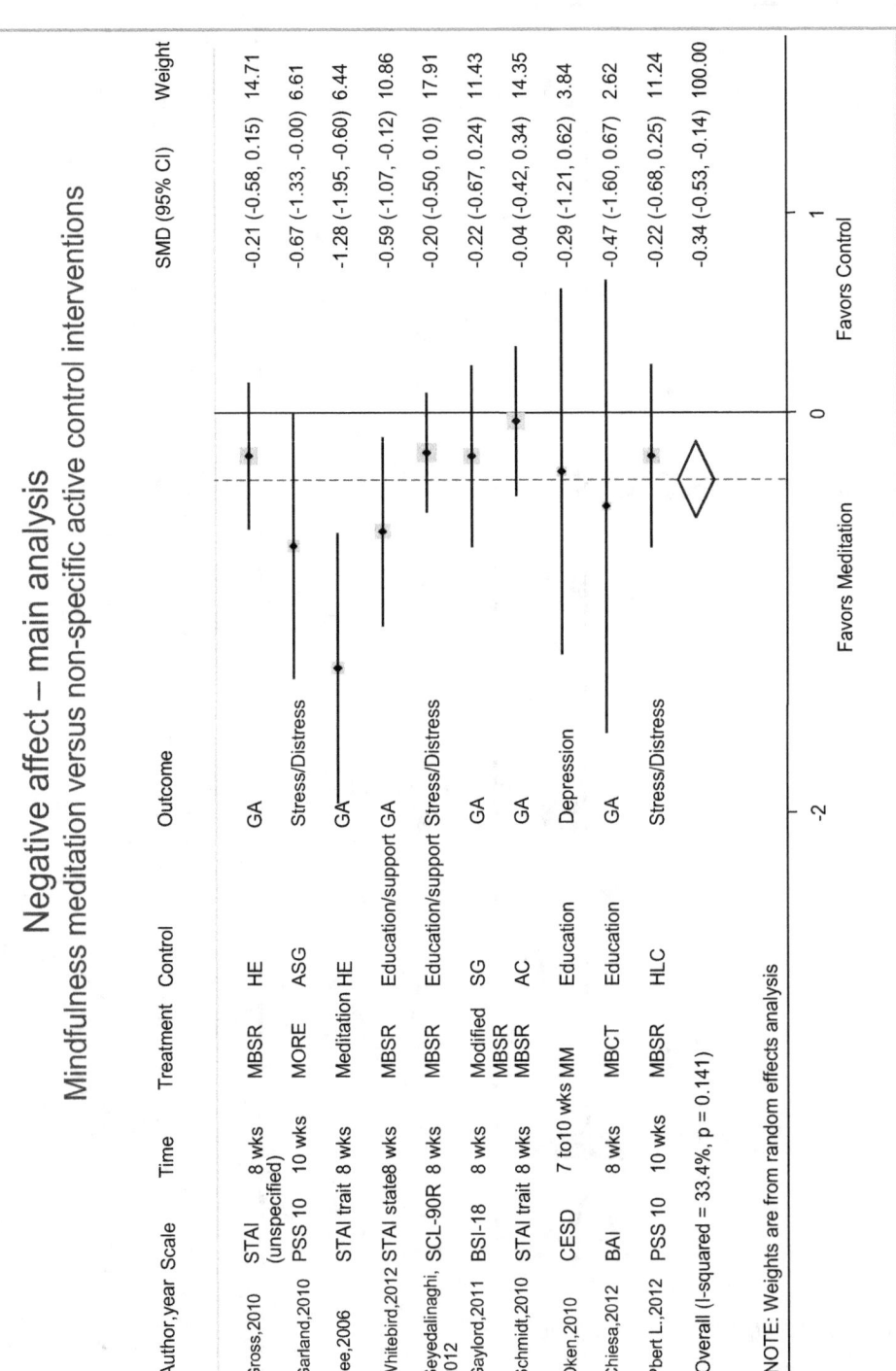

Notes: AC = Active Control; ASG = Alcohol Dependence Support Group; BAI=Beck Anxiety Inventory; BSI = Beck Stress Inventory; CESD = Center for Epidemiologic Studies Depression Scale; GA = General Anxiety; HE = Health Education; HLC = Healthy Living Course; MBCT = Mindfulness-based Cognitive Therapy; MBSR = Mindfulness-based Stress Reduction; MM = Mindfulness Meditation; MORE = Mindfulness-oriented Recovery Enhancement; PSS = Perceived Stress Scale; SCL = Symptom Checklist; SG = Support Group; STAI = State Trait Anxiety Inventory; PSS = Perceived Stress Scale; wks=weeks.

Figure 18. Relative difference between groups in the changes in measures of negative affect, in the mindfulness versus nonspecific active control studies (sensitivity analysis)

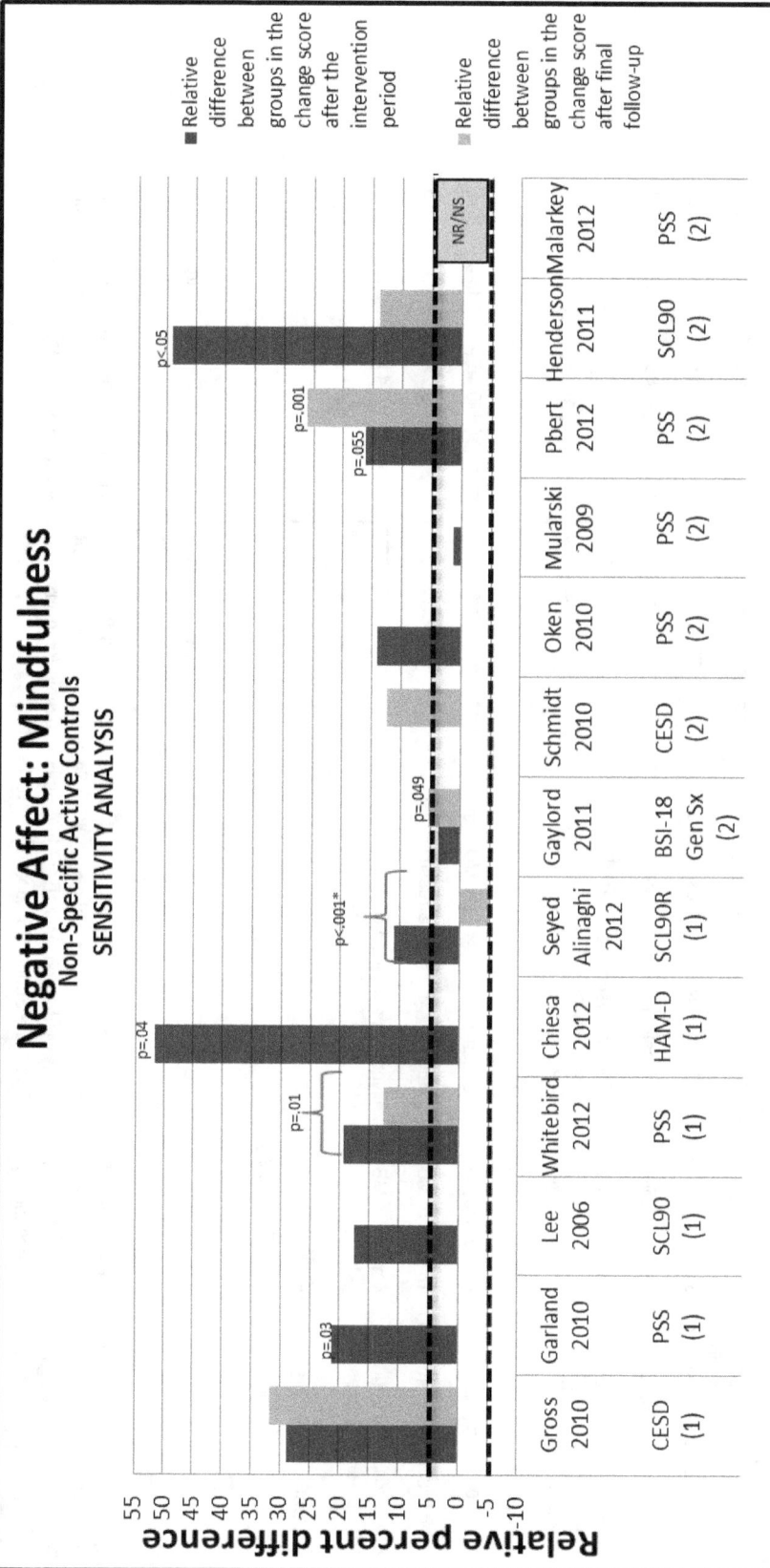

1. **Relative difference between groups in the change score.** This is a relative percent difference, using the baseline mean in the meditation group as the denominator. For example, if the meditation group improves from a 10 to 19 on a mental health scale and the control group improves from 11 to 16 on the same scale, the relative difference between groups in the change score is: $(((19-10)-(16-11))/10)\times 100 = 40\%$. The interpretation is that there is a 40% relative improvement on the mental health scale in the meditation group compared with the control group. See appendix E for absolute difference-in-change score values. Improvement in all scales is indicated in the positive direction. A positive relative percent difference means that the score improved more in the intervention group than in the control group
2. (1): Primary outcome. If the trial did not specify primary or secondary outcomes, this is either the outcome that the population was selected on or identified as a primary focus of the study. (2): Secondary outcome. If the trial did not specify primary or secondary outcomes, then this is not the outcome that the population was selected nor identified as a primary focus of the study.
3. NR/NS = Not Reported/Not significant. The trial measured this outcome and stated they were nonsignificant, and did not report actual results.
4. Black dotted lines from −5% to +5% indicate our criteria for no effect. It does not indicate statistical significance.
5. A p value above or below a bar indicates statistical significance reported in the original study publication. If there is no p value, the outcome was not significant in the original publication.
6. BSI-18 = Brief Symptom Inventory, General Symptom Severity Subscale; CESD=Center for Epidemiologic studies Depression Scale; HAM-D=Hamilton Psychiatric Rating Scale for Depression; STAI = State Trait Anxiety Inventory; PSS = Perceived Stress Scale; SCL90-R = Symptom Checklist 90 Depression subscale.

Figure 19. Meta-analysis of the effects of meditation programs on negative affect—sensitivity analysis (mindfulness meditation versus nonspecific active control interventions)

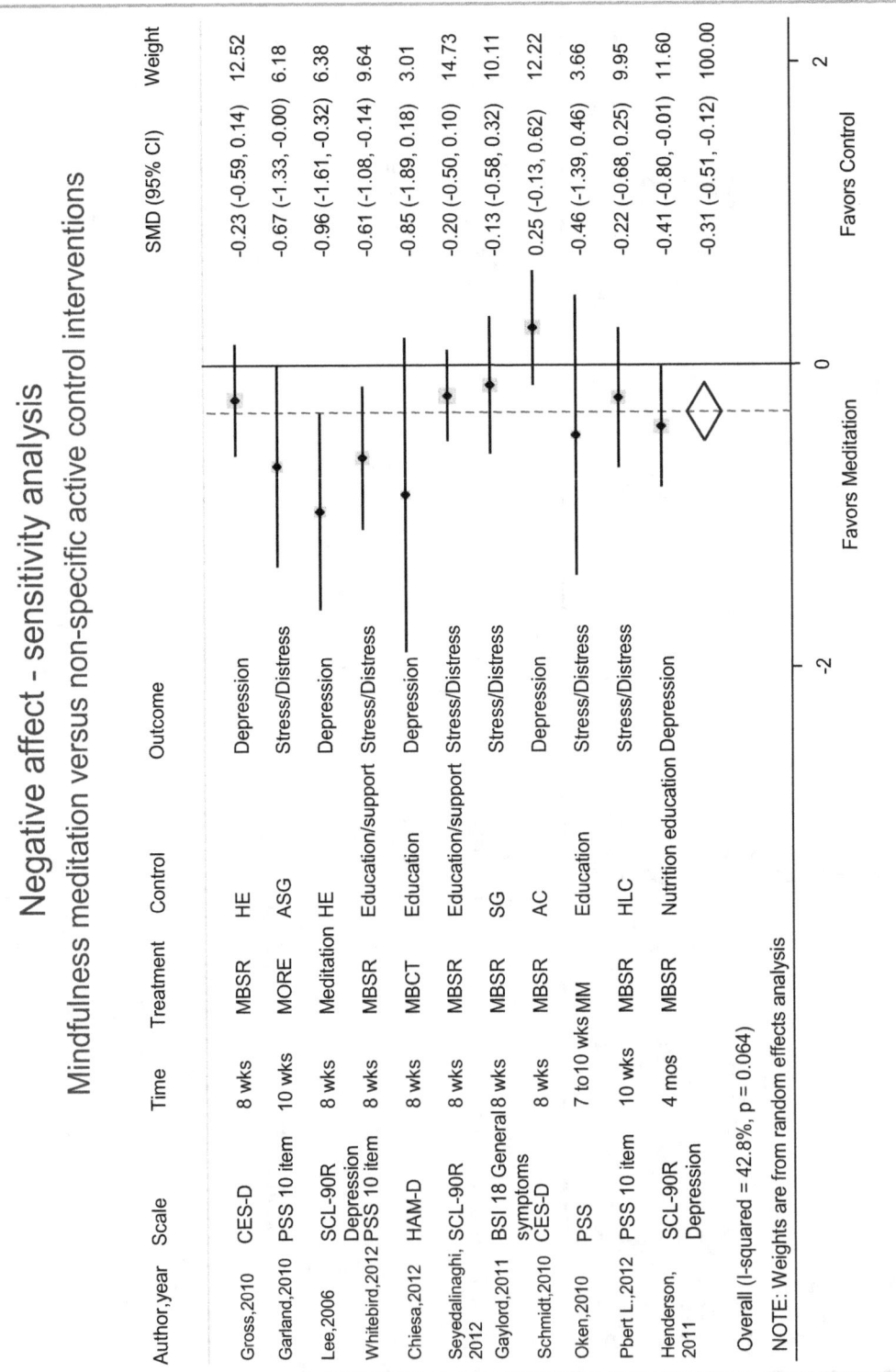

Notes: AC = Active Control; ASG = Alcohol Dependence Support Group; BSI = Beck Stress Inventory; CES-D = Center for Epidemiologic Studies Depression Scale; HE = Health Education; HLC = Healthy Living Course; HAM-D = Hamilton Psychiatric Rating Scale for depression; MBSR = Mindfulness-based Stress Reduction; MBCT = Mindfulness-based Cognitive Therapy; MM = Mindfulness Meditation; MORE = Mindfulness-oriented Recovery Enhancement; mos=Months; POMS = Profile of Mood States; PSS = Perceived Stress Scale; SCL = Symptom Checklist; SG = Support Group; wks = weeks.

Mantra Meditation Programs Versus <u>Nonspecific</u> Active Control

Five trials compared mantra meditation programs with nonspecific active controls, and evaluated a negative affect outcome (Table 11). Four were TM trials and one was other mantra meditation program. Three trials reported on anxiety and two on depression. The difference-in-change graphs show inconsistent results (Figure 20). We conducted a sensitivity analysis reversing the order of prioritization, prioritizing stress/distress over depression and depression over anxiety, to see if this would change our conclusions. The difference-in-change graph now showed consistently null results (Figure 21). A meta-analysis of the main outcomes for negative affect among mantra studies only replicated the anxiety meta-analysis (Figure 7) due to missing data on two of the trials that had a depression outcome. The meta-analysis of the sensitivity analysis showed a small nonsignificant overall effect (Figure 22).

The strength of evidence is insufficient that mantra programs have an effect on negative affect among various clinical populations when compared with a nonspecific active control. We based this rating on overall medium risk of bias, inconsistent results, indirect measures of negative affect, and imprecise estimates (Table 24).

Table 24. Grade of trials addressing the efficacy of mantra meditation programs on negative affect compared with nonspecific active controls among diverse populations

Number of Trials; Subjects	Domains Pertaining to Strength of Evidence				Magnitude of Effect and Strength of Evidence
	Risk of Bias	Consistency	Directness	Precision	
Negative Affect					Insufficient SOE of an effect
5; 438	Medium	Inconsistent	Indirect	Imprecise	−2.8% to +46.1% improvement

Note: SOE = Strength or Evidence

Figure 20. Relative difference between groups in the changes in measures of negative affect, in the mantra versus nonspecific active control studies

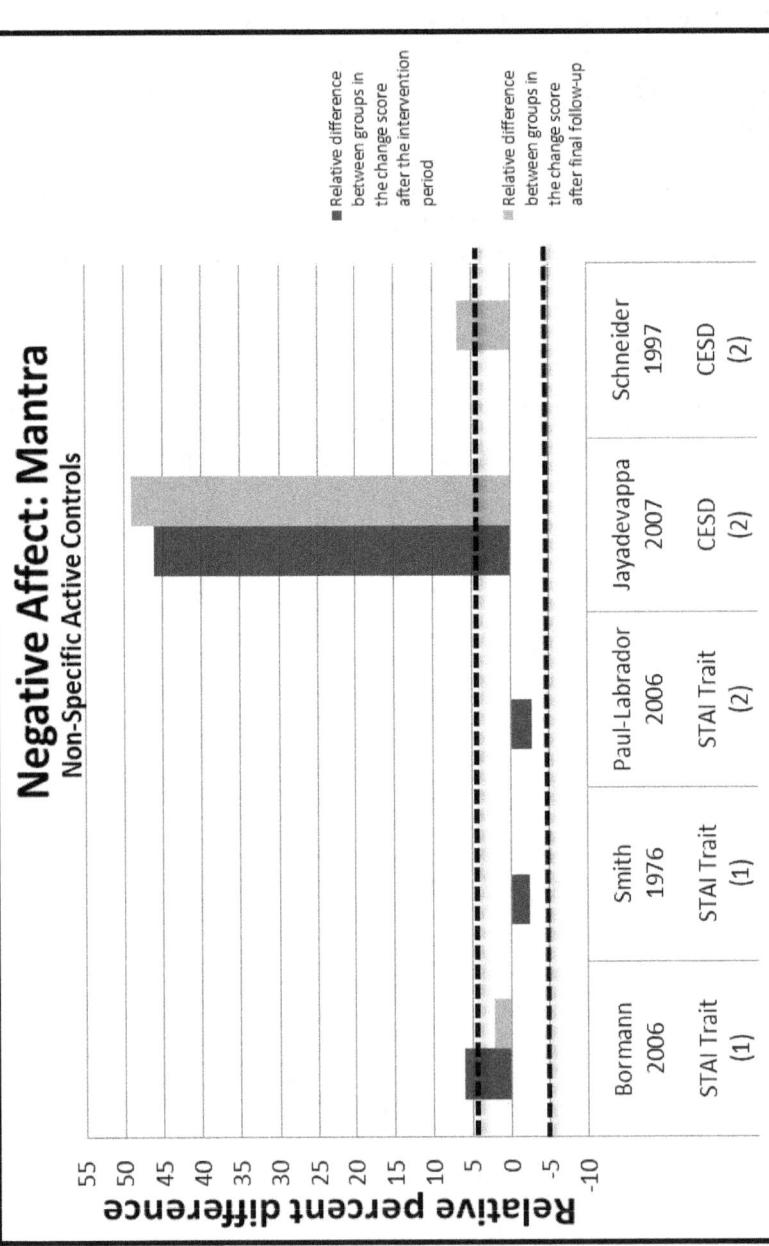

1. **Relative difference between groups in the change score.** This is a relative percent difference, using the baseline mean in the meditation group as the denominator. For example, if the meditation group improves from a 10 to 19 on a mental health scale and the control group improves from 11 to 16 on the same scale, the relative difference between groups in the change score is: $(((19-10)-(16-11))/10) \times 100 = 40\%$. The interpretation is that there is a 40% relative improvement on the mental health scale in the meditation group compared with the control group. See appendix E for absolute difference-in-change score values. Improvement in all scales is indicated in the positive direction. A positive relative percent difference means that the score improved more in the intervention group than in the control group.
2. (1): Primary outcome. If the trial did not specify primary or secondary outcomes, this is either the outcome that the population was selected on or identified as a primary focus of the study. (2): Secondary outcome. If the trial did not specify primary or secondary outcomes, then this is not the outcome that the population was selected nor identified as a primary focus of the study.
3. NR / NS = Not Reported/Not significant. The trial measured this outcome and stated they were nonsignificant, and did not report actual results.
4. Black dotted lines from −5% to +5% indicate our criteria for no effect. It does not indicate statistical significance.
5. A p value above or below a bar indicates statistical significance reported in the original study publication. If there is no p value, the outcome was not significant in the original publication.
6. CESD=Center for Epidemilogic studies Depression Scale; STAI = State Trait Anxiety Inventory; PSS = Perceived Stress Scale.

Figure 21. Relative difference between groups in the changes in measures of negative affect, in the mantra versus nonspecific active control studies (sensitivity analysis)

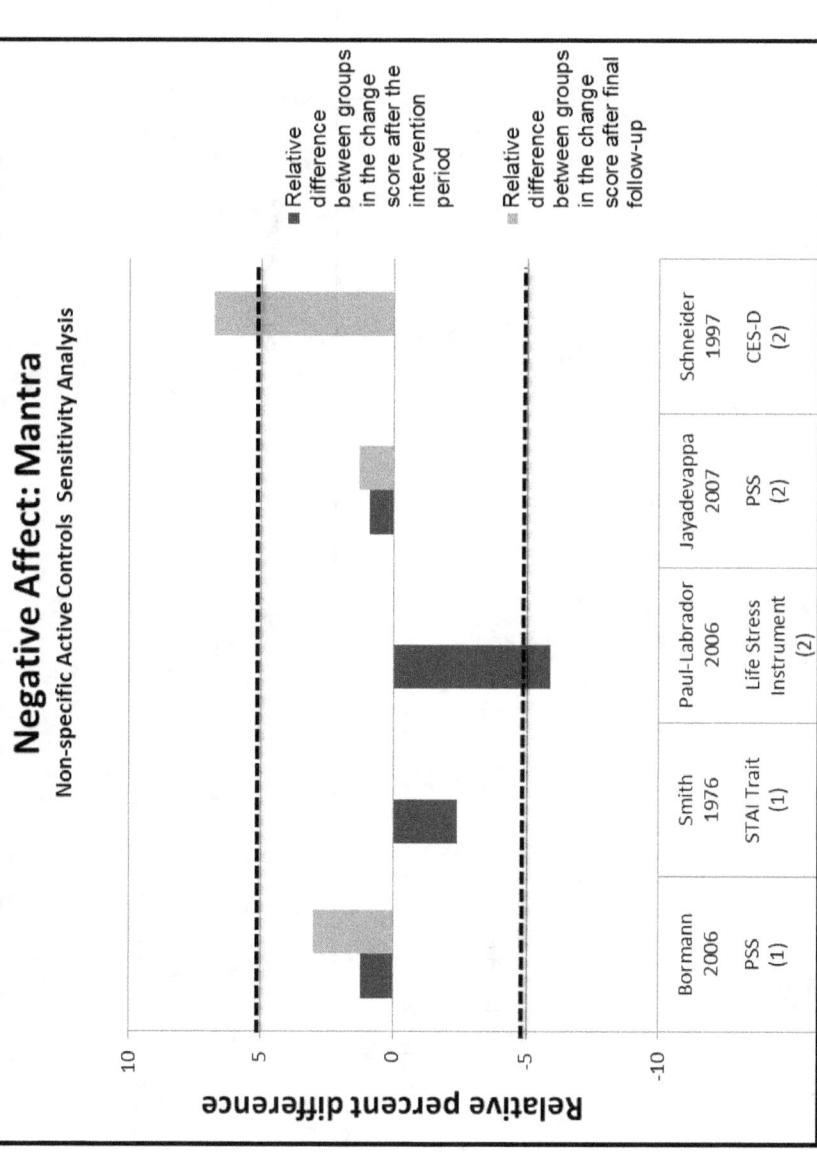

1. **Relative difference between groups in the change score.** This is a relative percent difference, using the baseline mean in the meditation group as the denominator. For example, if the meditation group improves from a 10 to 19 on a mental health scale and the control group improves from 11 to 16 on the same scale, the relative difference between groups in the change score is: $(((19-10)-(16-11))/10) \times 100 = 40\%$. The interpretation is that there is a 40% relative improvement on the mental health scale in the meditation group compared with the control group. See appendix E for absolute difference-in-change score values. Improvement in all scales is indicated in the positive direction. A positive relative percent difference means that the score improved more in the intervention group than in the control group
2. (1): Primary outcome. If the trial did not specify primary or secondary outcomes, then this is either the outcome that the population was selected on or identified as a primary focus of the study.
3. (2): Secondary outcome. If the trial did not specify primary or secondary outcomes, then this is not the outcome that the population was selected nor identified as a primary focus of the study.
4. Black dotted lines from −5% to +5% indicate our criteria for no effect. It does not indicate statistical significance.
5. A p value above or below a bar indicates statistical significance reported in the original study publication. If there is no p value with a bar, the outcome was not significant in the original study publication.
6. CESD=Center for Epidemilogic studies Depression Scale; STAI = State Trait Anxiety Inventory; PSS = Perceived Stress Scale.

Figure 22. Meta-analysis of the effects of mantra meditation programs on negative affect—sensitivity analysis (mantra vs. nonspecific active control interventions)

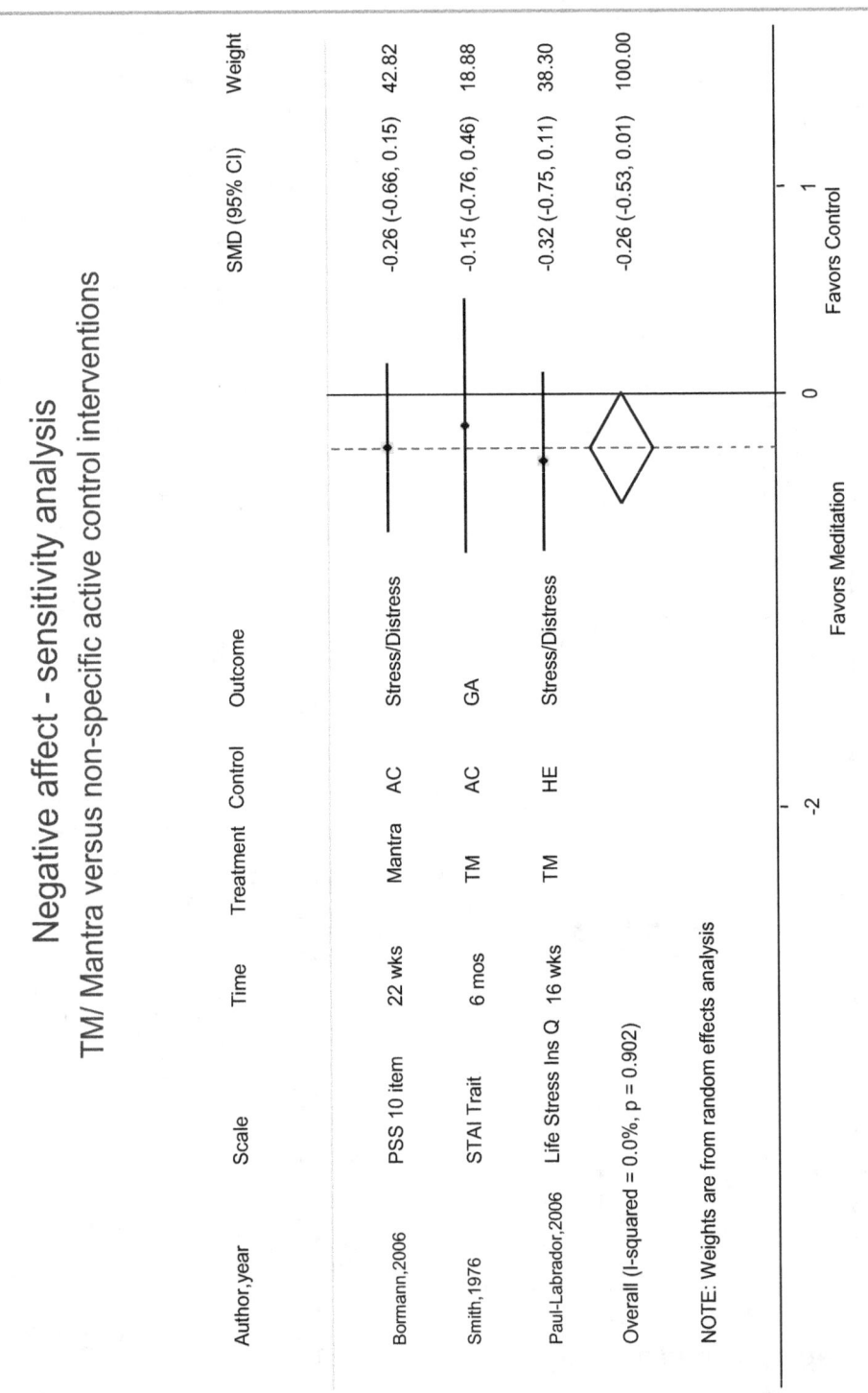

Note: AC = Active Control; HE=Health Education; GA = General Anxiety; mos = months; PSS = Perceived Stress Scale; STAI = State Trait Anxiety Inventory; TM = Transcendental Meditation; wks = weeks.

Positive Affect

Mindfulness Meditation Programs Versus Nonspecific Active Control

Three trials compared mindfulness meditation programs with nonspecific active controls, and evaluated positive affect as an outcome. They used differing populations, included a range of 18–137 patients, and were all of medium risk of bias (Table 12).

Henderson et al. randomized women with early-stage breast cancer (n=100) to MBSR or nonspecific active control.[57] The study used the Sense of Coherence Meaningfulness Subscale to measure subjective well-being as a secondary endpoint. At 4 months there was a statistically significant 6.8 percent improvement in mean Sense of Coherence Meaningfulness Subscale scores in the MBSR group as compared with the control group (p <0.05). However, this trial measured numerous outcomes and did not make any corrections for multiple comparisons. This trial had a medium risk of bias, provided 25 hours of training over 8 weeks, and did not specify whether it recommended home practice or not.

Gross et al. randomized solid organ transplant patients, post-surgery, (n=137) to MBSR versus health education.[54] The study used the Short Form-36 (SF-36) vitality score to measure improvement in positive mood as a secondary outcome. There were no differences between the groups at end of treatment. This trial provided 27 hours of training by a trained teacher, and unspecified amount of home practice over 8 weeks.

Chiesa et al. randomized patients with major depression (n=18) who failed to achieve remission after at least 8 weeks of antidepressant therapy, to either MBCT or nonspecific active control. The trial found a 54.6 percent reduction (p=.05) in the Psychological General Well-being Index. This trial had a medium risk of bias. It provided 16 hours of training over 8 weeks by a trained and certified teacher and had unspecified home practice.

Overall, the difference-in-change graphs show a small consistent effect of the mindfulness meditation programs on positive mood with one trial showing a small significant effect that diminishes with time, and another trial showing a large significant effect (Figures 23–24).

The strength of evidence is insufficient that mindfulness meditation program have an effect on positive affect when compared with a nonspecific active control. We based this rating on medium risk of bias, consistent findings, indirect measures, and imprecise estimates (Table 25).

Table 25. Grade of trials addressing the efficacy of mindfulness meditation programs on positive affect compared with nonspecific active controls among organ transplant recipients and breast cancer patients

Number of Trials; Subjects	Domains Pertaining to Strength of Evidence				Magnitude of Effect and Strength of Evidence
	Risk of Bias	Consistency	Directness	Precision	
Positive Affect					Insufficient SOE of an effect
3; 255	Medium	Consistent	Indirect	Imprecise	0.7% to 54.6% improvement

Note: SOE = Strength of Evidence

Figure 23. Relative difference between groups in the changes in measures of positive affect, in the mindfulness versus nonspecific active control/specific active control studies

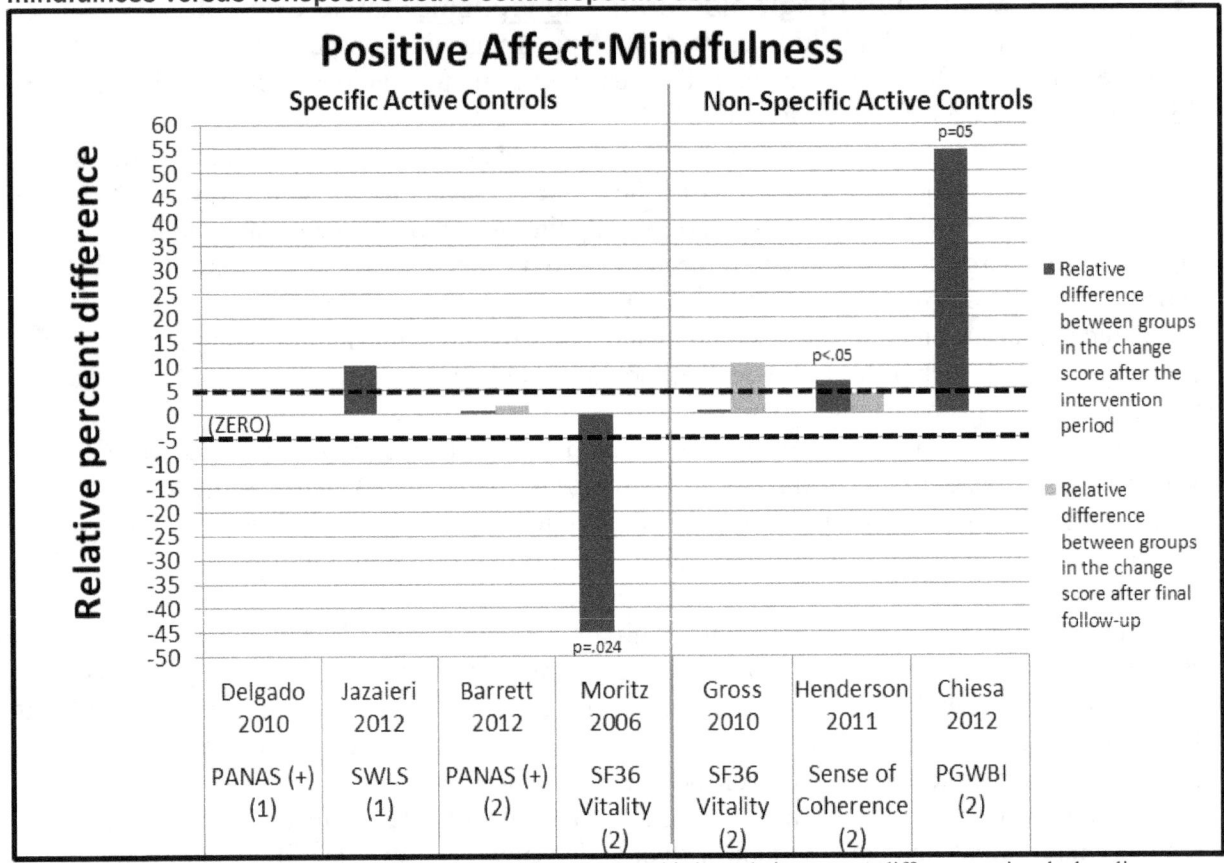

1. **Relative difference between groups in the change score**. This is a relative percent difference, using the baseline mean in the meditation group as the denominator. For example, if the meditation group improves from a 10 to 19 on a mental health scale and the control group improves from 11 to 16 on the same scale, the relative difference between groups in the change score is: $(((19-10)-(16-11))/10) \times 100 = 40\%$. The interpretation is that there is a 40% relative improvement on the mental health scale in the meditation group compared with the control group. See appendix E for absolute difference-in-change score values. Improvement in all scales is indicated in the positive direction. A positive relative percent difference means that the score improved more in the intervention group than in the control group
2. (1): Primary outcome. If the trial did not specify primary or secondary outcomes, this is either the outcome that the population was selected on or identified as a primary focus of the study. (2): Secondary outcome. If the trial did not specify primary or secondary outcomes, then this is not the outcome that the population was selected nor identified as a primary focus of the study.
3. NR/NS = Not Reported/Not significant. The trial measured this outcome and stated they were nonsignificant, and did not report actual results.
4. Black dotted lines from –5% to +5% indicate our criteria for no effect. It does not indicate statistical significance.
5. A p value above or below a bar indicates statistical significance reported in the original study publication. If there is no p value, the outcome was not significant in the original publication.
6. PANAS = Positive and Negative Affect Scale; PGWBI=Psychological General Well-being Index; SF-36 = Short Form-36; SWLS = Satisfaction with Life scale
7. Text describing results for comparisons with **specific** active controls for positive affect starts on page 97

Figure 24. Meta-analysis of the effects of meditation programs on positive affect with up to 4 months of followup

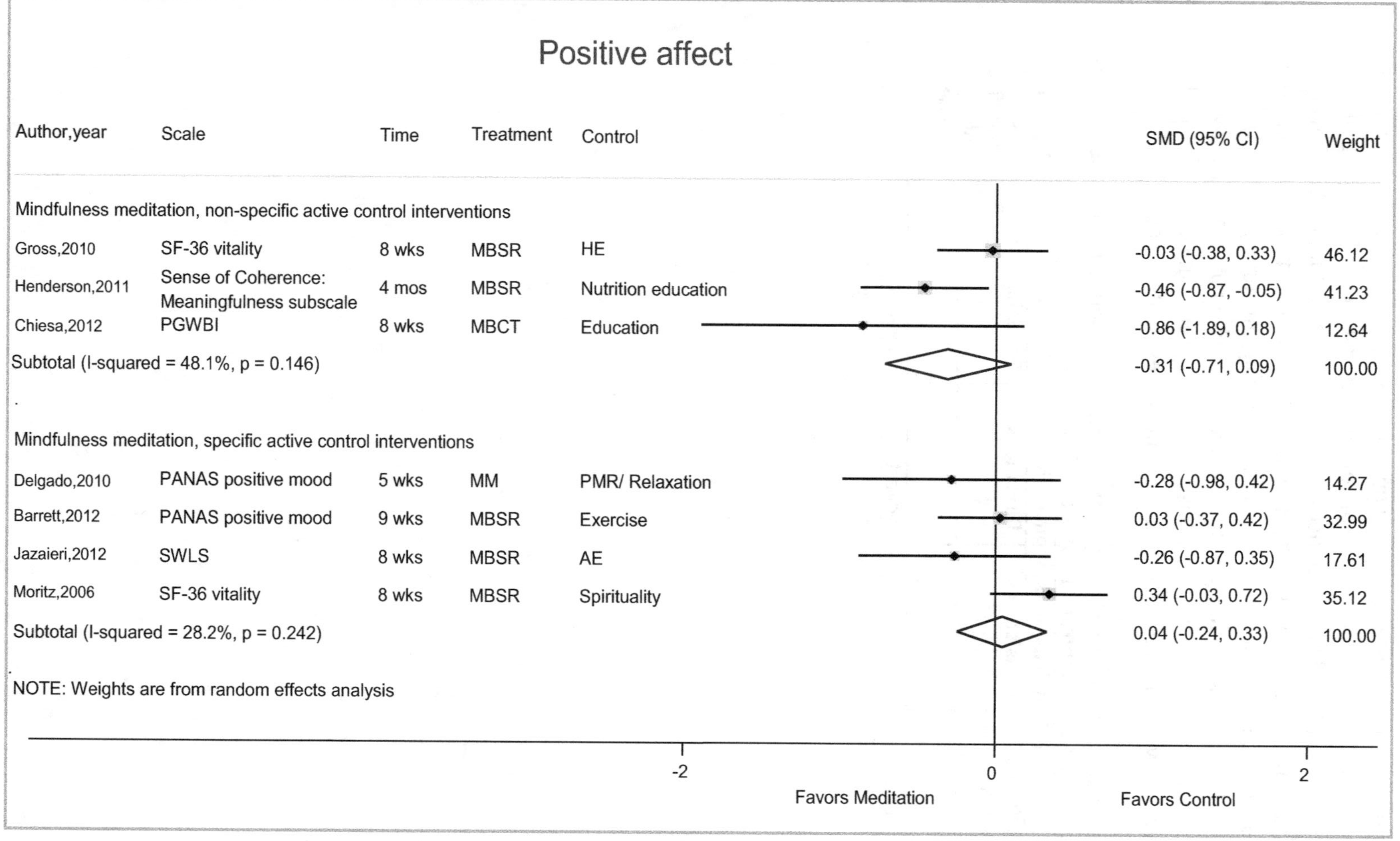

Positive affect

Author,year	Scale	Time	Treatment	Control	SMD (95% CI)	Weight
Mindfulness meditation, non-specific active control interventions						
Gross,2010	SF-36 vitality	8 wks	MBSR	HE	-0.03 (-0.38, 0.33)	46.12
Henderson,2011	Sense of Coherence: Meaningfulness subscale	4 mos	MBSR	Nutrition education	-0.46 (-0.87, -0.05)	41.23
Chiesa,2012	PGWBI	8 wks	MBCT	Education	-0.86 (-1.89, 0.18)	12.64
Subtotal (I-squared = 48.1%, p = 0.146)					-0.31 (-0.71, 0.09)	100.00
Mindfulness meditation, specific active control interventions						
Delgado,2010	PANAS positive mood	5 wks	MM	PMR/ Relaxation	-0.28 (-0.98, 0.42)	14.27
Barrett,2012	PANAS positive mood	9 wks	MBSR	Exercise	0.03 (-0.37, 0.42)	32.99
Jazaieri,2012	SWLS	8 wks	MBSR	AE	-0.26 (-0.87, 0.35)	17.61
Moritz,2006	SF-36 vitality	8 wks	MBSR	Spirituality	0.34 (-0.03, 0.72)	35.12
Subtotal (I-squared = 28.2%, p = 0.242)					0.04 (-0.24, 0.33)	100.00

NOTE: Weights are from random effects analysis

Favors Meditation / Favors Control

Notes: AE = Aerobic Exercise; HE = Health Education; HLC = Healthy Living Course; HAM-D = Hamilton Psychiatric Rating Scale for depression; MBSR = Mindfulness-based Stress Reduction; MBCT = Mindfulness-based Cognitive Therapy; MM = Mindfulness Meditation; mos=months; SF-36 = Short Form-36; SWLS = Satisfaction with Life Scale; PGWBI = Psychological General Well-being Index; PANAS = Positive and Negative Affect Score; wks = weeks.

Transcendental Meditation Versus <u>Nonspecific</u> Active Control

Jayadevappa et al. randomized CHF patients (n=23) to either 3 months of TM or health education, assessing positive mood as a secondary outcome using the SF-36 vitality subscale.[78] With 100 percent trial completion and a 95 percent compliance rate among the originally randomized subjects, this trial found no differences at 3 and 6 months (Figure 25). This trial had a low risk of bias, and provided 22.5 hours of training over 6 months by trained and certified teachers. It recommended up to 90 hours of home practice during this time (Table 12).

The strength of evidence is insufficient about the effects of TM on positive affect when compared with a nonspecific active control. We based this rating on a single low risk-of-bias study, unknown consistency, indirect measures, and imprecise estimates (Table 26).

Table 26. Grade of trials addressing the efficacy of transcendental meditation on positive affect compared with nonspecific active controls among cardiac patients

Number of Trials; Subjects	Domains Pertaining to Strength of Evidence				Magnitude of Effect and Strength of Evidence
	Risk of Bias	Consistency	Directness	Precision	
Positive Affect					Insufficient SOE of an effect
1; 23	Low	Unknown	Indirect	Imprecise	+2.4%

Note: SOE = Strength or Evidence; TM = Transcendental Meditation

Figure 25. Relative difference between groups in the changes in measures of positive affect, in the mantra versus nonspecific active control studies

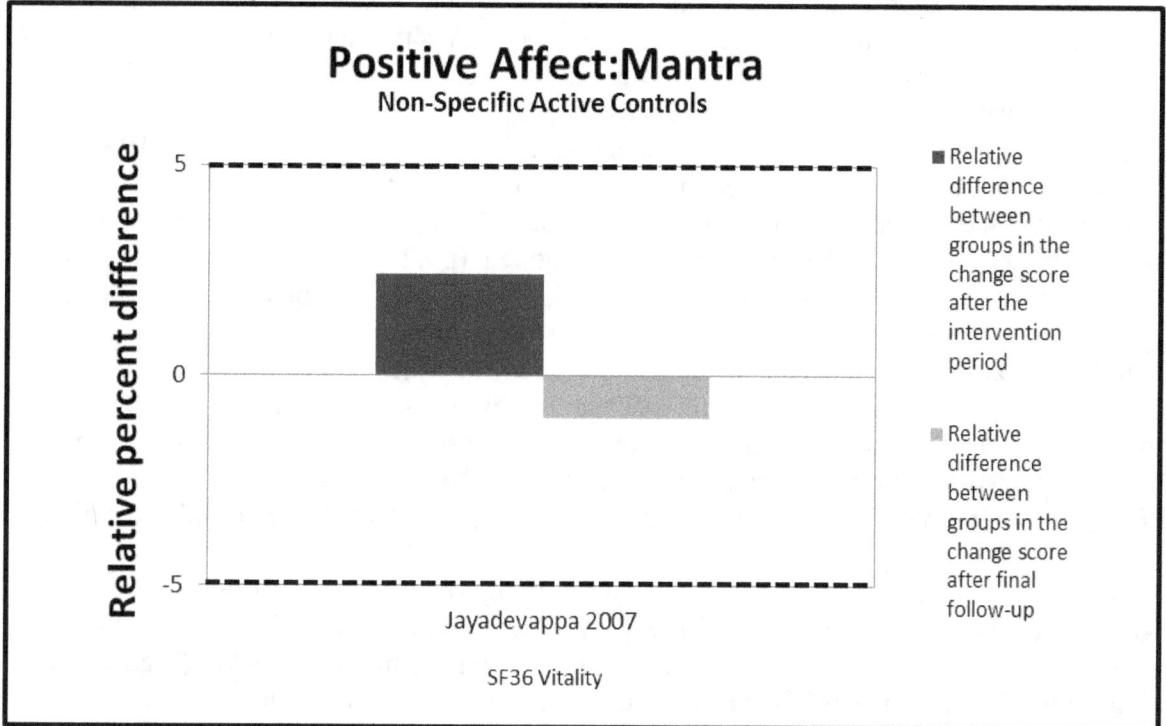

1. **Relative difference between groups in the change score**. This is a relative percent difference, using the baseline mean in the meditation group as the denominator. For example, if the meditation group improves from a 10 to 19 on a mental health scale and the control group improves from 11 to 16 on the same scale, the relative difference between groups in the change score is: (((19-10)-(16-11))/10)x100=40%. The interpretation is that there is a 40% relative improvement on the mental health scale in the meditation group compared with the control group. See appendix E for absolute difference-in-change score values. Improvement in all scales is indicated in the positive direction. A positive relative percent difference means that the score improved more in the intervention group than in the control group
2. (1): Primary outcome. If the trial did not specify primary or secondary outcomes, this is either the outcome that the population was selected on or identified as a primary focus of the study. (2): Secondary outcome. If the trial did not specify primary or secondary outcomes, then this is not the outcome that the population was selected nor identified as a primary focus of the study.
3. NR / NS = Not Reported/Not significant. The trial measured this outcome and stated they were nonsignificant, and did not report actual results.
4. Black dotted lines from −5% to +5% indicate our criteria for no effect. It does not indicate statistical significance.
5. A p value above or below a bar indicates statistical significance reported in the original study publication. If there is no p value, the outcome was not significant in the original publication.
6. SF-36=Short Form-36

Mental Component of Health-Related Quality of Life

Mindfulness Meditation Programs Versus <u>Nonspecific</u> Active Control

Pbert et al. randomized asthmatics to MBSR or education control (n=82), and specified asthma QOL as a primary outcome. It found a 6.2 percent (ns) and 26 percent (p=.002) improvement at 10 weeks and 12 months, respectively, in the emotional function domain of asthma quality of life. The trial provided 26 hours of training over 8 weeks with approximately 24 hours of recommended home practice, and had a low risk of bias. There was no information about the teachers (Table 13).

Whitebird et al. randomized patients who were caregivers of family members with dementia (n=78) to either MBSR or education support group. This trial did not specify primary or secondary outcomes, but the short form-12 (SF-12) mental component score was categorized as a primary focus of the study. The MBSR group showed a 28.4 and 24.3 percent reduction in perceived stress scores post-intervention and 6 months, respectively, (p<.001 for overall reductions) as compared with the education support group. This trial had a medium risk of bias, provided 25 hours of training over 8 weeks by a trained teacher, and had an average of 26.7 hours of homework completed by the participants.

Gross et al. randomized solid organ transplant patients, post-surgery, (n=137) to MBSR versus health education.[54] The trial used the SF-12 mental component score to measure improvement in the mental component of health-related QOL as a secondary outcome. There were no differences between the groups at end of treatment (p=.29). This trial provided 27 hours of training by a trained teacher, and had an unspecified amount of home practice over 8 weeks. This trial had medium risk of bias.

Mularski et al. randomized elderly patients, predominantly men, with moderate to severe chronic obstructive pulmonary disorder (n=49) to a mindfulness-based breathing therapy or a support group.[65] The trial used the Veterans Rand-36 to measure QOL as a secondary outcome. There was a nonsignificant 8.3 percent improvement in the Veterans Rand-36 scores in the MBBT group after 2 months. This trial suffered from a 42 percent attrition rate and had a high risk of bias.

The difference-in-change graphs suggested a small improvement for mindfulness meditation programs in the mental component of QOL when compared with nonspecific active controls (right side of Figure 26). The meta-analysis suggests a small nonsignificant effect (Figure 30)

The strength of evidence is low that mindfulness meditation programs improve the mental component of health-related QOL in various patients as compared with a nonspecific active control. We based this rating on overall medium risk of bias, consistent findings, direct measures, and imprecise estimates (Table 27).

Table 27. Grade of trials addressing the efficacy of mindfulness meditation programs on the mental component of health-related quality of life compared with nonspecific active controls among various patients

Number of Trials; Subjects	Domains Pertaining to Strength of Evidence				Magnitude of Effect and Strength of Evidence
	Risk of Bias	Consistency	Directness	Precision	
Mental health component of health-related QOL					Low SOE of an improvement
4; 346	Medium	Consistent	Direct	Imprecise	+5% to +28.4% improvement

Notes: SOE = Strength of Evidence; QOL = Quality of Life

Figure 26. Relative difference between groups in the changes in measures of mental component of health-related quality of life, in the mindfulness versus nonspecific active control/specific active control studies

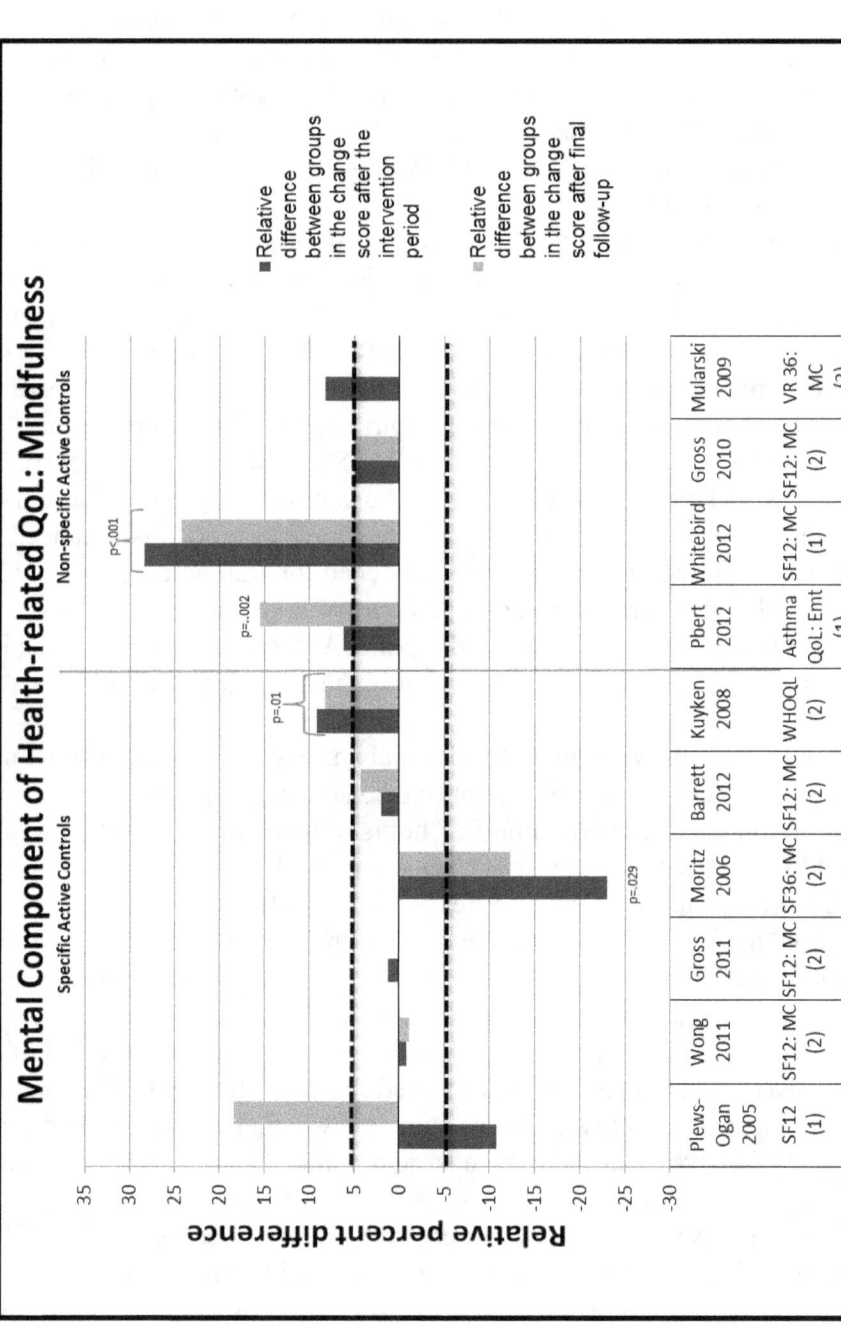

1. **Relative difference between groups in the change score.** This is a relative percent difference, using the baseline mean in the meditation group as the denominator. For example, if the meditation group improves from a 10 to 19 on a mental health scale and the control group improves from 11 to 16 on the same scale, the relative difference between groups in the change score is: (((19-10)−(16-11))/10)x100=40%. The interpretation is that there is a 40% relative improvement on the mental health scale in the meditation group compared with the control group. See appendix E for absolute difference-in-change score values. Improvement in all scales is indicated in the positive direction. A positive relative percent difference means that the score improved more in the intervention group than in the control group (1): Primary outcome. If the trial did not specify primary or secondary outcomes, this is either the outcome that the population was selected on or identified as a primary focus of the study. (2): Secondary outcome. If the trial did not specify primary or secondary outcomes, then this is not the outcome that the population was selected nor identified as a primary focus of the study.
2. NR/NS = Not Reported/Not significant. The trial measured this outcome and stated they were nonsignificant, and did not report actual results.
3. Black dotted lines from −5% to +5% indicate our criteria for no effect. It does not indicate statistical significance.
4. A p value above or below a bar indicates statistical significance reported in the original study publication. If there is no p value, the outcome was not significant in the original publication.
5. SF-12: MC = Short Form-12: Mental Component Score of Health-related Quality of Life; SF-36: MC = Short Form 36: Mental Component Score of Health-related Quality of Life; WHOQL = World Health Organization Quality of Life Assessment; VR36 = Veterans RAND 36 Item Health Survey.
6. Text describing results for comparisons with specific active controls for mental component of health-related quality of life starts on page 88

Comparisons With Specific Active Control

Anxiety

Mindfulness Meditation Programs Versus <u>Specific</u> Active Control

Nine trials evaluated a mindfulness meditation program against a specific active control for the outcome of anxiety (Table 8). Six trials used MBSR, one used MBCT, and two used mindfulness meditation. The control groups were heterogeneous including medications, spirituality interventions, exercise, and group therapies. Sample sizes ranged from 25–110. Two trials had a high risk of bias, five had a medium risk of bias, and two had a low risk of bias.

Wong et al.[74] randomized Chinese-speaking participants with chronic pain (n=99) to an 8-week MBSR program or a multidisciplinary pain intervention. The trial saw nonsignificant changes at 2 and 6 months post-intervention in the STAI state and trait scores. The profile of mood states (POMS) tension difference-in-change score showed the greatest change (11.5 percent) favoring MBSR, but was also nonsignificant.

Gross et al. randomized adults with primary chronic insomnia (n=30) to an 8-week MBSR program or an 8-week course of pharmacotherapy with eszopiclone.[55] At 2 and 5 months post-intervention, there were no significant changes in STAI state or trait scores in either group, but the directionality of difference-in-change point estimates favored the MBSR group.

Moritz et al. randomized people with mood disorders (n=165) recruited from primary care clinics to 8 weeks of either MBSR or an 8-week audio taped spirituality home trial program.[63] This trial evaluated the superiority of a spirituality program to MBSR, as opposed to other trials, using a comparative effectiveness design. MBSR was used as the control. They utilized a POMS score of 40 or greater as inclusion criteria, indicating a moderate degree of mood disturbance, and as a main outcome measure. Although groups appeared matched for amount of training (12 hours over 8 weeks), the spirituality group received up to 42 hours of home practice over that time and it is unclear whether the MBSR group received the same. At 8 weeks, the difference in the MBSR group from baseline was 39 percent lower than that in the spirituality group (p=0.007).

Koszycki et al.[58] randomized patients with generalized social anxiety disorder (n=53) to an 8-week course of MBSR or a 12-week course of group cognitive behavior therapy. MBSR received a maximum of 27.5 hours of training and a maximum of 28 hours of home practice over 8 weeks. Outcome measures included four scales of social anxiety, which favored group cognitive behavior therapy over MBSR: Liebowitz social anxiety-fear scale (p=.09), social anxiety-avoidance scale (p=.009), social phobia scale (p=.006), and social interaction scale (p=.057). Although the groups cognitive behavior therapy group ran for 4 weeks longer than MBSR, the total dose was similar (27.5 hours of training for MBSR vs. 30 hours for group cognitive behavior therapy). It remains unclear if it was the effect of the training over a longer period of time in the group cognitive behavior therapy arm that accounted for the differences. The analysis appeared to compare post-treatment scores only, and it was unclear whether they accounted for baseline differences in the analysis, given that there were large baseline differences between the groups.

Barrett et al.[85] randomized patients with a history of upper respiratory infections to MBSR or exercise (n=98). The trial provided about 20 hours of training by trained teachers, and approximately 42 hours of recommended homework over the 8-week training period. The STAI state score was a secondary outcome. The trial found no significant differences between the two arms.

Jazaieri et al.[87] randomized patients with social anxiety disorder to MBSR or exercise (n=56). The trial provided about 25 hours of training by trained teachers, and their participants performed an average of 28.3 hours of homework over the 8-week training period. Although they did not specify primary or secondary outcomes, the study characterized the Liebowitz social anxiety scale as a primary outcome since it was a primary focus of the study. The trial found a nonsignificant improvement of 6.2 percent, which worsened over time in the MBSR group as compared with exercise. This trial had a high risk of bias.

Philippot et al. randomized patients with tinnitus (n=30) to a 6-week modified MBCT program or progressive muscular relaxation training.[67] This trial used the STAI (unspecified) and found no statistically significant differences between-groups. It provided 13.5 hours of training and an unspecified amount of home practice. We rated it as medium risk of bias.

Delgado et al. randomized worriers (n=36) to 5 weeks of mindfulness meditation or progressive muscular relaxation, providing 10 hours of training and unspecified amount of home practice.[51] They found no significant differences in the STAI trait score, and had a medium risk of bias. Piet et al. randomized 26 patients with social phobia to MBCT or group cognitive behavior therapy.[68] They provided 16 hours of training and up to 28 hours of home practice over an 8-week period. This trial found no difference between the groups on the BAI However, the cognitive behavior therapy group was provided nearly double the amount of group training, 28 hours over 14 weeks, and this increased time and attention in the control group may not allow appropriate comparisons between the groups. This trial had a medium risk of bias.

The difference-in-change graphs showed inconsistent results (Figure 27). A meta-analysis of these trials showed nonsignificant effects around the null at end of treatment and end of study time points (Figures 6 and 7).

The strength of evidence is insufficient that mindfulness meditation programs have an effect on anxiety among various clinical populations when compared with a variety of specific active controls. We based this rating on overall medium risk of bias, inconsistent findings, directness of measures, and imprecise estimates (Table 28).

Table 28. Grade of trials addressing the efficacy of mindfulness meditation programs on anxiety compared with specific active controls among diverse populations

Number of Trials; Subjects	Domains Pertaining to Strength of Evidence				Magnitude of Effect and Strength of Evidence
	Risk of Bias	Consistency	Directness	Precision	
Anxiety					Insufficient SOE of an effect
9; 526	Medium	Inconsistent	Direct	Imprecise	−38.6 to +8.4%

Note: SOE = Strength of Evidence

Figure 27. Relative difference between groups in the changes in measures of general anxiety, in the mindfulness versus specific active control studies

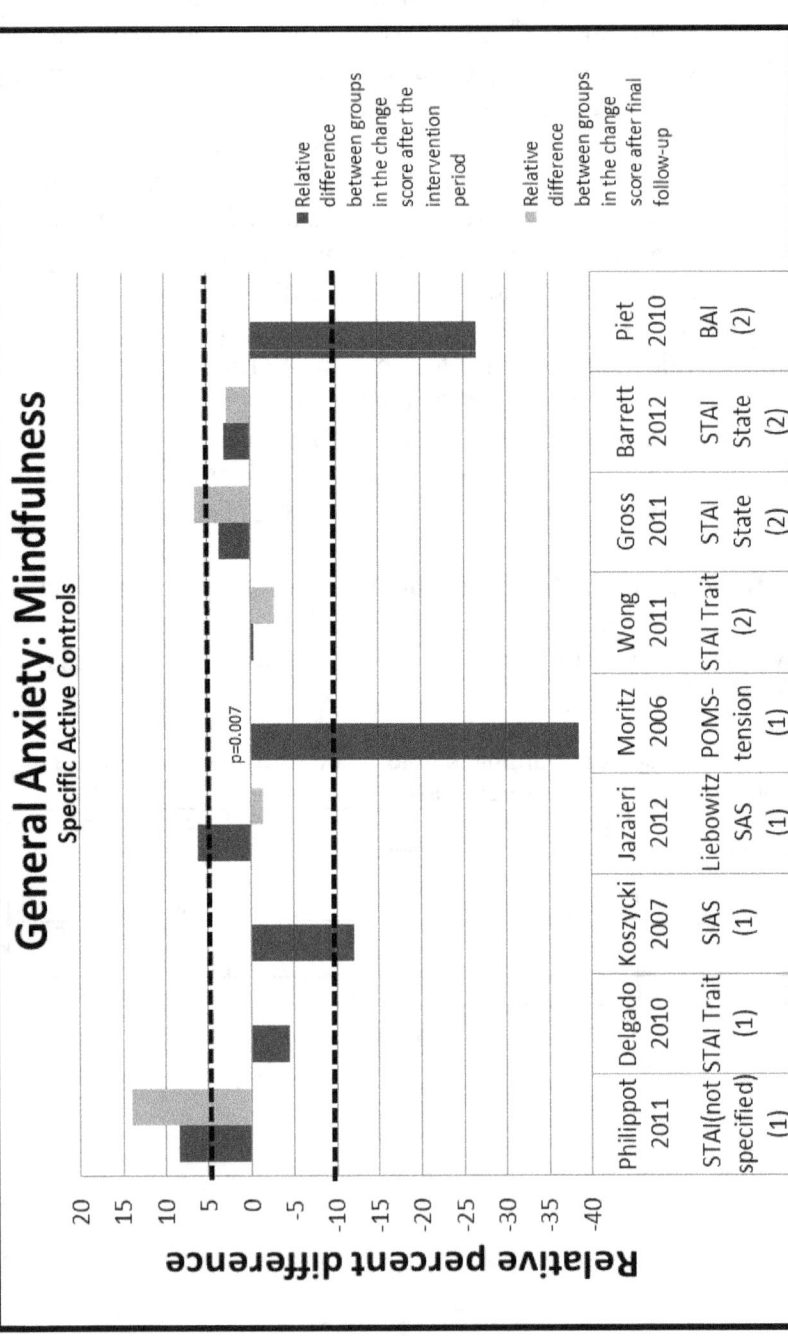

1. **Relative difference between groups in the change score.** This is a relative percent difference, using the baseline mean in the meditation group as the denominator. For example, if the meditation group improves from a 10 to 19 on a mental health scale and the control group improves from 11 to 16 on the same scale, the relative difference between groups in the change score is: (((19-10)−(16-11))/10)×100=40%. The interpretation is that there is a 40% relative improvement on the mental health scale in the meditation group compared with the control group. See appendix E for absolute difference-in-change score values. Improvement in all scales is indicated in the positive direction. A positive relative percent difference means that the score improved more in the intervention group than in the control group
2. (1): Primary outcome. If the trial did not specify primary or secondary outcomes, this is either the outcome that the population was selected on or identified as a primary focus of the study. (2): Secondary outcome. If the trial did not specify primary or secondary outcomes, then this is not the outcome that the population was selected nor identified as a primary focus of the study.
3. NR / NS = Not Reported/Not significant. The trial measured this outcome and stated they were nonsignificant, and did not report actual results.
4. Black dotted lines from −5% to +5% indicate our criteria for no effect. It does not indicate statistical significance.
5. A p value above or below a bar indicates statistical significance reported in the original study publication. If there is no p value, the outcome was not significant in the original publication.
6. BAI = Beck Anxiety Index; POMS = Profile of Mood States; SIAS = Social Interaction Scale; STAI = State Trait Anxiety Index.

Other Mantra Meditation Versus <u>Specific</u> Active Control

Lehrer et al. assigned anxious participants to clinically standardized meditation (n=23) or progressive muscular relaxation (n=19).[79] The program provided 7.5 hours of training and unspecified amount of home practice over 5 weeks (Table 8). Undergraduate and graduate students, with 4 months of training in the technique and no prior teaching experience, provided the training. Results on all four anxiety measures favored the progressive muscular relaxation group over the clinically standardized meditation group. For measures it used institute for personality and ability testing anxiety inventory, symptom checklist 90 anxiety subscale, and state trait anxiety index state and trait scales. At 6 weeks the differences were all nonsignificant, but ranged from 6–21 percent favoring the progressive muscular relaxation group (Figure 8).

The strength of evidence is insufficient about the effects of clinically standardized meditation on anxiety in an anxious population when compared with progressive muscular relaxation. We based this rating on a single study with medium risk of bias, unknown consistency, directness of measures, and imprecise estimates (Table 29).

Table 29. Grade of trials addressing the efficacy of clinically standardized meditation programs on anxiety compared with progressive muscle relaxation among anxious participants

Number of Trials; Subjects	Domains Pertaining to Strength of Evidence				Magnitude of Effect and Strength of Evidence at End of Intervention
	Risk of Bias	Consistency	Directness	Precision	
Anxiety					Insufficient SOE of an effect compared with PMR
1; 42	Medium	Unknown	Direct	Imprecise	−5.6% favoring PMR

Notes: SOE = Strength or Evidence; PMR = Progressive Muscle Relaxation

Depression

Mindfulness Meditation Programs Versus <u>Specific</u> Active Control

Eleven trials evaluated a mindfulness meditation programs against a specific active control for the outcome of depression (Table 9). Five trials compared MBSR to various specific active controls in diverse populations. Four trials compared MBCT to either antidepressant among depressed patients, cognitive behavior therapy among anxious patients, or progressive muscle relaxation among those suffering from tinnitus. One trial compared a mindfulness meditation program to progressive muscular relaxation and one trial compared a mindfulness meditation program to viniyoga. Four trials had a low risk of bias, five had a medium risk of bias, and two had a high risk of bias. Sample sizes ranged from 25–186.

Wong et al. randomized patients with chronic pain (n=99) in Hong Kong to MBSR or a multidisciplinary pain intervention.[74] The study used two scales to assess depression. It found a nonsignificant 10.7 percent improvement on the POMS-depression at 2 months, which maintained to 6 months. However, it found no difference in the Center for Epidemiologic Studies depression scale at 2 or 6 months. This trial had a low risk of bias, provided 27 hours of training, and an unspecified amount of home practice over 8 weeks. Its teachers were trained and had 5 years of experience teaching meditation.[74]

Gross et al. randomized people with insomnia (n=27) to MBSR or eszopiclone.[55] They found a 25.4 percent change in Center for Epidemiologic Studies depression scale favoring the drug at the end of 2 months, which increased to 42.2 percent at 5 months. Although these appeared to be large effects, the study reported the differences as not significant. This trial provided 26 hours of training and up to 36 hours of home practice over 8 weeks.

Koszyki et al. randomized patients with social anxiety disorder (n=53) to MBSR or group cognitive behavior therapy. The trial had a high risk of bias. They found a nonsignificant 5.3 percent difference favoring the cognitive behavior therapy group on the BDI II.[58]

Moritz et al. randomized patients with mood disorders (n=110) to a spirituality program versus MBSR.[63] In this trial, MBSR was the active control for the spirituality intervention. The spirituality intervention included a meditative component. It provided about 12 hours of training in both interventions over an 8-week period, with unspecified amount of home practice in the MBSR group. It provided up to 42 hours of home practice in the spirituality group. There was no information on teacher qualifications for MBSR. There was a significant 31.7 percent improvement on the POMS-depression scale in the spirituality program as compared with MBSR ($p<0.013$). This trial had a low risk of bias.

Jazaieri et al.[87] randomized patients with social anxiety disorder to MBSR or exercise (n=56). The trial provided about 25 hours of training by trained teachers, and their participants performed an average of 28.3 hours of homework over the 8-week training period. Although they did not specify primary or secondary outcomes, the study identified depression as a primary focus of the study. The trial found nonsignificant improvements of 22.8 and 14.2 percent at 8 weeks and 5 months, respectively, in the MBSR group as compared with exercise. The trial had a high risk of bias.

Segal et al. randomized depressed patients in acute remission to MBCT with tapering of antidepressant or maintenance antidepressant medication (n=53) to assess depression relapse. Relapse rates by 600 days were 46 percent for the antidepressant group and 38 percent for MBCT. This absolute 8 percent difference did not reach statistical significance. This trial had a low risk of bias. It provided 23 hours of training by trained and certified teachers, and recommended an unspecified amount of home practice.[71]

Kuyken et al. randomized patients with recurrent depression (n=123) who were in full or partial remission to either maintenance anti-depressant medication or MBCT with support to taper medication.[59] After 15 months, 60 percent of the antidepressant group had relapsed as compared with 47 percent in the MBCT group. This 13 percent absolute difference did not reach statistical significance. They also measured the Hamilton depression rating scores, which were 31.7 percent lower in the MBCT group at 3 months and 26.7 percent lower at 15 months ($p=.02$). On a third measure, the BDI II, the MBCT group showed a 14.6 percent reduction at 3 months and 15 percent reduction at 15 months compared with the antidepressant group. These differences did not reach statistical significance. Of note, 75 percent of the MBCT had discontinued their antidepressant by 6 months. This was a low risk-of-bias trial. It provided 24 hours of training and recommended up to 37.5 hours of home practice over an 8-week period. The teachers were trained and certified.

Piet et al. randomized young adults with social phobia (n=26) to either MBCT or group cognitive behavioral therapy in a crossover design with participants receiving both treatments.[68] We evaluated comparisons after the first intervention period only, before any crossover. They provided 16 hours of training and up to 28 hours of home practice over an 8-week period. This trial found a 24.3 percent nonsignificant change favoring the cognitive behavioral therapy group on the BDI-II. However, the cognitive behavioral therapy group received nearly doubles the amount of group training, 28 hours over 14 weeks, and this increased time and attention in the control group may not allow equivalent comparisons between the groups. This trial had a medium risk of bias.

Philippot et al. randomized patients with tinnitus (n=25) to a 6-week modified MBCT program or progressive relaxation training.[67] This trial used the BDI and found an insignificant 8.7 percent differences between groups at 6 weeks favoring mindfulness meditation. At 18 weeks this effect disappeared. This trial had a medium risk of bias and provided 13.5 hours of training with an unspecified amount of home practice.

Delgado et al. randomized female university students (n=32) who were worriers to 5 weeks of mindfulness meditation or progressive muscular relaxation, providing 10 hours of training and unspecified amount of home practice.[51] The study found a nonsignificant 13.3 percent improvement in the BDI in the mindfulness meditation group as compared with progressive muscular relaxation. This trial had a medium risk of bias.

Wolever et al. randomized stressed employees (n=186) to a mindfulness-at-work program or viniyoga for 12 weeks. Participants received 14 hours of training by trained teachers and unspecified amount of homework. Depression was a secondary outcome. The trial found a nonsignificant 8.5 percent improvement in the mindfulness group compared with control. This trial had a medium risk of bias.

The difference-in-change graphs show significant inconsistency (Figure 28). Two meta-analyses of results at the end of treatment and end of study show small nonsignificant effects slightly favoring meditation (Figures 10 and 11).

The strength of evidence is insufficient that mindfulness meditation programs have an effect on depressive symptoms among various clinical populations compared with a variety of specific active controls. We based this rating on overall medium risk of bias, inconsistent results, direct measures, and imprecise estimates (Table 30).

Table 30. Grade of trials addressing the efficacy of mindfulness meditation programs on depressive symptoms compared with specific active controls among diverse populations

Number of Trials; Subjects	Domains Pertaining to Strength of Evidence				Magnitude of Effect and Strength of Evidence
	Risk of Bias	Consistency	Directness	Precision	
Depressive Symptoms					Insufficient SOE of an effect
11; 821	Medium	Inconsistent	Direct	Imprecise	−31.7% to +22.8%

Note: SOE = Strength of Evidence

Figure 28. Relative difference between groups in the changes in measures of depression, in the mindfulness versus specific active control studies

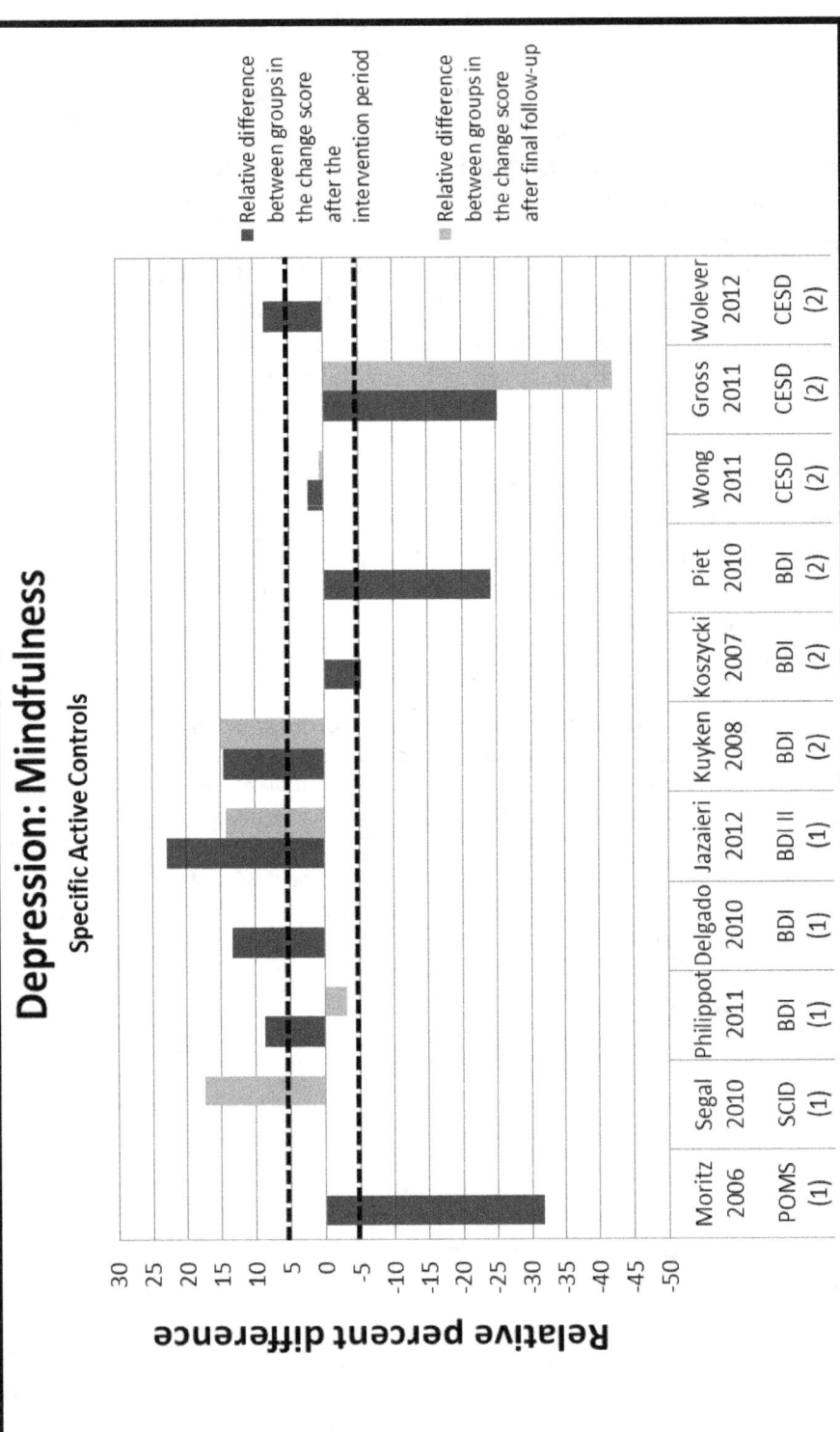

1. **Relative difference between groups in the change score.** This is a relative percent difference, using the baseline mean in the meditation group as the denominator. For example, if the meditation group improves from a 10 to 19 on a mental health scale and the control group improves from 11 to 16 on the same scale, the relative difference between groups in the change score is: $(((19-10)-(16-11))/10) \times 100 = 40\%$. The interpretation is that there is a 40% relative improvement on the mental health scale in the meditation group compared with the control group. See appendix E for absolute difference-in-change score values. Improvement in all scales is indicated in the positive direction. A positive relative percent difference means that the score improved more in the intervention group than in the control group
2. (1): Primary outcome. If the trial did not specify primary or secondary outcomes, this is either the outcome that the population was selected on or identified as a primary focus of the study. (2): Secondary outcome. If the trial did not specify primary or secondary outcomes, then this is not the outcome that the population was selected nor identified as a primary focus of the study.
3. NR / NS = Not Reported/Not significant. The trial measured this outcome and stated they were nonsignificant, and did not report actual results.
4. Black dotted lines from −5% to +5% indicate our criteria for no effect. It does not indicate statistical significance.
5. A p value above or below a bar indicates statistical significance reported in the original study publication. If there is no p value, the outcome was not significant in the original publication.
6. BDI = Beck Depression Inventory; CESD = Center for Epidemiologic Studies Depression Scale; POMS = Profile of Mood States; SCID = Structured Clinical Interview.

Other Mantra Meditation Versus <u>Specific</u> Active Control

Lehrer et al. assigned anxious participants to clinically standardized meditation or progressive muscular relaxation (n=42).[79] The program provided 7.5 hours of training and an unspecified amount of home practice over 5 weeks (Table 9). The trainers were undergraduate and graduate students with 4 months of training in the technique and no prior teaching experience. symptom checklist-90 depression scores favored the progressive muscular relaxation group over the clinically standardized meditation group. The difference-in-change scores were all nonsignificant, but ranged from 27.8 percent at 6 weeks to 7.8 percent at 6 months favoring the progressive muscular relaxation group (Figure 12).

The strength of evidence is insufficient that clinically standardized meditation has an effect on depressive symptoms in an anxious population compared with progressive muscular relaxation. We based this rating on a single study with medium risk of bias, unknown consistency, direct measures, and imprecise estimates (Table 31).

Table 31. Grade of trials addressing the efficacy of clinically standardized meditation programs on depression compared with progressive muscle relaxation among anxious participants

Number of Trials; Subjects	Domains Pertaining to Strength of Evidence				Magnitude of Effect and Strength of Evidence at End of Intervention
	Risk of Bias	Consistency	Directness	Precision	
Depressive Symptoms					Insufficient SOE of an effect
1; 42	Medium	Unknown	Direct	Imprecise	−27.8% favoring PMR

Notes: SOE = Strength of Evidence; PMR = Progressive Muscle Relaxation

Stress and Distress

Mindfulness Meditation Programs Versus <u>Specific</u> Active Control

Six mindfulness trials evaluated stress/distress as an outcome among populations with some form of emotional distress (Table 10). Delgado et al. randomized female university students (n=32) who had high scores on the Penn State worry questionnaire to 5 weeks of mindfulness meditation or progressive muscular relaxation, providing 10 hours of training and unspecified amount of home practice.[51] Scores on the positive and negative affect scale-negative mood were a primary focus of the trial, and were relatively unchanged at 5 weeks of intervention, and there was no difference between the two groups at the end of treatment. This trial had a medium risk of bias.

Moritz et al. randomized patients with mood disorders (n=110) to a spirituality program versus MBSR.[63] In this trial, MBSR was the active control. It provided about 12 hours of training in both interventions over an 8-week period. It provided up to 42 hours of home practice in the spirituality group and an unspecified amount of home practice in the MBSR group. There was no information on teacher qualifications for MBSR. This trial used two scales that assessed distress, which was a primary outcome for the trial. They found a 23.8 percent change favoring spirituality at 8 weeks (p=.034) on the POMS total mood disturbance score, and a 22.4 percent change favoring spirituality at 8 weeks (p=.0.34) on the SF-36 mental health subscale score. This trial had a low risk of bias. It is notable that this intervention included a meditative component, as well as breathing exercises that may resemble features of MBSR.

Piet et al. randomized young adults with social phobia (n=26) to MBCT or group cognitive behavioral therapy in a crossover design with participants receiving both treatments.[68] We evaluated comparisons after the first intervention period only, before any crossover. They provided 16 hours of training and up to 28 hours of home practice over an 8-week period. This trial found a 13.2 percent nonsignificant change favoring the cognitive behavior therapy group on the symptom checklist 90 global severity index. However, the cognitive behavior therapy group received nearly twice the amount of group training, 28 hours over 14 weeks, and this increased time and attention in the control arm may not allow equivalent comparisons between the groups. This trial had a medium risk of bias.

Jazaieri et al.[87] randomized patients with social anxiety disorder to MBSR or exercise (n=56). The trial provided about 25 hours of training by trained teachers, and their participants performed an average of 28.3 hours of homework over the 8-week training period. Although they did not specify primary or secondary outcomes, stress was identified as a primary focus of the study. The trial found a nonsignificant improvement of 17.6 percent in the perceived stress scale at 8 weeks in the MBSR group as compared with exercise. This trial had a high risk of bias.

Barrett et al.[85] randomized patients with a history of upper respiratory infections to MBSR or exercise (n=98). The trial provided about 20 hours of training by trained teachers, and approximately 42 hours of recommended homework over the 8-week training period. The perceived stress scale was a secondary outcome. The trial found no significant differences between the two arms. This trial was rated as medium risk of bias

Wolever et al. randomized stressed employees (n=186) to a mindfulness at work program or viniyoga for 12 weeks. Participants received 14 hours of training by trained teachers and unspecified amount of homework. Perceived stress was a primary outcome. The trial found no significant differences in the mindfulness group compared with control. This trial had a medium risk of bias.

The difference-in-change graphs showed inconsistent results (Figure 29). A meta-analysis suggested a nonsignificant null effect (Figure 14).

The strength of evidence is insufficient that mindfulness meditation programs affect improve distress among those with mood disturbance or symptoms of anxiety compared with a variety of specific active controls. We based this rating on overall medium risk of bias, inconsistent results, direct measures, and imprecise estimates (Table 32).

Table 32. Grade of trials addressing the efficacy of mindfulness meditation programs on distress compared with specific active controls among populations with emotional distress

Number of Trials; Subjects	Domains Pertaining to Strength of Evidence				Magnitude of Effect and Strength of Evidence
	Risk of Bias	Consistency	Directness	Precision	
Distress					Insufficient SOE of an effect on stress/distress
6; 508	Medium	Inconsistent	Direct	Imprecise	−23.8% to +17.6%

Note: SOE = Strength of Evidence

Figure 29. Relative difference between groups in the changes in measures of distress, in the mindfulness versus specific active control studies

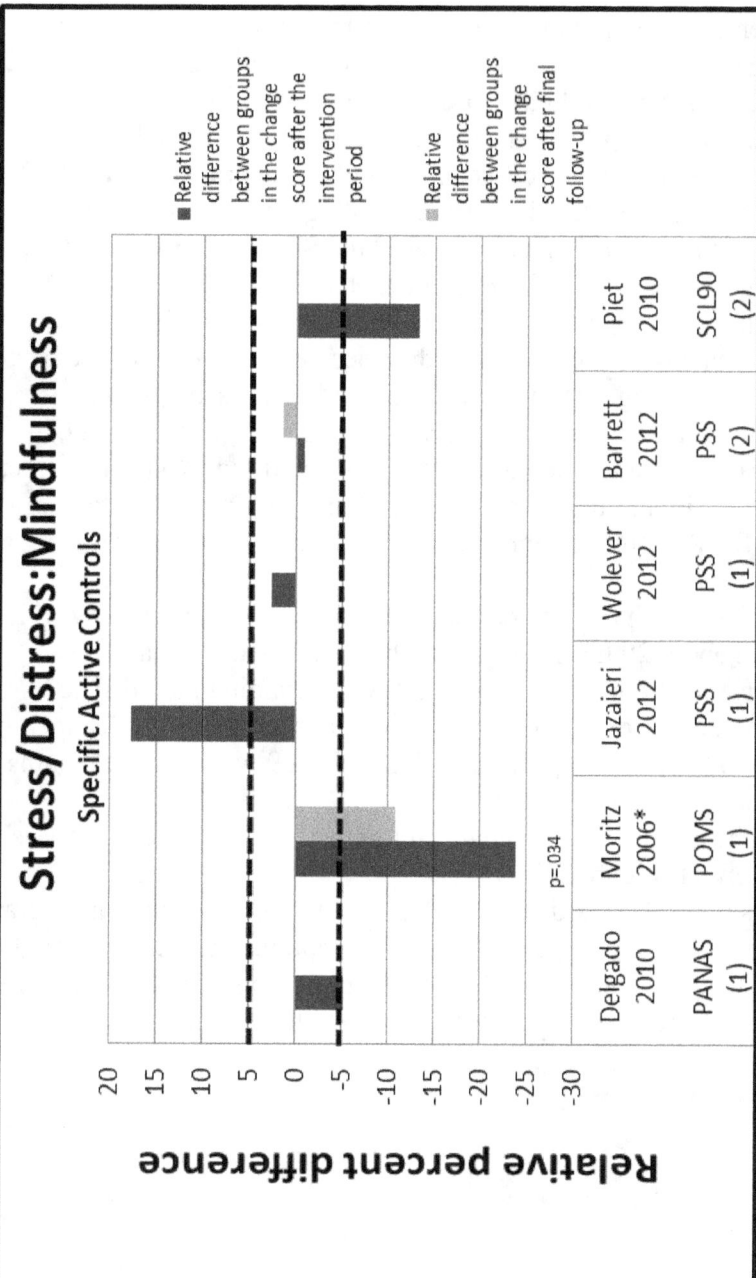

1. **Relative difference between groups in the change score.** This is a relative percent difference, using the baseline mean in the meditation group as the denominator. For example, if the meditation group improves from a 10 to 19 on a mental health scale and the control group improves from 11 to 16 on the same scale, the relative difference between groups in the change score is: $(((19-10)-(16-11))/10) \times 100 = 40\%$. The interpretation is that there is a 40% relative improvement on the mental health scale in the meditation group compared with the control group. See appendix E for absolute difference-in-change score values. Improvement in all scales is indicated in the positive direction. A positive relative percent difference means that the score improved more in the intervention group than in the control group
2. (1): Primary outcome. If the trial did not specify primary or secondary outcomes, this is either the outcome that the population was selected on or identified as a primary focus of the study. (2): Secondary outcome. If the trial did not specify primary or secondary outcomes, then this is not the outcome that the population was selected nor identified as a primary focus of the study.
3. NR / NS = Not Reported/Not significant. The trial measured this outcome and stated they were nonsignificant, and did not report actual results.
4. Black dotted lines from −5% to +5% indicate our criteria for no effect. It does not indicate statistical significance.
5. A p value above or below a bar indicates statistical significance reported in the original study publication. If there is no p value, the outcome was not significant in the original publication.
6. PANAS = Positive and Negative Affect Schedule; POMS = Profile of Mood States; PSS=Perceived Stress Scale; SCL90 = Symptom Checklist 90.

Positive Affect

Mindfulness Meditation Programs Versus <u>Specific</u> Active Control

Four trials evaluated the effect of mindfulness meditation programs compared with a specific active control on the outcome of positive affect (Table 12). Delgado et al. randomized female students (n=32) with high scores on the Pittsburgh sleep quality index (PSQI) to 5 weeks of either mindfulness training or progressive muscle relaxation training, providing 10 hours of training and unspecified amount of home practice.[51] The trial did not detect any within or between-group effects on the positive and negative affect schedule. This trial had a medium risk of bias.

Moritz et al. randomized patients with mood disorders (n=110) to a spirituality program versus MBSR.[63] In this trial, MBSR was the active control for the spirituality intervention they were testing. The trial selected participants with high scores on the POMS scale. The spirituality program had meditative components in it. It provided about 12 hours of training in both interventions over an 8-week period, with an unspecified amount of home practice in the MBSR group. It provided up to 42 hours of home practice in the spirituality group. There was no information on teacher qualifications for MBSR. The study used the SF-36 vitality score to measure improvement in positive affect as a secondary outcome. The SF-36 vitality scores were 45 percent greater for the spirituality group (p=.024). This trial had a low risk of bias.

Jazaieri et al.[87] randomized patients with social anxiety disorder to MBSR or exercise (n=56). The trial provided about 25 hours of training by trained teachers, and their participants performed an average of 28.3 hours of homework over the 8-week training period. Although they did not specify primary or secondary outcomes, positive affect was identified as a primary focus of the study. The trial found a nonsignificant improvement of 10.2 percent in the satisfaction with life scale at 8 weeks in the MBSR group as compared with exercise. This trial was rated as high risk of bias.

Barrett et al.[85] randomized patients with a history of upper respiratory infections to MBSR or exercise (n=98). The trial provided about 20 hours of training by trained teachers, and approximately 42 hours of recommended homework over the 8-week training period. The positive and negative affect scale was a secondary outcome. The trial found no significant differences between the two arms in the positive portion of this scale at 9 weeks and 5 months. This trial had a medium risk of bias.

The difference-in-change graphs showed inconsistent results (Figure 23). A meta-analysis showed a nonsignificant and null effect (Figure 24).

The strength of evidence is insufficient regarding the effect mindfulness meditation programs have on positive affect among those with a mood disturbance or symptoms of anxiety when compared with a variety of specific active controls. We based this rating on overall medium risk of bias, inconsistent findings, indirect measures, and imprecise estimates (Table 33).

Table 33. Grade of trials addressing the efficacy of mindfulness meditation programs on positive affect compared with progressive muscle relaxation or spirituality among various patients

Number of Trials; Subjects	Domains Pertaining to Strength of Evidence				Magnitude of Effect and Strength of Evidence
	Risk of Bias	Consistency	Directness	Precision	
Positive Affect					Insufficient SOE of an effect
4; 297	Medium	Inconsistent	Indirect	Imprecise	−45% to +10.2%

Notes: SOE = Strength or Evidence; MM = Mindfulness Meditation

Mental Component of Health-Related Quality of Life

Mindfulness Meditation Programs Versus Specific Active Control

Six trials evaluated the effect of mindfulness meditation programs compared with a specific active control on the outcome of the mental component of health-related QOL (Table 13). Five were MBSR trials and one was an MBCT trial. Three trials were low risk of bias, two medium, and one high. They used a variety of patient populations and specific active controls. Sample sizes ranged from 15–123.

Wong et al. randomized chronic pain patients (n=99) to an 8-week program in MBSR or multidisciplinary pain intervention.[74] The study used the validated Chinese SF-12 mental component subscale to measure QOL as a secondary outcome. There was no significant change in the scores between groups at 2 or 5 months. This trial had a low risk of bias, provided 27 hours of training and an unspecified amount of home practice over 8 weeks. Its teachers were trained and had 5 years of experience teaching meditation.[74]

Gross et al. randomized people with insomnia (n=27) to 8 weeks of MBSR versus pharmacotherapy for sleep (eszopiclone).[55] The trial used the SF-12 mental summary score to measure QOL as a secondary outcome. There was no significant change in SF-12 scores between the two groups. This trial provided 26 hours of training and up to 36 hours of home practice over 8 weeks. Its teachers were trained and certified.

Moritz et al. randomized patients with mood disorders (n=110) to a spirituality program versus MBSR.[63] In this trial, MBSR was the active control. It provided about 12 hours of training in both interventions over an 8-week period, with unspecified amount of home practice in the MBSR group. It provided up to 42 hours of home practice in the spirituality group. There was no information on teacher qualifications for MBSR. The trial used the SF-36 mental component survey to measure QOL as a secondary outcome. They found a 23 percent change favoring spirituality at 8 weeks (p=.029). This trial had a low risk of bias. It is notable that this intervention included a meditative component, as well as breathing exercises that may resemble features of MBSR.

Plews-Ogan et al. randomized people with chronic musculoskeletal pain (n=15) to 8 weeks of MBSR training or weekly massage.[69] The trial used the SF-12 mental health score to measure QOL as a primary endpoint. The difference-in-change point estimates were 10.8 percent favoring massage at 8 weeks and 18.4 percent favoring MBSR at 12 weeks. The trial did not calculate significance for difference-in-change estimates. This trial provided 20 hours of training over 8 weeks, and unspecified amount of home practice. There was no information on teacher qualifications. It had a high risk of bias.

Kuyken at al. randomized depressed patients at risk for relapse (n=123) to 8 weeks of MBCT and antidepressant tapering or maintenance antidepressant therapy.[59] The trials used the World

Health Organization quality of life instrument psychological subscale to measure QOL as a secondary outcome. At 3 months it found a 9.2 percent improvement in the MBCT group, which maintained at 15 months (p=.01). This trial provided 24 hours of training over 8 weeks by trained and certified instructors, and recommended up to 37.5 hours of home practice during that time. This trial had a low risk of bias.

Barrett et al.[85] randomized patients with a history of upper respiratory infections to MBSR or exercise (n=98). The trial provided about 20 hours of training by trained teachers, and approximately 42 hours of recommended homework over the 8-week training period. QOL was a secondary outcome. The trial found no significant differences between the two arms in the SF-12 mental component at 9 weeks and 5 months. This trial was rated as medium risk of bias.

The difference-in-change graphs showed inconsistent results (Figure 26). Meta-analysis showed a null and nonsignificant effect (Figure 30).

The strength of evidence is insufficient that mindfulness meditation program have an effect on the mental component of health-related quality of life among various clinical populations when compared with a variety of specific active controls. We based this rating on overall medium risk of bias, inconsistent findings, direct measures, and imprecise estimates (Table 34).

Table 34. Grade of trials addressing the efficacy of mindfulness meditation programs on the mental component of health-related quality of life compared with specific active controls among various populations

Number of Trials; Subjects	Domains Pertaining to Strength of Evidence				Magnitude of Effect and Strength of Evidence
	Risk of Bias	Consistency	Directness	Precision	
Mental Component of Health-Related Quality of Life					Insufficient SOE of an effect
6; 472	Medium	Inconsistent	Direct	Imprecise	−23% to +9.2%

Notes: SOE = Strength of Evidence; QOL = Quality of Life

Figure 30. Meta-analysis of the effects of meditation programs on the mental health component of health-related quality of life with up to 3 months of followup

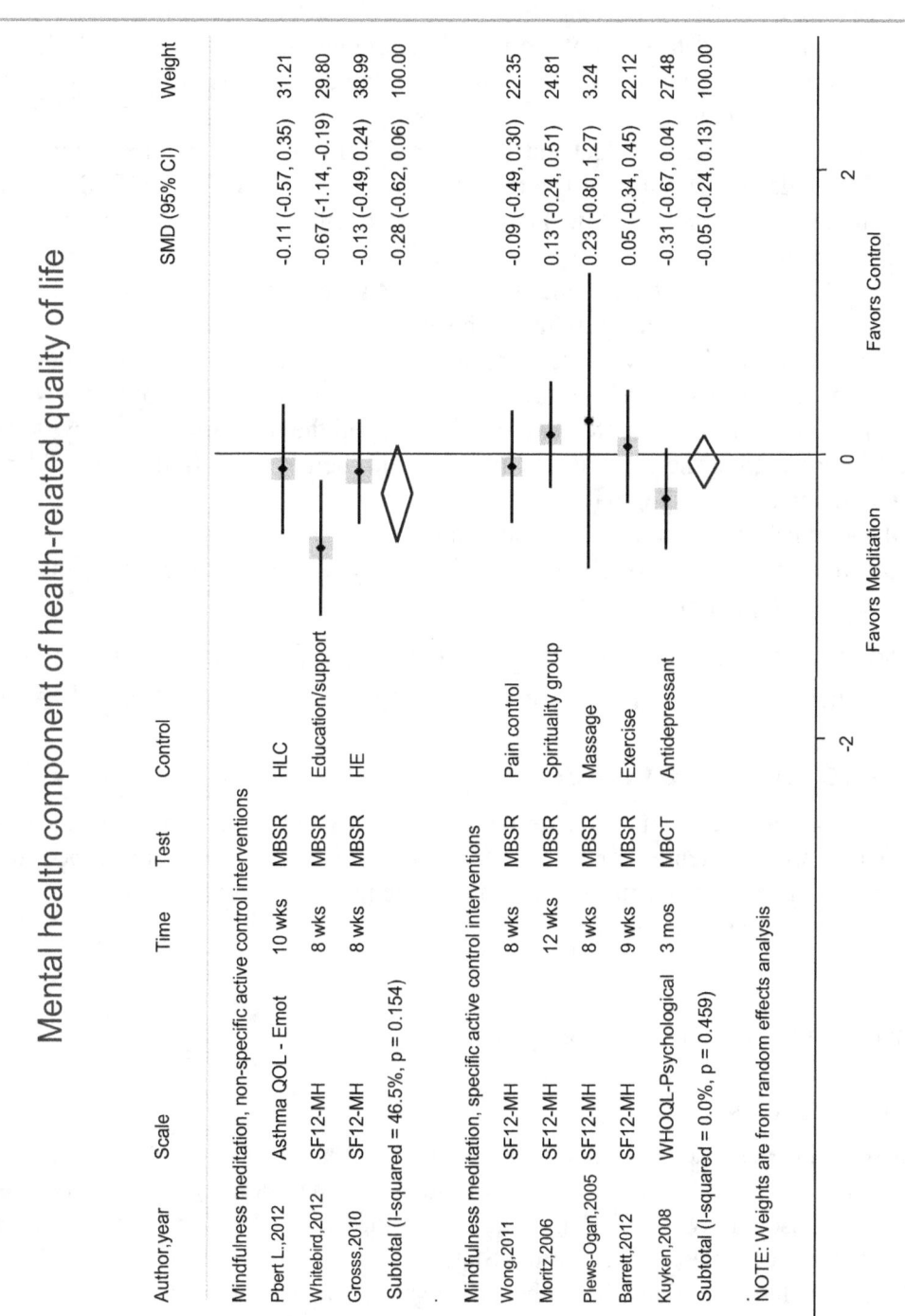

Notes: HE = Health Education; HLC = Healthy Living Course; MBSR = Mindfulness Based Stress Reduction; MBCT = Mindfulness-based Cognitive Therapy; SF-12: MH = Short Form-12: Mental Component Score of Health-related Quality of Life; Mental Component Score of Health-related Quality of Life; mos = months; WHOQL = World Health Organization Quality of Life Assessment; wks = weeks.

Applicability

Most of the trials that we included for this KQ took place in outpatient settings in the United States or Europe; two trials took place in Asia, and one in the Middle East. Almost all the trials listed some exclusion criteria which would apply to a large number of patients in an everyday internal medicine or primary care practice, including substance abuse, psychiatric disorder, or various medical disorders.

Regarding the population characteristics of the trials for this KQ, most of the trials did not specify the racial or ethnic characteristics of the included population. While about half the trials specified the educational characteristics of the study populations, the trials did not report other measures of socioeconomic status.

Although some of the trials for this KQ addressed a number of chronic medical conditions, including metabolic syndrome, chronic obstructive pulmonary disease, HIV, and CHF, the trials did not address a number of common medical conditions frequently found in medical practice, and often associated with anxiety, depression, stress, and distress, including diabetes, IBS, and opiate dependence. While half of the trials included patients with some form of mental health issue, a large number of them excluded patients with serious mental health conditions.

Thus, the findings for this KQ may be least applicable to patients with substance abuse, dementia, or other medical or psychiatric conditions excluded from the study populations. Given that the trials only substantially represented two continents, and the trials did not always specify the racial and ethnic makeup of the populations, it's unclear whether these findings would be applicable to more diverse patient populations.

Regarding the applicability of an intervention to a medical practice, both TM and mindfulness trials involved training for about 10–40 hours over several weeks, which makes them fairly practical in a typical outpatient setting.

Key Question 2. What are the efficacy and harms of meditation programs on attention among those with a clinical condition (medical or psychiatric)?

Key Points and Evidence Grades

- The strength of evidence is insufficient that mindfulness meditation programs have an effect on measures of attention among older caregivers compared with a nonspecific active control due to medium risk of bias in a single trial, unknown consistency, directness of measures, and imprecise estimates.

Harms

- We found no studies that reported on harms

Trial Characteristics

One RCT assessed the efficacy of a meditation program on attention as a component of their study. Oken et al. assessed the effects of a 7-week mindfulness meditation program on stress among caregivers of close relatives with dementia.[66] The study did not report the specific period of recruitment. The trial took place in the United States in an outpatient setting among a stressed population. The trial included participants with a score greater than 9 on the perceived stress scale and excluded individuals who were medically unstable, had significant cognitive dysfunction, significant visual impairment, or previous experience with stress-reduction classes[66] (Appendix E, Evidence Table E2).

Population Characteristics

The trial enrolled 31 dementia caregivers with a mean age range in the 60s.[66] Participants were predominantly female and greater than 90 percent were white (Appendix E).

Intervention Characteristics

The trial included three arms: a composite intervention based on MBSR/MBCT, which was compared with education (nonspecific active control), and to respite care.[66] The trial delivered all meditation interventions in a group format. The maximal training dose for was 9 hours delivered over 7 weeks. The trial used trained teachers but did not specify the amount of training or meditation experience. The trial recommended practice at home but did not specify the total duration and did not record actual amounts of training or home practice by the participants[66] (Appendix E).

Outcomes

The trial used the attentional network test as the measure of attention. The attentional network test is a computerized task for assessing various attention networks. This test requires participants indicate the direction of a target arrow that is accompanied on each side by two additional arrows. Occasionally, the target arrow is preceded by cues. The trial used a shortened version of this test that included only two attention conditions: cued/noncued and congruent/incongruent conditions, which present companion arrows in the same or opposite direction as the target arrow. The results included a conflict score, calculated as the reaction time difference between the incongruent and congruent conditions; and the alerting score, calculated as the reaction time difference between the noncued and cued conditions.

Attention

Mindfulness Meditation Programs Versus <u>Nonspecific</u> Active Control

The attentional network test alerting score for the meditation group was worse than for the education group at baseline. At 8 weeks post-intervention the meditation group improved its performance by doubling its score, resulting in an 81 percent increase from baseline compared with education.[66] This suggests an appropriate use of a cue by the meditation group to improve their performance from baseline to post-intervention. However, the data were highly skewed, and it is not apparent that the differences between meditation and education arms were statistically significant. There was a 15 percent nonsignificant difference among the groups on the attentional network test conflict score favoring mindfulness meditation (p=0.14).[66]

In summary, this trial had a medium risk of bias due to several factors including high attrition, allocation to groups was not concealed, and there was no intention-to-treat analysis. Overall, the strength of evidence is insufficient to comment on whether mindfulness meditation interventions improve attention among an older population compared with a nonspecific active control due to medium risk of bias, unknown consistency, directness of measures, and imprecision (Table 35).

The trial did not report on harms.

Table 35. Grade of trial addressing the efficacy of a meditation program on a measure of attention compared with a nonspecific active control among older caregivers

Condition; Number of Trials; Subjects	Domains Pertaining to Strength of Evidence				Magnitude of Effect and Strength of Evidence
	Risk of Bias	Consistency	Directness	Precision	
MM: Stressed Caregivers					Insufficient SOE of an effect on the Attention Network Score
1; 21	Medium	Unknown	Direct	Imprecise	15% to 81% favoring MM

Notes: SOE = Strength of Evidence; MM = Mindfulness Meditation

Applicability

The trial took place in the United States in an outpatient setting with predominantly female and predominantly white participants. The trial studied an older population of dementia caregivers without direct complaints of cognitive difficulties (i.e., attention). Therefore, these findings may not be applicable to other clinical populations where cognitive function is a reported concern (e.g., attention-deficit/hyperactivity disorder), and improvement (or lack thereof) on cognitive measures could provide more useful clinical information.

Key Question 3. What are the efficacy and harms of meditation programs on health-related behaviors affected by stress, specifically substance use, sleep, and eating, among those with a clinical condition (medical or psychiatric)?

Key Points and Evidence Grades

Comparisons With <u>Nonspecific</u> Active Controls

- The strength of evidence is insufficient about the effects of mindfulness meditation programs on sleep quality among a variety of populations when compared with a nonspecific active control. We based this rating on overall medium risk of bias, inconsistent findings, direct measures, and imprecise estimates.

Comparisons With <u>Specific</u> Active Controls

- The strength of evidence is insufficient that mindfulness programs have an effect on sleep when compared with exercise or eszopiclone. We based this rating on overall medium risk of bias, inconsistent results, directness of measures, and imprecise estimates.
- The strength of evidence is insufficient that mindfulness programs have an effect on eating compared with specific active controls. We based this rating on overall high risk of bias, consistent results, directness of measures, and imprecise estimates.
- The strength of evidence is insufficient that mindfulness meditation programs have an effect on substance use among smoking and alcoholic populations when compared with certain specific active controls. We based this rating on overall high risk of bias, inconsistent findings, direct measures, and imprecise estimates.
- The strength of evidence is low that mantra meditation programs do not reduce alcohol use among alcohol abusing populations when compared with intensive running or biofeedback. We based this rating on overall medium risk of bias, consistent findings, direct measures, and imprecise estimates.

Harms
- Four trials reported that they evaluated harms; none found any adverse events.

Trial Characteristics
Of the 13 trials that we included for this KQ,[49,50,54-56,61,62,66,70,73,80,84,85] 12 took place in the United States, while the other took place in Germany. Seven of these trials took place exclusively in an outpatient setting, two took place in an inpatient setting, and the remaining two trials had multiple locations. Only two of these trials explicitly reported the year of recruitment, and none of the trials reported the time period of recruitment.

All but two of these trials explicitly stated the length of treatment and timing of subsequent followup. Treatment ranged from 4–15 weeks, and followup ranged from none (i.e. treatment assessed at its end) to 18 months.

All 13 trials reported inclusion and exclusion criteria. One trial excluded individuals with chronic substance dependence. Five trials excluded subjects if they had unstable medical conditions. Eight other trials excluded patients due to psychiatric criteria. Three trials excluded due to severe cognitive dysfunction. Most trials excluded people with prior or recent experience in meditation.

Four of the 13 trials that we included in this review evaluated the effects of meditation on substance use: one related to cigarette smoking,[50] and three related to alcohol and drug use.[49,80,84] Two trials considered the effect of meditation on eating behaviors.[56,62] The remaining seven of the 13 included trials examined the effect of meditation programs on sleep[54,55,61,66,70,73,85] (Appendix E).

Population Characteristics
Seven trials took place in populations with chronic medical conditions;[54-56,61,62,70,85] four trials took place in populations with substance abuse;[49,50,80,84] and two trials targeted a population of caregivers under stress.[66,73] The percentage of female subjects totaled 30 percent or greater in 10 of the 13 trials,[50,54-56,61,62,66,70,73,85] with two of the 13 trials including female subjects exclusively.[56,70] The mean age of trial participants ranged from 24–67 years. Two of the 13 trials exhibited significant racial diversity in the subject populations.[50,84] Ten of the 13 trials provided information on the level of education completed by trial participants (Appendix E).

Intervention Characteristics
Of the four trials assessing the effects of meditation on substance use, two used mindfulness meditation based on mindfulness-based relapse prevention, with 9–12 hours of training over 4–9 weeks. Training and experience ranged from 12 years to greater than 13 years in mindfulness experience and social work, although there was no explicit mention of centralized training or certification. Another trial used clinically standardized meditation, a mantra-based concentrative meditation intervention taught by "experienced meditators," after which the group meditated together 3 times per week for the 8-week intervention.[80] One trial used a TM intervention taught by a certified instructor. Instruction used a seven-step process, followed by group meditations.[84] For the substance-use trials, comparisons included cognitive behavioral therapy treatment,[49] biofeedback,[84] smoking-cessation education,[50,76] and exercise.[80]

Two trials assessed eating in response to a mindfulness intervention. Hebert et al.,[56] assessing eating in breast cancer patients, compared a nutrition education program with a mindfulness-based program adapted from MBSR, while Miller et al.[62] assessed a mindfulness based eating program among diabetics.

All seven trials evaluating meditation for sleep evaluated either MBSR or an abbreviated derivative of MBSR.[54,55,61,66,70,73,85] Comparison treatments included pharmacotherapy for sleep[55], exercise[73,85] programs in relaxation,[70] or health education matched for time and attention.[54,66]

Only three of the 13 trials investigating stress-related behaviors measured adherence to home meditation practice[50,54,55] (Appendix E).

Outcomes

Mindfulness Meditation Programs Versus <u>Nonspecific</u> Active Control

Sleep

Four trials compared a mindfulness meditation program with a nonspecific active control on the outcome of sleep quality (Table 14). All four used the PSQI. Three had a medium risk of bias and one had a low risk of bias. Gross et al. randomized solid organ transplant recipients, post-surgery, (n=137) to either 8 weeks of MBSR or nonspecific active control.[54] The trial used the PSQI to measure sleep quality as a primary outcome. In a difference-in-change analysis, the MBSR group showed a 24.1 percent improvement in PSQI at 8 weeks, which further improved to 30.1 percent at 1 year (p=.02). This trial had a medium risk of bias. It provided 27 hours of training by a trained teacher and an unspecified amount of home practice over 8 weeks.

Schmidt et al. randomized women with fibromyalgia (n=109) to 8 weeks of MBSR or a nonspecific active control.[70] The study used the PSQI to measure sleep as a secondary endpoint and showed no difference between the arms. This trial provided 27 hours of training over 8 weeks by trained and certified teachers, and recommended up to 42 hours of home practice. It had a medium risk of bias.

Oken et al. randomized people who take care of elderly relatives with dementia (n=19) to 6 weeks of mindfulness meditation or a nonspecific active control.[66] The trial used the PSQI and Epworth sleepiness scale to measure sleep as a secondary outcome. This trial showed a 12.8 percent change on the Epworth sleepiness scale and a 3.4 percent change on the PSQI, both were nonsignificant and favored the control group. This trial had a medium risk of bias. It provided 9 hours of training over 7 weeks by a trained teacher and an unspecified amount of home practice.

Malarkey et al. randomized people who either had or were at risk for cardiovascular disease due to elevated C-Reactive protein levels (n=186) to mindfulness meditation or nonspecific active control.[61] It provided 9 hours of abbreviated MBSR training at work with approximately 18.5 hours of homework over 8 weeks. It measured sleep as a secondary outcome. At 8 weeks, the trial found no differences between the groups, but did not provide data for comparisons of the size of effect. This trial had a low risk of bias.

The difference-in-change graphs showed inconsistent results (Figure 31). A meta-analysis showed a small nonsignificant effect around the null (Figure 32). The strength of evidence is insufficient that mindfulness meditation programs have an effect on sleep quality among a variety of populations when compared with a nonspecific active control. We based this rating on trials of medium bias, inconsistent findings, direct measures, and imprecise estimates (Table 36).

Table 36. Grade of trials addressing the efficacy of mindfulness meditation program on sleep quality among various populations compared with a nonspecific active control

Number of Trials; Subjects	Domains Pertaining to Strength of Evidence				Magnitude of Effect and Strength of Evidence
	Risk of Bias	Consistency	Directness	Precision	
Sleep Quality					Insufficient SOE of an effect
4; 451	Medium	Inconsistent	Direct	Imprecise	−3.4% to 24.1%

Note: SOE = Strength of Evidence

Figure 31. Relative difference between groups in the changes in measures of sleep, in the mindfulness versus nonspecific/specific active control studies

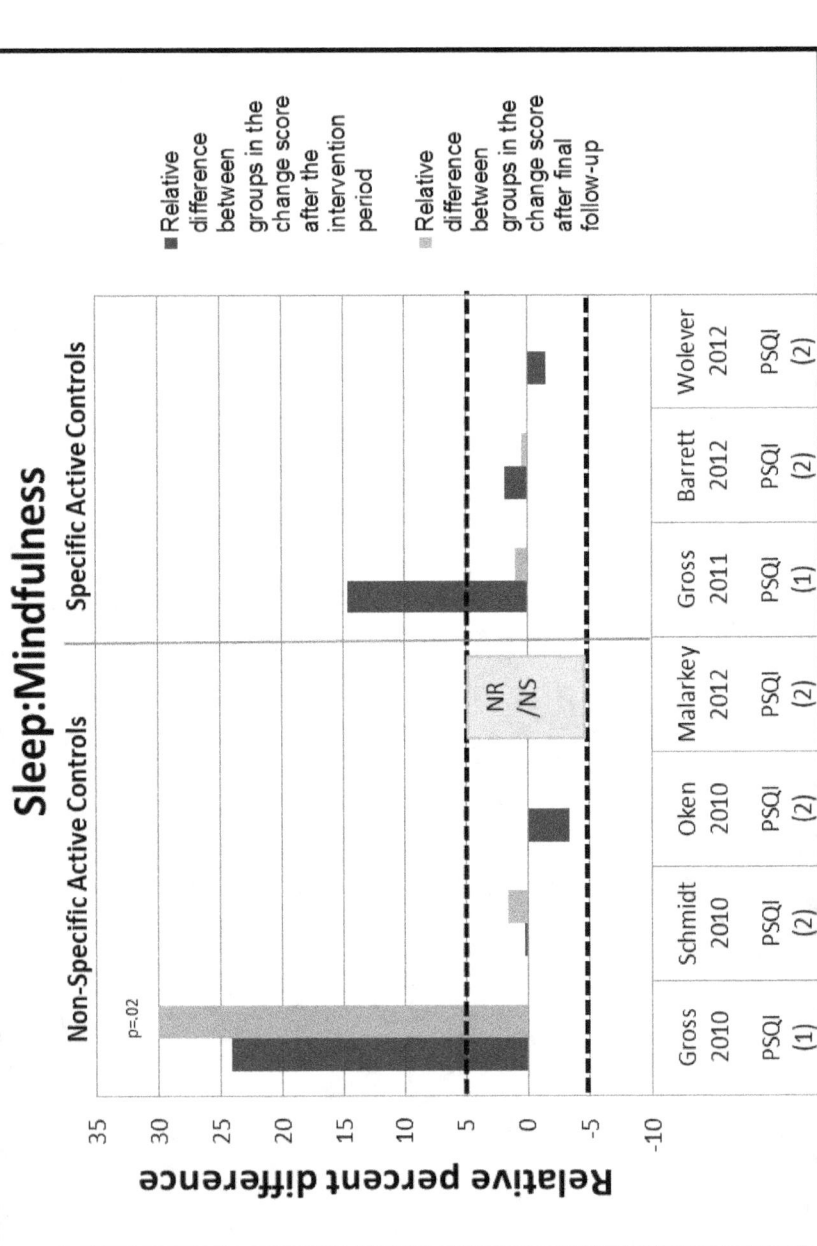

1. **Relative difference between groups in the change score.** This is a relative percent difference, using the baseline mean in the meditation group as the denominator. For example, if the meditation group improves from a 10 to 19 on a mental health scale and the control group improves from 11 to 16 on the same scale, the relative difference between groups in the change score is: (((19-10)-(16-11))/10)x100=40%. The interpretation is that there is a 40% relative improvement on the mental health scale in the meditation group compared with the control group. See appendix E for absolute difference-in-change score values. Improvement in all scales is indicated in the positive direction. A positive relative percent difference means that the score improved more in the intervention group than in the control group
2. (1): Primary outcome. If the trial did not specify primary or secondary outcomes, this is either the outcome that the population was selected on or identified as a primary focus of the study. (2): Secondary outcome. If the trial did not specify primary or secondary outcomes, then this is not the outcome that the population was selected nor identified as a primary focus of the study.
3. NR / NS = Not Reported/Not significant. The trial measured this outcome and stated they were nonsignificant, and did not report actual results.
4. Black dotted lines from −5% to +5% indicate our criteria for no effect. It does not indicate statistical significance.
5. A p value above or below a bar indicates statistical significance reported in the original study publication. If there is no p value, the outcome was not significant in the original publication.
6. PSQI = Pittsburgh Sleep Quality Index.

Figure 32. Meta-analysis of the effects of meditation programs on sleep with up to 3 months of followup

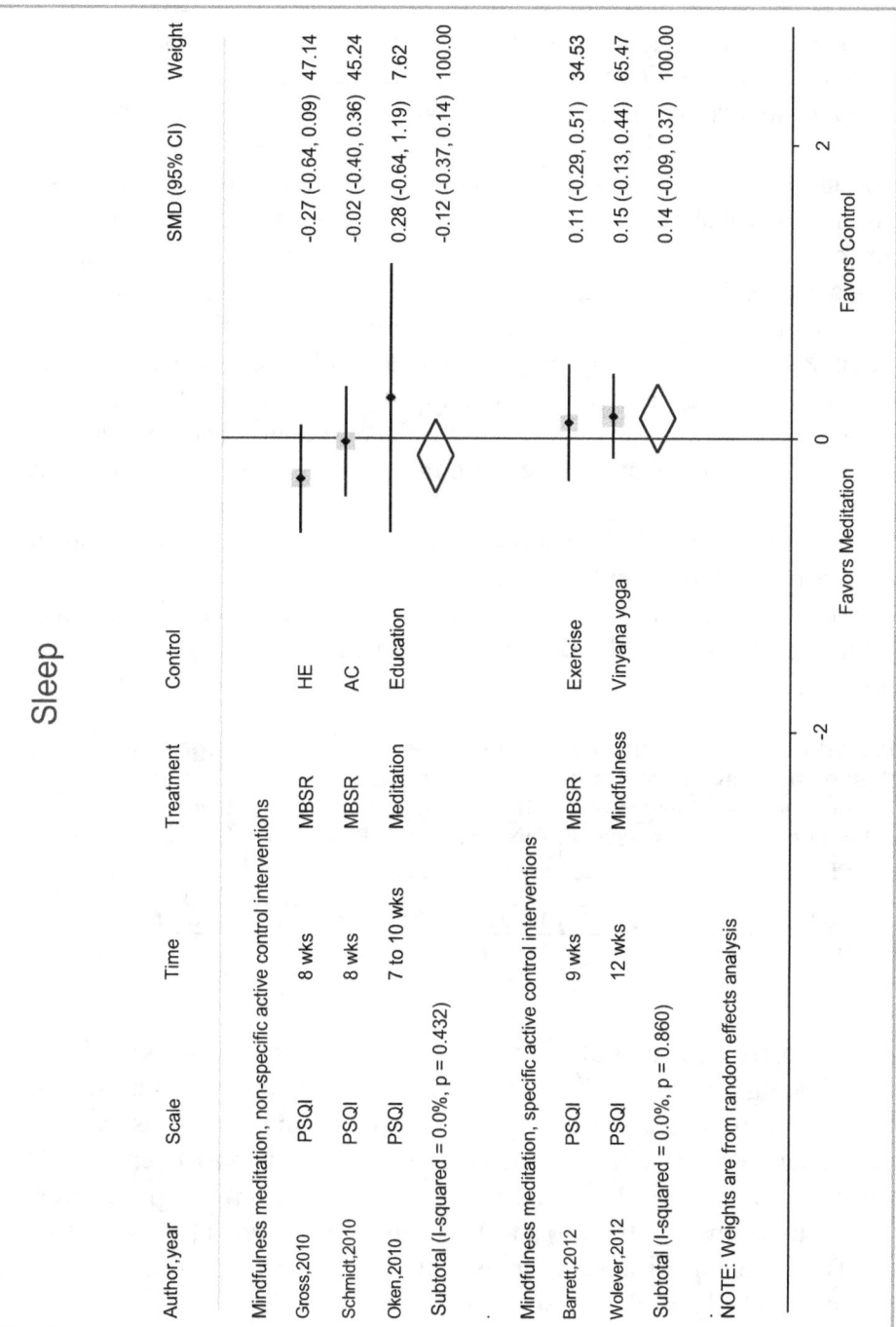

Notes: AC = Active Control; HE = Health Education; MBSR = Mindfulness Based Stress Reduction; PSQI = Pittsburgh Sleep Quality Index

Mindfulness Meditation Programs Versus <u>Specific</u> Active Control

Sleep

Three trials evaluated the effects of mindfulness meditation programs against a specific active control on the outcome of sleep (Table 14).[55,73,85] Gross et al. randomized people with insomnia (n=27) to MBSR or eszopiclone.[55] Sleep was a primary outcome. The study measured sleep time by wrist actigraphy. It measured overall sleep quality by the PSQI and insomnia severity index. Total sleep time and wake after sleep onset were not different between the groups, although it favored the eszopiclone group. The PSQI indicated a 14.7 percent improvement favoring the MBSR group, while the insomnia severity index showed a 15.5 percent improvement favoring the eszopiclone group. Both were nonsignificant. This trial provided 26 hours of training and up to 36 hours of home practice over 8 weeks. It had a medium risk of bias.

Barrett et al.[85] randomized patients with a history of upper respiratory infections to MBSR or exercise (n=98). The trial provided about 20 hours of training by trained teachers, and approximately 42 hours of recommended homework over the 8-week training period. Sleep quality was a secondary outcome. The trial found no significant differences between the two arms in the PSQI at 9 weeks and 5 months. This trial had a medium risk of bias.

Wolever et al. randomized stressed employees (n=186) to a mindfulness-at-work program or viniyoga for 12 weeks. Participants received 14 hours of training by trained teachers and unspecified amount of homework. Sleep quality was a secondary outcome. The trial found no significant differences in the PSQI in the mindfulness group compared with control. This trial had a medium risk of bias.

The difference-in-change graphs showed inconsistent results (Figure 31). A meta-analysis showed a nonsignificant result around the null (Figure 32). The strength of evidence is insufficient that mindfulness programs have an effect on sleep when compared with exercise or eszopiclone. We based this rating on overall medium risk of bias, inconsistent results, directness of measures, and imprecise estimates (Table 37).

Table 37. Grade of trials addressing the efficacy of mindfulness meditation programs on sleep quality compared with specific active controls in various populations

Number of Trials; Subjects	Domains Pertaining to Strength of Evidence				Magnitude of Effect and Strength of Evidence
	Risk of Bias	Consistency	Directness	Precision	
Sleep quality					Insufficient SOE of an effect
3; 311	Medium	Inconsistent	Direct	Imprecise	−1.5% to +14.7%

Note: SOE = Strength of Evidence.

Eating

Two trials evaluated the effects of mindfulness meditation programs against a specific active control on the outcome of eating (Table 14).[56,62] Hebert et al. evaluated the effects of MBSR compared with a nutrition education program among women with stage I or II breast cancer (n=106).[56] Ninety-five percent of the participants had complete diary data post-intervention (at 4 months) and 93 percent at 1 year. Women in the nutrition group had a significant 19.1 percent reduction in fat consumption at 4 months (p<.05) and 11.3 percent reduction at 1 year (p<.05) compared with MBSR. There were no differences in overall caloric consumption between groups at 4 months or 1 year. This trial had a medium risk of bias

Miller et al.[62] randomized diabetics to a mindfulness eating program versus the Smart Choices diabetes group self-management education program (n=52). This mindfulness program provided about 25 hours of training over 12 weeks and unspecified amount of homework. Total caloric consumption was a secondary outcome. The trial found a nonsignificant reduction of 14.9 and 10.4 percent at 3 and 6 months, respectively, compared with control. This trial had a high risk of bias.

The difference-in-change graphs show no improvement in the meditation arm in either trial compared with control (Figure 34). The strength of evidence is insufficient that mindfulness programs have an effect on eating compared with specific active controls. We based this rating on overall high risk of bias, consistent results, directness of measures, and imprecise estimates (Table 38).

Table 38. Grade of trials addressing the efficacy of mindfulness meditation programs on eating compared with specific active controls in diabetics and breast cancer populations

Number of Trials; Subjects	Domains Pertaining to Strength of Evidence				Magnitude of Effect and Strength of Evidence
	Risk of Bias	Consistency	Directness	Precision	
Eating					Insufficient SOE of an effect
2; 158	High	Consistent	Direct	Imprecise	−5.5% to −14.9%

Note: SOE = Strength of Evidence.

Substance Use

Two trials evaluated the effects of mindfulness meditation programs against a specific active control on the outcome of substance abuse (Table 14).[49,50]

Brewer et al. randomized smokers (N=71) to an 8-session, 4-week program of mindfulness meditation compared with a specific active control, the American Lung Association's freedom from smoking program.[50] The mindfulness meditation program is based on mindfulness-based relapse prevention and MBSR, and provided up to of 12 hours of meditation training by a single therapist with 13 years of experience with mindfulness meditation. While the freedom from smoking group reduced their cigarette use by 12 cigarettes/day, mindfulness meditation participants smoked 4.2 cigarettes/day less than the freedom from smoking program in a difference-in-change calculation (p=.008) at the end of the 4-week program. Mindfulness meditation participants had an absolute 21 percent higher levels of 1-week point-prevalence abstinence from smoking at 4 weeks (p=.06) and absolute 25 percent higher abstinence at 17-week followup (p=0.012). Additionally, within the mindfulness meditation group, both formal (p=0.019) and informal (p=0.01) mindfulness practice resulted in less cigarette use. This trial had a high risk of bias.[50] Overall, the strength of evidence is low to conclude that a 4-week mindfulness meditation program has an effect on smoking compared with a freedom from smoking program among smokers, due to high risk of bias, unknown consistency, directness of measures, and precise results.

Brewer et al. conducted a separate trial in which they randomized individuals with alcohol and/or cocaine abuse that were seeking outpatient treatment (n=24) to mindfulness meditation that consisted of mindfulness-based relapse prevention with cognitive behavioral therapy.[49] Following the treatment programs, there were no statistically significant differences in alcohol (p=.17) or cocaine (p=.09) use between groups. This trial provided 9 hours of training over 9 weeks by a teacher with 12 years of meditation experience, and did not report on whether it recommended any home practice. It had a 61 percent attrition rate and a high risk of bias.

The differences-in-change graphs showed inconsistent results (Figure 33). The strength of evidence is insufficient that mindfulness meditation programs have an effect on substance use among smoking and alcoholic populations when compared with certain specific active controls. We based this rating on overall high risk of bias, inconsistent findings, direct measures, and imprecise estimates (Table 39).

Table 39. Grade of trials addressing the efficacy of mindfulness meditation programs on substance use compared with specific active controls in smoking and alcoholic populations

Number of Trials; Subjects	Domains Pertaining to Strength of Evidence				Magnitude of Effect and Strength of Evidence
	Risk of Bias	Consistency	Directness	Precision	
substance use					Insufficient SOE of an effect
2; 95	High	Inconsistent	Direct	Imprecise	Null to +21% absolute improvement

Note: SOE = Strength of Evidence.

Figure 33. Relative difference between groups in the changes in measures of substance use/eating, in the mindfulness versus specific active control studies

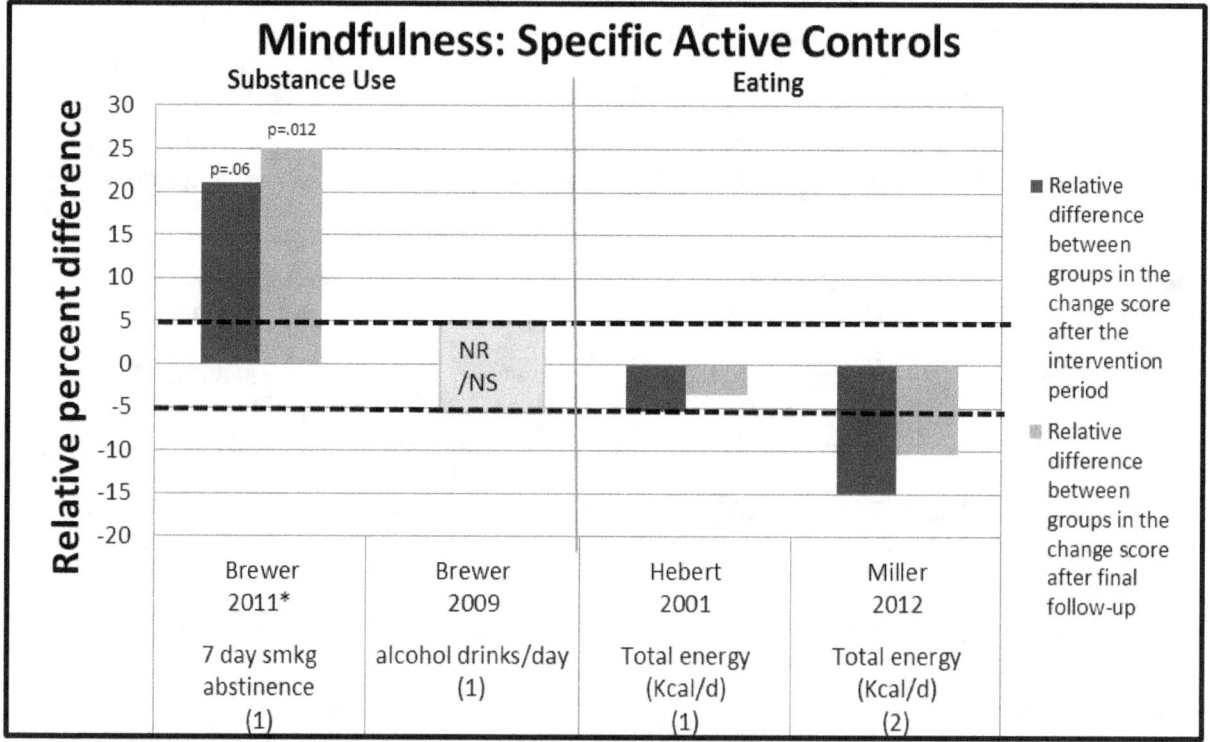

1. **Relative difference between groups in the change score.** This is a relative percent difference, using the baseline mean in the meditation group as the denominator. For example, if the meditation group improves from a 10 to 19 on a mental health scale and the control group improves from 11 to 16 on the same scale, the relative difference between groups in the change score is: (((19-10)-(16-11))/10)x100=40%. The interpretation is that there is a 40% relative improvement on the mental health scale in the meditation group compared with the control group. See appendix E for absolute difference-in-change score values. Improvement in all scales is indicated in the positive direction. A positive relative percent difference means that the score improved more in the intervention group than in the control group
2. (1): Primary outcome. If the trial did not specify primary or secondary outcomes, this is either the outcome that the population was selected on or identified as a primary focus of the study. (2): Secondary outcome. If the trial did not specify primary or secondary outcomes, then this is not the outcome that the population was selected nor identified as a primary focus of the study.
3. NR / NS = Not Reported/Not significant. The trial measured this outcome and stated they were nonsignificant, and did not report actual results.
4. Black dotted lines from −5% to +5% indicate our criteria for no effect. It does not indicate statistical significance.
5. A p value above or below a bar indicates statistical significance reported in the original study publication. If there is no p value, the outcome was not significant in the original publication.
6. Kcal/d = Kilocalorie per day.

Mantra Meditation Programs Versus <u>Specific</u> Active Control

Substance Use

Two trials used a mantra meditation programs to assess the effects on alcohol consumption against either an intensive running program among college students or biofeedback among recovering alcoholics (Table 14).[80,84] Murphy et al. randomized male college students who were heavy social drinkers (n=27) to an 8-week treatment programs in clinically standardized meditation or running.[80] The running group consumed 99.3 mL of ethanol less than the meditation group (p=.35). The meditation group received 8 hours of training over 8 weeks by a teacher with some experience in meditation, and up to 37.5 hour of home practice. The running group received 28 hours of training. This trial had a high risk of bias.

Taub et al. randomized alcoholics (n=87) in residential treatment program to TM or two different specific active control arms: biofeedback or neurotherapy. There was no difference in the percent of days abstinent from alcohol between the TM group and biofeedback. The TM group provided up to 19 hours of training over 4 weeks by certified teachers, and did not specify whether it recommended any amount of home practice. This trial had medium risk of bias.[84]

The difference-in-change graphs showed consistent results favoring control (Figure 34). The strength of evidence is low that mantra meditation programs do not reduce alcohol use among alcohol abusing populations when compared with intensive running or biofeedback. We based this rating on overall medium risk of bias, consistent findings, direct measures, and imprecise estimates (Table 40).

Table 40. Grade of trials addressing the efficacy and harms of mantra meditation programs on alcohol use among heavy alcohol drinkers compared with intensive running program or biofeedback

Number of Trials; Subjects	Domains Pertaining to Strength of Evidence				Magnitude of Effect and Strength of Evidence
	Risk of Bias	Consistency	Directness	Precision	
Alcohol use					Low SOE that alcohol use is not reduced
2; 145	Medium	consistent	Direct	Imprecise	−4.6% abstinence to −36.1% reduced consumption (both favoring control)

Notes: SOE = Strength of Evidence; CSM = Clinically Standardized Meditation; TM = Transcendental Meditation

Applicability

Twelve of 13 trials took place in the United States, so other regions might not find these findings applicable. Most of the trials took place in outpatient settings, so applicability to the inpatient setting is limited.

Regarding the population characteristics of the trials for this KQ, only two of 13 trials exhibited significant racial diversity in the study populations. Most of the trials excluded subjects from groups who might commonly be found in a medical practice, such as those with unstable medical conditions and psychiatric disorders.

Characteristics of the interventions represented in this KQ were diverse, making it difficult to foresee how these findings would be applicable to a similarly wide array of mindfulness practices under everyday clinical situations. For example, the trials did not specify the certification and training of instructors, and only a few trials specified the time spent in home training.

Figure 34. Relative difference between groups in the changes in measures of substance use, in the mantra versus nonspecific/specific active control studies

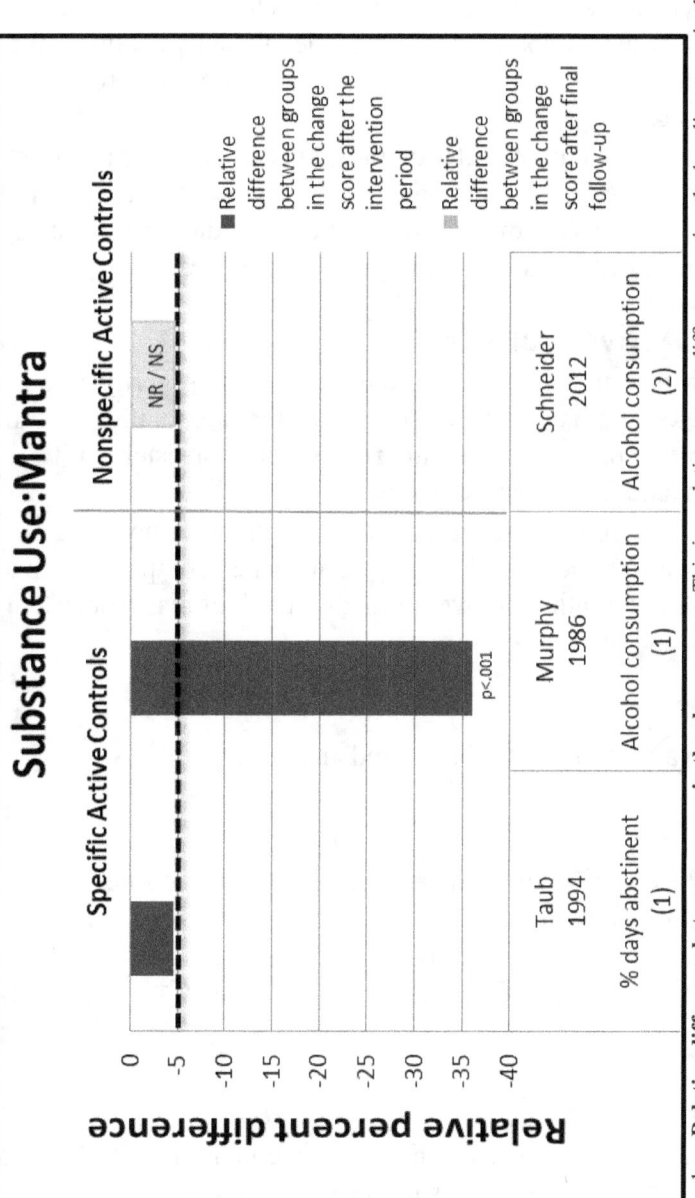

1. **Relative difference between groups in the change score.** This is a relative percent difference, using the baseline mean in the meditation group as the denominator. For example, if the meditation group improves from a 10 to 19 on a mental health scale and the control group improves from 11 to 16 on the same scale, the relative difference between groups in the change score is: $(((19-10)-(16-11))/10) \times 100 = 40\%$. The interpretation is that there is a 40% relative improvement on the mental health scale in the meditation group compared with the control group. See appendix E for absolute difference-in-change score values. Improvement in all scales is indicated in the positive direction. A positive relative percent difference means that the score improved more in the intervention group than in the control group
2. (1): Primary outcome. If the trial did not specify primary or secondary outcomes, this is either the outcome that the population was selected on or identified as a primary focus of the study. (2): Secondary outcome. If the trial did not specify primary or secondary outcomes, then this is not the outcome that the population was selected nor identified as a primary focus of the study.
3. NR / NS = Not Reported/Not significant. The trial measured this outcome and stated they were nonsignificant, and did not report actual results.
4. Black dotted lines from −5% to +5% indicate our criteria for no effect. It does not indicate statistical significance.
5. A p value above or below a bar indicates statistical significance reported in the original study publication. If there is no p value, the outcome was not significant in the original publication.

Key Question 4. What are the efficacy and harms of meditation programs on pain and weight among those with a clinical condition (medical or psychiatric)?

Key Points and Evidence Grades

Comparisons With <u>Nonspecific</u> Active Controls
- The strength of evidence is moderate that mindfulness meditation programs have a small improvement in pain severity among a variety of populations when compared with a nonspecific active control. We based this rating on trials with medium bias, consistent findings for a small positive effect, direct measures, and precise estimates.
- The strength of evidence is low that mantra meditation programs have no effect on pain severity among those with CHF when compared with a nonspecific active control. We based this rating on a single trial of low risk of bias, unknown consistency, direct measures, and imprecise estimates.
- The strength of evidence is low that mantra meditation programs do not have an effect on weight among diabetics, hypertensives, or those with coronary disease when compared with a nonspecific active control. We based this rating on overall medium risk of bias, consistent null findings, directness of measures, and imprecise estimates.

Comparisons With <u>Specific</u> Active Controls
- The strength of evidence is low that mindfulness has no effect on pain severity among those with chronic musculoskeletal pain or mood disturbance, compared with a specific active control. We based this rating on overall medium risk of bias, consistent null results, direct measures of pain, and imprecise estimates.
- The strength of evidence is low that mindfulness meditation programs do not have an effect on weight among breast cancer and chronic pain patients when compared with a specific active control. We based this rating on overall medium risk of bias, consistent results, directness of measures, and imprecise estimates.

Harms
- Four trials reported that they evaluated harms; none found any adverse events.

Trial Characteristics

We found 14 RCTs on this KQ. Eleven RCTs took place in the United States, one in Canada, one in Germany, and one in Hong Kong. All involved outpatients. Six trials did not report recruitment periods, the others were between 2000 and 2009. Trial duration ranged from 3 months to 9.3 years. All trials recruited only adults. Two recruited only females[53,70] (Appendix E).

Population Characteristics

Five of the trials recruited participants who reported a chronic pain condition[53,64,69,70,74] while nine used non-pain populations.[54,56,62,63,73,76-78,90] Two trials used general chronic pain patients of whom more than 95 percent had musculoskeletal pain,[69,74] while the other three used women with IBS (visceral pain), women with fibromyalgia (musculoskeletal pain), and patients with low back pain (also musculoskeletal pain). The sample size in trials that used a pain population ranged from 30–177. Two included only women.[53,70] The mean age was around 40–60 for these trials except for a trial that studied elderly low-back-pain patients,[64] who were, on average, 75 years old. Four trials reported ethnicity. In two, the majority of participants were white, and in the other two the entire population was black. Five trials reported education level. The percent that had completed high school ranged from 11–72 percent.[53,62,70,73,74] The majority of participants in the IBS trial had a college or graduate level education.[53] Among the non-pain population trials, participants were either solid organ transplant recipients,[54] patients, post-surgery, with psychological distress,[63] or African Americans with CHF.[78] Sample sizes ranged from 23–186 and included 30–80 percent women (Appendix Evidence Table E3).

Intervention Characteristics

Six trials used MBSR,[54,62,63,69,70,74] three used mindfulness meditation programs,[53,64,73] and four used TM.[76-78,90] While all trials used active controls, six of the mindfulness trials used a specific active control such as a multidisciplinary pain management program or massage. All others used a nonspecific active control to control for time, attention, and expectation, such as a health education group. All four of the TM programs used a nonspecific active control.

The studies typically conducted the mindfulness programs weekly for 1.5–2.5 hours over 8 weeks, and they ranged from 12–27 total hours of training. Although all of the trials indicated, in some form, that they recommended daily practice, only two of the trials specified the amount, recommending 45 minutes daily.[64,70] None of the trials reported on the actual amount of home practice in the meditation arm. Reports on instructor qualifications were lacking for most trials. Six of 10 mindfulness trials indicated that instructors had some training but only two gave enough information to suggest that the instructors had some kind of certification.[64,70] Only one trial reported on the personal meditation experience of the instructors,[64] and three trials reported an instructor's level of teaching experience.[70,74]

On average, the TM trials provided 1.5-hour sessions for seven consecutive days, and followup refresher meetings twice monthly for the first 3 months and then once monthly for the next 3 months. The trials did not give details of the followup meetings, but we estimated the duration at approximately 22.5 hours over a 6-month period, assuming the meetings were also 1.5 hours in length (an amount roughly similar to the mindfulness trials). They recommended approximately half-hour daily home practice for 6 months, which calculates to approximately 90 hours of home practice over 6 months. These trials reported a certified trainer without giving details of years of meditation or teaching experience.

Five trials measured weight changes.[77,56,62,76,90] Three were TM[77,76,90] and two used mindfulness meditation.[56,62] None of these trials reported details of hours of training, although we estimated the amount of training where some information was given. These trials gave little information on instructor qualifications or whether the participants performed home practice. The TM trials indicated their teachers were either trained or certified, and recommended between 30–40 minutes of daily meditation for the duration of their study, amounting to a total expected home practice dose of 90–120 hours over 6 months. None of the trials reported actual amounts of meditation (Appendix E).

Outcomes

Ascertainment of Outcomes (Scales)

Studies measured pain severity using the 11-point numerical rating scale for pain intensity or unpleasantness, perceived pain scale affective and sensory subscales, SF-36 bodily pain subscale, McGill pain questionnaire, and the IBS abdominal pain severity subscale. Studies measured weight in either pounds, kilograms, or body mass index (BMI) (Table 3).

Pain Severity

Mindfulness Meditation Program Versus a <u>Nonspecific</u> Active Control

Four trials evaluated MBSR against a nonspecific active control and assessed the outcome of pain severity (Table 15).[53,54,64,70] One trial evaluated visceral pain while the other three evaluated musculoskeletal pain. One trial had a low risk of bias, the remaining three had a medium risk of bias.

Gaylord et al. randomized women with IBS (n=75) to MBSR versus support program for women with IBS.[53] This was the only trial to assess visceral pain, and found a 30.6 percent reduction in abdominal pain severity in the MBSR group compared with control at 8 weeks; this maintained at 6 months (p=.015). This was a medium risk-of-bias trial that provided 23 hours of training and unspecified amount of home practice over 8 weeks.

Schmidt et al. randomized women with fibromyalgia (n=109) to 8 weeks of MBSR or a nonspecific active control.[70] The trial used perceived pain scale to measure pain severity as a secondary outcome. The perceived pain scale has affective and sensory subscales; the affective dimension measures the unpleasantness of the pain experience, whereas the sensory dimension measures the intensity of sensory qualities of the pain experience. There were no significant differences between the MBSR and control on either of the subscales (p=.18 for affective subscale, p=.60 for sensory subscale), although the meditation arm was favored by 5.7 percent for the sensory subscale. This trial provided 27 hours of training over 8 weeks by trained and certified teachers, and recommended up to 42 hours of home practice. It had a medium risk of bias.

Gross et al. randomized solid organ transplant patients, post-surgery, (n=137) to MBSR versus health education.[54] They found no change in the SF-36 bodily pain subscale within groups or between groups at 2 months or 1 year, although the meditation arm was favored by 5.1 percent. This trial provided 27 hours of training by a trained teacher, and unspecified amount of home practice over 8 weeks. This trial had medium risk of bias.

Morone et al. randomized older adults with chronic low back of moderate intensity (n=35) to MBSR or a health education program for 8 weeks.[64] They used two scales to assess pain severity: SF-36 pain subscale and McGill pain questionnaire current pain score. The MBSR group showed a nonsignificant 8.6 percent improvement in the SF-36 pain subscale at 8 weeks compared with control, but these differences disappeared at 6 months. There were no effects seen in the McGill pain questionnaire in a differences-in-change analysis. This trial provided 12 hours of training over 8 weeks by a teacher with 25 years of meditation experience and some teaching experience. The trial recommended up to 42 hours of home practice over the 8 weeks. This trial had a low risk of bias.

The difference-in-change graphs showed consistent small positive effects on pain severity (Figure 35). A meta-analysis showed a small statistically significant effect size favoring mindfulness meditation programs (Figure 36). The strength of evidence is moderate that mindfulness meditation programs have a small improvement in pain severity among a variety of populations when compared with a nonspecific active control. We based this rating on trials of medium bias, consistent findings for a small positive effect, direct measures, and precise estimates (Table 41).

Table 41. Grade of trials addressing the efficacy of mindfulness-based stress reduction on pain severity compared with nonspecific active controls among visceral pain, musculoskeletal pain, and organ transplant patients

Number of Trials; Subjects	Domains Pertaining to Strength of Evidence				Magnitude of Effect and Strength of Evidence
	Risk of bias	Consistency	Directness	Precision	
Pain Severity					Moderate SOE of an effect on pain severity
4; 341	Medium	Consistent	Direct	Precise	5.1% to 30.6% reduction in pain severity favoring MBSR

Notes: SOE = Strength of Evidence; MBSR = Mindfulness-based Stress Reduction

Figure 35. Relative difference between groups in the changes in measures of pain, in the mindfulness versus nonspecific active control studies

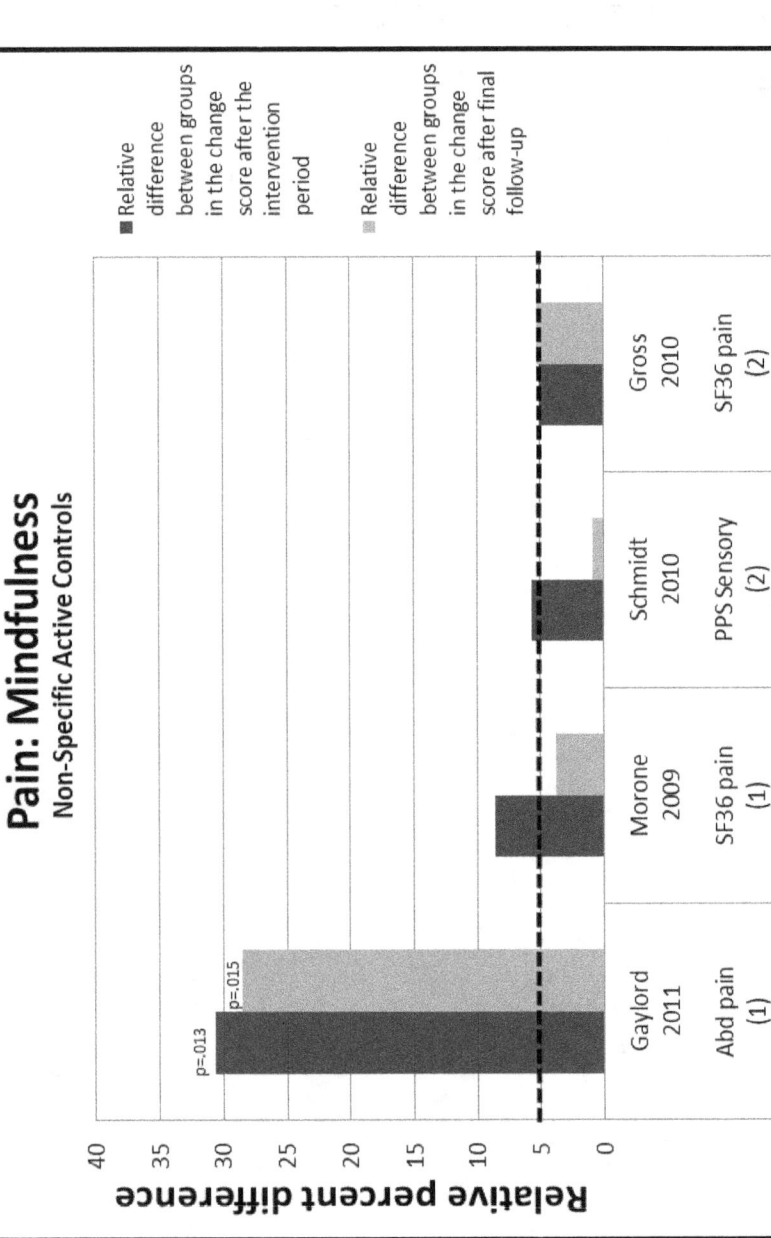

1. **Relative difference between groups in the change score**. This is a relative percent difference, using the baseline mean in the meditation group as the denominator. For example, if the meditation group improves from a 10 to 19 on a mental health scale and the control group improves from 11 to 16 on the same scale, the relative difference between groups in the change score is: (((19-10)-(16-11))/10)x100=40%. The interpretation is that there is a 40% relative improvement on the mental health scale in the meditation group compared with the control group. See appendix E for absolute difference-in-change score values. Improvement in all scales is indicated in the positive direction. A positive relative percent difference means that the score improved more in the intervention group than in the control group
2. (1): Primary outcome. If the trial did not specify primary or secondary outcomes, this is either the outcome that the population was selected on or identified as a primary focus of the study. (2): Secondary outcome. If the trial did not specify primary or secondary outcomes, then this is not the outcome that the population was selected nor identified as a primary focus of the study.
3. NR / NS = Not Reported/Not significant. The trial measured this outcome and stated they were nonsignificant, and did not report actual results.
4. Black dotted lines from –5% to +5% indicate our criteria for no effect. It does not indicate statistical significance.
5. A p value above or below a bar indicates statistical significance reported in the original study publication. If there is no p value, the outcome was not significant in the original publication.
6. Abd = Abdomen; PPS = Pain Perception (Sensory); SF-36 = Short Form-36.

Figure 36. Meta-analysis of the effects of meditation programs on pain severity with 8-12 weeks of followup

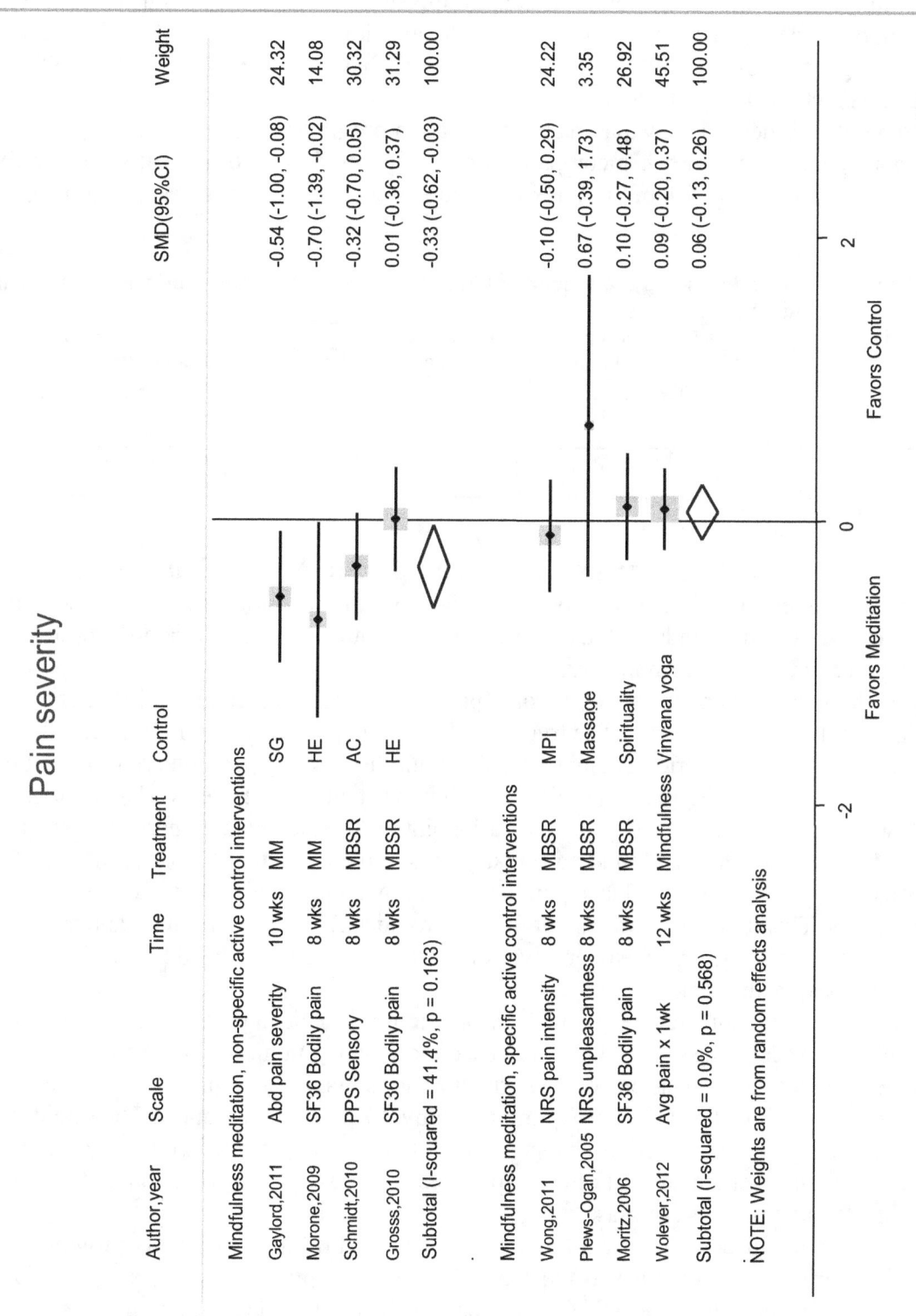

Notes: Abd = Abdomen; AC=Active Control; HE = Health Education; NRS = Numeric Rating Scale; MBSR = Mindfulness Based Stress Reduction; MM = Mindfulness Meditation; MPI= Multidisciplinary Pain Intervention; PPS = Pain Perception (Sensory); SF-36 = Short Form-36; SG = Support Group; wks = weeks

Transcendental Meditation Versus <u>Nonspecific</u> Active Control

One TM trial on African Americans with CHF assessed pain as a secondary outcome using the SF 36 pain subscale (n=23; Table 15).[78] With 100 percent trial completion and 95 percent compliance rate among the originally randomized subjects, there were no differences in the pain scores in both groups at 3 months. However, at 6 months the TM group showed an 18.4 percent improvement over health education (p=.08). This trial had a low risk of bias. It provided 22.5 hours of training over 6 months by trained and certified teachers and recommended up to 90 hours of home practice during this time.

The strength of evidence is low that mantra meditation programs have no effect on pain severity among those with CHF when compared with a nonspecific active control. We based this rating on a single trial of low risk of bias, unknown consistency, direct measures, and imprecise estimates (Table 42).

Table 42. Grade of trials addressing the efficacy of TM on pain severity compared with nonspecific active controls among cardiac patients

Number of Trials; Subjects	Domains Pertaining to Strength of Evidence				Magnitude of Effect and Strength of Evidence
	Risk of Bias	Consistency	Directness	Precision	
Pain Severity					Low SOE of no effect on pain severity
1; 23	Low	Unknown	Direct	Imprecise	−2.1% reduction in pain (favoring control)

Note: SOE = Strength Of Evidence

Mindfulness Meditation Programs Versus a Specific Active Control

Four trials assessed MBSR against a specific active control for the outcome of pain severity (Table 15). Two trials were conducted in chronic pain populations, one in a mood-disturbed population, and one in stressed employees.

Wong et al. randomized patients with chronic pain (n=99) in Hong Kong to MBSR or a multidisciplinary pain intervention.[74] The trial included participants who reported greater than or equal to 4/10 pain on the numerical rating scale. The multidisciplinary pain intervention group specifically excluded teaching of any mind-body techniques that might have overlapped with MBSR. Researchers powered this trial to detect a 1-point difference in the numerical rating scale between the two groups. The trial found no statistically significant difference between interventions. Both interventions reduced pain by approximately 0.5 points post treatment and 1 point at 6 months. This trial had a low risk of bias. It provided 27 hours of training and an unspecified amount of home practice over 8 weeks. Teachers were trained and had 5 years of experience teaching meditation.[74]

Plews-Ogan et al. randomized people with chronic musculoskeletal pain (n=15) to 8 weeks of MBSR training or weekly massage.[69] The study used the 11-point numerical rating scale for pain unpleasantness to measure pain as one of two primary endpoints. It found that the massage group improved 2.9 points while the MBSR group improved by 0.7 points at 2 months. The trial did not calculate significance for difference-in-change estimates. This trial provided 20 hours of training over 8 weeks, and unspecified amount of home practice. There was no information on teacher qualifications. It had a high risk of bias.

Moritz et al. randomized patients with mood disorders (n=110) to a spirituality program versus MBSR.[63] In this trial, MBSR was the active control. The spirituality intervention included a meditative component. It used the SF 36 bodily pain scale as a secondary outcome. In a difference-in-change estimate it found a nonsignificant 5.8 percent improvement in the spirituality group compared with the MBSR group. This trial provided about 12 hours of training in both interventions over an 8-week period, with unspecified amount of home practice in the MBSR group. It provided up to 42 hours of home practice in the spirituality group. There was no information on teacher qualifications for MBSR. This trial had a low risk of bias.

Wolever et al. randomized stressed employees (n=186) to a mindfulness-at-work program or viniyoga for 12 weeks. Participants received 14 hours of training by trained teachers and unspecified amount of homework. Pain was a secondary outcome. The trial found no improvement in the mindfulness group compared with control. This trial had a medium risk of bias.

The difference-in-change graphs showed consistent results favoring a null effect or the control group (Figure 37). A meta-analysis suggested a null effect (Figure 35). The strength of evidence is low that mindfulness has no effect on pain severity among those with chronic musculoskeletal pain or mood disturbance, compared with a specific active control. We based this rating on overall medium risk of bias, consistent null results, direct measures of pain, and imprecise estimates (Table 43).

Table 43. Grade of trials addressing the efficacy of mindfulness-based stress reduction on pain severity compared with specific active controls among chronic pain and mood disturbance patients

Number of Trials; Subjects	Domains Pertaining to Strength of Evidence				Magnitude of Effect and Strength of Evidence
	Risk of Bias	Consistency	Directness	Precision	
Pain Severity					Low SOE of no effect on pain severity
4; 410	Medium	Consistent	Direct	Imprecise	−0.6% to −31.9% favoring control

Note: SOE = Strength of Evidence

Figure 37. Relative difference between groups in the changes in measures of pain, in the mindfulness versus specific active control studies

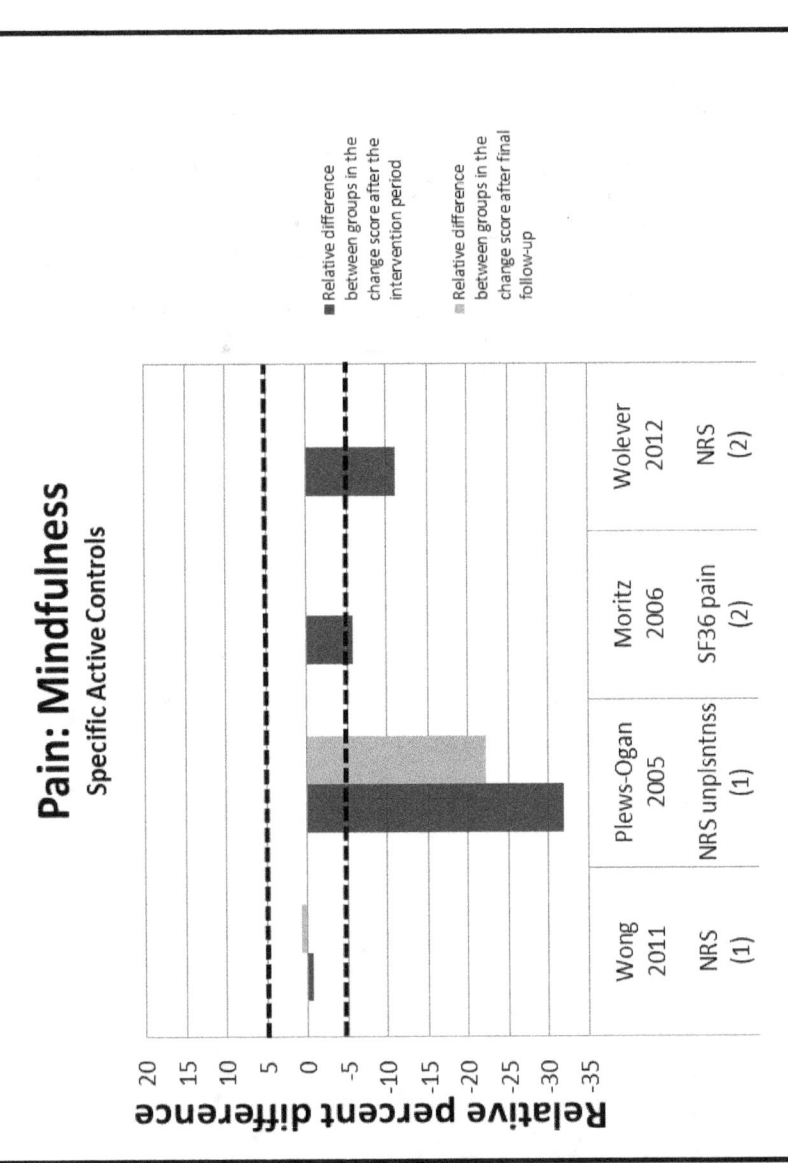

1. **Relative difference between groups in the change score.** This is a relative percent difference, using the baseline mean in the meditation group as the denominator. For example, if the meditation group improves from a 10 to 19 on a mental health scale and the control group improves from 11 to 16 on the same scale, the relative difference between groups in the change score is: (((19-10)-(16-11))/10)x100=40%. The interpretation is that there is a 40% relative improvement on the mental health scale in the meditation group compared with the control group. See appendix E for absolute difference-in-change score values. Improvement in all scales is indicated in the positive direction. A positive relative percent difference means that the score improved more in the intervention group than in the control group
2. (1): Primary outcome. If the trial did not specify primary or secondary outcomes, this is either the outcome that the population was selected on or identified as a primary focus of the study. (2): Secondary outcome. If the trial did not specify primary or secondary outcomes, then this is not the outcome that the population was selected nor identified as a primary focus of the study.
3. NR/NS = Not Reported/Not significant. The trial measured this outcome and stated they were nonsignificant, and did not report actual results.
4. Black dotted lines from −5% to +5% indicate our criteria for no effect. It does not indicate statistical significance.
5. A p value above or below a bar indicates statistical significance reported in the original study publication. If there is no p value, the outcome was not significant in the original publication.
6. NRS = Numeric Rating Scale; SF-36 = Short Form-36; unplsntnss = unpleasantness.

Weight

Mindfulness Meditation Programs Versus a <u>Specific</u> Active Control

Hebert et al. randomized women with early stage breast cancer (n=99) to MBSR versus nutrition education for 15 weeks (Table 16).[56] This trial found no difference in weight between the three groups at 4 or 12 months. This trial provided approximately 45 hours of training over 15 weeks, did not report on any teacher qualifications, and did not specify whether they recommended any home practice. This trial had a medium risk of bias.

Miller et al.[62] randomized diabetics to a mindfulness eating program versus the Smart Choices diabetes group self-management education program (n=52). This mindfulness program provided about 25 hours of training over 12 weeks and unspecified amount of homework. Weight loss was a primary outcome. The trial found no effect at 3 and 6 months compared with control. This trial had a high risk of bias.

The difference-in-change graphs showed consistent results favoring a null effect (Figure 38). The strength of evidence is low that mindfulness meditation programs do not have an effect on weight among breast cancer and chronic pain patients when compared with a specific active control. We based this rating on overall medium risk of bias, consistent results, directness of measures, and imprecise estimates (Table 44).

Table 44. Grade of trials addressing the efficacy of mindfulness-based stress reduction on weight among breast cancer and chronic pain patients compared with a specific active control

Number of Trials; Subjects	Domains Pertaining to Strength of Evidence				Magnitude of Effect and Strength of Evidence
	Risk of Bias	Consistency	Directness	Precision	
Weight					Low SOE of no effect on weight
2; 151	Medium	Consistent	Direct	Imprecise	1.1% weight loss to 1.7% weight gain in MBSR group

Notes: SOE = Strength of Evidence; MBSR = Mindfulness-based Stress Reduction

Transcendental Meditation Versus a <u>Nonspecific</u> Active Control

Three trials of TM evaluated weight as an outcome (Table 16). Elder et al. randomized adults with elevated HgA1c (n=54) to a TM program versus diabetes education classes[77]. There were no differences between the groups in weight loss (p=.26). This trial did not report on the amount of training provided or the duration of the training. It did specify it recommended about 90 hours of home practice over 6 months. The teachers were trained teachers of TM. This trial had a medium risk of bias.

Castillo-Richmond et al. conducted a trial of TM using a subsample from a larger randomized trial of TM on cardiovascular outcomes (n=60 of 170 from the original trial).[76] This trial found no difference in weight after 7 months between the groups (p=.48). This trial did not specify the amount of training provided, but did specify it recommended up to 120.6 hours of home practice over 7 months. The teachers had training and certification in the TM tradition. This trial had a high risk of bias, due largely to uncertain sampling methods from the primary trial.

Schneider et al.[90] randomized black adults with coronary artery disease to TM or health education. The study followed patients for an average of 5.4 years. The study estimated they received approximately 78 hours of training over this time by trained and certified teachers, along with approximately 1,310 hours of homework. After an average of 5.4 years, there were no differences in BMI between the two groups. This trial had a low risk of bias.

The difference-in-change graphs showed a consistent null effect on weight (Figure 38). The strength of evidence is low that mantra meditation programs do not have an effect on weight among diabetics, hypertensives, or those with coronary disease when compared with a nonspecific active control. We based this rating on overall medium risk of bias, consistent null findings, directness of measures, and imprecise estimates (Table 45).

Table 45. Grade of trials addressing the efficacy of meditation programs on weight among those with a clinical condition

Number of Trials; Subjects	Domains Pertaining to Strength of Evidence				Magnitude of Effect and Strength of Evidence
	Risk of Bias	Consistency	Directness	Precision	
Weight					Low SOE of no effect on weight
3; 297	Medium	Consistent	Direct	Imprecise	1.8% weight loss to 1.2% weight gain in TM group

Notes: SOE = Strength of Evidence; TM = Transcendental Meditation

Assessment of Potential Publication Bias

We could not conduct any reliable quantitative tests for publication bias since few studies were available for most outcomes, and we were unable to include all eligible studies in the meta-analysis due to missing data. Consequently, funnel plots were unlikely to provide much useful information regarding the possibility of publication bias. We reviewed the clinicaltrials.gov registration database to assess the number of trials that had been completed three or more years ago and that prespecified our outcomes but did not publish at all or did not publish all outcomes that were prespecified. We found 5 trials on clinicaltrials.gov that appeared to have been completed before Jan 1, 2010 that were published but did not publish the results of all outcomes they had prespecified on the registration Web site. We also found 9 trials that appeared to have been completed before January 1, 2010 but that we could not find any publication for, and had prespecified at least one of our outcomes. 10 registered trials had prespecified one or more KQ1 outcomes but did not publish them, 2 registered trials had prespecified attention as an outcome but did not publish, 5 registered trials prespecified one or more KQ3 outcomes but did not publish, and 5 registered trials prespecified one or more KQ4 outcomes but did not publish. For 8 of the 9 registered trials for which we could not find a publication, it was not possible to tell if those trials had actually been conducted or completed While examining for selective outcome reporting, we found one trial that selectively reported on positive outcomes. Among 109 outcomes in 41 trials, trials did not give enough information to calculate a relative difference-in-the-change score (our primary analysis) for six outcomes due to statistically insignificant findings. These are represented as solid grey boxes in the figures. Trials did not give enough information to conduct a meta-analysis on 16 outcomes. Our findings from the primary analysis are therefore less likely to be affected by publication bias than the meta-analysis.

Applicability

Eleven of 14 trials took place in the United States, the remainders took place in Canada, Germany, and Hong Kong, so that these findings might be inapplicable to patients or settings in other regions. All of the trials took place in outpatient settings, so these findings would not be applicable to the inpatient setting.

Regarding the population characteristics of the trials for this KQ, only one trial reported the racial or ethnic characteristics of its study population. In addition, these trials under represent younger patients (less than 45) and older patients (age greater than 80), making these findings less applicable to those groups. The most important proviso regarding the population characteristics is that the trials for this KQ were of two different kinds: those in populations with chronic pain, and those predominantly with another condition. Thus, the populations in these trials were heterogeneous as a group, making it difficult to identify the clinical populations for which these findings would be most applicable.

Characteristics of the interventions represented in this KQ were diverse, making it difficult to foresee how these findings would be applicable to a similarly wide array of mindfulness practices under everyday clinical situations. For example, only a few trials specified the certification and training of instructors or the time spent in home training.

Figure 38. Relative difference between groups in the changes in measures of weight, in the mindfulness/transcendental meditation versus specific/nonspecific active control studies

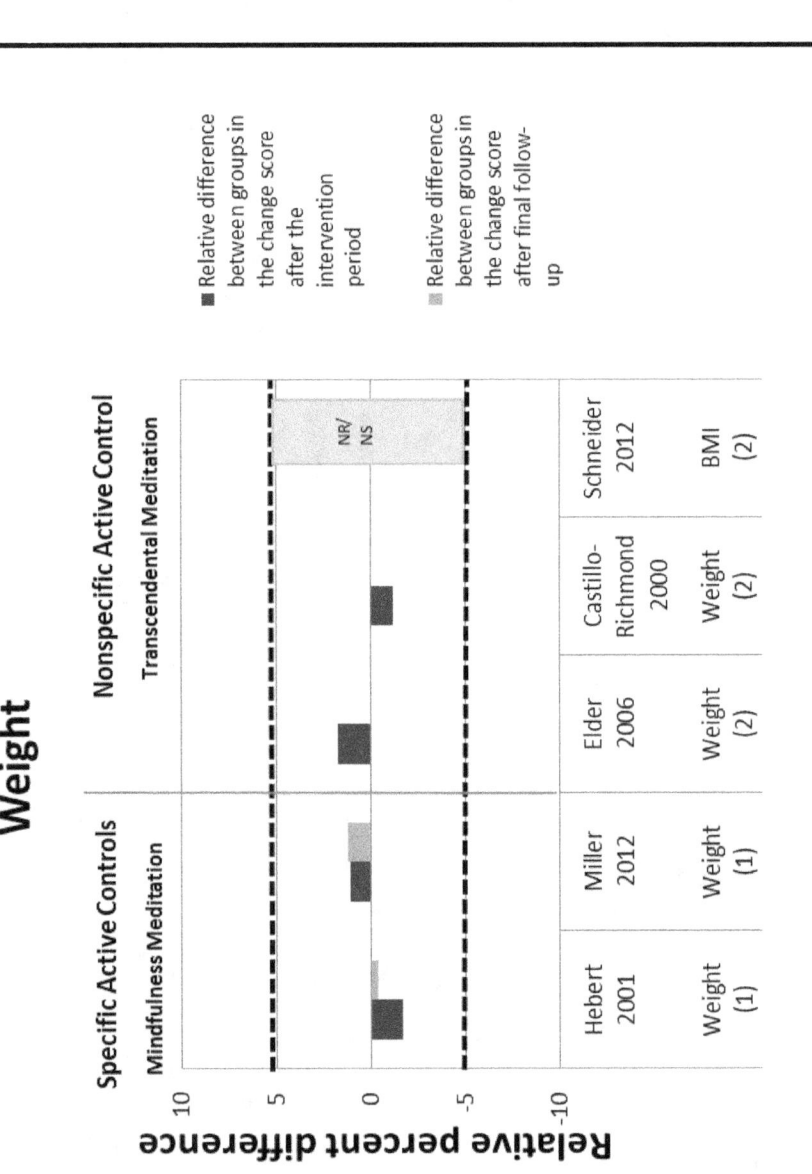

1. **Relative difference between groups in the change score.** This is a relative percent difference, using the baseline mean in the meditation group as the denominator. For example, if the meditation group improves from a 10 to 19 on a mental health scale and the control group improves from 11 to 16 on the same scale, the relative difference between groups in the change score is: (((19-10)−(16−11))/10)x100=40%. The interpretation is that there is a 40% relative improvement on the mental health scale in the meditation group compared with the control group. See appendix E for absolute difference-in-change score values. Improvement in all scales is indicated in the positive direction. A positive relative percent difference means that the score improved more in the intervention group than in the control group
2. (1): Primary outcome. If the trial did not specify primary or secondary outcomes, this is either the outcome that the population was selected on or identified as a primary focus of the study. (2): Secondary outcome. If the trial did not specify primary or secondary outcomes, then this is not the outcome that the population was selected nor identified as a primary focus of the study.
3. NR / NS = Not Reported/Not significant. The trial measured this outcome and stated they were nonsignificant, and did not report actual results.
4. Black dotted lines from −5% to +5% indicate our criteria for no effect. It does not indicate statistical significance.
5. A p value above or below a bar indicates statistical significance reported in the original study publication. If there is no p value, the outcome was not significant in the original publication.
6. Units of weight: kilograms (Hebert, 2001; Miller, 2012; Schneider,2012) and pounds (Elder, 2006; Castillo-Richmond, 2000).

Discussion

Forty-one randomized controlled trials (RCTs) reported in this review tested the effects of meditation programs in clinical conditions relative to active controls. Ten programs tested mantra meditation and 31 programs tested mindfulness meditation. Active control groups included both "nonspecific" controls as well as specific controls that offer an opportunity to examine the comparative effectiveness of meditation programs. Our review finds that the mantra meditation programs do not appear to improve any of the psychological stress and well-being outcomes we examined, but the strength of this evidence varies from low to insufficient. We find that the mindfulness meditation programs show small improvements in anxiety, depression, and pain with moderate strength of evidence, and small improvements in stress/distress, negative affect, and the mental-health component of health-related quality of life with low strength of evidence when compared to nonspecific active controls. The remaining outcomes had insufficient evidence to draw any level of conclusion for mindfulness meditation programs. We were unable to draw a high grade for either type of meditation program for any of the psychological stress and well-being outcomes. We also found no evidence for any harms, although few trials reported on this.

It is important to keep in mind the conceptual meanings of our different levels of strength of evidence. "High" strength of evidence indicates high confidence that the evidence reflects the true effect, and further research is very unlikely to change our confidence in the estimate of the effect. "Moderate" strength of evidence indicates moderate confidence that the evidence reflects the true effect, and further research may change our confidence in the estimate of the effect and may change the estimate. "Low" strength of evidence indicates low confidence that the evidence reflects the true effect, and further research is likely to change our confidence in the estimate of the effect and is likely to change the estimate. Finally "insufficient" strength of evidence indicates evidence is either unavailable or inadequate to draw a conclusion.

Before addressing each Key Question (KQ), there are some methodological aspects of this review that deserve comment.

First, our method purposely established a high standard for selecting RCTs by requiring the inclusion of an active control group that was matched for time and attention to the meditation program of interest. We elected to use this approach in order to add to what we have already learned from existing reviews of meditation, and to determine whether any comparative effectiveness conclusions could be drawn from the existing literature. This more rigorous approach supports the conclusion that meditation programs improve psychological stress and well-being in groups with clinical conditions; however, we find no evidence to support the differential effectiveness of meditation in comparison to other treatments for psychological stress and well-being.

Second, our two methods for reporting results—the difference-in-change graphs and the meta-analyses—provide different summaries of the studies included, each of which has strengths and weaknesses. Strengths of the difference-in-change approach include that it controls for baseline difference between groups and yields a change score on the outcome of interest that has the potential for determining clinical meaningfulness. Weaknesses of this approach include the absence of standards for determining clinical meaningfulness for most measures included in the meditation trials. Strengths of the meta-analysis include the empirical approach to summarizing and evaluating the magnitude and quality of the evidence. Weaknesses include the omission of some key papers due to the lack of outcome data available, and lack of adjustment for baseline differences.

And third, we selected an arbitrary cut-off of ±5 percent as the criteria for a difference in change over time indicating improvement of one group over another. This is a small difference for most measures of psychological stress and well-being and may be regarded by some readers as too liberal, especially if the outcome is clinically relevant (e.g., depression in people seeking care for depression). Since the findings reported in these papers generally do not report clinically meaningful outcomes (e.g., reduction in study participants meeting cut-offs for clinical syndromes), we selected a low threshold that could be universally applied to the heterogeneous group of measures included in these studies.

Key Question 1. What are the efficacy and harms of meditation programs on negative affect (e.g., anxiety, stress) and positive affect (e.g., well-being) among those with a clinical condition (medical or psychiatric)?

We found 32 trials for this KQ, including four evaluating TM, two evaluating other mantra meditation, and 26 evaluating mindfulness meditation. In general, we found no evidence that mantra meditation programs improve psychological stress and well-being. Mindfulness meditation programs improved multiple dimensions of negative affect, including anxiety, depression, and perceived stress/general distress, and the mental-health component of quality of life with a low to moderate strength of evidence when compared to a nonspecific active control. Well-being and positive mood are positive dimensions of mental health. While meditation programs generally seek to improve the positive dimensions of health, the available evidence from a very small number of studies did not show any effects on positive affect or well-being. Both analytic methods, the difference-in-change estimates (which accounted for baseline differences between groups) and the meta-analyses (which only compared end-line differences), generally showed consistent but small effects for anxiety, depression, and stress/distress. However, there are a number of observations that help interpret and give context to our conclusions.

The first observation is that there were very few mantra meditation programs included in our review. This significantly limited our ability to draw inferences about the effects of mantra meditation programs on psychological stress-related outcomes. Of the four TM trials, three were well-designed trials with low risk of bias that studied cardiac patients, while one had a high risk of bias and studied anxiety patients. Among the other mantra trials, both had a medium risk of bias. Based on the available evidence from these trials, we found no evidence that mantra meditation programs have an effect on psychological stress and well-being as compared to a nonspecific active control. These conclusions did not change when we evaluated TM separately from other mantra. Apart from the paucity of trials, another reason for seeing null results may also be due to the type of populations studied (e.g. 3 TM trials enrolled cardiac patients, while only 1 enrolled anxiety patients), and whether these study participants had high levels of a particular negative affect to begin with.

The second observation is that among mindfulness trials, the effects were significant for anxiety and marginally significant for depression at the end of treatment, and these effects continued to be significant at 3–6 months for both anxiety and depression. We did not conduct a meta-analysis of stress/distress at 8 weeks due to a concern for bias, and we did not have enough data to conduct a longer-term meta-analysis for stress/distress. The difference-in-change graphs for the trials comparing mindfulness meditation to nonspecific active controls show a relatively consistent improvement in stress/distress, which is consistent with a prior review by Chiesa et al., comparing MBSR to inactive controls.[16]

Third, when we combined each outcome that was a sub domain of negative affect (anxiety, depression, and stress/distress), we see a small and consistent signal that any domain of negative affect is improved in mindfulness programs when compared with a nonspecific active control. Since we could only include one outcome from any single trial, we prioritized anxiety over depression and depression over stress/distress for this analysis. When we conducted a sensitivity analysis reversing the prioritization of outcomes, we continued to find the same result.

Fourth, the effect sizes are small. However, they are fairly comparable with what would be expected from the use of an antidepressant in a primary care population. In a study using patient-level meta-analysis, Fournier et al. found that for patients with mild to moderate depressive symptoms, antidepressants had an effect size of 0.11 (−0.18, +0.41), while those with severe depression had an effect size of 0.17 (−0.08, +0.43) compared with placebo.[92] Over the course of 2–6 months, we find that mindfulness meditation program effect size estimates range from 0.22–0.40 for anxiety symptoms and 0.23–0.32 for depressive symptoms, and were statistically significant.

The fifth observation is that although there may be differences between trials for which these outcomes are a primary versus secondary focus, we did not find any evidence for this. While we did not conduct separate meta-analyses for primary versus secondary trials due to the small number of each, our analysis of the difference-in-change estimates did not suggest any difference. Some trials, in which an outcome was a primary focus, did not recruit based on high symptom levels of that outcome. Thus, the samples included in these trials more closely resemble a general primary care population, and there may not be room to measure an effect if symptom levels were low to start with (i.e. a "floor" effect).

Sixth, all of the findings favoring an improvement in outcomes among the mindfulness groups as compared to control were found only when the comparisons were made against a nonspecific active control. In each comparison that was made against a known treatment or therapy, mindfulness did not show superiority for any outcome. This was true for all comparisons among any form of meditation for any KQ. Out of 53 comparisons with a specific active control, we found only 2 that showed a statistically significant improvement: MBCT improved quality of life in comparison to antidepressant drug among depressed patientsand mindfulness therapy reduced cigarette consumption in comparison to the Freedom from Smoking program.[50] However, we also found five comparisons where the specific active control performed better, with statistically significant results, than the meditation programs. The comparisons with specific therapies led to highly inconsistent results for most outcomes (Figure 4b), and indicated that meditative therapies were no better than the specific therapies they were being compared to. These include such therapies as exercise, yoga, progressive muscle relaxation, cognitive behavioral therapy, and medications.

Seventh, some of our findings are inconsistent with previous reviews. For example, based on three trials we found no evidence that mindfulness-based cognitive therapy (MBCT) improves anxiety.[67,68,86] Previous reviews have concluded that MBCT is an effective intervention for anxiety or could provide some improvement in residual anxiety symptoms in some populations.[18,19] A strength of our methodology is the comparison of MBCT with nonspecific active controls, which suggests that the conclusions of earlier reviews may be due to nonspecific effects of treatment (e.g. time, attention, expectations for improvement) rather than effects specifically attributable to MBCT.

Finally, by delineating nonspecific and specific active controls, we hoped to derive some information about the comparative effectiveness of meditation programs. The heterogeneity of specific active treatments that these studies investigated makes it impossible to draw conclusions about inferiority or superiority of meditation programs. The studies in depression are notable, though, in examining the effects of MBCT during discontinuation of an antidepressant.[59,71] These two trials used a clinically important outcome of relapse rate among a depression population, compared MBCT with tapering of antidepressant medication to maintenance antidepressant medication, and found consistent absolute 8–13 percent reductions in relapse rates.[59,71] Both trials were rated as having low risk of bias. These findings warrant further investigation, and are generally consistent with prior reviews.[15,18,23]

Key Question 2. What are the efficacy and harms of meditation programs on attention among those with a clinical condition (medical or psychiatric)?

One RCT compared a meditation program to active control on the outcome of attention. There were no statistically significant differences between groups on the attentional network test. There were trends suggesting that the meditation program performed better than the nonspecific active control on this measure, although this did not reach statistical significance.

Of note, three previous reviews assessed the role of meditation programs on attention. A Cochrane review by Krisanaprakornkit et al.,[93] on meditation therapies for attention-deficit/hyperactivity disorder that included two mantra meditation trials, could not make any conclusions regarding the effectiveness of meditation programs for attention-deficit/hyperactivity disorder due to high risk of bias and small sample sizes. That review is not directly comparable to the current review, as the trial population is different (the previous review included children with attention-deficit/hyperactivity disorder) and each used different measures of attention. In addition, the previous review included four RCTs, two of which focused on yoga as the primary intervention, which was not included in the current review. Two additional systematic reviews assessed the effect of TM (Canter et al, 2003)[30] and mindfulness meditation programs (Chiesa 2010) on cognitive functioning, including the domain of attention. While the review by Canter et al. (2003) did not specify results pertaining to attention, the authors concluded that evidence does not support that TM has "a specific and cumulative effect on cognitive function." The review by Chiesa included 23 trials but only six RCTs, with the majority of the RCTs (4 of 6) conducted in healthy populations. Of note, the two trials on clinical populations did not include active controls and were, therefore, not included in the present review. The authors preliminarily concluded that mindfulness meditation programs were associated with improvements in attention, although the authors noted that limitations and variability in the trials requires further assessment. In conjunction with the current review, these findings further reiterate the need for more comprehensive trials with a variety of clinical populations (e.g., disorders where attention may be compromised) to provide a clearer understanding of the impact of meditation programs on attention.

Key Question 3. What are the efficacy and harms of meditation programs on health-related behaviors affected by stress, specifically substance use, sleep, and eating, among those with a clinical condition (medical or psychiatric)?

We included 13 trials for this KQ, four evaluating the effect of meditation on substance use,[49,50,80,84] two evaluating eating,[56,62] and seven evaluating sleep.[54,55,61,66,70,73,85] Overall, there is insufficient evidence to indicate that meditation programs alter health-related behaviors affected by stress.

Among the four trials evaluating substance use, all four were conducted in substance-using populations. Taken together, the trials of mindfulness and mantra meditation failed to provide sufficient evidence of benefit in reducing use of cigarettes or alcohol. Both trials of mindfulness failed to show an effect on reducing calorie consumption on breast cancer patients or diabetics.[56,62] Among the seven trials in which sleep was an outcome, only one used an insomnia population,[55] but failed to provide evidence of an effect on sleep time or quality. Four other trials, which assessed sleep as a secondary outcome among various clinical populations, had inconsistent results on sleep quality. However, results were significant for one trial in which sleep was a primary outcome.[54]

Our findings are consistent with past systematic reviews in this area, which have found insufficient evidence for the effects of meditation programs on health-related behaviors affected by stress among controlled studies. Zgierska et al. conducted a systematic review that included trials of a mindfulness-based intervention in patients with substance abuse.[26] It found no significant effect. Regarding eating disorders, Wanden (2011) conducted a systematic review that included articles considering mindfulness therapy as a treatment for eating disorders.[24] The authors stated that they found evidence of the effectiveness of mindfulness-based interventions for eating disorders. However, this review consisted of largely uncontrolled studies with an N of 1. The literature in this area is still in a preliminary state with regards to quality.

Winbush et al. evaluated seven trials on sleep, four of them uncontrolled, and concluded that the uncontrolled trials found an effect on sleep disturbance while the controlled trials did not find an effect.[25] This is also in line with the findings of this review.

Key Question 4. What are the efficacy and harms of meditation programs on pain and weight among those with a clinical condition (medical or psychiatric)?

We included 14 RCTs for this KQ. We found moderate strength of evidence that mindfulness-based stress reduction (MBSR) reduces pain severity to a small degree when compared with a nonspecific active control. We also found low strength of evidence that when MBSR was compared with various specific active controls including massage, MBSR was not superior in reducing pain severity. One TM trial did not find any improvement in pain severity, but was conducted in 23 patients with congestive heart failure and pain was a secondary outcome.

Among the trials evaluating pain, most evaluated musculoskeletal pain. Based on one study with large significant findings, there is a suggestion that MBSR may be useful for visceral pain. Gaylord et al. evaluated 75 women with irritable bowel syndrome and found a statistically significant 30 percent reduction in abdominal pain severity at 2 months that maintained at six months. Previous systematic reviews by Veehof et al. of trials for pain concluded an effect size of .37 for pain for MBSR and acceptance and commitment therapy, suggesting they were alternatives to cognitive behavior therapy.[94] A review by Bernardy et al. combined MBSR with a number of cognitive behavior therapy used on fibromyalgia patients and found that this group of interventions had no significant effects on pain among fibromyalgia patients.[27] Both included control and uncontrolled trials.

Two mindfulness trials evaluated weight as an outcome, and it was a primary outcome for both. Three TM trials evaluated weight as a secondary outcome. Due to consistently null results, there was low strength of evidence to suggest that TM or MBSR do not have an effect on weight.

Harm Outcomes for All Key Questions

Few trials reported on potential harms of meditation programs. Of the nine trials that reported on harms, none reported any harms of the intervention. One trial specified that they looked for toxicities of meditation to hematologic, renal, and liver markers and found none. The remaining eight trials did not specify the type of adverse event they were looking for. Seven reported that they found no significant adverse events, while one did not comment on adverse events. The remaining 32 trials did not report whether they monitored for adverse events.

Limitations of the Primary Studies

Although we collected information on amount of training provided in the meditation programs, the trials did not provide enough information to make use of that data. The studies generally did not provide enough information to allow us to draw any conclusions about how the effects of the interventions differed among subpopulations, such as racial-ethnic groups, elderly patients, or patients with specific medical or psychiatric conditions. The limited number of trials using various comparators among diverse populations also made using the available information on "dose" of meditation difficult. In addition, we could not rule out selective outcomes reporting and publication bias.

It may be that specific scales may be more relevant for a particular form of meditation. Many of the studies only assessed certain measures and the scales may have been limited in their ability to detect an effect. For example, there was only one measure of attention, and it's possible that this was not a sensitive measure for the populations assessed.

We intended to evaluate the effects of meditation programs on a broad range of medical and psychiatric conditions since psychological stress outcomes are not limited to any particular medical or psychiatric condition. Despite our focus on a subset of meditation programs tested in active controlled RCTs, we were unable to detect a specific effect of meditation on many outcomes, with the majority of our evidence grades being insufficient or low. This was mostly driven by two important evaluation criteria: the risk of bias and the inconsistencies in the body of evidence. The specific reasons for such inconsistencies may have included the differences in the particular clinical conditions, as well as the type of control groups used. When a study compared a meditation program to a specific active control, we could not easily compare these trials with those that used a nonspecific active control. We therefore separated these comparisons to be able to evaluate the effects against a relatively homogenous nonspecific active control group. Comparing trials that used one specific active control to another specific active control led to large inconsistencies that could be explained by differences in the control groups (Figures 26, 28–30, 32, 34–35, 38). The variations in sensitivities of scales that trials used to detect changes from the intervention, and the paucity of trials within each outcome domain, may have also contributed to the inconsistent findings. Another possibility is that there is no real effect of the programs on many of the outcomes that had inconsistent findings. While some of the outcomes were primary outcomes, many were secondary outcomes and the studies may not have been appropriately powered to detect changes in secondary outcomes.

Limitations of the Review

An important decision in setting up this review was the choice to examine only studies that randomized participants to a meditation program or an active control. We chose not to include observational studies or trials with nonactive controls because previews reviews have already examined these types of studies, this methodology increases risk of bias, and leaves questions regarding the specific effects of meditation on clinical outcomes. Observational studies have a particularly high risk of bias in this area of research because of problems such as self-selection of interventions (people are more likely to enroll in a meditation program if they believe in its benefits or have prior experience with meditation) and the use of largely self-reported outcome measures that can be easily biased by participants' beliefs in the benefits of meditation. In making this decision, we restricted our ability to examine longer-term outcomes, including potential harms of meditation. This is an intriguing issue in the literature, as various experts believe that the benefits of meditation increase with practice and may require years for meaningful, clinically relevant changes to occur. Also, because some meditation programs require behavior change and skill development, it is very likely that participants in observational studies are self-selected for personal characteristics that may not generalize to the larger population. This type of longitudinal observational study could be informative once the specific clinical efficacy of an intervention is established. Since the clinical efficacy of meditation programs remains in question, the validity of longitudinal observational studies remains limited.

We generally rated all self-reported outcomes as being direct except for measures of craving or sub measures of negative or positive affect. Some may consider the measures we rated as direct to be indirect, which would further lower the strength of evidence for such ratings. Our assessment of the risk of bias of these trials needs to be interpreted in the light of unique risk-of-bias issues for non-pharmacologic interventions where blinding of intervention is not possible. Thus, using blinded outcome assessors, even for self-report instruments, is one method that reduces risk of bias.

We did not rate the strength of evidence on publication bias. Our review of clinicaltrials.gov registration database did not provide sufficient information on the scales these trials used to measure outcomes, or on the types of controls they used. This did not allow us to verify whether a potentially applicable outcome could have been included in our review.

Stress outcomes encompass both psychological and biological markers, yet we focused only on the psychological markers. This may disappoint some readers and may have reduced the number of TM trials we included, since many recent trials have been more focused on physiologic markers of stress. However, we included studies with measures of psychological stress and well-being, even as secondary outcomes, and these contribute to the overall strength of our review. An interesting challenge for future work is raised by the findings of one particularly strong TM study. Paul-Labrador and colleagues[81] compared TM to a health education control condition in patients with congestive heart failure and found reductions in adjusted systolic blood pressure, heart rate variability, and insulin resistance in the absence of concurrent changes in anxiety, depression, or stress. Given the absence of changes in measures of psychological stress in this study, these authors postulate that meditation may alter the biologic stress response independently of psychological stress responses, a hypothesis that will need to be directly tested in future research.

In addition to limiting our focus to psychological stress and well-being outcomes, we also limited the types of meditation included. We chose not to include other eastern meditative traditions such as qi gong and yoga. These forms typically involve movement and published reports often do not clearly indicate whether the form practiced was purely or mostly meditative. In our initial review of papers for inclusion, we were unable to accurately identify qi gong trials that emphasized movement from those that did not. We also did not include studies in healthy populations.

We selected 5 percent difference in the outcome change scores as being potentially clinically significant and this decision needs to be interpreted in the context of heterogeneous scales reporting on various measures. The literature does not clearly define the appropriate threshold for what is clinically significant on most of these scales. There is variability across measures, and even for those measures that have clinical cut-offs (e.g., many measures of depression), studies rarely reported the change in proportion of study participants meeting these cut-offs following participation in the meditation programs. Some may consider a higher threshold as being clinically relevant. Another limitation is that our method of displaying the relative difference between groups in the change scores from different measurement scales did not take into consideration how the scales varied in the range of scores that were possible. However, we thought this simple method of displaying the data would make it easier for readers to understand the original data. Whenever possible, we also displayed the results using a meta-analysis of standardized mean differences that did account for differences between the measurement scales.

The personal characteristics of individuals (e.g. personality, spirituality, education, etc.) may influence their understanding and skill or abilities in performing meditation. Although trials appeared to recruit individuals with diverse conditions, we are unable to comment on whether individual characteristics of participants influence outcomes. For example, the studies generally did not provide enough information for us to determine whether the effectiveness of mindfulness meditation varied by race, ethnicity, or education.

While this review sought to assess the effectiveness of meditation programs above and beyond the nonspecific effects of time and attention, it did not assess the impact of the preferences of patients. Even though one therapy may not be better than another but is better than doing nothing, many patients may still prefer a particular therapy for personal or philosophical reasons. Further, by reviewing only trials with active controls, we rule out the possibility of an intervention which cultivates high expectations to have a useful effect, particularly when it comes with few to no harms and fits within a person's philosophical mindset.

Future Directions

Further research in meditation would benefit by addressing several methodological and conceptual issues.

First, all forms of meditation, including both mindfulness and mantra, imply that more time spent meditating will yield larger effects, especially in changing health outcomes including psychological stress and well being. Most forms, but not all, also present meditation as a skill in which skill development occurs over time and is most efficiently achieved by learning from an expert. Thus, more training with an expert and practice in daily life should lead to greater competency in the skill or practice, and greater competency or practice would presumably lead to better outcomes. When compared with other skills that require training, the amount of training in the trials we reviewed was quite small and generally offered over a fairly short period of time. Some of this is due to the challenging logistics of conducting RCTs, and some of this is due to the meditation programs tested (e.g., MBSR is a standardized 8-week program). There was little delineation on exactly what skill novice practitioners are acquiring, or measurement or validation that the skill was being practiced and applied. Given that meditation in its historical forms has been a long-term practice, consideration should be given to placing a greater emphasis on developing the skill. To facilitate this, we need better measurement tools. The currently available mindfulness scales have not been well validated and do not appear to distinguish different forms of meditation.[4] Thus, further work on the operationalization and measurement of mindfulness or the particular meditative skill is needed. For those meditation programs that do not believe they are training students in a skill, such as TM and certain mindfulness programs, there is still a need to be able to transparently assess whether a student has attained the mental state or is correctly executing the recommended mental activities (or absence of activities).

Second, trials need to document the amount of training clinicians provide and patients receive, as well as document the amount of home practice patients complete. This gives an indication of how effective the program is at delivering training, how adherent participants were with accepting the intervention, and, in turn, the likelihood these skills will actually be learned and developed by participants. With this type of data, analyses of "dosing" can address the question that remains unclear: how much is enough to accomplish each outcome of interest? As the literature develops and these dosing issues are addressed, RCTs may be indicated to test the effects of dosing on outcome. Amount of training interacts with time to followup and few trials in our review assessed long-term outcomes. One notable exception was the trial by Schneider et al., which followed patients for up to 9 years and assessed effects on mortality.[90] Additional high-quality studies with long-term followups are needed to fully examine the effects of "dosing" and the potential impact of meditation on objective indices of health including mortality.

Third, studies should report teacher qualifications in detail. A highly experienced teacher may have a very different effect than an inexperienced teacher, yet the current literature does not provide enough detail to examine this systematically. Given the numerous uncertainties and difficulties around definitions and measurement of skill in meditation programs, quantifying teacher experience and competence adds yet another level of uncertainty. However, the range of experience in meditation and competence as a teacher of this skill or practice likely plays a role in outcomes.

Fourth, the use of nonspecific active control allows one to infer on the effect of meditation when they are matched for time, attention, and expectancy. When using a specific active control, if one finds no statistically significant superiority over the control one is left with the issue of whether the meditation is equivalent to or not inferior to the control, or whether the trial was just underpowered to detect any difference. Conducting comparative effectiveness trials requires prior specification of the hypothesis (superiority, equivalence, non-inferiority), appropriate determination of the margins of clinical significance, and minimum importance difference.[95] In the case of equivalence and noninferiority trials, trials also need to have appropriate assay sensitivity. None of the trials showed statistically significant effects against a specific active control, nor did they appear adequately powered to assess noninferiority or equivalence. This leaves a lot of uncertainty in such trial designs.

Fifth, positive outcomes are a key focus of meditative practices. However, positive outcomes were not included as primary or even secondary outcomes for most trials. The few exceptions that we reviewed included measures of positive affect, sense of coherence, and vitality. Future studies should expand upon these domains. There are other domains such as self-efficacy, which we did not review, that may also be important outcomes.

Sixth, we were unable to review biologic markers of stress comprehensively for meditation programs, nor were we able to evaluate the effects of meditation programs that involve more movement such as yoga and qi gong, nor did we review the effects on healthy populations. Numerous trials have been conducted in these areas, and meditation research may benefit from a comprehensive review covering these areas. Such reviews would allow for a cross validation of psychological and biological outcomes.

Future trials should appropriately report key design characteristics to enable the assessment of risk of bias. Future trials should register the trial on a national register, standardize training by using trainers who meet specified criteria, specify primary and secondary outcomes *a priori*, power the trial based on the primary outcomes, use CONsolidated Standards of Reporting Trials recommendations for reporting results, and operationalize and measure the practice of meditation by study participants. However, an important part of the process of creating standardized meditation programs, when there is uncertainty around the effect or conceptualization of a particular program, is the innovation and testing of small changes to the existing programs in various contexts. We see this in the mindfulness trials and to a smaller degree in the mantra trials. While this adds a layer of complexity in synthesizing the results of these various programs, we do not intend to hinder the innovation of meditation researchers.

Conclusions

Our review shows that there is moderate strength of evidence that mindfulness meditation programs are beneficial for reducing pain severity, and there is low to moderate strength of evidence that mindfulness meditation programs may lead to improvement in dimensions of negative affect, including anxiety, depression, and perceived stress/general distress. Otherwise, much of the evidence was insufficient to address the comparisons for most of the questions. There were also too few trials of mantra meditation programs to draw meaningful conclusions. There may be many reasons for this lack of evidence.

First, while we sought to review the highest standards of behavioral RCTs, there was wide variation in risk of bias among these. Of 41 RCTs, we only rated 10 as low risk of bias. However, for studies where there is mostly a medium-to-high risk of bias, one might expect to see more positive results. We did not see this.

Second, many if not most studies appeared to be underpowered to find an effect, as we rated most of the studies as imprecise. While this is critical for the individual study, it may not matter as much for a systematic review where we are also concerned with the directionality of effect among numerous studies, irrespective of their statistical significance.

Third, we attempted to analyze the effect meditation programs have on certain domains of mental, emotional, and physical health that are affected by stress. These domains are heterogeneous and studies often report them on different scales, which make it more complicated to analyze. We found modest consistency in improvement on multiple domains of negative affect for mindfulness programs. However, we did not see an effect on positive affect. Due to the limited number of trials we reported, one should view these conclusions cautiously within the context of the particular population studied, type of meditation program used, and type of comparison used.

Fourth, for many outcomes, there was a dearth of adequate studies to draw detailed conclusions. For example, nearly all of the studies assessing pain focused on musculoskeletal pain populations. None assessed neuropathic pain, and only one assessed a visceral pain. We need further studies that better define what outcome is responsive to a particular meditation program.

Fifth, symptom levels may have been low to start with for many trials, not leaving much room to find a difference from an intervention. However, if one purpose of meditation interventions is to improve symptomatology at non-clinical levels, this issue may not be as relevant.

Sixth, the reasons for a lack of a significant reduction of stress-related health behavior outcomes may have to do with the way the research community conceptualizes meditation programs, the difficulties of acquiring such skills or meditative states, and the limited duration of RCTs. Historically, the general public did not conceptualize meditation as a quick fix toward anything. It was a skill or state one learns and practices over time to increase one's awareness; through this awareness one gains insight and understanding into the various subtleties of their existence. Training the mind in awareness, nonjudgementalness, or in the ability to become completely free of thoughts or other activity, are daunting accomplishments. While some meditators may feel that these are easy tasks to do, they likely overestimate their own skills due to a lack of awareness of the different degrees to which these tasks can be done or ability to objectively measure their own progress. Becoming an expert at simple skills such swimming, reading, or writing (which can be objectively measured by others) take a considerable amount of time, so it only follows that meditation would also take a long period of time to master. However many of the studies included in this review were short term (e.g., 2.5 hours a week for 8 weeks) and the participants likely did not achieve a level of expertise needed to improve outcomes that depend on a mastery of our mental and emotional processes. Trials of short duration and training may be insufficient to develop the meditative skills or states necessary to affect stress related outcomes in substantial ways.

References

1. The National Center for Complementary and Alternative Medicine (NCCAM) [Web Page]. http://nccam.nih.gov/ accessed on Jan 2012

2. Barnes PM, Bloom B, Nahin RL. Complementary and alternative medicine use among adults and children: United States, 2007. Natl Health Stat Report 2008; (12):1-23.

3. Goyal M, Haythornthwaite J, Levine D et al. Intensive meditation for refractory pain and symptoms. J Altern Complement Med 2010; 16(6):627-31.

4. Chiesa A, Malinowski P. Mindfulness-based approaches: are they all the same? J Clin Psychol 2011; 67(4):404-24.

5. Ospina MB, Bond TK, Karkhaneh M, Tjosvold L, Vandermeer B, Liang Y et al. Meditation Practices for Health: State of the Research. Evidence Report/Technology Assessment No. 155. (Prepared by the University of Alberta Evidence-based Practice Center under Contract No. 290-02-0023.) AHRQ Publication No. 07-E010. Rockville, MD: Agency for Healthcare Research and Quality. June 2007.

6. Travis F, Shear J. Focused attention, open monitoring and automatic self-transcending: Categories to organize meditations from Vedic, Buddhist and Chinese traditions. Conscious Cogn. 2010 Dec;19(4):1110-8

7. Bishop SR, Lau M, Shapiro S, et al. Mindfulness: A proposed operational definition. Clin Psychol Sci Prac. 2004;11:230-241.

8. Baer, R.A., Smith, G.T., Lykins, E., Button, D., Krietemeyer, J., Sauer, S., & Williams, J. (2008)..onstruct validity of the five facets mindfulness questionnaire in meditating and nonmeditating samples. Assessment, 15, 329342.

9. Baer, R.A., Walsh, E., & Lykins, E. (2009). Assessment of mindfulness. In F. Didonna (Ed.), Clinical handbook of mindfulness (pp. 153168). New York: Springer.

10. Malinowski, P. (2008). Mindfulness as psychological dimension: Concepts and applications. Irish Journal of Psychology, 29, 155166.

11. Chambers R GEAN. Mindful emotion regulation: An integrative review. Clin Psychol Rev 2009; 29(6):560-72.

12. Rapgay L, Bystrisky A. Classical mindfulness: an introduction to its theory and practice for clinical application. Ann N Y Acad Sci 2009; 1172:148-62.

13. Walach H. Review of "Effectiveness of Meditation in Healthcare." www.mum.edu/inmp/walach.html. Accessed February 17, 2012.

14. Orme-Johnson DW. Commentary on the AHRQ report on research on meditation practices in health. J Altern Complement Med 2008; 14(10):1215-21.

15. Bohlmeijer E, Prenger R, Taal E, Cuijpers P. The effects of mindfulness-based stress reduction therapy on mental health of adults with a chronic medical disease: a meta-analysis. J Psychosom Res 2010; 68(6):539-44.

16. Chiesa A, Serretti A. Mindfulness-based stress reduction for stress management in healthy people: a review and meta-analysis. J Altern Complement Med 2009; 15(5):593-600.

17. Chiesa A, Calati R, Serretti A. Does mindfulness training improve cognitive abilities? A systematic review of neuropsychological findings. ClinPsychol Rev 2011; 31(3):449-64.

18. Chiesa A, Serretti A. Mindfulness based cognitive therapy for psychiatric disorders: a systematic review and meta-analysis. Psychiatry Res 2011; 187(3):441-53.

19. Hofmann SG, Sawyer AT, Witt AA, Oh D.. The effect of mindfulness-based therapy on anxiety and depression: A meta-analytic review. J Consult Clin Psychol 2010; 78(2):169-83.

20. Krisanaprakornkit T, Ngamjarus C, Witoonchart C, Piyavhatkul N. Meditation therapies for attention-deficit/hyperactivity disorder (ADHD). Cochrane Database Syst Rev 2010; (6):CD006507.

21. Ledesma D, Kumano H. Mindfulness-based stress reduction and cancer: a meta-analysis. Psychooncology 2009; 18(6):571-9.

22. Matchim Y, Armer JM, Stewart BR. Mindfulness-based stress reduction among breast cancer survivors: a literature review and discussion. Oncol Nurs Forum 2011; 38(2):E61-71.

23. Piet J, Hougaard E. The effect of mindfulness-based cognitive therapy for prevention of relapse in recurrent major depressive disorder: a systematic review and meta-analysis. Clin Psychol Rev 2011; 31(6):1032-40.

24. Wanden-Berghe RG, Sanz-Valero J, Wanden-Berghe C. The application of mindfulness to eating disorders treatment: a systematic review. Eat Disord 2011; 19(1):34-48.

25. Winbush NY, Gross CR, Kreitzer MJ. The effects of mindfulness-based stress reduction on sleep disturbance: a systematic review. Explore (NY) 2007; 3(6):585-91.

26. Zgierska A, Rabago D, Chawla N, Kushner K, Koehler R, Marlatt A. Mindfulness meditation for substance use disorders: a systematic review. Subst Abus 2009; 30(4):266-94.

27. Bernardy K, Fuber N, Kollner V, Hauser W.. Efficacy of cognitive-behavioral therapies in fibromyalgia syndrome—a systematic review and metaanalysis of randomized controlled trials. J Rheumatol 2010; 37(10):1991-2005.

28. Rainforth MV, Schneider RH, Nidich SI, Gaylord-King C, Salerno JW, Anderson JW. Stress reduction programs in patients with elevated blood pressure: a systematic review and meta-analysis. Curr Hypertens Rep 2007; 9(6):520-8.

29. Anderson JW, Liu C, Kryscio RJ. Blood pressure response to transcendental meditation: a meta-analysis. Am J Hypertens 2008; 21(3):310-6.

30. Canter PH, Ernst E. The cumulative effects of Transcendental Meditation on cognitive function—a systematic review of randomised controlled trials. Wien Klin Wochenschr 2003; 115(21-22):758-66.

31. SO KT O-JD. Three randomized experiments on the longitudinal effects of the Transcendental Meditation technique on cognition. Intelligence 2001; 419-40.

32. Travis F GS, Stixrud W. ADHD, Brain Functioning, and Transcendental Meditation Practice. Mind & Brain, The Journal of Psychiatry 2011; 73-81.

33. Chen KW BCMEeal. Meditative therapies for reducing anxiety: a systematic review and meta-analysis of randomized controlled trials. Depress Anxiety 2012; 29(7):545-62.

34. Chambless DL, Hollon SD. Defining empirically supported therapies. J Consult Clin Psychol 1998; 66(1):7-18.

35. Hollon SD, Ponniah K. A review of empirically supported psychological therapies for mood disorders in adults. Depress Anxiety 2010; 27(10):891-932.

36. Moher D, Liberati A, Tetzlaff J, Altman DG, The PRISMA Group . Preferred Reporting Items for Systematic Reviews and Meta-Analyses: The PRISMA Statement. PLoS Med 6(7): e1000097.

37. Meditation Programs for Stress and Well-being—Research protocol [Web Page].

38. Google site http://translate.google.com

39. Bhogal SK, Teasell RW, Foley NC, Speechley MR. The PEDro scale provides a more comprehensive measure of methodological quality than the Jadad scale in stroke rehabilitation literature. J Clin Epidemiol 2005; 58(7):668-73.

40. Chambless DL, Ollendick TH. Empirically supported psychological interventions: controversies and evidence. Annu Rev Psychol 2001; 52:685-716.

41. Patient Reported Outcomes Measurement Information System (PROMIS®). www.nihpromis.org. Accessed August 10, 2011. [Web Page].

42. Cohen J. Statistical power analysis for the behavioral sciences. Hillsdale, NJ: L. Erlbaum Associates; 1988.

43. Lyubomirsky S, King L, Diener E. The benefits of frequent positive affect: does happiness lead to success? Psychol Bull 2005; 131(6):803-55.

44. Clark LA, Watson D. Tripartite model of anxiety and depression: psychometric evidence and taxonomic implications. J Abnorm Psychol 1991; 100(3):316-36.

45. Methods Guide for Effectiveness and Comparative Effectiveness Reviews. Rockville, MD: Agency for Healthcare Research and Quality; August 2007. AHRQ Publication No. 10(11)-EHC063-EF.

46. Higgins JP, Altman DG, Gotzsche PC et al. The Cochrane Collaboration's tool for assessing risk of bias in randomised trials. BMJ 2011; 343:d5928.

47. Higgins JPT, Green S, eds. Cochrane handbook for systematic reviews of Interventions Version 5.1.0. London: The Cochrane Collaboration; Updated March 2011. www.cochrane.org/training/cochrane-handbook. Accessed February 17, 2012.

48. Owens DK LKADeal. AHRQ series paper 5: grading the strength of a body of evidence when comparing medical interventions—agency for healthcare research and quality and the effective health-care program. J Clin Epidemiol 2010; 63(5):513-23.

49. Brewer JA, Sinha R, Chen JA et al. Mindfulness training and stress reactivity in substance abuse: results from a randomized, controlled stage I pilot study. Subst Abus 2009; 30(4):306-17.

50. Brewer JA, Mallik S, Babuscio TA et al. Mindfulness training for smoking cessation: Results from a randomized controlled trial. Drug Alcohol Depend 2011.

51. Delgado LC, Guerra P, Perakakis P, Vera MN, Reyes del Paso G, Vila J. Treating chronic worry: Psychological and physiological effects of a training programme based on mindfulness. Behav Res Ther 2010; 48(9):873-82.

52. Garland EL, Gaylord SA, Boettiger CA, Howard MO. Mindfulness training modifies cognitive, affective, and physiological mechanisms implicated in alcohol dependence: results of a randomized controlled pilot trial. J Psychoactive Drugs 2010; 42(2):177-92.

53. Gaylord SA, Palsson OS, Garland EL et al. Mindfulness training reduces the severity of irritable bowel syndrome in women: results of a randomized controlled trial. Am J Gastroenterol 2011; 106(9):1678-88.

54. Gross CR, Kreitzer MJ, Thomas W et al. Mindfulness-based stress reduction for solid organ transplant recipients: a randomized controlled trial. Altern Ther Health Med 2010; 16(5):30-8.

55. Gross CR, Kreitzer MJ, Reilly-Spong M et al. Mindfulness-based stress reduction versus pharmacotherapy for chronic primary insomnia: a randomized controlled clinical trial. Explore (NY) 2011; 7(2):76-87.

56. Hebert JR, Ebbeling CB, Olendzki BC et al. Change in women's diet and body mass following intensive intervention for early-stage breast cancer. J Am Diet Assoc 2001; 101(4):421-31.

57. Henderson VP, Clemow L, Massion AO, Hurley TG, Druker S, Hebert JR. The effects of mindfulness-based stress reduction on psychosocial outcomes and quality of life in early-stage breast cancer patients: a randomized trial. Breast Cancer Res Treat 2011.

58. Koszycki D, Benger M, Shlik J, Bradwejn J. Randomized trial of a meditation-based stress reduction program and cognitive behavior therapy in generalized social anxiety disorder. Behav Res Ther 2007; 45(10):2518-26.

59. Kuyken W, Byford S, Taylor RS et al. Mindfulness-based cognitive therapy to prevent relapse in recurrent depression. J Consult Clin Psychol 2008; 76(6):966-78.

60. Lee SH, Ahn SC, Lee YJ, Choi TK, Yook KH, Suh SY. Effectiveness of a meditation-based stress management program as an adjunct to pharmacotherapy in patients with anxiety disorder. J Psychosom Res 2007; 62(2):189-95.

61. Malarkey WB, Jarjoura D, Klatt M. Workplace based mindfulness practice and inflammation: A randomized trial. Brain Behav Immun 2012.

62. Miller CK, Kristeller JL, Headings A, Nagaraja H, Miser WF. Comparative Effectiveness of a Mindful Eating Intervention to a Diabetes Self-Management Intervention among Adults with Type 2 Diabetes: A Pilot Study. J Acad Nutr Diet 2012; 112(11):1835-42.

63. Moritz S, Quan H, Rickhi B et al. A home study-based spirituality education program decreases emotional distress and increases quality of life—a randomized, controlled trial. Altern Ther Health Med 2006; 12(6):26-35.

64. Morone NE, Rollman BL, Moore CG, Li Q, Weiner DK. A mind-body program for older adults with chronic low back pain: results of a pilot study. Pain Med 2009; 10(8):1395-407.

65. Mularski RA, Munjas BA, Lorenz KA et al. Randomized controlled trial of mindfulness-based therapy for dyspnea in chronic obstructive lung disease. J Altern Complement Med 2009; 15(10):1083-90.

66. Oken BS, Fonareva I, Haas M et al. Pilot controlled trial of mindfulness meditation and education for dementia caregivers. J Altern Complement Med 2010; 16(10):1031-8.

67. Philippot P, Nef F, Clauw L, Romree M, Segal Z. A Randomized Controlled Trial of Mindfulness-Based Cognitive Therapy for Treating Tinnitus. Clin Psychol Psychother 2011.

68. Piet J, Hougaard E, Hecksher MS, Rosenberg NK. A randomized pilot study of mindfulness-based cognitive therapy and group cognitive-behavioral therapy for young adults with social phobia. Scand J Psychol 2010; 51(5):403-10.

69. Plews-Ogan M, Owens JE, Goodman M, Wolfe P, Schorling J. A pilot study evaluating mindfulness-based stress reduction and massage for the management of chronic pain. J Gen Intern Med 2005; 20(12):1136-8.

70. Schmidt S, Grossman P, Schwarzer B, Jena S, Naumann J, Walach H. Treating fibromyalgia with mindfulness-based stress reduction: results from a 3-armed randomized controlled trial. Pain 2011; 152(2):361-9.

71. Segal ZV, Bieling P, Young T et al. Antidepressant monotherapy vs sequential pharmacotherapy and mindfulness-based cognitive therapy, or placebo, for relapse prophylaxis in recurrent depression. Arch Gen Psychiatry 2010; 67(12):1256-64.

72. Whitebird RR, Kreitzer M, Crain AL, Lewis BA, Hanson LR, Enstad CJ. Mindfulness-Based Stress Reduction for Family Caregivers: A Randomized Controlled Trial. Gerontologist 2012.

73. Wolever RQ, Bobinet KJ, McCabe K et al. Effective and viable mind-body stress reduction in the workplace: a randomized controlled trial. J Occup Health Psychol 2012; 17(2):246-58.

74. Wong SY, Chan FW, Wong RL et al. Comparing the Effectiveness of Mindfulness-based Stress Reduction and Multidisciplinary Intervention Programs for Chronic Pain: A Randomized Comparative Trial. Clin J Pain 2011; 27(8):724-34.

75. Bormann JE, Gifford AL, Shively M et al. Effects of spiritual mantram repetition on HIV outcomes: a randomized controlled trial. J Behav Med 2006; 29(4):359-76.

76. Castillo-Richmond A, Schneider RH, Alexander CN et al. Effects of stress reduction on carotid atherosclerosis in hypertensive African Americans. Stroke 2000; 31(3):568-73.

77. Elder C, Aickin M, Bauer V, Cairns J, Vuckovic N. Randomized trial of a whole-system ayurvedic protocol for type 2 diabetes. Altern Ther Health Med 2006; 12(5):24-30.

78. Jayadevappa R, Johnson JC, Bloom BS et al. Effectiveness of transcendental meditation on functional capacity and quality of life of African Americans with congestive heart failure: a randomized control study Ethn Dis. 2007 Summer;17(3):595. Ethnicity & Disease 2007; 17(1):72-7.

79. Lehrer PM. Progressive relaxation and meditation: A study of psychophysiological and therapeutic differences between two techniques. Behav Res Ther 1983; 21(6):651-62.

80. Murphy TJ, Pagano RR, Marlatt GA. Lifestyle modification with heavy alcohol drinkers: effects of aerobic exercise and meditation. Addict Behav 1986; 11(2):175-86.

81. Paul-Labrador M, Polk D, Dwyer JH et al. Effects of a randomized controlled trial of transcendental meditation on components of the metabolic syndrome in subjects with coronary heart disease. Arch Intern Med 2006; 166(11):1218-24.

82. Sheppard II WD, Staggers Jr. FJ, John L. The effects of a stress management program in a high security government agency. 1997; 10(4):341-50.

83. Smith JC. Psychotherapeutic effects of transcendental meditation with controls for expectation of relief and daily sitting. J Consult Clin Psychol 1976; 44(4):630-7.

84. Taub E, Steiner SS, Weingarten E, Walton KG. Effectiveness of broad spectrum approaches to relapse prevention in severe alcoholism: A long-term, randomized, controlled trial of Transcendental Meditation, EMG biofeedback and electronic neurotherapy. Alcoholism Treatment Quarterly 1994; 11(1-2):187-220.

85. Barrett B, Hayney MS, Muller D et al. Meditation or exercise for preventing acute respiratory infection: a randomized controlled trial. Ann Fam Med 2012; 10(4):337-46.

86. Chiesa A, Mandelli L, Serretti A. Mindfulness-based cognitive therapy versus psycho-education for patients with major depression who did not achieve remission following antidepressant treatment: a preliminary analysis. J Altern Complement Med 2012; 18(8):756-60.

87. Jazaieri H, Goldin PR, Werner K, Ziv M, Gross JJ. A Randomized Trial of MBSR Versus Aerobic Exercise for Social Anxiety Disorder. J Clin Psychol 2012.

88. Pbert L, Madison JM, Druker S et al. Effect of mindfulness training on asthma quality of life and lung function: A randomised controlled trial. 2012; 67(9):769-76.

89. SeyedAlinaghi S, Jam S, Foroughi M et al. Randomized controlled trial of mindfulness-based stress reduction delivered to human immunodeficiency virus-positive patients in Iran: effects on CD4[sup]+[/sup] T lymphocyte count and medical and psychological symptoms. Psychosom Med 2012; 74(6):620-7.

90. Schneider RH, Grim CE, Rainforth MV et al. Stress Reduction in the Secondary Prevention of Cardiovascular Disease: Randomized, Controlled Trial of Transcendental Meditation and Health Education in Blacks. (1941-7705 (Electronic). 1941-7713 (Linking)).

91. Pipe TB, Bortz JJ, Dueck A, Pendergast D, Buchda V, Summers J. Nurse leader mindfulness meditation program for stress management: a randomized controlled trial. J Nurs Adm 2009; 39(3):130-7.

92. Fournier JC, DeRubeis RJ, Hollon SD, et al. Antidepressant drug effects and depression severity: a patient-level meta-analysis. JAMA. Jan 6 2010;303(1):47-53.

93. Krisanaprakornkit T, Krisanaprakornkit W, Piyavhatkul N, Laopaiboon M. Meditation therapy for anxiety disorders. Cochrane Database Syst Rev 2006; (1):CD004998.

94. Veehof MM, Oskam MJ, Schreurs KM, Bohlmeijer ET. Acceptance-based interventions for the treatment of chronic pain: a systematic review and meta-analysis. Pain 2011; 152(3):533-42.

95. Treadwell JR, Singh S, Talati R, et al. A Framework for "Best Evidence" Approaches in Systematic Reviews. Methods Research Report (Prepared by the ECRI Institute Evidence-based Practice Center under Contract No. HHSA 290-2007-10063-I). Rockville, MD: Agency for Healthcare Research and Quality; June 2011. AHRQ Publication No. 11-EHC046-EF.

Appendix A. Abbreviations and Glossary of Terms

Table A1. Abbreviations and acronyms

Abbreviation/Acronym	Explanation
AC	Active Control
ASG	Alcohol dependence Support Group
BAI	Beck Anxiety Index
BDI	Beck Depression Inventory
BSI	Brief Symptom Inventory
CBGT	Cognitive Behavioral Group Therapy
CESD	Center for Epidemiologic Studies Depression Scale
CHF	Congestive heart failure
COPD	Chronic obstructive pulmonary disease
CSM	Clinically Standardized Meditation
FFS	Freedom From Smoking Treatment
HE	Health Education
IBS	irritable bowel syndrome
IPAT	Institute for Personality and Ability Testing
Kcal/d	Kilocalorie per day
LSQ	Life Stress Ins Q
M-ADM	Maintenance Antidepressant Mono-Therapy
MBBT	Mindfulness-based Breathing Therapy
MBCT	Mindfulness-based Cognitive Therapy
MBRP	Mindfulness-based Relapse Prevention
MBSR	Mindfulness Based Stress Reduction
MG	Mindfulness Group/Mindfulness Treatment Group
MORE	Mindfulness-oriented Recovery Enhancement
MP	Meditation Program
MPI	Multidisciplinary Pain Intervention
MT	Mindfulness Training
NE	Nutrition Education
NEP	Nutrition Education Program
NP	Not Provided
NRS	Numeric Rating Scale
OM	Other Mantra (any mantra program other than TM)
P+CL	Placebo Plus Clinical Management
PANAS	Positive and Negative Affect Scale/Schedule
PANAS-N	Positive and Negative Affect Scale—Negative mood
PCT	Pharmacotherapy
POMS	Profile of Mood States
PMR	Progressive muscular relaxation
PPS	Pain Perception (Sensory)
PSQL	Pittsburgh Sleep Quality Index
PSS	Perceived Stress Scale
RG	Relaxation Treatment Group
RL	Progressive Muscle Relaxation Group
SCID	Structured Clinical Interview
SCL	Symptom Checklist
SCL90	Symptom Checklist 90
SCL90-GSI	Symptom Checklist 90 Global Severity Index
SF12:MC	Short Form-12: Mental Component Score of Health-related Quality of Life
SF36	Short Form-36
SF36:MC	Short Form 36: Mental Component Score of Health-related Quality of Life
SG	Support Group
SIAS	Social Interaction Scale
SP	Spiritual Meditation Group
SRDS	Self-rating Depression Scale
STAI	State Trait Anxiety Index

Abbreviation/Acronym	Explanation
TM	Transcendental Meditation
VR36	Veterans RAND 36 Item Health Survey
WHOQL	World Health Organization Quality of Life Assessment

Appendix Table A2. Glossary

Term	Definition
Affect	A clinical term that refers to emotion or mood. It can be positive, such as the feeling of well-being, or negative, such as anxiousness, depression, or stress. Studies usually measure affect through self-reported questionnaires designed to gauge how much someone experiences a particular affect.
Attrition	A reduction in sample size due to withdrawal of study participants
Difference in change	An analytic strategy that factors in baseline measurements of both the treatment group and control group in examining the effect of a treatment.
Intent-to-treat (ITT)	An analytic strategy that includes all patients based on their original assignment in a randomized controlled trial. This allows for more accurate assessment of the effectiveness of an intervention as everyone who is initially randomized is included in the analysis, regardless of their completion of the trial.
Mantra meditation	Any mantra meditation program, including transcendental meditation (TM), Clinically standardized meditation, or other mantra-based program
Meta-analysis	A statistical method of combining results from a group of research findings in order to determine patterns and an overall effect size (i.e., strength of a relationship).
Mindfulness meditation	Any mindfulness meditation program, including mindfulness-based stress reduction (MBSR), mindfulness-based cognitive therapy (MBCT), or other variation
Modified mindfulness program	Any mindfulness program that has used a variation of MBSR or other Buddhist-based mindfulness technique
Nonspecific active control	A nonspecific active control only matches time and attention, and is not a known therapy
Other Mantra	Any mantra program other than transcendental meditation (TM)
Percent difference in change	Percent change that the difference in change (see above) represents from baseline.
Randomization	A process whereby participants in a research study are assigned to a treatment(s) or control group(s) by chance (i.e., there is an equal possibility that they will be assigned to either group(s)). This allows for equal allocation of factors that may impact study results (e.g., age, gender, race, etc.) in each group.
Scale	An instrument to measure something. Examples include the Perceived Stress Scale or the SF 36 Mental Health subscale.
Specific active control	A specific active control compares the intervention to another known therapy, such as progressive muscle relaxation.
Standardized mean difference	A statistic in meta-analysis when studies that assess an outcome using a variety of measures are made standard on a scale for a more direct comparison.

Appendix B. Detailed Search Strategies

PubMed
meditation[mh] OR meditat*[tiab] OR mindful*[tiab] OR transcendental Meditation[mh] OR "transcendental Meditation"[tiab] OR "mindfulness-based cognitive therapy"[tiab] OR "MBCT"[tiab] OR "mindfulness-based stress reduction"[tiab] OR "MBSR"[tiab] OR Vipassana[tiab] OR zen[tiab] OR Qi-gong[tiab] OR Qigong[tiab] OR Chi kung[tiab] OR Tai Chi[tiab] OR TaiChi[tiab] OR tai ji[mh] OR Yoga[mh] OR yoga[tiab] OR Yogic[tiab] OR dhyana[tiab] OR asana[tiab] OR pranayama[tiab] OR sudarshan[tiab]

CINAHL
TI meditat* OR SU meditation OR TI mindful* OR SU mindfulness OR TI "transcendental Meditation" OR SU transcendental Meditation OR TI "mindfulness-based cognitive therapy" OR TI "MBCT" OR TI "mindfulness-based stress reduction" OR TI "MBSR" OR TI Vipassana OR TI zen OR TI Qigong OR TI Qi gong OR SU Qigong OR TI Chi kung OR TI Tai Chi OR TI TaiChi OR SU Tai Chi OR TI Yoga OR SU yoga OR TI dhyana OR TI asana OR TI pranayama OR TI sudarshan

PsycINFO
TI meditat* OR SU meditation OR TI mindful* OR SU mindfulness OR TI "transcendental Meditation" OR SU transcendental Meditation OR TI "mindfulness-based cognitive therapy" OR TI "MBCT" OR TI "mindfulness-based stress reduction" OR TI "MBSR" OR TI Vipassana OR TI zen OR TI Qigong OR TI Qi gong OR SU Qigong OR TI Chi kung OR TI Tai Chi OR TI TaiChi OR SU Tai Chi OR TI Yoga OR SU yoga OR TI dhyana OR TI asana OR TI pranayama OR TI sudarshan

PsycARTICLES
TI meditat* OR SU meditation OR TI mindful* OR SU mindfulness OR TI "transcendental Meditation" OR SU transcendental Meditation OR TI "mindfulness-based cognitive therapy" OR TI "MBCT" OR TI "mindfulness-based stress reduction" OR TI "MBSR" OR TI Vipassana OR TI zen OR TI Qigong OR TI Qi gong OR SU Qigong OR TI Chi kung OR TI Tai Chi OR TI TaiChi OR SU Tai Chi OR TI Yoga OR SU yoga OR TI dhyana OR TI asana OR TI pranayama OR TI sudarshan

Scopus
(KEY(meditation) OR TITLE(meditation) OR KEY(mindfulness) OR TITLE(mindfulness) OR TITLE("transcendental Meditation") OR TITLE("mindfulness-based cognitive therapy") OR TITLE("MBCT") OR TITLE("mindfulness-based stress reduction") OR TITLE("MBSR") OR KEY(yoga) OR TITLE(yoga) OR TITLE-ABS-KEY(vipassana) OR TITLE-ABS-KEY(tai chi) OR TITLE-ABS-KEY(qigong) OR TITLE-ABS-KEY(chi kung) OR TITLE-ABS-KEY(dhyana) OR TITLE-ABS-KEY(asana) OR TITLE-ABS-KEY(pranayama) OR TITLE-ABS-KEY(sudarshan))

Cochrane

ID	Search
#1	(meditation):ti,ab,kw
#2	MeSH descriptor Meditation, this term only
#3	(meditation):ti or (meditation):kw
#4	(#2 OR #3)
#5	MeSH descriptor Tai Ji explode tree 1
#6	MeSH descriptor Yoga explode tree 1
#7	(#4 OR #5 OR #6)
#8	(Vipassana):ti or (Vipassana):kw or (zen):ti or (zen):kw or (Qigong):ti
#9	(#7 OR #8)
#10	"Tai Chi":ti or "Tai Chi":kw or (yoga):ti or (yoga):kw or (dhyana):kw
#11	(#9 OR #10)
#12	(Qigong):kw or (asana):ti or (asana):kw or (pranayama):ti or (pranayama):kw
#13	(#11 OR #12)

Embase

'meditation'/exp/mj OR meditat*:ab,ti OR mindful*:ab,ti OR transcendental AND meditation:ab,ti OR 'transcendental meditation':ab,ti OR 'mindfulness-based cognitive therapy':ab,ti OR 'mbct':ab,ti OR 'mindfulness-based stress reduction':ab,ti OR 'mbsr':ab,ti OR vipassana:ab,ti OR zen:ab,ti OR 'qi gong':ab,ti OR qigong:ab,ti OR chi AND kung:ab,ti OR tai AND chi:ab,ti OR taichi:ab,ti OR tai AND ji:ab,ti OR yoga:ab,ti OR yogic:ab,ti OR dhyana:ab,ti OR asana:ab,ti OR pranayama:ab,ti OR sudarshan:ab,ti AND [humans]/lim

AMED

Meditation (TI) OR Meditation (Sh) OR Mindfulness (TI) OR Mindfulness (Sh) OR Transcendental Meditation (TI) OR Transcendental Meditation (Sh) OR Mindfulness-based cognitive therapy (TI) OR Mindfulness-based cognitive therapy (Sh) OR MBCT (TI) OR MBCT (Sh) OR Mindfulness-Based Stress Reduction(TI) OR Mindfulness-Based Stress Reduction (Sh) OR MBSR (TI) OR MBSR (Sh) OR Vipassana (TI) OR Vipassana (Sh) OR Zen (TI) OR Zen (Sh) OR Qi-gong(TI) OR Qi-gong (Sh) OR Qigong(TI) OR Qigong (Sh) OR Chi kung (TI) OR Chi kung (Sh) OR Tai Chi(TI) OR Tai Chi(Sh) OR TaiChi(TI) OR TaiChi (Sh) OR Tai ji(TI) OR Tai ji(Sh) OR Yoga (TI) OR Yoga(Sh) OR Yogic(TI) OR Yogic(Sh) OR Dhyana(TI) OR Dhyana(Sh) OR Asana(TI) OR Asana(Sh) OR Pranayama(TI) OR Pranayama(Sh) OR Surdarshan(TI) OR Surdarshan(Sh)

Appendix C. Screening Forms

Title—Abstract Review
Selected—No

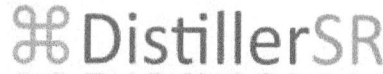 dsleicher

Project Meditation (Switch) User mreuben (My Settings)
Messages 3 new

Live Support | User Guide

Review | Datarama | Reports | References | Forms | Manage Levels | Users | Project | Logout

Refid: 12, Skateboards: Are they really perilous? A retrospective study from a district hospital.
Rethnam U, Yesupalan RS, Sinha A.

[Submit Form] and go to [ ] or Skip to Next

1. **Does this article POTENTIALLY apply to ANY of the key questions?**

   ⦿ NO, this article DOES NOT apply to any of the Key Questions (check all of the following reasons that apply)

   ☐ No original data (systematic reviews, editorial, commentary, letters, meta-analysis)
   ☐ Other meditation form-DBT,ACT,CBT, IMBT
   ☐ Study only includes children, adolescent(0-18years)
   ☐ No Control group
   ☐ Not Randomized
   ☐ Not relevant to key questions
   ☐ Other   [   ]

   ○ Yes, this article may apply to the key questions
   ○ Unclear-get it for article review

Please click below to see:
key questions

[Submit Form] and go to [ ] or Skip to Next

**Article Review
Selected—Yes**

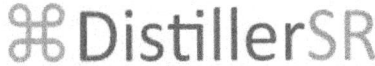 dsleicher

Project	Meditation (Switch) User mreuben (My Settings)
Messages	3 new

Live Support | User Guide

Review | Datarama | Reports | References | Forms | Manage Levels | Users | Project | Logout

Refid: 12, Skateboards: Are they really perilous? A retrospective study from a district hospital.
Rethnam U, Yesupalan RS, Sinha A.

[SubmitPart] and go to [   ] or Skip to Next

1. Is this article in **English**:

   ⊙ Yes
   ○ No

2. **Does this article POTENTIALLY apply to ANY of the key questions?**

   ○ NO, this article DOES NOT apply to any of the Key Questions (check all of the following reasons that apply)
   ⊙ Yes, this article may apply to the key questions

Please select the type of meditation (choose **ALL** that apply):

☐ Yoga
☐ Tai Chi
☐ Qi Gong
☐ Mindfulness Meditation
☐ TM
☐ Other [   ]

Does this study address sleep or substance use outcomes:

○ Yes
○ No
Clear Response

Please select the **Population type:**

○ Healthy
○ Clinical - Please specify: [   ]

Please select the **control type**:

○ Wait list or Usual care only
○ Active control or Other active treatment

Comments:
[   ]

[SubmitPart] and go to [   ] or Skip to Next

**Article Review
Selected—No**

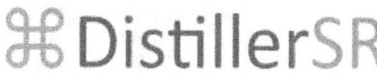

Project	Meditation (Switch) User mreuben (My Settings)
Messages	3 new

Live Support | User Guide

Review | Datarama | Reports | References | Forms | Manage Levels | Users | Project | Logout

---

Refid: 12, Skateboards: Are they really perilous? A retrospective study from a district hospital.
Rethnam U, Yesupalan RS, Sinha A.

[SubmitForm] and go to [ ] or Skip to Next

1. Is this article in **English**:

   ○ Yes
   ⊙ No

2. **Does this article POTENTIALLY apply to ANY of the key questions?**

   ⊙ NO, this article DOES NOT apply to any of the Key Questions (check all of the following reasons that apply)

   ☐ No original data (systematic reviews, editorial, commentary, letters, meta-analysis)
   ☐ Meeting abstracts
   ☐ Other meditation form -DBT, ACT, CBT, IMBT
   ☐ Study only includes children, adolescent(0-18years)
   ☐ No Control group
   ☐ Not Randomized
   ☐ Not relevant to key questions
   ☐ Movement-based meditation -Yoga, TaiChi, Qi Gong
   ☐ Other   [   ]

   ○ Yes, this article may apply to the key questions

Comments:
[   ]

[SubmitForm] and go to [ ] or Skip to Next

Study Characteristics
Selected—Yes

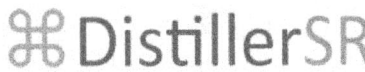

| Project | Meditation (Switch) | User | mreuben (My Settings) |
| Messages | 3 new | | |

Live Support   User Guide

Review | Datarama | Reports | References | Forms | Manage Levels | Users | Project | Logout

Refid: 12, Skateboards: Are they really perilous? A retrospective study from a district hospital.
Rethnam U, Yesupalan RS, Sinha A.

[Submit Form] and go to [   ] or Skip to Next

1. After full review of this article, does it apply to, and contain abstractable data to answer any key questions?

   ⦿ Yes
   ○ No -please provide reason [   ]

2. Where did the study occur? (Check all that apply)

   ○ United States
   ○ Canada
   ○ United Kingdom
   ○ Japan
   ○ China
   ○ India
   ○ Multi-national Europe
   ○ Worldwide
   ○ Other (specify): [   ]
   ○ Not reported

3. Study setting

   ○ Outpatient
   ○ Inpatient
   ○ Meditation center
   ○ Other -please specify [   ]

Recruitment/Enrollment

   ☐ Start Year [   ]
   ☐ End Year [   ]
   ☐ Not Reported [   ]

5. Total duration of study (including training and participants follow-up)

   ○ Please specify: [   ]
   ○ Not Reported

Please specify Inclusion/Exclusion criteria for all populations

Age (specify)

○ Inclusion [ ] ○ Exclusion [ ] ○ Not Reported

Understands English
○ Inclusion [ ] ○ Exclusion [ ] ○ Not Reported

Substance use or dependence
○ Inclusion [ ] ○ Exclusion [ ] ○ Not Reported

Significant psychiatric condition - please specify
○ Inclusion [ ] ○ Exclusion [ ] ○ Not Reported

Significant medical condition - please specify
○ Inclusion [ ] ○ Exclusion [ ] ○ Not Reported

Already trained in or currently practices meditation/ stress reduction technique
○ Inclusion [ ] ○ Exclusion [ ] ○ Not Reported

Other please specify
○ Inclusion [ ] ○ Exclusion [ ] ○ Not Reported

Other please specify
○ Inclusion [ ] ○ Exclusion [ ] Clear Response

Other please specify
○ Inclusion [ ] ○ Exclusion [ ] ○ Not Reported

Other please specify
○ Inclusion [ ] ○ Exclusion [ ] Clear Response

Other please specify
○ Inclusion [ ] ○ Exclusion [ ] Clear Response

Other please specify
○ Inclusion [ ] ○ Exclusion [ ] ○ Not Reported

Other please specify
○ Inclusion [ ] ○ Exclusion [ ] Clear Response

Other please specify
○ Inclusion [ ] ○ Exclusion [ ] ○ Not Reported

Other please specify
○ Inclusion [ ] ○ Exclusion [ ] Clear Response

Other please specify
○ Inclusion [ ]   ○ Exclusion [ ]   Clear Response

Other please specify
○ Inclusion [ ]   ○ Exclusion [ ]   Clear Response

Other please specify
○ Inclusion [ ]   ○ Exclusion [ ]   Clear Response

R2 only: If you are reviewing R1 data entry, enter you initials when you have completed the audit

[Submit Form] and go to [ ] or Skip to Next

Study Characteristics
Selected—No

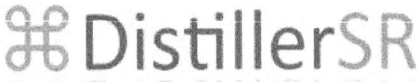

Project: Meditation (Switch) User: mreuben (My Settings)
Messages: 3 new

Live Support | User Guide

Review | Datarama | Reports | References | Forms | Manage Levels | Users | Project | Logout

Refid: 12, Skateboards: Are they really perilous? A retrospective study from a district hospital.
Rethnam U, Yesupalan RS, Sinha A.

[Submit Form] and go to [ ] or Skip to Next

1. After full review of this article, does it apply to, and contain abstractable data to answer any key questions?

○ Yes
⦿ No -please provide reason [ ]

R2 only: If you are reviewing R1 data entry, enter you initials when you have completed the audit

[Submit Form] and go to [ ] or Skip to Next

**Participant Characteristics
Selected—Reported**

32. Race/ethnicity
◉ Reported

	Overall Group	Arm 1 (Meditation)	Arm 2	Arm 3	Arm 4	Arm 5	Arm 6
White, non-Hispanic	33. ☐ n ☐ %	34. ☐ n ☐ %	35. ☐ n ☐ %	36. ☐ n ☐ %	37. ☐ n ☐ %	38. ☐ n ☐ %	39. ☐ n ☐ %
Black, non-Hispanic	40. ☐ n ☐ %	41. ☐ n ☐ %	42. ☐ n ☐ %	43. ☐ n ☐ %	44. ☐ n ☐ %	45. ☐ n ☐ %	46. ☐ n ☐ %
Latino/Hispanic	47. ☐ n ☐ %	48. ☐ n ☐ %	49. ☐ n ☐ %	50. ☐ n ☐ %	51. ☐ n ☐ %	52. ☐ n ☐ %	53. ☐ n ☐ %
Asian/Pacific Islander	54. ☐ n ☐ %	55. ☐ n ☐ %	56. ☐ n ☐ %	57. ☐ n ☐ %	58. ☐ n ☐ %	59. ☐ n ☐ %	60. ☐ n ☐ %
American Indian/Alaska Native	61. ☐ n ☐ %	62. ☐ n ☐ %	63. ☐ n ☐ %	64. ☐ n ☐ %	65. ☐ n ☐ %	66. ☐ n ☐ %	67. ☐ n ☐ %
Other	69. ☐ n ☐ %	70. ☐ n ☐ %	71. ☐ n ☐ %	72. ☐ n ☐ %	73. ☐ n ☐ %	74. ☐ n ☐ %	75. ☐ n ☐ %
Other	77. ☐ n ☐ %	78. ☐ n ☐ %	79. ☐ n ☐ %	80. ☐ n ☐ %	81. ☐ n ☐ %	82. ☐ n ☐ %	83. ☐ n ☐ %
Other	85. ☐ n ☐ %	86. ☐ n ☐ %	87. ☐ n ☐ %	88. ☐ n ☐ %	89. ☐ n ☐ %	90. ☐ n ☐ %	91. ☐ n ☐ %

○ not reported

92. Education
◉ Reported

	Overall Group	Arm 1 (Meditation)	Arm 2	Arm 3	Arm 4	Arm 5	Arm 6
< High School	93. ☐ n ☐ %	94. ☐ n ☐ %	95. ☐ n ☐ %	96. ☐ n ☐ %	97. ☐ n ☐ %	98. ☐ n ☐ %	99. ☐ n ☐ %
Completed High School	100. ☐ n ☐ %	101. ☐ n ☐ %	102. ☐ n ☐ %	103. ☐ n ☐ %	104. ☐ n ☐ %	105. ☐ n ☐ %	106. ☐ n ☐ %
College Degree	107. ☐ n ☐ %	108. ☐ n ☐ %	109. ☐ n ☐ %	110. ☐ n ☐ %	111. ☐ n ☐ %	112. ☐ n ☐ %	113. ☐ n ☐ %

Post-graduate Degree	114. ☐ n ☐ %	115. ☐ n ☐ %	116. ☐ n ☐ %	117. ☐ n ☐ %	118. ☐ n ☐ %	119. ☐ n ☐ %	120. ☐ n ☐ %
Years of education	121. ☐ mean ☐ median ☐ min ☐ max	122. ☐ mean ☐ median ☐ min ☐ max	123. ☐ mean ☐ median ☐ min ☐ max	124. ☐ mean ☐ median ☐ min ☐ max	125. ☐ mean ☐ median ☐ min ☐ max	126. ☐ mean ☐ median ☐ min ☐ max	127. ☐ mean ☐ median ☐ min ☐ max
Other	129. ☐ n ☐ %	130. ☐ n ☐ %	131. ☐ n ☐ %	132. ☐ n ☐ %	133. ☐ n ☐ %	134. ☐ n ☐ %	135. ☐ n ☐ %
Other	137. ☐ n ☐ %	138. ☐ n ☐ %	139. ☐ n ☐ %	140. ☐ n ☐ %	141. ☐ n ☐ %	142. ☐ n ☐ %	143. ☐ n ☐ %
Other	145. ☐ n ☐ %	146. ☐ n ☐ %	147. ☐ n ☐ %	148. ☐ n ☐ %	149. ☐ n ☐ %	150. ☐ n ☐ %	151. ☐ n ☐ %

○ not reported

152. BMI

○ reported

Overall Group	Arm 1 (Meditation)	Arm 2	Arm 3	Arm 4	Arm 5	Arm 6
153. ☐ mean ☐ Median ☐ Range	154. ☐ mean ☐ Median ☐ Range	155. ☐ mean ☐ Median ☐ Range	156. ☐ mean ☐ Median ☐ Range	157. ☐ mean ☐ Median ☐ Range	158. ☐ mean ☐ median ☐ range	159. ☐ mean ☐ median ☐ range

○ not reported

160. Weight

○ reported

Overall Group	Arm 1 (Meditation)	Arm 2	Arm 3	Arm 4	Arm 5	Arm 6
161. ☐ mean ☐ Median ☐ Range	162. ☐ mean ☐ Median ☐ Range	163. ☐ mean ☐ Median ☐ Range	164. ☐ mean ☐ Median ☐ Range	165. ☐ mean ☐ Median ☐ Range	166. ☐ mean ☐ median ☐ range	167. ☐ mean ☐ median ☐ range

○ not reported

168. If any of above characteristics differs by group, please describe

169. R2 only: if you are reviewing R1 data entry, enter your initials when you have completed the audit

DistillerSR

[Submit Form] and go to [ ] or Skip to Next

Intervention Characteristics
Arm A

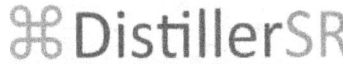

ritu.sharma

Project	Meditation (Switch) User mreuben (My Settings)
Messages	3 new

Live Support | User Guide

Review | Datarama | Reports | References | Forms | Manage Levels | Users | Project | Logout

Refid: 12, Skateboards: Are they really perilous? A retrospective study from a district hospital.
Rethnam U, Yesupalan RS, Sinha A.

[Submit Form] and go to [ ] or Skip to Next
This is a "multi-form" meaning you can fill out the same form multiple time (i.e., a different set of data is entered for each study arms."

1. Please select the arm and specify

⊙ Arm A(Meditation)
   Please select the intervention
   ○ MBSR
   ○ MBCT
   ○ Vipassana
   ○ Zen
   ○ Mantra Meditation
   ○ TM
   ○ Meditative prayer
   ○ Sahaj yoga
   ○ Dhyan yoga
   ○ Other (e.g. composite interventions) - please specify [ ]
   Clear Response

3. Delivery of Intervention
   ☐ Group
   ☐ Individual
   ☐ Other-please specify [ ]

Frequency of Traning Intervention (how many times per day/week)

4. How many times	5. Per day/week
○ Once	○ Daily
○ Twice	○ Weekly
○ Other - please specify [ ]	○ Biweekly
	○ Monthly
	○ Other-please specify [ ]

Duration of Intervention

6.	7.
☐ Number of sessions [ ]	○ Length of time per session (hrs) [ ]
☐ Not Reported	○ Not Reported
☐ Other/additional sessions - please specify [ ]	

Total Duration of Training

8.	9.
☐ Total numbers of weeks [ ]	☐ Total hours [ ]
☐ Not Reported	☐ Not Reported
☐ Other - please specify [ ]	

Detail of Trainers

10. Number of trainers	11. Did a trained meditation instructor(s) deliver the intervention	12. Qualifications of Trainers	13. Year of meditation/teaching experience
☐ Enter number of trainers [ ] ☐ Not Reported	○ Yes ○ No ○ Not Reported	○ Certified ○ Not Certified ○ Not Reported ○ Other [ ]	☐ Years of meditation practice [ ] ☐ Years of teaching experience [ ] ☐ Other-Please Specify [ ] ☐ Not Reported

Frequency of HOME PRACTICE (how many times per day/week)

14. How many times	15. Per day/week
○ Once ○ Twice ○ Other - please specify [ ] ○ Not Reported	○ Daily ○ Weekly ○ Biweekly ○ Monthly ○ Other-please specify [ ] ○ Not Reported Clear Response

16. How much time per home session in minutes

- ○ 5 minutes
- ○ 10 minutes
- ○ 15 minutes
- ○ Other - please specify [ ]
- ○ Not Reported

17. Total home practice (hrs)

- ☐ Total number of hrs [ ]
- ☐ Not Reported

○ Arm B-specify
○ Arm C-specify
○ Arm D -Usual Care

37. R2 only: if you are reviewing R1 data entry, enter your initials when you have completed the audit

[ ]

[Submit Form] and go to [ ] or Skip to Next

Intervention Arm B (same for Arm C)

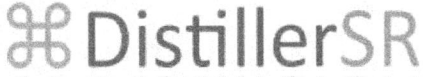
ritu.sharma

| Project | Meditation (Switch) | User | mreuben (My Settings) |
| Messages | 3 new | | |

Live Support | User Guide

Review | Datarama | Reports | References | Forms | Manage Levels | Users | Project | Logout

---

Refid: 12, Skateboards: Are they really perilous? A retrospective study from a district hospital.
Rethnam U, Yesupalan RS, Sinha A.

[Submit Form] and go to [   ] or Skip to Next

This is a "multi-form" meaning you can fill out the same form multiple time (i.e., a different set of data is entered for each study arms."

1. Please select the arm and specify

   ○ Arm A (Meditation)
   ● Arm B - specify
      Delivery of Intervention - Arm B

      ○ Group
      ○ Individual
      ○ Other - please specify [   ]

   Frequency of Traning Intervention (how many times per day/week) - ARM B

19. How many times	20. Per day/week
○ Once	○ Daily
○ Twice	○ Weekly
○ Other - please specify [ ]	○ Biweekly
	○ Monthly
	○ Other - please specify [ ]

   Duration of Intervention - ARM B

21.	22.
☐ Number of sessions [ ]	☐ Length of time per session (hrs) [ ]
☐ Other/additional sessions - please specify [ ]	☐ Not Reported
☐ Not Reported	

   Total Duration of Training - ARM B

23.	24.
☐ Total numbers of weeks [ ]	☐ Total hours [ ]
☐ Other - please specify [ ]	☐ Not Reported
☐ Not Reported	

DistillerSR

Detail of Trainers -ARM B

25. What were the qualifications of the trainer for this ARM B?

- ○ Certified
- ○ Not Certified
- ○ Not Reported
- ○ Other [ ]

Frequency of HOME PRACTICE (how many times per day/week) -ARM B

26. Was any home practice/work done in the comparison group?

- ○ Matched to 1st Arm
- ○ Not Matched to 1st Arm
- ○ Other - please specify [ ]
- ○ Not Reported

○ Arm C-specify
○ Arm D -Usual Care

37. R2 only: if you are reviewing R1 data entry, enter your initials when you have completed the audit

[ ]

[Submit Form] and go to [ ] or Skip to Next

Intervention Arm D (Usual Care)

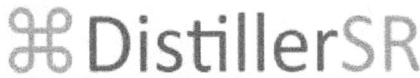

ritu.sharma

Project	Meditation (Switch) User mreuben (My Settings)
Messages	3 new

Live Support | User Guide

Review | Datarama | Reports | References | Forms | Manage Levels | Users | Project | Logout

Refid: 12, Skateboards: Are they really perilous? A retrospective study from a district hospital.
Rethnam U, Yesupalan RS, Sinha A.

[Submit Form] and go to [ ] or Skip to Next

This is a "multi-form" meaning you can fill out the same form multiple time (i.e., a different set of data is entered for each study arms."

1. Please select the arm and specify

   ○ Arm A (Meditation)
   ○ Arm B - specify [ ]
   ○ Arm C - specify [ ]
   ⦿ Arm D - Usual Care
      Comments for Usual Care
      [ ]

37. R2 only: if you are reviewing R1 data entry, enter your initials when you have completed the audit

[ ]

[Submit Form] and go to [ ] or Skip to Next

Outcomes for KQ 1
Anxiety Scales

DistillerSR

⌘ DistillerSR

ritu.sharma

| Project | Meditation (Switch) | User | mreuben (My Settings) |
| Messages | 3 new | | |

Live Support | User Guide

Review | Dataforms | Reports | References | Forms | Manage Levels | Users | Project | Logout

Refid: 12, Skateboards: Are they really perilous? A retrospective study from a district hospital.
Rethnam U, Yesupalan RS, Sinha A.

[Submit Form] and go to [ ] or Skip to Next

Please submit one form per outcome

1. This study does not apply to KQ1

☐ No

KQ 1: What are the efficacy and harms of Meditation Programs on negative affect (e.g. anxiety, stress) and positive affect (e.g. well being) among those with a clinical condition (medical or psychiatric)?

Please select the outcome and outcome measure for KQ1

2. Outcome

◉ Anxiety
Outcome Scales - Anxiety

○ BAI [ ]
○ HADS [ ]
○ Penn State Worry Questionnaire [ ]
○ State Trait Anxiety Inventory [ ]
○ SCL-90 subscale [ ]
○ BSI-18 subscale [ ]
○ POMS tension anxiety [ ]
○ Other - please specify [ ]
Clear Response

○ Depression
○ Stress
○ General Distress
○ Subjective well being
○ Harms
Clear Response

TABLE 1: Measures of association

ARM A - Please specify	Outcome measures at **baseline**	Outcome measures **at end of treatment**	Outcome measures **at last followup**
[ ]	☐ N [ ]	☐ N [ ]	☐ N [ ]
	☐ At Baseline	☐ Enter TIME [ ]	☐ Enter TIME [ ]
	☐ Mean [ ]	☐ Mean [ ]	☐ Mean [ ]
	☐ Standard Deviation [ ]	☐ Standard Deviation [ ]	☐ Standard Deviation [ ]
	☐ CI OR pvalue (specify) [ ]	☐ CI or pvalue (specify) [ ]	☐ CI or pvalue (specify) [ ]
	☐ RR or OR(specify) [ ]	☐ RR or OR(specify) [ ]	☐ RR or OR(specify) [ ]
	☐ Hazard Ratio [ ]	☐ Hazard Ratio [ ]	☐ Hazard Ratio [ ]
	☐ Other - please specify [ ]	☐ Other - please specify [ ]	☐ Other - please specify [ ]
ARM B - Please specify	Outcome measures at **baseline**	Outcome measures **at end of treatment**	Outcome measures **at last followup**
[ ]	☐ N [ ]	☐ N [ ]	☐ N [ ]
	☐ At Baseline	☐ Enter TIME [ ]	☐ Enter TIME [ ]
	☐ Mean [ ]	☐ Mean [ ]	☐ Mean [ ]
	☐ Standard Deviation [ ]	☐ Standard Deviation [ ]	☐ Standard Deviation [ ]
	☐ CI OR pvalue (specify) [ ]	☐ CI or pvalue (specify) [ ]	☐ CI or pvalue (specify) [ ]
	☐ RR or OR(specify) [ ]	☐ RR or OR(specify) [ ]	☐ RR or OR(specify) [ ]
	☐ Hazard Ratio [ ]		

		☐ Other - please specify		☐ Hazard Ratio		☐ Hazard Ratio	
				☐ Other - please specify		☐ Other - please specify	
ARM C-Please specify		Outcome measures at **baseline**		Outcome measures **at end of treatment**		Outcome measures **at last followup**	
		☐ N		☐ N		☐ N	
		☐ At Baseline		☐ Enter TIME		☐ Enter TIME	
		☐ Mean		☐ Mean		☐ Mean	
		☐ Standard Deviation		☐ Standard Deviation		☐ Standard Deviation	
		☐ CI OR pvalue (specify)		☐ CI or pvalue (specify)		☐ CI or pvalue (specify)	
		☐ RR or OR(specify)		☐ RR or OR(specify)		☐ RR or OR(specify)	
		☐ Hazard Ratio		☐ Hazard Ratio		☐ Hazard Ratio	
		☐ Other - please specify		☐ Other - please specify		☐ Other - please specify	
ARM D-Please specify		Outcome measures at **baseline**		Outcome measures **at end of treatment**		Outcome measures **at last followup**	
		☐ N		☐ N		☐ N	
		☐ At Baseline		☐ Enter TIME		☐ Enter TIME	
		☐ Mean		☐ Mean		☐ Mean	
		☐ Standard Deviation		☐ Standard Deviation		☐ Standard Deviation	
		☐ CI OR pvalue (specify)		☐ CI or pvalue (specify)		☐ CI or pvalue (specify)	
		☐ RR or OR(specify)		☐ RR or OR(specify)		☐ RR or OR(specify)	
		☐ Hazard Ratio		☐ RR or OR(specify)		☐ RR or OR(specify)	
		☐ Other - please specify		☐ Hazard Ratio		☐ Hazard Ratio	
				☐ Other - please specify		☐ Other - please specify	

TABLE 2: Mean difference from baseline

24. Arm A (Meditation)	25. Total N in ARM	26. Outcomes measures at **END OF TREATMENT**		27. Outcomes measures at **LAST FOLLOWUP**	
		☐ Enter TIME		☐ Enter TIME	
		☐ Mean		☐ Mean	
		☐ Standard Error		☐ Standard Error	
		☐ 95% CI		☐ 95% CI	
		☐ Risk difference		☐ Risk difference	
		☐ P-value		☐ P-value	
		☐ Hazard Ratio		☐ Hazard Ratio	
		☐ Other-pelase specify		☐ Other-pelase specify	
28. Arm B - please specify	29. Total N in ARM	30. Outcomes measures at **END OF TREATMENT**		31. Outcomes measures at **LAST FOLLOWUP**	
		☐ Enter TIME		☐ Enter TIME	
		☐ Mean		☐ Mean	
		☐ Standard Error		☐ Standard Error	
		☐ 95% CI		☐ 95% CI	
		☐ Risk difference		☐ Risk difference	
		☐ P-value		☐ P-value	
		☐ Hazard Ratio		☐ Hazard Ratio	
		☐ Other-pelase specify		☐ Other-pelase specify	
32. Arm C - please specify	33. Total N in ARM	34. Outcomes measures at **END OF TREATMENT**		35. Outcomes measures at **LAST FOLLOWUP**	
		☐ Enter TIME		☐ Enter TIME	
		☐ Mean		☐ Mean	
		☐ Standard Error		☐ Standard Error	
		☐ 95% CI		☐ 95% CI	
		☐ Risk difference		☐ Risk difference	
		☐ P-value		☐ P-value	
		☐ Hazard Ratio		☐ Hazard Ratio	
		☐ Other-pelase specify		☐ Other-pelase specify	

57. Groups compared	58. Outcomes measures at **END OF TREATMENT**	59. Outcomes measures at **LAST FOLLOWUP**
○ A vs. B ○ A vs. C ○ A vs. D ○ Other - please specify [ ] Clear Response	☐ Enter TIME [ ] ☐ Mean [ ] ☐ Standard Error [ ] ☐ 95% CI [ ] ☐ Risk difference [ ] ☐ P-value [ ] ☐ Hazard Ratio [ ] ☐ Other-pelase specify [ ]	☐ Enter TIME [ ] ☐ Mean [ ] ☐ Standard Error [ ] ☐ 95% CI [ ] ☐ Risk difference [ ] ☐ P-value [ ] ☐ Hazard Ratio [ ] ☐ Other-pelase specify [ ]
60. Groups compared	61. Outcomes measures at **END OF TREATMENT**	62. Outcomes measures at **LAST FOLLOWUP**
○ A vs. B ○ A vs. C ○ A vs. D ○ Other - please specify [ ] Clear Response	☐ Enter TIME [ ] ☐ Mean [ ] ☐ Standard Error [ ] ☐ 95% CI [ ] ☐ Risk difference [ ] ☐ P-value [ ] ☐ Hazard Ratio [ ] ☐ Other-pelase specify [ ]	☐ Enter TIME [ ] ☐ Mean [ ] ☐ Standard Error [ ] ☐ 95% CI [ ] ☐ Risk difference [ ] ☐ P-value [ ] ☐ Hazard Ratio [ ] ☐ Other-pelase specify [ ]
63. Groups compared	64. Outcomes measures at **END OF TREATMENT**	65. Outcomes measures at **LAST FOLLOWUP**
○ A vs. B ○ A vs. C ○ A vs. D ○ Other - please specify [ ] Clear Response	☐ Enter TIME [ ] ☐ Mean [ ] ☐ Standard Error [ ] ☐ 95% CI [ ] ☐ Risk difference [ ] ☐ P-value [ ] ☐ Hazard Ratio [ ] ☐ Other-pelase specify [ ]	☐ Enter TIME [ ] ☐ Mean [ ] ☐ Standard Error [ ] ☐ 95% CI [ ] ☐ Risk difference [ ] ☐ P-value [ ] ☐ Hazard Ratio [ ] ☐ Other-pelase specify [ ]
66. Groups compared	67. Outcomes measures at **END OF TREATMENT**	68. Outcomes measures at **LAST FOLLOWUP**
○ A vs. B ○ A vs. C ○ A vs. D ○ Other - please specify [ ] Clear Response	☐ Enter TIME [ ] ☐ Mean [ ] ☐ Standard Error [ ] ☐ 95% CI [ ] ☐ Risk difference [ ] ☐ P-value [ ] ☐ Hazard Ratio [ ] ☐ Other-pelase specify [ ]	☐ Enter TIME [ ] ☐ Mean [ ] ☐ Standard Error [ ] ☐ 95% CI [ ] ☐ Risk difference [ ] ☐ P-value [ ] ☐ Hazard Ratio [ ] ☐ Other-pelase specify [ ]

Adverse Events

69. **Were any adverse events reported?**

☐ The paper specified that there were no AEs
☐ Paper reported on an AE - please specify [ ]
☐ Paper did not mention anything about an AE

70. Comments:

[ ]

[Submit Form] and go to [ ] or Skip to Next

Outcomes for KQ1
Depression Scales

DistillerSR

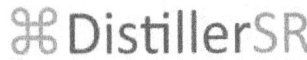

ritu.sharma

Project   Meditation (Switch)   User mreuben (My Settings)
Messages 3 new

Live Support   User Guide

| Review | Datarama | Reports | References | Forms | Manage Levels | Users | Project | Logout |

Refid: 12, Skateboards: Are they really perilous? A retrospective study from a district hospital.
Rethnam U, Yesupalan RS, Sinha A.

[Submit Form] and go to [   ] or Skip to Next

Please submit one form per outcome

1. This study does not apply to KQ1

☐ No

KQ 1: What are the efficacy and harms of Meditation Programs on negative affect (e.g. anxiety, stress) and positive affect (e.g. well being) among those with a clinical condition (medical or psychiatric)?

Please select the outcome and outcome measure for KQ1

2. Outcome

○ Anxiety
● Depression
  Outcome Scales-Depression
  ○ BDI [   ]
  ○ Hospital Anxiety and Depression Scale [   ]
  ○ SCL-90 subscale [   ]
  ○ BSI-18 subscale [   ]
  ○ Other - please specify [   ]
  Clear Response

○ Stress
○ General Distress
○ Subjective well being
○ Harms
Clear Response

TABLE 1: Measures of association

ARM A - Please specify	Outcome measures at **baseline**	Outcome measures **at end of treatment**	Outcome measures **at last followup**
[ ]	☐ N [ ] ☐ At Baseline [ ] ☐ Mean [ ] ☐ Standard Deviation [ ] ☐ CI OR pvalue (specify) [ ] ☐ RR or OR(specify) [ ] ☐ Hazard Ratio [ ] ☐ Other - please specify [ ]	☐ N [ ] ☐ Enter TIME [ ] ☐ Mean [ ] ☐ Standard Deviation [ ] ☐ CI or pvalue (specify) [ ] ☐ RR or OR(specify) [ ] ☐ Hazard Ratio [ ] ☐ Other - please specify [ ]	☐ N [ ] ☐ Enter TIME [ ] ☐ Mean [ ] ☐ Standard Deviation [ ] ☐ CI or pvalue (specify) [ ] ☐ RR or OR(specify) [ ] ☐ Hazard Ratio [ ] ☐ Other - please specify [ ]
ARM B - Please specify	Outcome measures at **baseline**	Outcome measures **at end of treatment**	Outcome measures **at last followup**
[ ]	☐ N [ ] ☐ At Baseline [ ] ☐ Mean [ ] ☐ Standard Deviation [ ] ☐ CI OR pvalue (specify) [ ] ☐ RR or OR(specify) [ ] ☐ Hazard Ratio [ ] ☐ Other - please specify [ ]	☐ N [ ] ☐ Enter TIME [ ] ☐ Mean [ ] ☐ Standard Deviation [ ] ☐ CI or pvalue (specify) [ ] ☐ RR or OR(specify) [ ] ☐ Hazard Ratio [ ] ☐ Other - please specify [ ]	☐ N [ ] ☐ Enter TIME [ ] ☐ Mean [ ] ☐ Standard Deviation [ ] ☐ CI or pvalue (specify) [ ] ☐ RR or OR(specify) [ ] ☐ Hazard Ratio [ ] ☐ Other - please specify [ ]
ARM C - Please specify	Outcome measures at **baseline**	Outcome measures **at end of treatment**	Outcome measures **at last followup**

	☐ N	☐ N	☐ N
	☐ At Baseline	☐ Enter TIME	☐ Enter TIME
	☐ Mean	☐ Mean	☐ Mean
	☐ Standard Deviation	☐ Standard Deviation	☐ Standard Deviation
	☐ CI OR pvalue (specify)	☐ CI or pvalue (specify)	☐ CI or pvalue (specify)
	☐ RR or OR(specify)	☐ RR or OR(specify)	☐ RR or OR(specify)
	☐ Hazard Ratio	☐ Hazard Ratio	☐ Hazard Ratio
	☐ Other - please specify	☐ Other - please specify	☐ Other - please specify
ARM D- Please specify	Outcome measures at **baseline**	Outcome measures **at end of treatment**	Outcome measures **at last followup**
	☐ N	☐ N	☐ N
	☐ At Baseline	☐ Enter TIME	☐ Enter TIME
	☐ Mean	☐ Mean	☐ Mean
	☐ Standard Deviation	☐ Standard Deviation	☐ Standard Deviation
	☐ CI OR pvalue (specify)	☐ CI or pvalue (specify)	☐ CI or pvalue (specify)
	☐ RR or OR(specify)	☐ RR or OR(specify)	☐ RR or OR(specify)
	☐ Hazard Ratio	☐ Hazard Ratio	☐ Hazard Ratio
	☐ Other - please specify	☐ Other - please specify	☐ Other - please specify

TABLE 2: Mean difference from baseline

24. Arm A (Meditation)	25. Total N in ARM	26. Outcomes measures at **END OF TREATMENT**	27. Outcomes measures at **LAST FOLLOWUP**
		☐ Enter TIME	☐ Enter TIME
		☐ Mean	☐ Mean
		☐ Standard Error	☐ Standard Error
		☐ 95% CI	☐ 95% CI
		☐ Risk difference	☐ Risk difference
		☐ P-value	☐ P-value
		☐ Hazard Ratio	☐ Hazard Ratio
		☐ Other-pelase specify	☐ Other-pelase specify
28. Arm B - please specify	29. Total N in ARM	30. Outcomes measures at **END OF TREATMENT**	31. Outcomes measures at **LAST FOLLOWUP**
		☐ Enter TIME	☐ Enter TIME
		☐ Mean	☐ Mean
		☐ Standard Error	☐ Standard Error
		☐ 95% CI	☐ 95% CI
		☐ Risk difference	☐ Risk difference
		☐ P-value	☐ P-value
		☐ Hazard Ratio	☐ Hazard Ratio
		☐ Other-pelase specify	☐ Other-pelase specify
32. Arm C - please specify	33. Total N in ARM	34. Outcomes measures at **END OF TREATMENT**	35. Outcomes measures at **LAST FOLLOWUP**
		☐ Enter TIME	☐ Enter TIME
		☐ Mean	☐ Mean
		☐ Standard Error	☐ Standard Error
		☐ 95% CI	☐ 95% CI
		☐ Risk difference	☐ Risk difference
		☐ P-value	☐ P-value
		☐ Hazard Ratio	☐ Hazard Ratio
		☐ Other-pelase specify	☐ Other-pelase specify
36. Arm D- please specify	37. Total N in ARM	38. Outcomes measures at **END OF TREATMENT**	39. Outcomes measures at **LAST FOLLOWUP**
		☐ Enter TIME	☐ Enter TIME
		☐ Mean	☐ Mean

			☐ Standard Error ☐ 95% CI ☐ Risk difference ☐ P-value ☐ Hazard Ratio ☐ Other-pelase specify	☐ Standard Error ☐ 95% CI ☐ Risk difference ☐ P-value ☐ Hazard Ratio ☐ Other-pelase specify

TABLE 3: Mean difference between groups

Arm A (Meditation) Vs. Arm B	40. Total N in ARM ☐ Total N in Arm A ☐ Total N in Arm B ☐ Total N in both arms	41. Outcome At BASELINE ☐ At Baseline ☐ Mean ☐ Standard Error ☐ 95% CI ☐ Risk difference ☐ P-value ☐ Hazard Ratio ☐ Other-pelase specify	42. Outcomes at END OF TREATMENT ☐ Enter TIME ☐ Mean ☐ Standard Error ☐ 95% CI ☐ Risk difference ☐ P-value ☐ Hazard Ratio ☐ Other-pelase specify	43. Outcomes at LAST FOLLOWUP ☐ Enter TIME ☐ Mean ☐ Standard Error ☐ 95% CI ☐ Risk difference ☐ P-value ☐ Hazard Ratio ☐ Other-pelase specify
Arm A (Meditation) Vs. Arm C	44. Total N in ARM ☐ Total N in Arm A ☐ Total N in Arm C ☐ Total N in both arms	45. Outcomes at BASELINE ☐ At Baseline ☐ Mean ☐ Standard Error ☐ 95% CI ☐ Risk difference ☐ P-value ☐ Hazard Ratio ☐ Other-pelase specify	46. Outcomes at END OF TREATMENT ☐ Enter TIME ☐ Mean ☐ Standard Error ☐ 95% CI ☐ Risk difference ☐ P-value ☐ Hazard Ratio ☐ Other-pelase specify	47. Outcomes at LAST FOLLOWUP ☐ Enter TIME ☐ Mean ☐ Standard Error ☐ 95% CI ☐ Risk difference ☐ P-value ☐ Hazard Ratio ☐ Other-pelase specify
Arm A (Meditation) Vs. Arm D	48. Total N in ARM ☐ Total N in Arm A ☐ Total N in Arm D ☐ Total N in both arms	49. Outcomes at BASELINE ☐ At Baseline ☐ Mean ☐ Standard Error ☐ 95% CI ☐ Risk difference ☐ P-value ☐ Hazard Ratio ☐ Other-pelase specify	50. Outcomes at END OF TREATMENT ☐ Enter TIME ☐ Mean ☐ Standard Error ☐ 95% CI ☐ Risk difference ☐ P-value ☐ Hazard Ratio ☐ Other-pelase specify	51. Outcomes at LAST FOLLOWUP ☐ Enter TIME ☐ Mean ☐ Standard Error ☐ 95% CI ☐ Risk difference ☐ P-value ☐ Hazard Ratio ☐ Other-pelase specify
52. Other please spcify	53. Total N in ARM ☐ Total N in Arm ☐ Total N in Arm ☐ Total N in both arms	54. Outcomes at BASELINE ☐ At Baseline ☐ Mean ☐ Standard Error ☐ 95% CI ☐ Risk difference ☐ P-value ☐ Hazard Ratio ☐ Other-pelase specify	55. Outcomes at END OF TREATMENT ☐ Enter TIME ☐ Mean ☐ Standard Error ☐ 95% CI ☐ Risk difference ☐ P-value ☐ Hazard Ratio ☐ Other-pelase specify	56. Outcomes at LAST FOLLOWUP ☐ Enter TIME ☐ Mean ☐ Standard Error ☐ 95% CI ☐ Risk difference ☐ P-value ☐ Hazard Ratio ☐ Other-pelase specify

TABLE 4: Diff-in-diff

57. Groups compared	58. Outcomes measures at END OF TREATMENT	59. Outcomes measures at LAST FOLLOWUP
○ A vs. B ○ A vs. C ○ A vs. D	☐ Enter TIME ☐ Mean	☐ Enter TIME ☐ Mean

DistillerSR

	☐ Standard Error	☐ Standard Error
○ Other - please specify	☐ 95% CI	☐ 95% CI
Clear Response	☐ Risk difference	☐ Risk difference
	☐ P-value	☐ P-value
	☐ Hazard Ratio	☐ Hazard Ratio
	☐ Other-pelase specify	☐ Other-pelase specify

60. Groups compared	61. Outcomes measures at **END OF TREATMENT**	62. Outcomes measures at **LAST FOLLOWUP**
○ A vs. B	☐ Enter TIME	☐ Enter TIME
○ A vs. C	☐ Mean	☐ Mean
○ A vs. D	☐ Standard Error	☐ Standard Error
○ Other - please specify	☐ 95% CI	☐ 95% CI
Clear Response	☐ Risk difference	☐ Risk difference
	☐ P-value	☐ P-value
	☐ Hazard Ratio	☐ Hazard Ratio
	☐ Other-pelase specify	☐ Other-pelase specify

63. Groups compared	64. Outcomes measures at **END OF TREATMENT**	65. Outcomes measures at **LAST FOLLOWUP**
○ A vs. B	☐ Enter TIME	☐ Enter TIME
○ A vs. C	☐ Mean	☐ Mean
○ A vs. D	☐ Standard Error	☐ Standard Error
○ Other - please specify	☐ 95% CI	☐ 95% CI
Clear Response	☐ Risk difference	☐ Risk difference
	☐ P-value	☐ P-value
	☐ Hazard Ratio	☐ Hazard Ratio
	☐ Other-pelase specify	☐ Other-pelase specify

66. Groups compared	67. Outcomes measures at **END OF TREATMENT**	68. Outcomes measures at **LAST FOLLOWUP**
○ A vs. B	☐ Enter TIME	☐ Enter TIME
○ A vs. C	☐ Mean	☐ Mean
○ A vs. D	☐ Standard Error	☐ Standard Error
○ Other - please specify	☐ 95% CI	☐ 95% CI
Clear Response	☐ Risk difference	☐ Risk difference
	☐ P-value	☐ P-value
	☐ Hazard Ratio	☐ Hazard Ratio
	☐ Other-pelase specify	☐ Other-pelase specify

Adverse Events

69. **Were any adverse events reported?**

☐ The paper specified that there were no AEs
☐ Paper reported on an AE - please specify
☐ Paper did not mention anything about an AE

70. Comments:

[Submit Form] and go to [ ] or Skip to Next

Outcomes for KQ1
Scales for Stress

DistillerSR

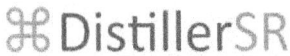

ritu.sharma

Project: Meditation (Switch) User: mreuben (My Settings)
Messages: 3 new

Live Support | User Guide

Review | Datarama | Reports | References | Forms | Manage Levels | Users | Project | Logout

Refid: 12, Skateboards: Are they really perilous? A retrospective study from a district hospital.
Rethnam U, Yesupalan RS, Sinha A.

[Submit Form] and go to [ ] or Skip to Next

Please submit one form per outcome

1. **This study does not apply to KQ1**
   - ☐ No

KQ 1: What are the efficacy and harms of Meditation Programs on negative affect (e.g. anxiety, stress) and positive affect (e.g. well being) among those with a clinical condition (medical or psychiatric)?

Please select the outcome and outcome measure for KQ1

2. Outcome
   - ○ Anxiety
   - ○ Depression
   - ⦿ Stress
     Outcome Scales - Stress
     - ○ PSS
     - ○ Calgary Symptoms of Stress Inventory (c-sosi)
     - ○ Other- please specify
     Clear Response
   - ○ General Distress
   - ○ Subjective well being
   - ○ Harms
   Clear Response

TABLE 1: Measures of association

ARM A - Please specify	Outcome measures at baseline	Outcome measures at end of treatment	Outcome measures at last followup
	☐ N ☐ At Baseline ☐ Mean ☐ Standard Deviation ☐ CI OR pvalue (specify) ☐ RR or OR(specify) ☐ Hazard Ratio ☐ Other - please specify	☐ N ☐ Enter TIME ☐ Mean ☐ Standard Deviation ☐ CI or pvalue (specify) ☐ RR or OR(specify) ☐ Hazard Ratio ☐ Other - please specify	☐ N ☐ Enter TIME ☐ Mean ☐ Standard Deviation ☐ CI or pvalue (specify) ☐ RR or OR(specify) ☐ Hazard Ratio ☐ Other - please specify
ARM B - Please specify	Outcome measures at baseline	Outcome measures at end of treatment	Outcome measures at last followup
	☐ N ☐ At Baseline ☐ Mean ☐ Standard Deviation ☐ CI OR pvalue (specify) ☐ RR or OR(specify) ☐ Hazard Ratio ☐ Other - please specify	☐ N ☐ Enter TIME ☐ Mean ☐ Standard Deviation ☐ CI or pvalue (specify) ☐ RR or OR(specify) ☐ Hazard Ratio ☐ Other - please specify	☐ N ☐ Enter TIME ☐ Mean ☐ Standard Deviation ☐ CI or pvalue (specify) ☐ RR or OR(specify) ☐ Hazard Ratio ☐ Other - please specify
ARM C - Please specify	Outcome measures at baseline	Outcome measures at end of treatment	Outcome measures at last followup
	☐ N ☐ At Baseline	☐ N ☐ Enter TIME	☐ N ☐ Enter TIME

		☐ Mean		☐ Mean		☐ Mean	
		☐ Standard Deviation		☐ Standard Deviation		☐ Standard Deviation	
		☐ CI OR pvalue (specify)		☐ CI or pvalue (specify)		☐ CI or pvalue (specify)	
		☐ RR or OR(specify)		☐ RR or OR(specify)		☐ RR or OR(specify)	
		☐ Hazard Ratio		☐ Hazard Ratio		☐ Hazard Ratio	
		☐ Other - please specify		☐ Other - please specify		☐ Other - please specify	
ARM D-Please specify		Outcome measures at **baseline**		Outcome measures **at end of treatment**		Outcome measures **at last followup**	
		☐ N		☐ N		☐ N	
		☐ At Baseline		☐ Enter TIME		☐ Enter TIME	
		☐ Mean		☐ Mean		☐ Mean	
		☐ Standard Deviation		☐ Standard Deviation		☐ Standard Deviation	
		☐ CI OR pvalue (specify)		☐ CI or pvalue (specify)		☐ CI or pvalue (specify)	
		☐ RR or OR(specify)		☐ RR or OR(specify)		☐ RR or OR(specify)	
		☐ Hazard Ratio		☐ Hazard Ratio		☐ Hazard Ratio	
		☐ Other - please specify		☐ Other - please specify		☐ Other - please specify	

TABLE 2: Mean difference from baseline

24. Arm A (Meditation)	25. Total N in ARM	26. Outcomes measures at **END OF TREATMENT**		27. Outcomes measures at **LAST FOLLOWUP**	
		☐ Enter TIME		☐ Enter TIME	
		☐ Mean		☐ Mean	
		☐ Standard Error		☐ Standard Error	
		☐ 95% CI		☐ 95% CI	
		☐ Risk difference		☐ Risk difference	
		☐ P-value		☐ P-value	
		☐ Hazard Ratio		☐ Hazard Ratio	
		☐ Other-pelase specify		☐ Other-pelase specify	
28. Arm B - please specify	29. Total N in ARM	30. Outcomes measures at **END OF TREATMENT**		31. Outcomes measures at **LAST FOLLOWUP**	
		☐ Enter TIME		☐ Enter TIME	
		☐ Mean		☐ Mean	
		☐ Standard Error		☐ Standard Error	
		☐ 95% CI		☐ 95% CI	
		☐ Risk difference		☐ Risk difference	
		☐ P-value		☐ P-value	
		☐ Hazard Ratio		☐ Hazard Ratio	
		☐ Other-pelase specify		☐ Other-pelase specify	
32. Arm C - please specify	33. Total N in ARM	34. Outcomes measures at **END OF TREATMENT**		35. Outcomes measures at **LAST FOLLOWUP**	
		☐ Enter TIME		☐ Enter TIME	
		☐ Mean		☐ Mean	
		☐ Standard Error		☐ Standard Error	
		☐ 95% CI		☐ 95% CI	
		☐ Risk difference		☐ Risk difference	
		☐ P-value		☐ P-value	
		☐ Hazard Ratio		☐ Hazard Ratio	
		☐ Other-pelase specify		☐ Other-pelase specify	
36. Arm D- please specify	37. Total N in ARM	38. Outcomes measures at **END OF TREATMENT**		39. Outcomes measures at **LAST FOLLOWUP**	
		☐ Enter TIME		☐ Enter TIME	
		☐ Mean		☐ Mean	
		☐ Standard Error		☐ Standard Error	

| | | ☐ 95% CI
☐ Risk difference
☐ P-value
☐ Hazard Ratio
☐ Other-pelase specify | ☐ 95% CI
☐ Risk difference
☐ P-value
☐ Hazard Ratio
☐ Other-pelase specify |

TABLE 3: Mean difference between groups

		41. Outcome At BASELINE	42. Outcomes at END OF TREATMENT	43. Outcomes at LAST FOLLOWUP
Arm A (Meditation) Vs. Arm B	40. Total N in ARM ☐ Total N in Arm A ☐ Total N in Arm B ☐ Total N in both arms	☐ At Baseline ☐ Mean ☐ Standard Error ☐ 95% CI ☐ Risk difference ☐ P-value ☐ Hazard Ratio ☐ Other-pelase specify	☐ Enter TIME ☐ Mean ☐ Standard Error ☐ 95% CI ☐ Risk difference ☐ P-value ☐ Hazard Ratio ☐ Other-pelase specify	☐ Enter TIME ☐ Mean ☐ Standard Error ☐ 95% CI ☐ Risk difference ☐ P-value ☐ Hazard Ratio ☐ Other-pelase specify
Arm A (Meditation) Vs. Arm C	44. Total N in ARM ☐ Total N in Arm A ☐ Total N in Arm C ☐ Total N in both arms	45. Outcomes at BASELINE ☐ At Baseline ☐ Mean ☐ Standard Error ☐ 95% CI ☐ Risk difference ☐ P-value ☐ Hazard Ratio ☐ Other-pelase specify	46. Outcomes at END OF TREATMENT ☐ Enter TIME ☐ Mean ☐ Standard Error ☐ 95% CI ☐ Risk difference ☐ P-value ☐ Hazard Ratio ☐ Other-pelase specify	47. Outcomes at LAST FOLLOWUP ☐ Enter TIME ☐ Mean ☐ Standard Error ☐ 95% CI ☐ Risk difference ☐ P-value ☐ Hazard Ratio ☐ Other-pelase specify
Arm A (Meditation) Vs. Arm D	48. Total N in ARM ☐ Total N in Arm A ☐ Total N in Arm D ☐ Total N in both arms	49. Outcomes at BASELINE ☐ At Baseline ☐ Mean ☐ Standard Error ☐ 95% CI ☐ Risk difference ☐ P-value ☐ Hazard Ratio ☐ Other-pelase specify	50. Outcomes at END OF TREATMENT ☐ Enter TIME ☐ Mean ☐ Standard Error ☐ 95% CI ☐ Risk difference ☐ P-value ☐ Hazard Ratio ☐ Other-pelase specify	51. Outcomes at LAST FOLLOWUP ☐ Enter TIME ☐ Mean ☐ Standard Error ☐ 95% CI ☐ Risk difference ☐ P-value ☐ Hazard Ratio ☐ Other-pelase specify
52. Other please spcify	53. Total N in ARM ☐ Total N in Arm ☐ Total N in Arm ☐ Total N in both arms	54. Outcomes at BASELINE ☐ At Baseline ☐ Mean ☐ Standard Error ☐ 95% CI ☐ Risk difference ☐ P-value ☐ Hazard Ratio ☐ Other-pelase specify	55. Outcomes at END OF TREATMENT ☐ Enter TIME ☐ Mean ☐ Standard Error ☐ 95% CI ☐ Risk difference ☐ P-value ☐ Hazard Ratio ☐ Other-pelase specify	56. Outcomes at LAST FOLLOWUP ☐ Enter TIME ☐ Mean ☐ Standard Error ☐ 95% CI ☐ Risk difference ☐ P-value ☐ Hazard Ratio ☐ Other-pelase specify

TABLE 4: Diff-in-diff

57. Groups compared	58. Outcomes measures at END OF TREATMENT	59. Outcomes measures at LAST FOLLOWUP
○ A vs. B ○ A vs. C ○ A vs. D ○ Other - please specify	☐ Enter TIME ☐ Mean ☐ Standard Error	☐ Enter TIME ☐ Mean ☐ Standard Error

Outcomes for KQ1
Scales for General Distress

DistillerSR

⌘ DistillerSR

ritu.sharma

Project	Meditation (Switch) User mreuben (My Settings)
Messages	3 new

Live Support | User Guide

Review | Datarama | Reports | References | Forms | Manage Levels | Users | Project | Logout

Refid: 12, Skateboards: Are they really perilous? A retrospective study from a district hospital.
Rethnam U, Yesupalan RS, Sinha A.

[Submit Form] and go to [   ] or Skip to Next

Please submit one form per outcome

1. This study does not apply to KQ1

   ☐ No

KQ 1: What are the efficacy and harms of Meditation Programs on negative affect (e.g. anxiety, stress) and positive affect (e.g. well being) among those with a clinical condition (medical or psychiatric)?

Please select the outcome and outcome measure for KQ1

2. Outcome

   ○ Anxiety
   ○ Depression
   ○ Stress
   ◉ General Distress

   Outcome Scales - General Distress

   ○ SCL - 90 total score [   ]
   ○ HADS [   ]
   ○ BSI - 18 general severity [   ]
   ○ Other - please specify [   ]
   Clear Response

   ○ Subjective well being
   ○ Harms
   Clear Response

TABLE 1: Measures of association

ARM A -Please specify	Outcome measures at <u>baseline</u>	Outcome measures <u>at end of treatment</u>	Outcome measures <u>at last followup</u>
[ ]	☐ N [ ] ☐ At Baseline ☐ Mean [ ] ☐ Standard Deviation [ ] ☐ CI OR pvalue (specify) ☐ RR or OR(specify) [ ] ☐ Hazard Ratio ☐ Other - please specify	☐ N [ ] ☐ Enter TIME [ ] ☐ Mean [ ] ☐ Standard Deviation [ ] ☐ CI or pvalue (specify) [ ] ☐ RR or OR(specify) [ ] ☐ Hazard Ratio ☐ Other - please specify [ ]	☐ N [ ] ☐ Enter TIME [ ] ☐ Mean [ ] ☐ Standard Deviation [ ] ☐ CI or pvalue (specify) [ ] ☐ RR or OR(specify) [ ] ☐ Hazard Ratio ☐ Other - please specify [ ]
ARM B -Please specify	Outcome measures at <u>baseline</u>	Outcome measures <u>at end of treatment</u>	Outcome measures <u>at last followup</u>
[ ]	☐ N [ ] ☐ At Baseline ☐ Mean [ ] ☐ Standard Deviation [ ] ☐ CI OR pvalue (specify) ☐ RR or OR(specify) [ ] ☐ Hazard Ratio ☐ Other - please specify	☐ N [ ] ☐ Enter TIME [ ] ☐ Mean [ ] ☐ Standard Deviation [ ] ☐ CI or pvalue (specify) [ ] ☐ RR or OR(specify) [ ] ☐ Hazard Ratio ☐ Other - please specify [ ]	☐ N [ ] ☐ Enter TIME [ ] ☐ Mean [ ] ☐ Standard Deviation [ ] ☐ CI or pvalue (specify) [ ] ☐ RR or OR(specify) [ ] ☐ Hazard Ratio ☐ Other - please specify [ ]
ARM C-Please specify	Outcome measures at <u>baseline</u>	Outcome measures <u>at end of treatment</u>	Outcome measures <u>at last followup</u>
	☐ N	☐ N	☐ N

		Outcome measures at baseline		Outcome measures at end of treatment		Outcome measures at last followup	
		☐ At Baseline		☐ Enter TIME		☐ Enter TIME	
		☐ Mean		☐ Mean		☐ Mean	
		☐ Standard Deviation		☐ Standard Deviation		☐ Standard Deviation	
		☐ CI OR pvalue (specify)		☐ CI or pvalue (specify)		☐ CI or pvalue (specify)	
		☐ RR or OR(specify)		☐ RR or OR(specify)		☐ RR or OR(specify)	
		☐ Hazard Ratio		☐ Hazard Ratio		☐ Hazard Ratio	
		☐ Other - please specify		☐ Other - please specify		☐ Other - please specify	
ARM D-Please specify		Outcome measures at baseline		Outcome measures at end of treatment		Outcome measures at last followup	
		☐ N		☐ N		☐ N	
		☐ At Baseline		☐ Enter TIME		☐ Enter TIME	
		☐ Mean		☐ Mean		☐ Mean	
		☐ Standard Deviation		☐ Standard Deviation		☐ Standard Deviation	
		☐ CI OR pvalue (specify)		☐ CI or pvalue (specify)		☐ CI or pvalue (specify)	
		☐ RR or OR(specify)		☐ RR or OR(specify)		☐ RR or OR(specify)	
		☐ Hazard Ratio		☐ Hazard Ratio		☐ Hazard Ratio	
		☐ Other - please specify		☐ Other - please specify		☐ Other - please specify	

TABLE 2: Mean difference from baseline

24. Arm A (Meditation)	25. Total N in ARM	26. Outcomes measures at **END OF TREATMENT**	27. Outcomes measures at **LAST FOLLOWUP**
		☐ Enter TIME	☐ Enter TIME
		☐ Mean	☐ Mean
		☐ Standard Error	☐ Standard Error
		☐ 95% CI	☐ 95% CI
		☐ Risk difference	☐ Risk difference
		☐ P-value	☐ P-value
		☐ Hazard Ratio	☐ Hazard Ratio
		☐ Other-pelase specify	☐ Other-pelase specify
28. Arm B - please specify	29. Total N in ARM	30. Outcomes measures at **END OF TREATMENT**	31. Outcomes measures at **LAST FOLLOWUP**
		☐ Enter TIME	☐ Enter TIME
		☐ Mean	☐ Mean
		☐ Standard Error	☐ Standard Error
		☐ 95% CI	☐ 95% CI
		☐ Risk difference	☐ Risk difference
		☐ P-value	☐ P-value
		☐ Hazard Ratio	☐ Hazard Ratio
		☐ Other-pelase specify	☐ Other-pelase specify
32. Arm C - please specify	33. Total N in ARM	34. Outcomes measures at **END OF TREATMENT**	35. Outcomes measures at **LAST FOLLOWUP**
		☐ Enter TIME	☐ Enter TIME
		☐ Mean	☐ Mean
		☐ Standard Error	☐ Standard Error
		☐ 95% CI	☐ 95% CI
		☐ Risk difference	☐ Risk difference
		☐ P-value	☐ P-value
		☐ Hazard Ratio	☐ Hazard Ratio
		☐ Other-pelase specify	☐ Other-pelase specify
36. Arm D- please specify	37. Total N in ARM	38. Outcomes measures at **END OF TREATMENT**	39. Outcomes measures at **LAST FOLLOWUP**
		☐ Enter TIME	☐ Enter TIME
		☐ Mean	☐ Mean

	☐ Standard Error	☐ Standard Error
○ Other - please specify	☐ 95% CI	☐ 95% CI
Clear Response	☐ Risk difference	☐ Risk difference
	☐ P-value	☐ P-value
	☐ Hazard Ratio	☐ Hazard Ratio
	☐ Other-pelase specify	☐ Other-pelase specify
60. Groups compared	**61. Outcomes measures at END OF TREATMENT**	**62. Outcomes measures at LAST FOLLOWUP**
○ A vs. B	☐ Enter TIME	☐ Enter TIME
○ A vs. C	☐ Mean	☐ Mean
○ A vs. D	☐ Standard Error	☐ Standard Error
○ Other - please specify	☐ 95% CI	☐ 95% CI
Clear Response	☐ Risk difference	☐ Risk difference
	☐ P-value	☐ P-value
	☐ Hazard Ratio	☐ Hazard Ratio
	☐ Other-pelase specify	☐ Other-pelase specify
63. Groups compared	**64. Outcomes measures at END OF TREATMENT**	**65. Outcomes measures at LAST FOLLOWUP**
○ A vs. B	☐ Enter TIME	☐ Enter TIME
○ A vs. C	☐ Mean	☐ Mean
○ A vs. D	☐ Standard Error	☐ Standard Error
○ Other - please specify	☐ 95% CI	☐ 95% CI
Clear Response	☐ Risk difference	☐ Risk difference
	☐ P-value	☐ P-value
	☐ Hazard Ratio	☐ Hazard Ratio
	☐ Other-pelase specify	☐ Other-pelase specify
66. Groups compared	**67. Outcomes measures at END OF TREATMENT**	**68. Outcomes measures at LAST FOLLOWUP**
○ A vs. B	☐ Enter TIME	☐ Enter TIME
○ A vs. C	☐ Mean	☐ Mean
○ A vs. D	☐ Standard Error	☐ Standard Error
○ Other - please specify	☐ 95% CI	☐ 95% CI
Clear Response	☐ Risk difference	☐ Risk difference
	☐ P-value	☐ P-value
	☐ Hazard Ratio	☐ Hazard Ratio
	☐ Other-pelase specify	☐ Other-pelase specify

Adverse Events

69. Were any adverse events reported?
☐ The paper specified that there were no AEs
☐ Paper reported on an AE - please specify
☐ Paper did not mention anything about an AE

70. Comments:

[Submit Form] and go to [ ] or Skip to Next

Outcomes for KQ1
Scales for Subjective Well-Being

DistillerSR

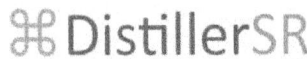

ritu.sharma

Project   Meditation (Switch)   User   mreuben (My Settings)
Messages   3 new

Live Support   User Guide

| Review | Datarama | Reports | References | Forms | Manage Levels | Users | Project | Logout |

Refid: 12, Skateboards: Are they really perilous? A retrospective study from a district hospital.
Rethnam U, Yesupalan RS, Sinha A.

[Submit Form] and go to [ ] or Skip to Next

Please submit one form per outcome

1. This study does not apply to KQ1

☐ No

KQ 1: What are the efficacy and harms of Meditation Programs on negative affect (e.g. anxiety, stress) and positive affect (e.g. well being) among those with a clinical condition (medical or psychiatric)?

Please select the outcome and outcome measure for KQ1

2. Outcome

○ Anxiety
○ Depression
○ Stress
○ General Distress
◉ Subjective well being

   Outcome Scales - Subjective well being

   ○ SF-12 mental component [   ]
   ○ Other - please specify   [   ]
   Clear Response

○ Harms
Clear Response

TABLE 1: Measures of association

ARM A -Please specify	Outcome measures at **baseline**	Outcome measures **at end of treatment**	Outcome measures **at last followup**
	☐ N [ ] ☐ At Baseline [ ] ☐ Mean [ ] ☐ Standard Deviation [ ] ☐ CI OR pvalue (specify) [ ] ☐ RR or OR(specify) [ ] ☐ Hazard Ratio [ ] ☐ Other - please specify [ ]	☐ N [ ] ☐ Enter TIME [ ] ☐ Mean [ ] ☐ Standard Deviation [ ] ☐ CI or pvalue (specify) [ ] ☐ RR or OR(specify) [ ] ☐ Hazard Ratio [ ] ☐ Other - please specify [ ]	☐ N [ ] ☐ Enter TIME [ ] ☐ Mean [ ] ☐ Standard Deviation [ ] ☐ CI or pvalue (specify) [ ] ☐ RR or OR(specify) [ ] ☐ Hazard Ratio [ ] ☐ Other - please specify [ ]
ARM B -Please specify	Outcome measures at **baseline**	Outcome measures **at end of treatment**	Outcome measures **at last followup**
	☐ N [ ] ☐ At Baseline [ ] ☐ Mean [ ] ☐ Standard Deviation [ ] ☐ CI OR pvalue (specify) [ ] ☐ RR or OR(specify) [ ] ☐ Hazard Ratio [ ] ☐ Other - please specify [ ]	☐ N [ ] ☐ Enter TIME [ ] ☐ Mean [ ] ☐ Standard Deviation [ ] ☐ CI or pvalue (specify) [ ] ☐ RR or OR(specify) [ ] ☐ Hazard Ratio [ ] ☐ Other - please specify [ ]	☐ N [ ] ☐ Enter TIME [ ] ☐ Mean [ ] ☐ Standard Deviation [ ] ☐ CI or pvalue (specify) [ ] ☐ RR or OR(specify) [ ] ☐ Hazard Ratio [ ] ☐ Other - please specify [ ]
ARM C-Please specify	Outcome measures at **baseline**	Outcome measures **at end of treatment**	Outcome measures **at last followup**
	☐ N [ ] ☐ At Baseline [ ] ☐ Mean [ ]	☐ N [ ] ☐ Enter TIME [ ] ☐ Mean [ ]	☐ N [ ] ☐ Enter TIME [ ] ☐ Mean [ ]

		Standard Deviation		Standard Deviation		Standard Deviation	
		☐ CI OR pvalue (specify)		☐ CI or pvalue (specify)		☐ CI or pvalue (specify)	
		☐ RR or OR(specify)		☐ RR or OR(specify)		☐ RR or OR(specify)	
		☐ Hazard Ratio		☐ Hazard Ratio		☐ Hazard Ratio	
		☐ Other - please specify		☐ Other - please specify		☐ Other - please specify	
ARM D-Please specify		Outcome measures at **baseline**		Outcome measures **at end of treatment**		Outcome measures **at last followup**	
		☐ N		☐ N		☐ N	
		☐ At Baseline		☐ Enter TIME		☐ Enter TIME	
		☐ Mean		☐ Mean		☐ Mean	
		☐ Standard Deviation		☐ Standard Deviation		☐ Standard Deviation	
		☐ CI OR pvalue (specify)		☐ CI or pvalue (specify)		☐ CI or pvalue (specify)	
		☐ RR or OR(specify)		☐ RR or OR(specify)		☐ RR or OR(specify)	
		☐ Hazard Ratio		☐ Hazard Ratio		☐ Hazard Ratio	
		☐ Other - please specify		☐ Other - please specify		☐ Other - please specify	

TABLE 2: Mean difference from baseline

24. Arm A (Meditation)	25. Total N in ARM	26. Outcomes measures at **END OF TREATMENT**		27. Outcomes measures at **LAST FOLLOWUP**	
		☐ Enter TIME		☐ Enter TIME	
		☐ Mean		☐ Mean	
		☐ Standard Error		☐ Standard Error	
		☐ 95% CI		☐ 95% CI	
		☐ Risk difference		☐ Risk difference	
		☐ P-value		☐ P-value	
		☐ Hazard Ratio		☐ Hazard Ratio	
		☐ Other-pelase specify		☐ Other-pelase specify	
28. Arm B - please specify	29. Total N in ARM	30. Outcomes measures at **END OF TREATMENT**		31. Outcomes measures at **LAST FOLLOWUP**	
		☐ Enter TIME		☐ Enter TIME	
		☐ Mean		☐ Mean	
		☐ Standard Error		☐ Standard Error	
		☐ 95% CI		☐ 95% CI	
		☐ Risk difference		☐ Risk difference	
		☐ P-value		☐ P-value	
		☐ Hazard Ratio		☐ Hazard Ratio	
		☐ Other-pelase specify		☐ Other-pelase specify	
32. Arm C - please specify	33. Total N in ARM	34. Outcomes measures at **END OF TREATMENT**		35. Outcomes measures at **LAST FOLLOWUP**	
		☐ Enter TIME		☐ Enter TIME	
		☐ Mean		☐ Mean	
		☐ Standard Error		☐ Standard Error	
		☐ 95% CI		☐ 95% CI	
		☐ Risk difference		☐ Risk difference	
		☐ P-value		☐ P-value	
		☐ Hazard Ratio		☐ Hazard Ratio	
		☐ Other-pelase specify		☐ Other-pelase specify	
36. Arm D- please specify	37. Total N in ARM	38. Outcomes measures at **END OF TREATMENT**		39. Outcomes measures at **LAST FOLLOWUP**	
		☐ Enter TIME		☐ Enter TIME	
		☐ Mean		☐ Mean	
		☐ Standard Error		☐ Standard Error	
		☐ 95% CI		☐ 95% CI	

DistillerSR

			☐ Risk difference		☐ Risk difference	
			☐ P-value		☐ P-value	
			☐ Hazard Ratio		☐ Hazard Ratio	
			☐ Other-pelase specify		☐ Other-pelase specify	

TABLE 3: Mean difference between groups

Arm A (Meditation) Vs. Arm B	40. Total N in ARM	41. Outcome At BASELINE	42. Outcomes at END OF TREATMENT	43. Outcomes at LAST FOLLOWUP
	☐ Total N in Arm A ☐ Total N in Arm B ☐ Total N in both arms	☐ At Baseline ☐ Mean ☐ Standard Error ☐ 95% CI ☐ Risk difference ☐ P-value ☐ Hazard Ratio ☐ Other-pelase specify	☐ Enter TIME ☐ Mean ☐ Standard Error ☐ 95% CI ☐ Risk difference ☐ P-value ☐ Hazard Ratio ☐ Other-pelase specify	☐ Enter TIME ☐ Mean ☐ Standard Error ☐ 95% CI ☐ Risk difference ☐ P-value ☐ Hazard Ratio ☐ Other-pelase specify
Arm A (Meditation) Vs. Arm C	44. Total N in ARM	45. Outcomes at BASELINE	46. Outcomes at END OF TREATMENT	47. Outcomes at LAST FOLLOWUP
	☐ Total N in Arm A ☐ Total N in Arm C ☐ Total N in both arms	☐ At Baseline ☐ Mean ☐ Standard Error ☐ 95% CI ☐ Risk difference ☐ P-value ☐ Hazard Ratio ☐ Other-pelase specify	☐ Enter TIME ☐ Mean ☐ Standard Error ☐ 95% CI ☐ Risk difference ☐ P-value ☐ Hazard Ratio ☐ Other-pelase specify	☐ Enter TIME ☐ Mean ☐ Standard Error ☐ 95% CI ☐ Risk difference ☐ P-value ☐ Hazard Ratio ☐ Other-pelase specify
Arm A (Meditation) Vs. Arm D	48. Total N in ARM	49. Outcomes at BASELINE	50. Outcomes at END OF TREATMENT	51. Outcomes at LAST FOLLOWUP
	☐ Total N in Arm A ☐ Total N in Arm D ☐ Total N in both arms	☐ At Baseline ☐ Mean ☐ Standard Error ☐ 95% CI ☐ Risk difference ☐ P-value ☐ Hazard Ratio ☐ Other-pelase specify	☐ Enter TIME ☐ Mean ☐ Standard Error ☐ 95% CI ☐ Risk difference ☐ P-value ☐ Hazard Ratio ☐ Other-pelase specify	☐ Enter TIME ☐ Mean ☐ Standard Error ☐ 95% CI ☐ Risk difference ☐ P-value ☐ Hazard Ratio ☐ Other-pelase specify
52. Other please spcify	53. Total N in ARM	54. Outcomes at BASELINE	55. Outcomes at END OF TREATMENT	56. Outcomes at LAST FOLLOWUP
	☐ Total N in Arm ☐ Total N in Arm ☐ Total N in both arms	☐ At Baseline ☐ Mean ☐ Standard Error ☐ 95% CI ☐ Risk difference ☐ P-value ☐ Hazard Ratio ☐ Other-pelase specify	☐ Enter TIME ☐ Mean ☐ Standard Error ☐ 95% CI ☐ Risk difference ☐ P-value ☐ Hazard Ratio ☐ Other-pelase specify	☐ Enter TIME ☐ Mean ☐ Standard Error ☐ 95% CI ☐ Risk difference ☐ P-value ☐ Hazard Ratio ☐ Other-pelase specify

TABLE 4: Diff-in-diff

57. Groups compared	58. Outcomes measures at END OF TREATMENT	59. Outcomes measures at LAST FOLLOWUP
○ A vs. B ○ A vs. C ○ A vs. D ○ Other - please specify Clear Response	☐ Enter TIME ☐ Mean ☐ Standard Error ☐ 95% CI	☐ Enter TIME ☐ Mean ☐ Standard Error ☐ 95% CI

	☐ Risk difference	☐ Risk difference	
	☐ P-value	☐ P-value	
	☐ Hazard Ratio	☐ Hazard Ratio	
	☐ Other-pelase specify	☐ Other-pelase specify	
60. Groups compared ○ A vs. B ○ A vs. C ○ A vs. D ○ Other - please specify [ ] Clear Response	61. Outcomes measures at **END OF TREATMENT** ☐ Enter TIME ☐ Mean ☐ Standard Error ☐ 95% CI ☐ Risk difference ☐ P-value ☐ Hazard Ratio ☐ Other-pelase specify	62. Outcomes measures at **LAST FOLLOWUP** ☐ Enter TIME ☐ Mean ☐ Standard Error ☐ 95% CI ☐ Risk difference ☐ P-value ☐ Hazard Ratio ☐ Other-pelase specify	
63. Groups compared ○ A vs. B ○ A vs. C ○ A vs. D ○ Other - please specify [ ] Clear Response	64. Outcomes measures at **END OF TREATMENT** ☐ Enter TIME ☐ Mean ☐ Standard Error ☐ 95% CI ☐ Risk difference ☐ P-value ☐ Hazard Ratio ☐ Other-pelase specify	65. Outcomes measures at **LAST FOLLOWUP** ☐ Enter TIME ☐ Mean ☐ Standard Error ☐ 95% CI ☐ Risk difference ☐ P-value ☐ Hazard Ratio ☐ Other-pelase specify	
66. Groups compared ○ A vs. B ○ A vs. C ○ A vs. D ○ Other - please specify [ ] Clear Response	67. Outcomes measures at **END OF TREATMENT** ☐ Enter TIME ☐ Mean ☐ Standard Error ☐ 95% CI ☐ Risk difference ☐ P-value ☐ Hazard Ratio ☐ Other-pelase specify	68. Outcomes measures at **LAST FOLLOWUP** ☐ Enter TIME ☐ Mean ☐ Standard Error ☐ 95% CI ☐ Risk difference ☐ P-value ☐ Hazard Ratio ☐ Other-pelase specify	

Adverse Events

69. **Were any adverse events reported?**

☐ The paper specified that there were no AEs
☐ Paper reported on an AE - please specify [ ]
☐ Paper did not mention anything about an AE

70. Comments:

[ ]

[Submit Form] and go to [ ] or Skip to Next

Outcomes for KQ 1—Harms

DistillerSR

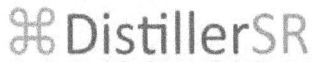

Refid: 12, Skateboards: Are they really perilous? A retrospective study from a district hospital.
Rethnam U, Yesupalan RS, Sinha A.

Submit Form and go to [ ] or Skip to Next

Please submit one form per outcome

1. This study does not apply to KQ1
   ☐ No

KQ 1: What are the efficacy and harms of Meditation Programs on negative affect (e.g. anxiety, stress) and positive affect (e.g. well being) among those with a clinical condition (medical or psychiatric)?

Please select the outcome and outcome measure for KQ1

2. Outcome
   ○ Anxiety
   ○ Depression
   ○ Stress
   ○ General Distress
   ○ Subjective well being
   ⦿ Harms
   Clear Response

TABLE 1: Measures of association

ARM A - Please specify	Outcome measures at baseline	Outcome measures at end of treatment	Outcome measures at last followup
	☐ N ☐ At Baseline ☐ Mean ☐ Standard Deviation ☐ CI OR pvalue (specify) ☐ RR or OR (specify) ☐ Hazard Ratio ☐ Other - please specify	☐ N ☐ Enter TIME ☐ Mean ☐ Standard Deviation ☐ CI or pvalue (specify) ☐ RR or OR (specify) ☐ Hazard Ratio ☐ Other - please specify	☐ N ☐ Enter TIME ☐ Mean ☐ Standard Deviation ☐ CI or pvalue (specify) ☐ RR or OR (specify) ☐ Hazard Ratio ☐ Other - please specify
ARM B - Please specify	Outcome measures at baseline	Outcome measures at end of treatment	Outcome measures at last followup
	☐ N ☐ At Baseline ☐ Mean ☐ Standard Deviation ☐ CI OR pvalue (specify) ☐ RR or OR (specify) ☐ Hazard Ratio ☐ Other - please specify	☐ N ☐ Enter TIME ☐ Mean ☐ Standard Deviation ☐ CI or pvalue (specify) ☐ RR or OR (specify) ☐ Hazard Ratio ☐ Other - please specify	☐ N ☐ Enter TIME ☐ Mean ☐ Standard Deviation ☐ CI or pvalue (specify) ☐ RR or OR (specify) ☐ Hazard Ratio ☐ Other - please specify
ARM C - Please specify	Outcome measures at baseline	Outcome measures at end of treatment	Outcome measures at last followup
	☐ N ☐ At Baseline ☐ Mean ☐ Standard Deviation ☐ CI OR pvalue (specify) ☐ RR or OR (specify) ☐ Hazard Ratio	☐ N ☐ Enter TIME ☐ Mean ☐ Standard Deviation ☐ CI or pvalue (specify) ☐ RR or OR (specify) ☐ Hazard Ratio	☐ N ☐ Enter TIME ☐ Mean ☐ Standard Deviation ☐ CI or pvalue (specify) ☐ RR or OR (specify) ☐ Hazard Ratio

DistillerSR

ARM D-Please specify	Outcome measures at baseline	Outcome measures at end of treatment	Outcome measures at last followup
	☐ Other - please specify	☐ Other - please specify	☐ Other - please specify
	☐ N ☐ At Baseline ☐ Mean ☐ Standard Deviation ☐ CI OR pvalue (specify) ☐ RR or OR(specify) ☐ Hazard Ratio ☐ Other - please specify	☐ N ☐ Enter TIME ☐ Mean ☐ Standard Deviation ☐ CI or pvalue (specify) ☐ RR or OR(specify) ☐ Hazard Ratio ☐ Other - please specify	☐ N ☐ Enter TIME ☐ Mean ☐ Standard Deviation ☐ CI or pvalue (specify) ☐ RR or OR(specify) ☐ Hazard Ratio ☐ Other - please specify

TABLE 2: Mean difference from baseline

24. Arm A (Meditation)	25. Total N in ARM	26. Outcomes measures at END OF TREATMENT	27. Outcomes measures at LAST FOLLOWUP
		☐ Enter TIME ☐ Mean ☐ Standard Error ☐ 95% CI ☐ Risk difference ☐ P-value ☐ Hazard Ratio ☐ Other-pelase specify	☐ Enter TIME ☐ Mean ☐ Standard Error ☐ 95% CI ☐ Risk difference ☐ P-value ☐ Hazard Ratio ☐ Other-pelase specify
28. Arm B - please specify	29. Total N in ARM	30. Outcomes measures at END OF TREATMENT	31. Outcomes measures at LAST FOLLOWUP
		☐ Enter TIME ☐ Mean ☐ Standard Error ☐ 95% CI ☐ Risk difference ☐ P-value ☐ Hazard Ratio ☐ Other-pelase specify	☐ Enter TIME ☐ Mean ☐ Standard Error ☐ 95% CI ☐ Risk difference ☐ P-value ☐ Hazard Ratio ☐ Other-pelase specify
32. Arm C - please specify	33. Total N in ARM	34. Outcomes measures at END OF TREATMENT	35. Outcomes measures at LAST FOLLOWUP
		☐ Enter TIME ☐ Mean ☐ Standard Error ☐ 95% CI ☐ Risk difference ☐ P-value ☐ Hazard Ratio ☐ Other-pelase specify	☐ Enter TIME ☐ Mean ☐ Standard Error ☐ 95% CI ☐ Risk difference ☐ P-value ☐ Hazard Ratio ☐ Other-pelase specify
36. Arm D- please specify	37. Total N in ARM	38. Outcomes measures at END OF TREATMENT	39. Outcomes measures at LAST FOLLOWUP
		☐ Enter TIME ☐ Mean ☐ Standard Error ☐ 95% CI ☐ Risk difference ☐ P-value ☐ Hazard Ratio ☐ Other-pelase specify	☐ Enter TIME ☐ Mean ☐ Standard Error ☐ 95% CI ☐ Risk difference ☐ P-value ☐ Hazard Ratio ☐ Other-pelase specify

TABLE 3: Mean difference between groups

Arm A (Meditation) Vs. Arm B	40. Total N in ARM	41. Outcome At BASELINE	42. Outcomes at END OF TREATMENT	43. Outcomes at LAST FOLLOWUP
	☐ Total N in Arm A ☐ Total N in Arm B ☐ Total N in both arms	☐ At Baseline ☐ Mean ☐ Standard Error ☐ 95% CI ☐ Risk difference ☐ P-value ☐ Hazard Ratio ☐ Other-pelase specify	☐ Enter TIME ☐ Mean ☐ Standard Error ☐ 95% CI ☐ Risk difference ☐ P-value ☐ Hazard Ratio ☐ Other-pelase specify	☐ Enter TIME ☐ Mean ☐ Standard Error ☐ 95% CI ☐ Risk difference ☐ P-value ☐ Hazard Ratio ☐ Other-pelase specify
Arm A (Meditation) Vs. Arm C	44. Total N in ARM	45. Outcomes at BASELINE	46. Outcomes at END OF TREATMENT	47. Outcomes at LAST FOLLOWUP
	☐ Total N in Arm A ☐ Total N in Arm C ☐ Total N in both arms	☐ At Baseline ☐ Mean ☐ Standard Error ☐ 95% CI ☐ Risk difference ☐ P-value ☐ Hazard Ratio ☐ Other-pelase specify	☐ Enter TIME ☐ Mean ☐ Standard Error ☐ 95% CI ☐ Risk difference ☐ P-value ☐ Hazard Ratio ☐ Other-pelase specify	☐ Enter TIME ☐ Mean ☐ Standard Error ☐ 95% CI ☐ Risk difference ☐ P-value ☐ Hazard Ratio ☐ Other-pelase specify
Arm A (Meditation) Vs. Arm D	48. Total N in ARM	49. Outcomes at BASELINE	50. Outcomes at END OF TREATMENT	51. Outcomes at LAST FOLLOWUP
	☐ Total N in Arm A ☐ Total N in Arm D ☐ Total N in both arms	☐ At Baseline ☐ Mean ☐ Standard Error ☐ 95% CI ☐ Risk difference ☐ P-value ☐ Hazard Ratio ☐ Other-pelase specify	☐ Enter TIME ☐ Mean ☐ Standard Error ☐ 95% CI ☐ Risk difference ☐ P-value ☐ Hazard Ratio ☐ Other-pelase specify	☐ Enter TIME ☐ Mean ☐ Standard Error ☐ 95% CI ☐ Risk difference ☐ P-value ☐ Hazard Ratio ☐ Other-pelase specify
52. Other please spcify	53. Total N in ARM	54. Outcomes at BASELINE	55. Outcomes at END OF TREATMENT	56. Outcomes at LAST FOLLOWUP
	☐ Total N in Arm ☐ Total N in Arm ☐ Total N in both arms	☐ At Baseline ☐ Mean ☐ Standard Error ☐ 95% CI ☐ Risk difference ☐ P-value ☐ Hazard Ratio ☐ Other-pelase specify	☐ Enter TIME ☐ Mean ☐ Standard Error ☐ 95% CI ☐ Risk difference ☐ P-value ☐ Hazard Ratio ☐ Other-pelase specify	☐ Enter TIME ☐ Mean ☐ Standard Error ☐ 95% CI ☐ Risk difference ☐ P-value ☐ Hazard Ratio ☐ Other-pelase specify

TABLE 4: Diff-in-diff

67. Groups compared	58. Outcomes measures at END OF TREATMENT	59. Outcomes measures at LAST FOLLOWUP
○ A vs. B ○ A vs. C ○ A vs. D ○ Other - please specify Clear Response	☐ Enter TIME ☐ Mean ☐ Standard Error ☐ 95% CI ☐ Risk difference ☐ P-value ☐ Hazard Ratio ☐ Other-pelase specify	☐ Enter TIME ☐ Mean ☐ Standard Error ☐ 95% CI ☐ Risk difference ☐ P-value ☐ Hazard Ratio ☐ Other-pelase specify

DistillerSR

60. Groups compared	61. Outcomes measures at **END OF TREATMENT**	62. Outcomes measures at **LAST FOLLOWUP**
○ A vs. B ○ A vs. C ○ A vs. D ○ Other - please specify [ ] Clear Response	☐ Enter TIME [ ] ☐ Mean [ ] ☐ Standard Error [ ] ☐ 95% CI [ ] ☐ Risk difference [ ] ☐ P-value [ ] ☐ Hazard Ratio [ ] ☐ Other-pelase specify [ ]	☐ Enter TIME [ ] ☐ Mean [ ] ☐ Standard Error [ ] ☐ 95% CI [ ] ☐ Risk difference [ ] ☐ P-value [ ] ☐ Hazard Ratio [ ] ☐ Other-pelase specify [ ]
63. Groups compared	64. Outcomes measures at **END OF TREATMENT**	65. Outcomes measures at **LAST FOLLOWUP**
○ A vs. B ○ A vs. C ○ A vs. D ○ Other - please specify [ ] Clear Response	☐ Enter TIME [ ] ☐ Mean [ ] ☐ Standard Error [ ] ☐ 95% CI [ ] ☐ Risk difference [ ] ☐ P-value [ ] ☐ Hazard Ratio [ ] ☐ Other-pelase specify [ ]	☐ Enter TIME [ ] ☐ Mean [ ] ☐ Standard Error [ ] ☐ 95% CI [ ] ☐ Risk difference [ ] ☐ P-value [ ] ☐ Hazard Ratio [ ] ☐ Other-pelase specify [ ]
66. Groups compared	67. Outcomes measures at **END OF TREATMENT**	68. Outcomes measures at **LAST FOLLOWUP**
○ A vs. B ○ A vs. C ○ A vs. D ○ Other - please specify [ ] Clear Response	☐ Enter TIME [ ] ☐ Mean [ ] ☐ Standard Error [ ] ☐ 95% CI [ ] ☐ Risk difference [ ] ☐ P-value [ ] ☐ Hazard Ratio [ ] ☐ Other-pelase specify [ ]	☐ Enter TIME [ ] ☐ Mean [ ] ☐ Standard Error [ ] ☐ 95% CI [ ] ☐ Risk difference [ ] ☐ P-value [ ] ☐ Hazard Ratio [ ] ☐ Other-pelase specify [ ]

Adverse Events

69. Were any adverse events reported?
   ☐ The paper specified that there were no AEs
   ☐ Paper reported on an AE - please specify [ ]
   ☐ Paper did not mention anything about an AE

70. Comments:
   [ ]

[Submit Form] and go to [ ] or Skip to Next

Outcomes for KQ 2

DistillerSR

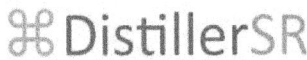

ritu.sharma

Project Meditation (Switch) User mreuben (My Settings)
Messages 3 new

Live Support | User Guide

Review | Datarama | Reports | References | Forms | Manage Levels | Users | Project | Logout

Refid: 12, Skateboards: Are they really perilous? A retrospective study from a district hospital.
Rethnam U, Yesupalan RS, Sinha A.

[Submit Form] and go to [ ] or Skip to Next

Please submit one form per outcome

1. This study does not apply to KQ2

☐ No

KQ 2: What are the efficacy and harms of Meditation Programs on attention among those with a clinical condition (medical or psychiatric)?

Please select the outcome and outcome measure for KQ 2

2. Outcome

- ○ Attentional Bias
- ⊙ Associate Learning subtest
- ○ Word Fluency subtest
- ○ Overlearned Verbal Task (OVT)
- ○ Stroop Color-Word Interference Test (CW1T)
- ○ Cognitive scale of the Cognitive-Somatic Anxiety Questionnaire
- ○ Cognitive Interference Questionnaire
- ○ Attentional Interference Scale
- ○ Letter Cancellation Test
- ○ Trail making Test; Ruff
- ○ Digits Forward / Backward
- ○ Harms
- ○ Other- please specify

Clear Response

TABLE 1: Measures of association

ARM A - Please specify	Outcome measures at baseline	Outcome measures at end of treatment	Outcome measures at last followup
	☐ N ☐ At Baseline ☐ Mean ☐ Standard Deviation ☐ CI OR pvalue (specify) ☐ RR or OR(specify) ☐ Hazard Ratio ☐ Other - please specify	☐ N ☐ Enter TIME ☐ Mean ☐ Standard Deviation ☐ CI or pvalue (specify) ☐ RR or OR(specify) ☐ Hazard Ratio ☐ Other - please specify	☐ N ☐ Enter TIME ☐ Mean ☐ Standard Deviation ☐ CI or pvalue (specify) ☐ RR or OR(specify) ☐ Hazard Ratio ☐ Other - please specify
ARM B - Please specify	Outcome measures at baseline	Outcome measures at end of treatment	Outcome measures at last followup
	☐ N ☐ At Baseline ☐ Mean ☐ Standard Deviation ☐ CI OR pvalue (specify) ☐ RR or OR(specify) ☐ Hazard Ratio ☐ Other - please specify	☐ N ☐ Enter TIME ☐ Mean ☐ Standard Deviation ☐ CI or pvalue (specify) ☐ RR or OR(specify) ☐ Hazard Ratio ☐ Other - please specify	☐ N ☐ Enter TIME ☐ Mean ☐ Standard Deviation ☐ CI or pvalue (specify) ☐ RR or OR(specify) ☐ Hazard Ratio ☐ Other - please specify

DistillerSR

ARM C-Please specify	Outcome measures at baseline	Outcome measures at end of treatment	Outcome measures at last followup
	☐ N ☐ At Baseline ☐ Mean ☐ Standard Deviation ☐ CI OR pvalue (specify) ☐ RR or OR(specify) ☐ Hazard Ratio ☐ Other - please specify	☐ N ☐ Enter TIME ☐ Mean ☐ Standard Deviation ☐ CI or pvalue (specify) ☐ RR or OR(specify) ☐ Hazard Ratio ☐ Other - please specify	☐ N ☐ Enter TIME ☐ Mean ☐ Standard Deviation ☐ CI or pvalue (specify) ☐ RR or OR(specify) ☐ Hazard Ratio ☐ Other - please specify
ARM D-Please specify	Outcome measures at baseline	Outcome measures at end of treatment	Outcome measures at last followup
	☐ N ☐ At Baseline ☐ Mean ☐ Standard Deviation ☐ CI OR pvalue (specify) ☐ RR or OR(specify) ☐ Hazard Ratio ☐ Other - please specify	☐ N ☐ Enter TIME ☐ Mean ☐ Standard Deviation ☐ CI or pvalue (specify) ☐ RR or OR(specify) ☐ Hazard Ratio ☐ Other - please specify	☐ N ☐ Enter TIME ☐ Mean ☐ Standard Deviation ☐ CI or pvalue (specify) ☐ RR or OR(specify) ☐ Hazard Ratio ☐ Other - please specify

TABLE 2: Mean difference from baseline

19. Arm A (Meditation)	20. Total N in ARM	21. Outcomes measures at END OF TREATMENT	22. Outcomes measures at LAST FOLLOWUP
		☐ Enter TIME ☐ Mean ☐ Standard Error ☐ 95% CI ☐ Risk difference ☐ P-value ☐ Hazard Ratio ☐ Other-pelase specify	☐ Enter TIME ☐ Mean ☐ Standard Error ☐ 95% CI ☐ Risk difference ☐ P-value ☐ Hazard Ratio ☐ Other-pelase specify
23. Arm B - please specify	24. Total N in ARM	25. Outcomes measures at END OF TREATMENT	26. Outcomes measures at LAST FOLLOWUP
		☐ Enter TIME ☐ Mean ☐ Standard Error ☐ 95% CI ☐ Risk difference ☐ P-value ☐ Hazard Ratio ☐ Other-pelase specify	☐ Enter TIME ☐ Mean ☐ Standard Error ☐ 95% CI ☐ Risk difference ☐ P-value ☐ Hazard Ratio ☐ Other-pelase specify
27. Arm C - please specify	28. Total N in ARM	29. Outcomes measures at END OF TREATMENT	30. Outcomes measures at LAST FOLLOWUP
		☐ Enter TIME ☐ Mean ☐ Standard Error ☐ 95% CI ☐ Risk difference ☐ P-value ☐ Hazard Ratio ☐ Other-pelase specify	☐ Enter TIME ☐ Mean ☐ Standard Error ☐ 95% CI ☐ Risk difference ☐ P-value ☐ Hazard Ratio ☐ Other-pelase specify
31. Arm D- please specify	32. Total N in ARM	33. Outcomes measures at END OF TREATMENT	34. Outcomes measures at LAST FOLLOWUP
		☐ Enter TIME	☐ Enter TIME

Outcomes for KQ 3
Scales for Substance Use

Refid: 12, Skateboards: Are they really perilous? A retrospective study from a district hospital.
Rethnam U, Yesupalan RS, Sinha A.

Please submit one form per outcome

1. **This study does not apply to KQ3**
   ☐ No

KQ 3: What are the efficacy and harms of Meditation Programs on health-related behaviors affected by stress, specifically substance use, sleep, and eating, among those with a clinical condition (medical or psychiatric)?

Please select the outcome and outcome measure for KQ3

2. Outcome
   - ◉ Substance use
     Outcome Scales - Substance use
     - ○ Self-reported smoking (cigs/day)
     - ○ Self-reported abstinence
     - ○ Carbon monoxide (CO)
     - ○ Penn Alcohol Craving Scale
     - ○ Impaired Alcohol response inhibition scale
     - ○ % days of substance use
     - ○ drug/alcohol craving
     - ○ Other - please specify
     Clear Response
   - ○ Sleep
   - ○ Eating
   - ○ Harms
   Clear Response

TABLE 1: Measures of association

ARM A - Please specify	Outcome measures at **baseline**	Outcome measures **at end of treatment**	Outcome measures **at last followup**
	☐ N	☐ N	☐ N
	☐ At Baseline	☐ Enter TIME	☐ Enter TIME
	☐ Mean	☐ Mean	☐ Mean
	☐ Standard Deviation	☐ Standard Deviation	☐ Standard Deviation
	☐ CI OR pvalue (specify)	☐ CI or pvalue (specify)	☐ CI or pvalue (specify)
	☐ RR or OR(specify)	☐ RR or OR(specify)	☐ RR or OR(specify)
	☐ Hazard Ratio	☐ Hazard Ratio	☐ Hazard Ratio
	☐ Other - please specify	☐ Other - please specify	☐ Other - please specify
ARM B - Please specify	Outcome measures at **baseline**	Outcome measures **at end of treatment**	Outcome measures **at last followup**
	☐ N	☐ N	☐ N
	☐ At Baseline	☐ Enter TIME	☐ Enter TIME
	☐ Mean	☐ Mean	☐ Mean
	☐ Standard Deviation	☐ Standard Deviation	☐ Standard Deviation
	☐ CI OR pvalue (specify)	☐ CI or pvalue (specify)	☐ CI or pvalue (specify)
	☐ RR or OR(specify)	☐ RR or OR(specify)	☐ RR or OR(specify)
	☐ Hazard Ratio	☐ Hazard Ratio	☐ Hazard Ratio
	☐ Other - please specify	☐ Other - please specify	☐ Other - please specify

ARM C-Please specify	Outcome measures at baseline	Outcome measures at end of treatment	Outcome measures at last followup
	☐ N ☐ At Baseline ☐ Mean ☐ Standard Deviation ☐ CI OR pvalue (specify) ☐ RR or OR(specify) ☐ Hazard Ratio ☐ Other - please specify	☐ N ☐ Enter TIME ☐ Mean ☐ Standard Deviation ☐ CI or pvalue (specify) ☐ RR or OR(specify) ☐ Hazard Ratio ☐ Other - please specify	☐ N ☐ Enter TIME ☐ Mean ☐ Standard Deviation ☐ CI or pvalue (specify) ☐ RR or OR(specify) ☐ Hazard Ratio ☐ Other - please specify
ARM D-Please specify	Outcome measures at baseline	Outcome measures at end of treatment	Outcome measures at last followup
	☐ N ☐ At Baseline ☐ Mean ☐ Standard Deviation ☐ CI OR pvalue (specify) ☐ RR or OR(specify) ☐ Hazard Ratio ☐ Other - please specify	☐ N ☐ Enter TIME ☐ Mean ☐ Standard Deviation ☐ CI or pvalue (specify) ☐ RR or OR(specify) ☐ Hazard Ratio ☐ Other - please specify	☐ N ☐ Enter TIME ☐ Mean ☐ Standard Deviation ☐ CI or pvalue (specify) ☐ RR or OR(specify) ☐ Hazard Ratio ☐ Other - please specify

TABLE 2: Mean difference from baseline

22. Arm A (Meditation)	23. Total N in ARM	24. Outcomes measures at END OF TREATMENT	25. Outcomes measures at LAST FOLLOWUP
		☐ Enter TIME ☐ Mean ☐ Standard Error ☐ 95% CI ☐ Risk difference ☐ P-value ☐ Hazard Ratio ☐ Other-pelase specify	☐ Enter TIME ☐ Mean ☐ Standard Error ☐ 95% CI ☐ Risk difference ☐ P-value ☐ Hazard Ratio ☐ Other-pelase specify
26. Arm B - please specify	27. Total N in ARM	28. Outcomes measures at END OF TREATMENT	29. Outcomes measures at LAST FOLLOWUP
		☐ Enter TIME ☐ Mean ☐ Standard Error ☐ 95% CI ☐ Risk difference ☐ P-value ☐ Hazard Ratio ☐ Other-pelase specify	☐ Enter TIME ☐ Mean ☐ Standard Error ☐ 95% CI ☐ Risk difference ☐ P-value ☐ Hazard Ratio ☐ Other-pelase specify
30. Arm C - please specify	31. Total N in ARM	32. Outcomes measures at END OF TREATMENT	33. Outcomes measures at LAST FOLLOWUP
		☐ Enter TIME ☐ Mean ☐ Standard Error ☐ 95% CI ☐ Risk difference ☐ P-value ☐ Hazard Ratio ☐ Other-pelase specify	☐ Enter TIME ☐ Mean ☐ Standard Error ☐ 95% CI ☐ Risk difference ☐ P-value ☐ Hazard Ratio ☐ Other-pelase specify
34. Arm D- please specify	35. Total N in ARM	36. Outcomes measures at END OF TREATMENT	37. Outcomes measures at LAST FOLLOWUP

DistillerSR

		☐ Enter TIME ☐ Mean ☐ Standard Error ☐ 95% CI ☐ Risk difference ☐ P-value ☐ Hazard Ratio ☐ Other-pelase specify	☐ Enter TIME ☐ Mean ☐ Standard Error ☐ 95% CI ☐ Risk difference ☐ P-value ☐ Hazard Ratio ☐ Other-pelase specify

TABLE 3: Mean difference between groups

Arm A (Meditation) Vs. Arm B	38. Total N in ARM ☐ Total N in Arm A ☐ Total N in Arm B ☐ Total N in both arms	39. Outcome At BASELINE ☐ At Baseline ☐ Mean ☐ Standard Error ☐ 95% CI ☐ Risk difference ☐ P-value ☐ Hazard Ratio ☐ Other-pelase specify	40. Outcomes at END OF TREATMENT ☐ Enter TIME ☐ Mean ☐ Standard Error ☐ 95% CI ☐ Risk difference ☐ P-value ☐ Hazard Ratio ☐ Other-pelase specify	41. Outcomes at LAST FOLLOWUP ☐ Enter TIME ☐ Mean ☐ Standard Error ☐ 95% CI ☐ Risk difference ☐ P-value ☐ Hazard Ratio ☐ Other-pelase specify
Arm A (Meditation) Vs. Arm C	42. Total N in ARM ☐ Total N in Arm A ☐ Total N in Arm C ☐ Total N in both arms	43. Outcomes at BASELINE ☐ At Baseline ☐ Mean ☐ Standard Error ☐ 95% CI ☐ Risk difference ☐ P-value ☐ Hazard Ratio ☐ Other-pelase specify	44. Outcomes at END OF TREATMENT ☐ Enter TIME ☐ Mean ☐ Standard Error ☐ 95% CI ☐ Risk difference ☐ P-value ☐ Hazard Ratio ☐ Other-pelase specify	45. Outcomes at LAST FOLLOWUP ☐ Enter TIME ☐ Mean ☐ Standard Error ☐ 95% CI ☐ Risk difference ☐ P-value ☐ Hazard Ratio ☐ Other-pelase specify
Arm A (Meditation) Vs. Arm D	46. Total N in ARM ☐ Total N in Arm A ☐ Total N in Arm D ☐ Total N in both arms	47. Outcomes at BASELINE ☐ At Baseline ☐ Mean ☐ Standard Error ☐ 95% CI ☐ Risk difference ☐ P-value ☐ Hazard Ratio ☐ Other-pelase specify	48. Outcomes at END OF TREATMENT ☐ Enter TIME ☐ Mean ☐ Standard Error ☐ 95% CI ☐ Risk difference ☐ P-value ☐ Hazard Ratio ☐ Other-pelase specify	49. Outcomes at LAST FOLLOWUP ☐ Enter TIME ☐ Mean ☐ Standard Error ☐ 95% CI ☐ Risk difference ☐ P-value ☐ Hazard Ratio ☐ Other-pelase specify
50. Other please spcify	51. Total N in ARM ☐ Total N in Arm ☐ Total N in Arm ☐ Total N in both arms	52. Outcomes at BASELINE ☐ At Baseline ☐ Mean ☐ Standard Error ☐ 95% CI ☐ Risk difference ☐ P-value ☐ Hazard Ratio ☐ Other-pelase specify	53. Outcomes at END OF TREATMENT ☐ Enter TIME ☐ Mean ☐ Standard Error ☐ 95% CI ☐ Risk difference ☐ P-value ☐ Hazard Ratio ☐ Other-pelase specify	54. Outcomes at LAST FOLLOWUP ☐ Enter TIME ☐ Mean ☐ Standard Error ☐ 95% CI ☐ Risk difference ☐ P-value ☐ Hazard Ratio ☐ Other-pelase specify

TABLE 4: Diff-in-diff

55. Groups compared	56. Outcomes measures at END OF TREATMENT	57. Outcomes measures at LAST FOLLOWUP

Outcomes for KQ 3
Scales for Sleep

DistillerSR

⌘ DistillerSR

ritu.sharma

Project: Meditation (Switch) User: mreuben (My Settings)
Messages: 3 new

Live Support | User Guide

Review ▾ | Datastore | Reports ▾ | References ▾ | Forms ▾ | Manage Levels ▾ | Users ▾ | Project ▾ | Logout

Refid: 12, Skateboards: Are they really perilous? A retrospective study from a district hospital.
Rethnam U, Yesupalan RS, Sinha A.

[Submit Form] and go to [ ] or Skip to Next

Please submit one form per outcome

1. This study does not apply to KQ3
☐ No

KQ 3: What are the efficacy and harms of Meditation Programs on health-related behaviors affected by stress, specifically substance use, sleep, and eating, among those with a clinical condition (medical or psychiatric)?

Please select the outcome and outcome measure for KQ3

2. Outcome
○ Substance use
⦿ Sleep
   Outcome Scales-Sleep
   ○ Total sleep time -Please specify if its coming from DIARY or ACTIGRAPHY
   ○ Sleep onset latency -Please specify if its coming from DIARY or ACTIGRAPHY
   ○ Wake after sleep onset -Please specify if its coming from DIARY or ACTIGRAPHY
   ○ sleep efficiency -Please specify if its coming from DIARY or ACTIGRAPHY
   ○ Pittsburgh Sleep Quality Index (PSQI)
   ○ Abridged PSQI
   ○ Insomnia severity index
   ○ Other- please specify
   Clear Response
○ Eating
○ Harms
Clear Response

TABLE 1: Measures of association

ARM A - Please specify	Outcome measures at **baseline**	Outcome measures **at end of treatment**	Outcome measures **at last followup**
	☐ N	☐ N	☐ N
	☐ At Baseline	☐ Enter TIME	☐ Enter TIME
	☐ Mean	☐ Mean	☐ Mean
	☐ Standard Deviation	☐ Standard Deviation	☐ Standard Deviation
	☐ CI OR pvalue (specify)	☐ CI or pvalue (specify)	☐ CI or pvalue (specify)
	☐ RR or OR(specify)	☐ RR or OR(specify)	☐ RR or OR(specify)
	☐ Hazard Ratio	☐ Hazard Ratio	☐ Hazard Ratio
	☐ Other - please specify	☐ Other - please specify	☐ Other - please specify
ARM B - Please specify	Outcome measures at **baseline**	Outcome measures **at end of treatment**	Outcome measures **at last followup**
	☐ N	☐ N	☐ N
	☐ At Baseline	☐ Enter TIME	☐ Enter TIME
	☐ Mean	☐ Mean	☐ Mean
	☐ Standard Deviation	☐ Standard Deviation	☐ Standard Deviation
	☐ CI OR pvalue (specify)	☐ CI or pvalue (specify)	☐ CI or pvalue (specify)
	☐ RR or OR(specify)	☐ RR or OR(specify)	☐ RR or OR(specify)
	☐ Hazard Ratio	☐ Hazard Ratio	☐ Hazard Ratio
	☐ Other - please specify	☐ Other - please specify	☐ Other - please specify

https://systematic-review.ca/Submit/RenderForm.php?id=13&hide_abstract=1 [6/14/2012 2:57:33 PM]

ARM C-Please specify	Outcome measures at **baseline**	Outcome measures **at end of treatment**	Outcome measures **at last followup**
	☐ N ☐ At Baseline ☐ Mean ☐ Standard Deviation ☐ CI OR pvalue (specify) ☐ RR or OR(specify) ☐ Hazard Ratio ☐ Other - please specify	☐ N ☐ Enter TIME ☐ Mean ☐ Standard Deviation ☐ CI or pvalue (specify) ☐ RR or OR(specify) ☐ Hazard Ratio ☐ Other - please specify	☐ N ☐ Enter TIME ☐ Mean ☐ Standard Deviation ☐ CI or pvalue (specify) ☐ RR or OR(specify) ☐ Hazard Ratio ☐ Other - please specify
ARM D-Please specify	Outcome measures at **baseline**	Outcome measures **at end of treatment**	Outcome measures **at last followup**
	☐ N ☐ At Baseline ☐ Mean ☐ Standard Deviation ☐ CI OR pvalue (specify) ☐ RR or OR(specify) ☐ Hazard Ratio ☐ Other - please specify	☐ N ☐ Enter TIME ☐ Mean ☐ Standard Deviation ☐ CI or pvalue (specify) ☐ RR or OR(specify) ☐ Hazard Ratio ☐ Other - please specify	☐ N ☐ Enter TIME ☐ Mean ☐ Standard Deviation ☐ CI or pvalue (specify) ☐ RR or OR(specify) ☐ Hazard Ratio ☐ Other - please specify

TABLE 2: Mean difference from baseline

22. Arm A (Meditation)	23. Total N in ARM	24. Outcomes measures at **END OF TREATMENT**	25. Outcomes measures at **LAST FOLLOWUP**
		☐ Enter TIME ☐ Mean ☐ Standard Error ☐ 95% CI ☐ Risk difference ☐ P-value ☐ Hazard Ratio ☐ Other-pelase specify	☐ Enter TIME ☐ Mean ☐ Standard Error ☐ 95% CI ☐ Risk difference ☐ P-value ☐ Hazard Ratio ☐ Other-pelase specify
26. Arm B - please specify	27. Total N in ARM	28. Outcomes measures at **END OF TREATMENT**	29. Outcomes measures at **LAST FOLLOWUP**
		☐ Enter TIME ☐ Mean ☐ Standard Error ☐ 95% CI ☐ Risk difference ☐ P-value ☐ Hazard Ratio ☐ Other-pelase specify	☐ Enter TIME ☐ Mean ☐ Standard Error ☐ 95% CI ☐ Risk difference ☐ P-value ☐ Hazard Ratio ☐ Other-pelase specify
30. Arm C - please specify	31. Total N in ARM	32. Outcomes measures at **END OF TREATMENT**	33. Outcomes measures at **LAST FOLLOWUP**
		☐ Enter TIME ☐ Mean ☐ Standard Error ☐ 95% CI ☐ Risk difference ☐ P-value ☐ Hazard Ratio ☐ Other-pelase specify	☐ Enter TIME ☐ Mean ☐ Standard Error ☐ 95% CI ☐ Risk difference ☐ P-value ☐ Hazard Ratio ☐ Other-pelase specify
34. Arm D- please specify	35. Total N in ARM	36. Outcomes measures at **END OF TREATMENT**	37. Outcomes measures at **LAST FOLLOWUP**

		☐ Enter TIME	☐ Enter TIME
		☐ Mean	☐ Mean
		☐ Standard Error	☐ Standard Error
		☐ 95% CI	☐ 95% CI
		☐ Risk difference	☐ Risk difference
		☐ P-value	☐ P-value
		☐ Hazard Ratio	☐ Hazard Ratio
		☐ Other-pelase specify	☐ Other-pelase specify

TABLE 3: Mean difference between groups

	38. Total N in ARM	39. Outcome At BASELINE	40. Outcomes at END OF TREATMENT	41. Outcomes at LAST FOLLOWUP
Arm A (Meditation) Vs. Arm B	☐ Total N in Arm A ☐ Total N in Arm B ☐ Total N in both arms	☐ At Baseline ☐ Mean ☐ Standard Error ☐ 95% CI ☐ Risk difference ☐ P-value ☐ Hazard Ratio ☐ Other-pelase specify	☐ Enter TIME ☐ Mean ☐ Standard Error ☐ 95% CI ☐ Risk difference ☐ P-value ☐ Hazard Ratio ☐ Other-pelase specify	☐ Enter TIME ☐ Mean ☐ Standard Error ☐ 95% CI ☐ Risk difference ☐ P-value ☐ Hazard Ratio ☐ Other-pelase specify
	42. Total N in ARM	43. Outcomes at BASELINE	44. Outcomes at END OF TREATMENT	45. Outcomes at LAST FOLLOWUP
Arm A (Meditation) Vs. Arm C	☐ Total N in Arm A ☐ Total N in Arm C ☐ Total N in both arms	☐ At Baseline ☐ Mean ☐ Standard Error ☐ 95% CI ☐ Risk difference ☐ P-value ☐ Hazard Ratio ☐ Other-pelase specify	☐ Enter TIME ☐ Mean ☐ Standard Error ☐ 95% CI ☐ Risk difference ☐ P-value ☐ Hazard Ratio ☐ Other-pelase specify	☐ Enter TIME ☐ Mean ☐ Standard Error ☐ 95% CI ☐ Risk difference ☐ P-value ☐ Hazard Ratio ☐ Other-pelase specify
	46. Total N in ARM	47. Outcomes at BASELINE	48. Outcomes at END OF TREATMENT	49. Outcomes at LAST FOLLOWUP
Arm A (Meditation) Vs. Arm D	☐ Total N in Arm A ☐ Total N in Arm D ☐ Total N in both arms	☐ At Baseline ☐ Mean ☐ Standard Error ☐ 95% CI ☐ Risk difference ☐ P-value ☐ Hazard Ratio ☐ Other-pelase specify	☐ Enter TIME ☐ Mean ☐ Standard Error ☐ 95% CI ☐ Risk difference ☐ P-value ☐ Hazard Ratio ☐ Other-pelase specify	☐ Enter TIME ☐ Mean ☐ Standard Error ☐ 95% CI ☐ Risk difference ☐ P-value ☐ Hazard Ratio ☐ Other-pelase specify
50. Other please spcify	51. Total N in ARM	52. Outcomes at BASELINE	53. Outcomes at END OF TREATMENT	54. Outcomes at LAST FOLLOWUP
	☐ Total N in Arm ☐ Total N in Arm ☐ Total N in both arms	☐ At Baseline ☐ Mean ☐ Standard Error ☐ 95% CI ☐ Risk difference ☐ P-value ☐ Hazard Ratio ☐ Other-pelase specify	☐ Enter TIME ☐ Mean ☐ Standard Error ☐ 95% CI ☐ Risk difference ☐ P-value ☐ Hazard Ratio ☐ Other-pelase specify	☐ Enter TIME ☐ Mean ☐ Standard Error ☐ 95% CI ☐ Risk difference ☐ P-value ☐ Hazard Ratio ☐ Other-pelase specify

TABLE 4: Diff-in-diff

55. Groups compared	56. Outcomes measures at END OF TREATMENT	57. Outcomes measures at LAST FOLLOWUP

DistillerSR

○ A vs. B ○ A vs. C ○ A vs. D ○ Other - please specify [ ] Clear Response	☐ Enter TIME [ ] ☐ Mean [ ] ☐ Standard Error [ ] ☐ 95% CI [ ] ☐ Risk difference [ ] ☐ P-value [ ] ☐ Hazard Ratio [ ] ☐ Other-pelase specify [ ]	☐ Enter TIME [ ] ☐ Mean [ ] ☐ Standard Error [ ] ☐ 95% CI [ ] ☐ Risk difference [ ] ☐ P-value [ ] ☐ Hazard Ratio [ ] ☐ Other-pelase specify [ ]
58. Groups compared ○ A vs. B ○ A vs. C ○ A vs. D ○ Other - please specify [ ] Clear Response	59. Outcomes measures at **END OF TREATMENT** ☐ Enter TIME [ ] ☐ Mean [ ] ☐ Standard Error [ ] ☐ 95% CI [ ] ☐ Risk difference [ ] ☐ P-value [ ] ☐ Hazard Ratio [ ] ☐ Other-pelase specify [ ]	60. Outcomes measures at **LAST FOLLOWUP** ☐ Enter TIME [ ] ☐ Mean [ ] ☐ Standard Error [ ] ☐ 95% CI [ ] ☐ Risk difference [ ] ☐ P-value [ ] ☐ Hazard Ratio [ ] ☐ Other-pelase specify [ ]
61. Groups compared ○ A vs. B ○ A vs. C ○ A vs. D ○ Other - please specify [ ] Clear Response	62. Outcomes measures at **END OF TREATMENT** ☐ Enter TIME [ ] ☐ Mean [ ] ☐ Standard Error [ ] ☐ 95% CI [ ] ☐ Risk difference [ ] ☐ P-value [ ] ☐ Hazard Ratio [ ] ☐ Other-pelase specify [ ]	63. Outcomes measures at **LAST FOLLOWUP** ☐ Enter TIME [ ] ☐ Mean [ ] ☐ Standard Error [ ] ☐ 95% CI [ ] ☐ Risk difference [ ] ☐ P-value [ ] ☐ Hazard Ratio [ ] ☐ Other-pelase specify [ ]
64. Groups compared ○ A vs. B ○ A vs. C ○ A vs. D ○ Other - please specify [ ] Clear Response	65. Outcomes measures at **END OF TREATMENT** ☐ Enter TIME [ ] ☐ Mean [ ] ☐ Standard Error [ ] ☐ 95% CI [ ] ☐ Risk difference [ ] ☐ P-value [ ] ☐ Hazard Ratio [ ] ☐ Other-pelase specify [ ]	66. Outcomes measures at **LAST FOLLOWUP** ☐ Enter TIME [ ] ☐ Mean [ ] ☐ Standard Error [ ] ☐ 95% CI [ ] ☐ Risk difference [ ] ☐ P-value [ ] ☐ Hazard Ratio [ ] ☐ Other-pelase specify [ ]

67. Comments:
[ ]

[Submit Form] and go to [ ] or Skip to Next

Outcomes for KQ 3
Scales for Eating

DistillerSR

⌘ DistillerSR

ritu.sharma

Project	Meditation (Switch) User mreuben (My Settings)
Messages	3 new

Live Support | User Guide

Review ▾ | Datarama | Reports ▾ | References ▾ | Forms ▾ | Manage Levels ▾ | Users ▾ | Project ▾ | Logout

Refid: 12, Skateboards: Are they really perilous? A retrospective study from a district hospital.
Rethnam U, Yesupalan RS, Sinha A.

[Submit Form] and go to [ ] or Skip to Next

Please submit one form per outcome

1. **This study does not apply to KQ3**
   ☐ No

KQ 3: What are the efficacy and harms of Meditation Programs on health-related behaviors affected by stress, specifically substance use, sleep, and eating, among those with a clinical condition (medical or psychiatric)?

Please select the outcome and outcome measure for KQ3

2. **Outcome**
   ○ Substance use
   ○ Sleep
   ⦿ Eating
   Outcome Scales - Eating
   ○ General food craving questionnaire, subdomains [ ]
   ○ Self reported dietary inventory [ ]
   ○ 7 day diet recall [ ]
   ○ Other-please specify [ ]
   Clear Response

   ○ Harms
   Clear Response

TABLE 1: Measures of association

ARM A - Please specify	Outcome measures at **baseline**		Outcome measures **at end of treatment**		Outcome measures **at last followup**	
[ ]	☐ N	[ ]	☐ N	[ ]	☐ N	[ ]
	☐ At Baseline		☐ Enter TIME	[ ]	☐ Enter TIME	[ ]
	☐ Mean	[ ]	☐ Mean	[ ]	☐ Mean	[ ]
	☐ Standard Deviation	[ ]	☐ Standard Deviation	[ ]	☐ Standard Deviation	[ ]
	☐ CI OR pvalue (specify)	[ ]	☐ CI or pvalue (specify)	[ ]	☐ CI or pvalue (specify)	[ ]
	☐ RR or OR(specify)	[ ]	☐ RR or OR(specify)	[ ]	☐ RR or OR(specify)	[ ]
	☐ Hazard Ratio	[ ]	☐ Hazard Ratio	[ ]	☐ Hazard Ratio	[ ]
	☐ Other - please specify	[ ]	☐ Other - please specify	[ ]	☐ Other - please specify	[ ]
ARM B - Please specify	Outcome measures at **baseline**		Outcome measures **at end of treatment**		Outcome measures **at last followup**	
[ ]	☐ N	[ ]	☐ N	[ ]	☐ N	[ ]
	☐ At Baseline		☐ Enter TIME	[ ]	☐ Enter TIME	[ ]
	☐ Mean	[ ]	☐ Mean	[ ]	☐ Mean	[ ]
	☐ Standard Deviation	[ ]	☐ Standard Deviation	[ ]	☐ Standard Deviation	[ ]
	☐ CI OR pvalue (specify)	[ ]	☐ CI or pvalue (specify)	[ ]	☐ CI or pvalue (specify)	[ ]
	☐ RR or OR(specify)	[ ]	☐ RR or OR(specify)	[ ]	☐ RR or OR(specify)	[ ]
	☐ Hazard Ratio	[ ]	☐ Hazard Ratio	[ ]	☐ Hazard Ratio	[ ]
	☐ Other - please specify	[ ]	☐ Other - please specify	[ ]	☐ Other - please specify	[ ]
ARM C - Please specify	Outcome measures at **baseline**		Outcome measures **at end of treatment**		Outcome measures **at last followup**	
[ ]	☐ N	[ ]	☐ N	[ ]	☐ N	[ ]
	☐ At Baseline		☐ Enter TIME	[ ]	☐ Enter TIME	[ ]

DistillerSR

		☐ Mean	☐ Mean	☐ Mean
		☐ Standard Deviation	☐ Standard Deviation	☐ Standard Deviation
		☐ CI OR pvalue (specify)	☐ CI or pvalue (specify)	☐ CI or pvalue (specify)
		☐ RR or OR(specify)	☐ RR or OR(specify)	☐ RR or OR(specify)
		☐ Hazard Ratio	☐ Hazard Ratio	☐ Hazard Ratio
		☐ Other - please specify	☐ Other - please specify	☐ Other - please specify
ARM D-Please specify		Outcome measures at **baseline**	Outcome measures **at end of treatment**	Outcome measures **at last followup**
		☐ N	☐ N	☐ N
		☐ At Baseline	☐ Enter TIME	☐ Enter TIME
		☐ Mean	☐ Mean	☐ Mean
		☐ Standard Deviation	☐ Standard Deviation	☐ Standard Deviation
		☐ CI OR pvalue (specify)	☐ CI or pvalue (specify)	☐ CI or pvalue (specify)
		☐ RR or OR(specify)	☐ RR or OR(specify)	☐ RR or OR(specify)
		☐ Hazard Ratio	☐ Hazard Ratio	☐ Hazard Ratio
		☐ Other - please specify	☐ Other - please specify	☐ Other - please specify

TABLE 2: Mean difference from baseline

22. Arm A (Meditation)	23. Total N in ARM	24. Outcomes measures at **END OF TREATMENT**	25. Outcomes measures at **LAST FOLLOWUP**
		☐ Enter TIME	☐ Enter TIME
		☐ Mean	☐ Mean
		☐ Standard Error	☐ Standard Error
		☐ 95% CI	☐ 95% CI
		☐ Risk difference	☐ Risk difference
		☐ P-value	☐ P-value
		☐ Hazard Ratio	☐ Hazard Ratio
		☐ Other-pelase specify	☐ Other-pelase specify
26. Arm B - please specify	27. Total N in ARM	28. Outcomes measures at **END OF TREATMENT**	29. Outcomes measures at **LAST FOLLOWUP**
		☐ Enter TIME	☐ Enter TIME
		☐ Mean	☐ Mean
		☐ Standard Error	☐ Standard Error
		☐ 95% CI	☐ 95% CI
		☐ Risk difference	☐ Risk difference
		☐ P-value	☐ P-value
		☐ Hazard Ratio	☐ Hazard Ratio
		☐ Other-pelase specify	☐ Other-pelase specify
30. Arm C - please specify	31. Total N in ARM	32. Outcomes measures at **END OF TREATMENT**	33. Outcomes measures at **LAST FOLLOWUP**
		☐ Enter TIME	☐ Enter TIME
		☐ Mean	☐ Mean
		☐ Standard Error	☐ Standard Error
		☐ 95% CI	☐ 95% CI
		☐ Risk difference	☐ Risk difference
		☐ P-value	☐ P-value
		☐ Hazard Ratio	☐ Hazard Ratio
		☐ Other-pelase specify	☐ Other-pelase specify
34. Arm D- please specify	35. Total N in ARM	36. Outcomes measures at **END OF TREATMENT**	37. Outcomes measures at **LAST FOLLOWUP**
		☐ Enter TIME	☐ Enter TIME
		☐ Mean	☐ Mean
		☐ Standard Error	☐ Standard Error
		☐ 95% CI	☐ 95% CI

DistillerSR

		☐ Risk difference		☐ Risk difference	
		☐ P-value		☐ P-value	
		☐ Hazard Ratio		☐ Hazard Ratio	
		☐ Other-pelase specify		☐ Other-pelase specify	

TABLE 3: Mean difference between groups

Arm A (Meditation) Vs. Arm B	38. Total N in ARM	39. Outcome At BASELINE	40. Outcomes at END OF TREATMENT	41. Outcomes at LAST FOLLOWUP
	☐ Total N in Arm A	☐ At Baseline	☐ Enter TIME	☐ Enter TIME
	☐ Total N in Arm B	☐ Mean	☐ Mean	☐ Mean
	☐ Total N in both arms	☐ Standard Error	☐ Standard Error	☐ Standard Error
		☐ 95% CI	☐ 95% CI	☐ 95% CI
		☐ Risk difference	☐ Risk difference	☐ Risk difference
		☐ P-value	☐ P-value	☐ P-value
		☐ Hazard Ratio	☐ Hazard Ratio	☐ Hazard Ratio
		☐ Other-pelase specify	☐ Other-pelase specify	☐ Other-pelase specify
Arm A (Meditation) Vs. Arm C	42. Total N in ARM	43. Outcomes at BASELINE	44. Outcomes at END OF TREATMENT	45. Outcomes at LAST FOLLOWUP
	☐ Total N in Arm A	☐ At Baseline	☐ Enter TIME	☐ Enter TIME
	☐ Total N in Arm C	☐ Mean	☐ Mean	☐ Mean
	☐ Total N in both arms	☐ Standard Error	☐ Standard Error	☐ Standard Error
		☐ 95% CI	☐ 95% CI	☐ 95% CI
		☐ Risk difference	☐ Risk difference	☐ Risk difference
		☐ P-value	☐ P-value	☐ P-value
		☐ Hazard Ratio	☐ Hazard Ratio	☐ Hazard Ratio
		☐ Other-pelase specify	☐ Other-pelase specify	☐ Other-pelase specify
Arm A (Meditation) Vs. Arm D	46. Total N in ARM	47. Outcomes at BASELINE	48. Outcomes at END OF TREATMENT	49. Outcomes at LAST FOLLOWUP
	☐ Total N in Arm A	☐ At Baseline	☐ Enter TIME	☐ Enter TIME
	☐ Total N in Arm D	☐ Mean	☐ Mean	☐ Mean
	☐ Total N in both arms	☐ Standard Error	☐ Standard Error	☐ Standard Error
		☐ 95% CI	☐ 95% CI	☐ 95% CI
		☐ Risk difference	☐ Risk difference	☐ Risk difference
		☐ P-value	☐ P-value	☐ P-value
		☐ Hazard Ratio	☐ Hazard Ratio	☐ Hazard Ratio
		☐ Other-pelase specify	☐ Other-pelase specify	☐ Other-pelase specify
50. Other please spcify	51. Total N in ARM	52. Outcomes at BASELINE	53. Outcomes at END OF TREATMENT	54. Outcomes at LAST FOLLOWUP
	☐ Total N in Arm	☐ At Baseline	☐ Enter TIME	☐ Enter TIME
	☐ Total N in Arm	☐ Mean	☐ Mean	☐ Mean
	☐ Total N in both arms	☐ Standard Error	☐ Standard Error	☐ Standard Error
		☐ 95% CI	☐ 95% CI	☐ 95% CI
		☐ Risk difference	☐ Risk difference	☐ Risk difference
		☐ P-value	☐ P-value	☐ P-value
		☐ Hazard Ratio	☐ Hazard Ratio	☐ Hazard Ratio
		☐ Other-pelase specify	☐ Other-pelase specify	☐ Other-pelase specify

TABLE 4: Diff-in-diff

55. Groups compared	56. Outcomes measures at END OF TREATMENT	57. Outcomes measures at LAST FOLLOWUP
○ A vs. B	☐ Enter TIME	☐ Enter TIME
○ A vs. C	☐ Mean	☐ Mean
○ A vs. D	☐ Standard Error	☐ Standard Error
○ Other - please specify	☐ 95% CI	☐ 95% CI
Clear Response		

Outcomes for KQ 3—Harms

DistillerSR

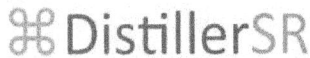

Refid: 12, Skateboards: Are they really perilous? A retrospective study from a district hospital.
Rethnam U, Yesupalan RS, Sinha A.

Please submit one form per outcome

1. This study does not apply to KQ3

  ☐ No

KQ 3: What are the efficacy and harms of Meditation Programs on health-related behaviors affected by stress, specifically substance use, sleep, and eating, among those with a clinical condition (medical or psychiatric)?

Please select the outcome and outcome measure for KQ3

2. Outcome

  ○ Substance use
  ○ Sleep
  ○ Eating
  ⦿ Harms
  Clear Response

TABLE 1: Measures of association

ARM A - Please specify	Outcome measures at **baseline**	Outcome measures **at end of treatment**	Outcome measures **at last followup**
	☐ N	☐ N	☐ N
	☐ At Baseline	☐ Enter TIME	☐ Enter TIME
	☐ Mean	☐ Mean	☐ Mean
	☐ Standard Deviation	☐ Standard Deviation	☐ Standard Deviation
	☐ CI OR pvalue (specify)	☐ CI or pvalue (specify)	☐ CI or pvalue (specify)
	☐ RR or OR(specify)	☐ RR or OR(specify)	☐ RR or OR(specify)
	☐ Hazard Ratio	☐ Hazard Ratio	☐ Hazard Ratio
	☐ Other - please specify	☐ Other - please specify	☐ Other - please specify
ARM B - Please specify	Outcome measures at **baseline**	Outcome measures **at end of treatment**	Outcome measures **at last followup**
	☐ N	☐ N	☐ N
	☐ At Baseline	☐ Enter TIME	☐ Enter TIME
	☐ Mean	☐ Mean	☐ Mean
	☐ Standard Deviation	☐ Standard Deviation	☐ Standard Deviation
	☐ CI OR pvalue (specify)	☐ CI or pvalue (specify)	☐ CI or pvalue (specify)
	☐ RR or OR(specify)	☐ RR or OR(specify)	☐ RR or OR(specify)
	☐ Hazard Ratio	☐ Hazard Ratio	☐ Hazard Ratio
	☐ Other - please specify	☐ Other - please specify	☐ Other - please specify
ARM C - Please specify	Outcome measures at **baseline**	Outcome measures **at end of treatment**	Outcome measures **at last followup**
	☐ N	☐ N	☐ N
	☐ At Baseline	☐ Enter TIME	☐ Enter TIME
	☐ Mean	☐ Mean	☐ Mean
	☐ Standard Deviation	☐ Standard Deviation	☐ Standard Deviation
	☐ CI OR pvalue (specify)	☐ CI or pvalue (specify)	☐ CI or pvalue (specify)
	☐ RR or OR(specify)	☐ RR or OR(specify)	☐ RR or OR(specify)
	☐ Hazard Ratio	☐ Hazard Ratio	☐ Hazard Ratio
	☐ Other - please specify	☐ Other - please specify	☐ Other - please specify

ARM D-Please specify	Outcome measures at **baseline**	Outcome measures **at end of treatment**	Outcome measures **at last followup**
	☐ N ☐ At Baseline ☐ Mean ☐ Standard Deviation ☐ CI OR pvalue (specify) ☐ RR or OR(specify) ☐ Hazard Ratio ☐ Other - please specify	☐ N ☐ Enter TIME ☐ Mean ☐ Standard Deviation ☐ CI or pvalue (specify) ☐ RR or OR(specify) ☐ Hazard Ratio ☐ Other - please specify	☐ N ☐ Enter TIME ☐ Mean ☐ Standard Deviation ☐ CI or pvalue (specify) ☐ RR or OR(specify) ☐ Hazard Ratio ☐ Other - please specify

TABLE 2: Mean difference from baseline

22. Arm A (Meditation)	23. Total N in ARM	24. Outcomes measures at **END OF TREATMENT**	25. Outcomes measures at **LAST FOLLOWUP**
		☐ Enter TIME ☐ Mean ☐ Standard Error ☐ 95% CI ☐ Risk difference ☐ P-value ☐ Hazard Ratio ☐ Other-pelase specify	☐ Enter TIME ☐ Mean ☐ Standard Error ☐ 95% CI ☐ Risk difference ☐ P-value ☐ Hazard Ratio ☐ Other-pelase specify
26. Arm B - please specify	27. Total N in ARM	28. Outcomes measures at **END OF TREATMENT**	29. Outcomes measures at **LAST FOLLOWUP**
		☐ Enter TIME ☐ Mean ☐ Standard Error ☐ 95% CI ☐ Risk difference ☐ P-value ☐ Hazard Ratio ☐ Other-pelase specify	☐ Enter TIME ☐ Mean ☐ Standard Error ☐ 95% CI ☐ Risk difference ☐ P-value ☐ Hazard Ratio ☐ Other-pelase specify
30. Arm C - please specify	31. Total N in ARM	32. Outcomes measures at **END OF TREATMENT**	33. Outcomes measures at **LAST FOLLOWUP**
		☐ Enter TIME ☐ Mean ☐ Standard Error ☐ 95% CI ☐ Risk difference ☐ P-value ☐ Hazard Ratio ☐ Other-pelase specify	☐ Enter TIME ☐ Mean ☐ Standard Error ☐ 95% CI ☐ Risk difference ☐ P-value ☐ Hazard Ratio ☐ Other-pelase specify
34. Arm D- please specify	35. Total N in ARM	36. Outcomes measures at **END OF TREATMENT**	37. Outcomes measures at **LAST FOLLOWUP**
		☐ Enter TIME ☐ Mean ☐ Standard Error ☐ 95% CI ☐ Risk difference ☐ P-value ☐ Hazard Ratio ☐ Other-pelase specify	☐ Enter TIME ☐ Mean ☐ Standard Error ☐ 95% CI ☐ Risk difference ☐ P-value ☐ Hazard Ratio ☐ Other-pelase specify

TABLE 3: Mean difference between groups

DistillerSR

○ A vs. C ○ A vs. D ○ Other - please specify [ ] Clear Response	☐ Mean [ ] ☐ Standard Error [ ] ☐ 95% CI [ ] ☐ Risk difference [ ] ☐ P-value [ ] ☐ Hazard Ratio [ ] ☐ Other-pelase specify [ ]	☐ Mean [ ] ☐ Standard Error [ ] ☐ 95% CI [ ] ☐ Risk difference [ ] ☐ P-value [ ] ☐ Hazard Ratio [ ] ☐ Other-pelase specify [ ]
61. Groups compared ○ A vs. B ○ A vs. C ○ A vs. D ○ Other - please specify [ ] Clear Response	**62. Outcomes measures at END OF TREATMENT** ☐ Enter TIME [ ] ☐ Mean [ ] ☐ Standard Error [ ] ☐ 95% CI [ ] ☐ Risk difference [ ] ☐ P-value [ ] ☐ Hazard Ratio [ ] ☐ Other-pelase specify [ ]	**63. Outcomes measures at LAST FOLLOWUP** ☐ Enter TIME [ ] ☐ Mean [ ] ☐ Standard Error [ ] ☐ 95% CI [ ] ☐ Risk difference [ ] ☐ P-value [ ] ☐ Hazard Ratio [ ] ☐ Other-pelase specify [ ]
64. Groups compared ○ A vs. B ○ A vs. C ○ A vs. D ○ Other - please specify [ ] Clear Response	**65. Outcomes measures at END OF TREATMENT** ☐ Enter TIME [ ] ☐ Mean [ ] ☐ Standard Error [ ] ☐ 95% CI [ ] ☐ Risk difference [ ] ☐ P-value [ ] ☐ Hazard Ratio [ ] ☐ Other-pelase specify [ ]	**66. Outcomes measures at LAST FOLLOWUP** ☐ Enter TIME [ ] ☐ Mean [ ] ☐ Standard Error [ ] ☐ 95% CI [ ] ☐ Risk difference [ ] ☐ P-value [ ] ☐ Hazard Ratio [ ] ☐ Other-pelase specify [ ]

67. Comments:
[   ]

[Submit Form] and go to [   ] or Skip to Next

Outcomes for KQ 4
Scales for Pain

DistillerSR

Refid: 12, Skateboards: Are they really perilous? A retrospective study from a district hospital.
Rethnam U, Yesupalan RS, Sinha A.

Please submit one form per outcome

1. This study does not apply to KQ4
   ☐ No

KQ 4: What are the efficacy and harms of Meditation Programs on pain and weight among those with a clinical condition (medical or psychiatric)?

Please select the outcome and outcome measure for KQ 4

2. Outcome
   ◉ Pain (intensity, interference, unpleasantness)

   Pain (intensity, interference, unpleasantness) outcome scales
   - ○ Pain intensity
   - ○ Pain interference
   - ○ SF 36 pain subscale
   - ○ Pain perception scale (PPS), including subdomains
   - ○ Roland-Morris Disability Questionnaire (RMDQ)
   - ○ Visual Analogue Scale (VAS) for pain
   - ○ Neuropathic pain scale
   - ○ Other - please specify

   Clear Response

   ○ Weight
   ○ Harms
   Clear Response

TABLE 1: Measures of association

ARM A - Please specify	Outcome measures at **baseline**	Outcome measures **at end of treatment**	Outcome measures **at last followup**
	☐ N	☐ N	☐ N
	☐ At Baseline	☐ Enter TIME	☐ Enter TIME
	☐ Mean	☐ Mean	☐ Mean
	☐ Standard Deviation	☐ Standard Deviation	☐ Standard Deviation
	☐ CI OR pvalue (specify)	☐ CI or pvalue (specify)	☐ CI or pvalue (specify)
	☐ RR or OR(specify)	☐ RR or OR(specify)	☐ RR or OR(specify)
	☐ Hazard Ratio	☐ Hazard Ratio	☐ Hazard Ratio
	☐ Other - please specify	☐ Other - please specify	☐ Other - please specify
ARM B - Please specify	Outcome measures at **baseline**	Outcome measures **at end of treatment**	Outcome measures **at last followup**
	☐ N	☐ N	☐ N
	☐ At Baseline	☐ Enter TIME	☐ Enter TIME
	☐ Mean	☐ Mean	☐ Mean
	☐ Standard Deviation	☐ Standard Deviation	☐ Standard Deviation
	☐ CI OR pvalue (specify)	☐ CI or pvalue (specify)	☐ CI or pvalue (specify)
	☐ RR or OR(specify)	☐ RR or OR(specify)	☐ RR or OR(specify)
	☐ Hazard Ratio	☐ Hazard Ratio	☐ Hazard Ratio
	☐ Other - please specify	☐ Other - please specify	☐ Other - please specify
ARM C - Please specify	Outcome measures at **baseline**	Outcome measures **at end of treatment**	Outcome measures **at last followup**

		☐ Standard Error ☐ 95% CI ☐ Risk difference ☐ P-value ☐ Hazard Ratio ☐ Other-pelase specify	☐ Standard Error ☐ 95% CI ☐ Risk difference ☐ P-value ☐ Hazard Ratio ☐ Other-pelase specify

TABLE 3: Mean difference between groups

Arm A (Meditation) Vs. Arm B	37. Total N in ARM ☐ Total N in Arm A ☐ Total N in Arm B ☐ Total N in both arms	38. Outcome At BASELINE ☐ At Baseline ☐ Mean ☐ Standard Error ☐ 95% CI ☐ Risk difference ☐ P-value ☐ Hazard Ratio ☐ Other-pelase specify	39. Outcomes at END OF TREATMENT ☐ Enter TIME ☐ Mean ☐ Standard Error ☐ 95% CI ☐ Risk difference ☐ P-value ☐ Hazard Ratio ☐ Other-pelase specify	40. Outcomes at LAST FOLLOWUP ☐ Enter TIME ☐ Mean ☐ Standard Error ☐ 95% CI ☐ Risk difference ☐ P-value ☐ Hazard Ratio ☐ Other-pelase specify
Arm A (Meditation) Vs. Arm C	41. Total N in ARM ☐ Total N in Arm A ☐ Total N in Arm C ☐ Total N in both arms	42. Outcomes at BASELINE ☐ At Baseline ☐ Mean ☐ Standard Error ☐ 95% CI ☐ Risk difference ☐ P-value ☐ Hazard Ratio ☐ Other-pelase specify	43. Outcomes at END OF TREATMENT ☐ Enter TIME ☐ Mean ☐ Standard Error ☐ 95% CI ☐ Risk difference ☐ P-value ☐ Hazard Ratio ☐ Other-pelase specify	44. Outcomes at LAST FOLLOWUP ☐ Enter TIME ☐ Mean ☐ Standard Error ☐ 95% CI ☐ Risk difference ☐ P-value ☐ Hazard Ratio ☐ Other-pelase specify
Arm A (Meditation) Vs. Arm D	45. Total N in ARM ☐ Total N in Arm A ☐ Total N in Arm D ☐ Total N in both arms	46. Outcomes at BASELINE ☐ At Baseline ☐ Mean ☐ Standard Error ☐ 95% CI ☐ Risk difference ☐ P-value ☐ Hazard Ratio ☐ Other-pelase specify	47. Outcomes at END OF TREATMENT ☐ Enter TIME ☐ Mean ☐ Standard Error ☐ 95% CI ☐ Risk difference ☐ P-value ☐ Hazard Ratio ☐ Other-pelase specify	48. Outcomes at LAST FOLLOWUP ☐ Enter TIME ☐ Mean ☐ Standard Error ☐ 95% CI ☐ Risk difference ☐ P-value ☐ Hazard Ratio ☐ Other-pelase specify
49. Other please spcify	50. Total N in ARM ☐ Total N in Arm ☐ Total N in Arm ☐ Total N in both arms	51. Outcomes at BASELINE ☐ At Baseline ☐ Mean ☐ Standard Error ☐ 95% CI ☐ Risk difference ☐ P-value ☐ Hazard Ratio ☐ Other-pelase specify	52. Outcomes at END OF TREATMENT ☐ Enter TIME ☐ Mean ☐ Standard Error ☐ 95% CI ☐ Risk difference ☐ P-value ☐ Hazard Ratio ☐ Other-pelase specify	53. Outcomes at LAST FOLLOWUP ☐ Enter TIME ☐ Mean ☐ Standard Error ☐ 95% CI ☐ Risk difference ☐ P-value ☐ Hazard Ratio ☐ Other-pelase specify

TABLE 4: Diff-in-diff

54. Groups compared ○ A vs. B ○ A vs. C	55. Outcomes measures at END OF TREATMENT ☐ Enter TIME	56. Outcomes measures at LAST FOLLOWUP ☐ Enter TIME

Outcomes for KQ 4
Scales for Weight

DistillerSR

⌘ DistillerSR

ritu.sharma

Project: Meditation (Switch) User: mreuben (My Settings)
Messages: 3 new

Review | Dataoma | Reports | References | Forms | Manage Levels | Users | Project | Logout

Refid: 12, Skateboards: Are they really perilous? A retrospective study from a district hospital.
Rethnam U, Yesupalan RS, Sinha A.

[Submit Form] and go to [ ] or Skip to Next

Please submit one form per outcome

1. This study does not apply to KQ4
☐ No

KQ 4: What are the efficacy and harms of Meditation Programs on pain and weight among those with a clinical condition (medical or psychiatric)?

Please select the outcome and outcome measure for KQ 4

2. Outcome
○ Pain (intensity, interference, unpleasantness)
◉ Weight
   Weight outcome scales
     ○ Weight [ ]
     ○ BMI [ ]
     ○ Other - please specify [ ]
     Clear Response

○ Harms
Clear Response

TABLE 1: Measures of association

ARM A - Please specify	Outcome measures at **baseline**	Outcome measures **at end of treatment**	Outcome measures **at last followup**
[ ]	☐ N [ ] ☐ At Baseline ☐ Mean [ ] ☐ Standard Deviation [ ] ☐ CI OR pvalue (specify) [ ] ☐ RR or OR(specify) [ ] ☐ Hazard Ratio [ ] ☐ Other - please specify [ ]	☐ N [ ] ☐ Enter TIME [ ] ☐ Mean [ ] ☐ Standard Deviation [ ] ☐ CI or pvalue (specify) [ ] ☐ RR or OR(specify) [ ] ☐ Hazard Ratio [ ] ☐ Other - please specify [ ]	☐ N [ ] ☐ Enter TIME [ ] ☐ Mean [ ] ☐ Standard Deviation [ ] ☐ CI or pvalue (specify) [ ] ☐ RR or OR(specify) [ ] ☐ Hazard Ratio [ ] ☐ Other - please specify [ ]
ARM B - Please specify	Outcome measures at **baseline**	Outcome measures **at end of treatment**	Outcome measures **at last followup**
[ ]	☐ N [ ] ☐ At Baseline ☐ Mean [ ] ☐ Standard Deviation [ ] ☐ CI OR pvalue (specify) [ ] ☐ RR or OR(specify) [ ] ☐ Hazard Ratio [ ] ☐ Other - please specify [ ]	☐ N [ ] ☐ Enter TIME [ ] ☐ Mean [ ] ☐ Standard Deviation [ ] ☐ CI or pvalue (specify) [ ] ☐ RR or OR(specify) [ ] ☐ Hazard Ratio [ ] ☐ Other - please specify [ ]	☐ N [ ] ☐ Enter TIME [ ] ☐ Mean [ ] ☐ Standard Deviation [ ] ☐ CI or pvalue (specify) [ ] ☐ RR or OR(specify) [ ] ☐ Hazard Ratio [ ] ☐ Other - please specify [ ]
ARM C - Please specify	Outcome measures at **baseline**	Outcome measures **at end of treatment**	Outcome measures **at last followup**
[ ]	☐ N [ ] ☐ At Baseline ☐ Mean [ ] ☐ Standard Deviation [ ] ☐ CI OR pvalue (specify)	☐ N [ ] ☐ Enter TIME [ ] ☐ Mean [ ] ☐ Standard Deviation	☐ N [ ] ☐ Enter TIME [ ] ☐ Mean [ ] ☐ Standard Deviation

		☐ RR or OR(specify) ☐ Hazard Ratio ☐ Other - please specify	☐ CI or pvalue (specify) ☐ RR or OR(specify) ☐ Hazard Ratio ☐ Other - please specify	☐ CI or pvalue (specify) ☐ RR or OR(specify) ☐ Hazard Ratio ☐ Other - please specify
ARM D-Please specify	Outcome measures at **baseline** ☐ N ☐ At Baseline ☐ Mean ☐ Standard Deviation ☐ CI OR pvalue (specify) ☐ RR or OR(specify) ☐ Hazard Ratio ☐ Other - please specify		Outcome measures **at end of treatment** ☐ N ☐ Enter TIME ☐ Mean ☐ Standard Deviation ☐ CI or pvalue (specify) ☐ RR or OR(specify) ☐ Hazard Ratio ☐ Other - please specify	Outcome measures **at last followup** ☐ N ☐ Enter TIME ☐ Mean ☐ Standard Deviation ☐ CI or pvalue (specify) ☐ RR or OR(specify) ☐ Hazard Ratio ☐ Other - please specify

TABLE 2: Mean difference from baseline

21. Arm A (Meditation)	22. Total N in ARM	23. Outcomes measures at **END OF TREATMENT**	24. Outcomes measures at **LAST FOLLOWUP**
		☐ Enter TIME ☐ Mean ☐ Standard Error ☐ 95% CI ☐ Risk difference ☐ P-value ☐ Hazard Ratio ☐ Other-pelase specify	☐ Enter TIME ☐ Mean ☐ Standard Error ☐ 95% CI ☐ Risk difference ☐ P-value ☐ Hazard Ratio ☐ Other-pelase specify
25. Arm B - please specify	26. Total N in ARM	27. Outcomes measures at **END OF TREATMENT**	28. Outcomes measures at **LAST FOLLOWUP**
		☐ Enter TIME ☐ Mean ☐ Standard Error ☐ 95% CI ☐ Risk difference ☐ P-value ☐ Hazard Ratio ☐ Other-pelase specify	☐ Enter TIME ☐ Mean ☐ Standard Error ☐ 95% CI ☐ Risk difference ☐ P-value ☐ Hazard Ratio ☐ Other-pelase specify
29. Arm C - please specify	30. Total N in ARM	31. Outcomes measures at **END OF TREATMENT**	32. Outcomes measures at **LAST FOLLOWUP**
		☐ Enter TIME ☐ Mean ☐ Standard Error ☐ 95% CI ☐ Risk difference ☐ P-value ☐ Hazard Ratio ☐ Other-pelase specify	☐ Enter TIME ☐ Mean ☐ Standard Error ☐ 95% CI ☐ Risk difference ☐ P-value ☐ Hazard Ratio ☐ Other-pelase specify
33. Arm D - please specify	34. Total N in ARM	35. Outcomes measures at **END OF TREATMENT**	36. Outcomes measures at **LAST FOLLOWUP**
		☐ Enter TIME ☐ Mean ☐ Standard Error ☐ 95% CI ☐ Risk difference ☐ P-value	☐ Enter TIME ☐ Mean ☐ Standard Error ☐ 95% CI ☐ Risk difference ☐ P-value

| | ☐ Hazard Ratio | ☐ Hazard Ratio |
| | ☐ Other-pelase specify | ☐ Other-pelase specify |

57. Groups compared	58. Outcomes measures at **END OF TREATMENT**	59. Outcomes measures at **LAST FOLLOWUP**
○ A vs. B ○ A vs. C ○ A vs. D ○ Other - please specify Clear Response	☐ Enter TIME ☐ Mean ☐ Standard Error ☐ 95% CI ☐ Risk difference ☐ P-value ☐ Hazard Ratio ☐ Other-pelase specify	☐ Enter TIME ☐ Mean ☐ Standard Error ☐ 95% CI ☐ Risk difference ☐ P-value ☐ Hazard Ratio ☐ Other-pelase specify
60. Groups compared	61. Outcomes measures at **END OF TREATMENT**	62. Outcomes measures at **LAST FOLLOWUP**
○ A vs. B ○ A vs. C ○ A vs. D ○ Other - please specify Clear Response	☐ Enter TIME ☐ Mean ☐ Standard Error ☐ 95% CI ☐ Risk difference ☐ P-value ☐ Hazard Ratio ☐ Other-pelase specify	☐ Enter TIME ☐ Mean ☐ Standard Error ☐ 95% CI ☐ Risk difference ☐ P-value ☐ Hazard Ratio ☐ Other-pelase specify
63. Groups compared	64. Outcomes measures at **END OF TREATMENT**	65. Outcomes measures at **LAST FOLLOWUP**
○ A vs. B ○ A vs. C ○ A vs. D ○ Other - please specify Clear Response	☐ Enter TIME ☐ Mean ☐ Standard Error ☐ 95% CI ☐ Risk difference ☐ P-value ☐ Hazard Ratio ☐ Other-pelase specify	☐ Enter TIME ☐ Mean ☐ Standard Error ☐ 95% CI ☐ Risk difference ☐ P-value ☐ Hazard Ratio ☐ Other-pelase specify

66. Comments:

[Submit Form] and go to [ ] or Skip to Next

Outcomes for KQ 4—Harms

DistillerSR

Refid: 12, Skateboards: Are they really perilous? A retrospective study from a district hospital.
Rethnam U, Yesupalan RS, Sinha A.

Please submit one form per outcome

1. **This study does not apply to KQ4**

   ☐ No

KQ 4: What are the efficacy and harms of Meditation Programs on pain and weight among those with a clinical condition (medical or psychiatric)?

Please select the outcome and outcome measure for KQ 4

2. Outcome

   ○ Pain (intensity, interference, unpleasantness)
   ○ Weight
   ⊙ Harms
   Clear Response

TABLE 1: Measures of association

ARM A - Please specify	Outcome measures at baseline	Outcome measures at end of treatment	Outcome measures at last followup
	☐ N	☐ N	☐ N
	☐ At Baseline	☐ Enter TIME	☐ Enter TIME
	☐ Mean	☐ Mean	☐ Mean
	☐ Standard Deviation	☐ Standard Deviation	☐ Standard Deviation
	☐ CI OR pvalue (specify)	☐ CI or pvalue (specify)	☐ CI or pvalue (specify)
	☐ RR or OR(specify)	☐ RR or OR(specify)	☐ RR or OR(specify)
	☐ Hazard Ratio	☐ Hazard Ratio	☐ Hazard Ratio
	☐ Other - please specify	☐ Other - please specify	☐ Other - please specify
ARM B - Please specify	Outcome measures at baseline	Outcome measures at end of treatment	Outcome measures at last followup
	☐ N	☐ N	☐ N
	☐ At Baseline	☐ Enter TIME	☐ Enter TIME
	☐ Mean	☐ Mean	☐ Mean
	☐ Standard Deviation	☐ Standard Deviation	☐ Standard Deviation
	☐ CI OR pvalue (specify)	☐ CI or pvalue (specify)	☐ CI or pvalue (specify)
	☐ RR or OR(specify)	☐ RR or OR(specify)	☐ RR or OR(specify)
	☐ Hazard Ratio	☐ Hazard Ratio	☐ Hazard Ratio
	☐ Other - please specify	☐ Other - please specify	☐ Other - please specify
ARM C - Please specify	Outcome measures at baseline	Outcome measures at end of treatment	Outcome measures at last followup
	☐ N	☐ N	☐ N
	☐ At Baseline	☐ Enter TIME	☐ Enter TIME
	☐ Mean	☐ Mean	☐ Mean
	☐ Standard Deviation	☐ Standard Deviation	☐ Standard Deviation
	☐ CI OR pvalue (specify)	☐ CI or pvalue (specify)	☐ CI or pvalue (specify)
	☐ RR or OR(specify)	☐ RR or OR(specify)	☐ RR or OR(specify)
	☐ Hazard Ratio	☐ Hazard Ratio	☐ Hazard Ratio
	☐ Other - please specify	☐ Other - please specify	☐ Other - please specify
ARM D - Please specify	Outcome measures at baseline	Outcome measures at end of treatment	Outcome measures at last followup

DistillerSR

| | ☐ N
☐ At Baseline
☐ Mean
☐ Standard Deviation
☐ CI OR pvalue (specify)
☐ RR or OR(specify)
☐ Hazard Ratio
☐ Other - please specify | | ☐ N
☐ Enter TIME
☐ Mean
☐ Standard Deviation
☐ CI or pvalue (specify)
☐ RR or OR(specify)
☐ Hazard Ratio
☐ Other - please specify | | ☐ N
☐ Enter TIME
☐ Mean
☐ Standard Deviation
☐ CI or pvalue (specify)
☐ RR or OR(specify)
☐ Hazard Ratio
☐ Other - please specify | |

TABLE 2: Mean difference from baseline

21. Arm A (Meditation)	22. Total N in ARM	23. Outcomes measures at **END OF TREATMENT**	24. Outcomes measures at **LAST FOLLOWUP**
		☐ Enter TIME ☐ Mean ☐ Standard Error ☐ 95% CI ☐ Risk difference ☐ P-value ☐ Hazard Ratio ☐ Other-pelase specify	☐ Enter TIME ☐ Mean ☐ Standard Error ☐ 95% CI ☐ Risk difference ☐ P-value ☐ Hazard Ratio ☐ Other-pelase specify
25. Arm B - please specify	26. Total N in ARM	27. Outcomes measures at **END OF TREATMENT**	28. Outcomes measures at **LAST FOLLOWUP**
		☐ Enter TIME ☐ Mean ☐ Standard Error ☐ 95% CI ☐ Risk difference ☐ P-value ☐ Hazard Ratio ☐ Other-pelase specify	☐ Enter TIME ☐ Mean ☐ Standard Error ☐ 95% CI ☐ Risk difference ☐ P-value ☐ Hazard Ratio ☐ Other-pelase specify
29. Arm C - please specify	30. Total N in ARM	31. Outcomes measures at **END OF TREATMENT**	32. Outcomes measures at **LAST FOLLOWUP**
		☐ Enter TIME ☐ Mean ☐ Standard Error ☐ 95% CI ☐ Risk difference ☐ P-value ☐ Hazard Ratio ☐ Other-pelase specify	☐ Enter TIME ☐ Mean ☐ Standard Error ☐ 95% CI ☐ Risk difference ☐ P-value ☐ Hazard Ratio ☐ Other-pelase specify
33. Arm D- please specify	34. Total N in ARM	35. Outcomes measures at **END OF TREATMENT**	36. Outcomes measures at **LAST FOLLOWUP**
		☐ Enter TIME ☐ Mean ☐ Standard Error ☐ 95% CI ☐ Risk difference ☐ P-value ☐ Hazard Ratio ☐ Other-pelase specify	☐ Enter TIME ☐ Mean ☐ Standard Error ☐ 95% CI ☐ Risk difference ☐ P-value ☐ Hazard Ratio ☐ Other-pelase specify

TABLE 3: Mean difference between groups

Arm A (Meditation) Vs. Arm B	37. Total N in ARM	38. Outcome **At BASELINE**	39. Outcomes at **END OF TREATMENT**	40. Outcomes at **LAST FOLLOWUP**
		☐ At Baseline		

DistillerSR

	☐ Total N in Arm A ☐ Total N in Arm B ☐ Total N in both arms	☐ Mean ☐ Standard Error ☐ 95% CI ☐ Risk difference ☐ P-value ☐ Hazard Ratio ☐ Other-pelase specify	☐ Enter TIME ☐ Mean ☐ Standard Error ☐ 95% CI ☐ Risk difference ☐ P-value ☐ Hazard Ratio ☐ Other-pelase specify	☐ Enter TIME ☐ Mean ☐ Standard Error ☐ 95% CI ☐ Risk difference ☐ P-value ☐ Hazard Ratio ☐ Other-pelase specify
Arm A (Meditation) Vs. Arm C	41. Total N in ARM ☐ Total N in Arm A ☐ Total N in Arm C ☐ Total N in both arms	42. Outcomes at **BASELINE** ☐ At Baseline ☐ Mean ☐ Standard Error ☐ 95% CI ☐ Risk difference ☐ P-value ☐ Hazard Ratio ☐ Other-pelase specify	43. Outcomes at **END OF TREATMENT** ☐ Enter TIME ☐ Mean ☐ Standard Error ☐ 95% CI ☐ Risk difference ☐ P-value ☐ Hazard Ratio ☐ Other-pelase specify	44. Outcomes at **LAST FOLLOWUP** ☐ Enter TIME ☐ Mean ☐ Standard Error ☐ 95% CI ☐ Risk difference ☐ P-value ☐ Hazard Ratio ☐ Other-pelase specify
Arm A (Meditation) Vs. Arm D	45. Total N in ARM ☐ Total N in Arm A ☐ Total N in Arm D ☐ Total N in both arms	46. Outcomes at **BASELINE** ☐ At Baseline ☐ Mean ☐ Standard Error ☐ 95% CI ☐ Risk difference ☐ P-value ☐ Hazard Ratio ☐ Other-pelase specify	47. Outcomes at **END OF TREATMENT** ☐ Enter TIME ☐ Mean ☐ Standard Error ☐ 95% CI ☐ Risk difference ☐ P-value ☐ Hazard Ratio ☐ Other-pelase specify	48. Outcomes at **LAST FOLLOWUP** ☐ Enter TIME ☐ Mean ☐ Standard Error ☐ 95% CI ☐ Risk difference ☐ P-value ☐ Hazard Ratio ☐ Other-pelase specify
49. Other please spcify	50. Total N in ARM ☐ Total N in Arm ☐ Total N in Arm ☐ Total N in both arms	51. Outcomes at **BASELINE** ☐ At Baseline ☐ Mean ☐ Standard Error ☐ 95% CI ☐ Risk difference ☐ P-value ☐ Hazard Ratio ☐ Other-pelase specify	52. Outcomes at **END OF TREATMENT** ☐ Enter TIME ☐ Mean ☐ Standard Error ☐ 95% CI ☐ Risk difference ☐ P-value ☐ Hazard Ratio ☐ Other-pelase specify	53. Outcomes at **LAST FOLLOWUP** ☐ Enter TIME ☐ Mean ☐ Standard Error ☐ 95% CI ☐ Risk difference ☐ P-value ☐ Hazard Ratio ☐ Other-pelase specify

TABLE 4: Diff-in-diff

54. Groups compared	55. Outcomes measures at **END OF TREATMENT**	56. Outcomes measures at **LAST FOLLOWUP**
○ A vs. B ○ A vs. C ○ A vs. D ○ Other - please specify Clear Response	☐ Enter TIME ☐ Mean ☐ Standard Error ☐ 95% CI ☐ Risk difference ☐ P-value ☐ Hazard Ratio ☐ Other-pelase specify	☐ Enter TIME ☐ Mean ☐ Standard Error ☐ 95% CI ☐ Risk difference ☐ P-value ☐ Hazard Ratio ☐ Other-pelase specify
57. Groups compared	58. Outcomes measures at **END OF TREATMENT**	59. Outcomes measures at **LAST FOLLOWUP**
○ A vs. B ○ A vs. C ○ A vs. D	☐ Enter TIME ☐ Mean	☐ Enter TIME ☐ Mean

Risk of Bias

DistillerSR

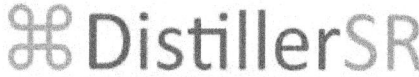   ritu.sharma

Project   Meditation (Switch)   User   mreuben (My Settings)
Messages   3 new

Live Support   User Guide

| Review | Datarama | Reports | References | Forms | Manage Levels | Users | Project | Logout |

Refid: 12, Skateboards: Are they really perilous? A retrospective study from a district hospital.
Rethnam U, Yesupalan RS, Sinha A.

[SubmitForm] and go to [   ] or Skip to Next

Selection Bias

Was the method of randomization described in the paper?

○ Yes
○ No
Clear Response

Did they use a random number generator or table?

○ Yes
○ No
○ Not Reported
Clear Response

Was allocation concealed?

○ Yes
○ No
○ Not Reported
Clear Response

Performance Bias:

Was the control matched for time and attention by the instructors?

○ >=75%
○ < 75%
○ Unclear
Clear Response

Was credibility of the control evaluated?

○ Yes
○ No
Clear Response

Was the credibility comparable?

○ Yes
○ No
○ Not Reported
Clear Response

Attrition Bias:

DistillerSR

Was there a description of withdrawals and dropouts?

○ Yes
○ No
Clear Response

Was attrition >20% at the end of treatment (calculate from total N randomized)?

○ Yes
○ No
Clear Response

Was intent-to-treat (RANDOMIZED = ANALYZED) analysis used? They must impute noncompleter or other missing data in order to say "YES"

○ Yes
○ No
Clear Response

Detection Bias:

Were those who collected data on the participants blind to the allocation?

○ Yes
○ No
○ Not Reported
Clear Response

Reporting Bias:

Were their primary and secondary outcomes specified?

○ Yes
○ No
Clear Response

Comments, including any potential ERRORS IN REPORTING notes:

[Submit Form] and go to [   ] or Skip to Next

Appendix D. Excluded Studies

Appendix D lists studies that were excluded from this review, categorized by reason for exclusion and alphabetized.

No Original Data

Biofeedback and meditation have little effect on high blood pressure. AHRQ Research Activities 1993; (171):4-5.

Yoga may help improve women's sexual function. Harv Womens Health Watch 2010; 17(8):7.

Carefully performed yoga may help with chronic back pain. Mayo Clin Health Lett 2010; 28(5):4.

Daily 12-minute meditation can improve cognition, memory, & attention. Journal of Gerontological Nursing 2010; 36(6):5.

Retraction. Preliminary study of the effects of Tai Chi and Qigong medical exercise on indicators of metabolic syndrome and glycaemic control in adults with raised blood glucose levels. Br J Sports Med 2010; 44(8):608.

Ades PA, Wu G. Benefits of tai chi in chronic heart failure: body or mind? Am J Med 2004; 117(8):611-2.

Aickin M. Does T'ai Chi Chuan improve health-related quality of life in elderly patients? [1]. 2007; 13(10):1053.

Anon. Influence of mindfulness meditation on assisted reproduction treatment programmes. Human Reproduction (Oxford, England) 2003; 18 suppl 1:207-8.

Anon. Meditation-based treatment for binge-eating disorder. Http://Www.Clinicaltrials.Gov 2003.

Anon. Meditation or education for Alzheimer caregivers or meditation for Alzheimer caregivers. Http://Www.Clinicaltrials.Gov 2007.

Anon. Mindfulness meditation as a rehabilitation strategy for persons with schizophrenia. Http://Wwwclinicaltrialsgov 2009.

Arana D. The practice of mindfulness meditation to alleviate the symptoms of chronic shyness and social anxiety. Dissertation Abstracts International 2006; 67(5-B):2822.

Arcari P. Efficacy of a workplace smoking cessation program: mindfulness meditation vs cognitive-behavioral interventions. Boston College, 1996.

Aron A, Aron EN. The transcendental meditation program's effect on addictive behavior. Addict Behav 1980; 5(1):3-12.

Asare F, Simren M. Mindfulness-based stress reduction in patients with irritable bowel syndrome. Aliment Pharmacol Ther 2011; 34(5):578-9; author reply 579-80.

Asberg M, Skold C, Wahlberg K, Nygren A. [Mindfulness meditation--an old fashion method for stress relief]. Lakartidningen 2006; 103(42):3174-7.

Barnes VA. Reduced cardiovascular and all-cause mortality in older African Americans practicing the Transcendental Meditation [dissertation]. Dissertation Abstracts International 1997; 57(8-B).

Barrows K. The application of mindfulness to HIV. Focus 2006; 21(8):1-5.

Battle CL, Uebelacker LA, Howard M, Castaneda M. Prenatal yoga and depression during pregnancy. Birth 2010; 37(4):353-4.

Bauer-Wu S. Mindfulness meditation. Oncology (Williston Park) 2010; 24(10 Suppl):36-40.

Benson H, Malvea BP, Graham JR. Physiologic correlates of meditation and their clinical effects in headache: an ongoing investigation. Headache 1973; 13(1):23-4.

Bijlani RL. Influence of yoga on brain and behaviour: facts and speculations. Indian J Physiol Pharmacol 2004; 48(1):1-5.

Blomberg M. [Training for improved body awareness and relaxation for stress management]. Lakartidningen 2004; 101(15-16):1398-400.

Boudette R. Integrating mindfulness into the therapy hour. Eat Disord 2011; 19(1):108-15.

Bower JE. Management of cancer-related fatigue. Clin Adv Hematol Oncol 2006; 4(11):828-9.

Bowman K. Commentary on "Loving-kindness meditation for chronic low back pain". J Holist Nurs 2005; 23(3):305-9.

Brown KD, Koziol JA, Lotz M. A yoga-based exercise program to reduce the risk of falls in seniors: a pilot and feasibility study. J Altern Complement Med 2008; 14(5):454-7.

Buhle J, Wager TD. Does meditation training lead to enduring changes in the anticipation and experience of pain? Pain 2010; 150(3):382-3.

Butler LD, Spiegel D. Meditation and hypnosis for chronic depressed mood. Controlled-Trials.Com 2006.

Campbell C. Re: The effectiveness of yoga for the improvement of well-being and resilience to stress in the workplace. Scand J Work Environ Health 2011; 37(1):80.

Campbell RJ, Brantley J. Being mindful of change: a technique to reduce stress amid change. J AHIMA 2011; 82(8):36-9.

Canter P, Jayadevappa R. Is transcendental meditation effective in congestive heart failure? Focus on Alternative & Complementary Therapies 2007; 12(3):199-201.

Carlisle TW. Effects of the transcendental meditation program on Psychological, health, social, and behavioral indicators of stress reduction and Human Resource development in the indian workplace. Dissertation Abstracts International 2005; 65(12-A):4629.

Cashman K, Halpern M. Transcendental meditation and individual development. NLN Publ 1977; (16-1674):70-6.

Chalmers R. Transcendental meditation does not predispose to epilepsy. Med Hypotheses 2005; 65(3):624-5.

Chang J, Chiung W. Effect of meditation on music performance anxiety. Dissertation Abstracts International 2001; 62(5-A):1765.

Chen HL, Liu K, You QS. Attention should be paid to preventing knee injury in tai chi exercise. Inj Prev 2011; 17(4):286-7.

Cheng TO. Tai Chi for chronic heart failure. Int J Cardiol 2006; 110(1):96.

Cheng TO. Tai Chi: the Chinese ancient wisdom of an ideal exercise for cardiac patients. Int J Cardiol 2007; 117(3):293-5.

Chiesa A, Brambilla P, Serretti A. Neuro-imaging of mindfulness meditations: implications for clinical practice. Epidemiol Psychiatr Sci 2011; 20(2):205-10.

Danusantoso H, Heijnen L. Tai Chi Chuan for people with haemophilia. Haemophilia 2001; 7(4):437-9.

Delmonte MM. Physiological concomitants of meditation practice. Int J Psychosom 1984; 31(4):23-36.

Dillbeck MC. The application of the transcendental meditation program to corrections. International Journal of Comparative and Applied Criminal Justice 1987; 1(11):111-32.

Dosh SA. The treatment of adults with essential hypertension. J. Fam. Pract. 2002; 51(1):74-80.

Eliopoulos C. Integrative care--health benefits of Tai Chi. Director 2001; 9(4):138-9.

Eliopoulos C. Integrative care--take a deep breath and stretch ... benefits of yoga in LTC. Director 2004; 12(2):114-5.

Epstein-Lubow GP, Miller IW, McBee L. Mindfulness training for caregivers. Psychiatr Serv 2006; 57(3):421.

Evans AT, Hadler NM. Yoga improved function and reduced symptoms of chronic low-back pain more than a self-care book. ACP J Club 2006; 145(1):16.

Evans S, Cousins L, Tsao JC, Sternlieb B, Zeltzer LK. Protocol for a randomized controlled study of Iyengar yoga for youth with irritable bowel syndrome. Trials 2011; 12:15.

Evans S, Cousins L, Tsao JC, Subramanian S, Sternlieb B, Zeltzer LK. A randomized controlled trial examining Iyengar yoga for young adults with rheumatoid arthritis: a study protocol. Trials 2011; 12:19.

Fehr TG. Transcendental meditation may prevent partial epilepsy. Med Hypotheses 2006; 67(6):1462-3.

Freret N, Ricci L, Murphy S. Recruiting and screening older, transitional to frail adults in congregate living facilities. Appl Nurs Res 2003; 16(2):118-25.

Garcia-Trujillo Mr, De Rivera Jlg. Physiological Changes Induced By Meditation And Deep Relaxation: Cambios Fisiologicos Durante Los Ejercicios De Meditacion Y Relajacion Profunda. 1992; 13(6-7):57-63.

Garland SN, Carlson LE, Antle MC, Samuels C, Campbell T. I-CAN SLEEP: rationale and design of a non-inferiority RCT of Mindfulness-based Stress Reduction and Cognitive Behavioral Therapy for the treatment of Insomnia in CANcer survivors. Contemp Clin Trials 2011; 32(5):747-54.

Gokal R, Shillito L, Maharaj SR. Positive impact of yoga and pranayam on obesity, hypertension, blood sugar, and cholesterol: a pilot assessment. J Altern Complement Med 2007; 13(10):1056-7.

Gorczynski P, Faulkner G. Exercise therapy for schizophrenia (Brief record). Schizophrenia Bulletin 2010; 36(4):665-6.

Grandinetti NS, Schneider R, Chang H, Ricketts L, Toomey M. The transcendental meditation program and cardiovascular disease in native Hawaiins. Journal of Psychosomatic Research 2003; 55:144.

Grant JA, Rainville P. Hypnosis and meditation: similar experiential changes and shared brain mechanisms. Med Hypotheses 2005; 65(3):625-6.

Graves N, Krepcho M, Mayo HG, Hill J. Clinical inquiries. Does yoga speed healing for patients with low back pain? J Fam Pract 2004; 53(8):661-2.

Greenfield RH. Blowing off steam: Mindfulness and COPD. 2010; 13(3):34-6.

Greenfield RH. "Qigong show"-MQ for cancer patients. 2010; 13(1):11-2.

Hankey A, McCrum S. Qigong: life energy and a new science of life. J Altern Complement Med 2006; 12(9):841-2.

Heidenreich T, Tuin I, Pflug B, Michal M, Michalak J. Mindfulness-based cognitive therapy for persistent insomnia: A pilot study [2]. 2006; 75(3):188-9.

Immink M. A yoga and meditation program to improve physical function, mood and quality of life in individuals with chronic stroke hemiparesis. Australian New Zealand Clinical Trials Registry (ANZCTR) Http://Www.Anzctr.Org.Au/ 2009.

Jackson C. Pilates and yoga: holistic practices that are perfect together. Holist Nurs Pract 2011; 25(5):225-30.

Jaseja H. A brief study of a possible relation of epilepsy association with meditation. Med Hypotheses 2006; 66(5):1036-7.

Jaseja H. Meditation and epilepsy: the ongoing debate. Med Hypotheses 2007; 68(4):916-7.

Kamiya K. Keratectasia, Rubbing, Yoga, Weightlifting, and Intraocular Pressure. Cornea 2010.

Kemp C A. Qigong as a therapeutic intervention with older adults (Provisional abstract). Journal of Holistic Nursing 2004; 22(4):351-73.

Kepner J. Yoga research and Richard Freeman. Altern Ther Health Med 2004; 10(4):14.

Khianman B, Pattanittum P, Thinkhamrop J, Lumbiganon P. Relaxation therapy for preventing and treating preterm labour. 2008; (4).

Krishnamurthy M, Telles S. Effects of Yoga and an Ayurveda preparation on gait, balance and mobility in older persons. Med Sci Monit 2007; 13(12):LE19-20.

Kugler JE. Meditation and the electroencephalogram. Electroencephalogr Clin Neurophysiol Suppl 1982; (35):391-8.

Liem T. Osteopathy and Hatha Yoga: Osteopathie und (Hatha-)Yoga. 2009; 10(1):21-7.

Lin MR, Hwang HF, Wang YW, Chang SH, Wolf SL. Community-based tai chi and its effect on injurious falls, balance, gait, and fear of falling in older people. Phys Ther 2006; 86(9):1189-201.

Maki PM. New data on mindfulness-based stress reduction for hot flashes: how do alternative therapies compare with selective serotonin reuptake inhibitors? Menopause 2011; 18(6):596-8.

Manikonda P, Stoerk S, Toegel S et al. Influence of non-pharmacological treatment (contemplative meditation and breathing technique) on stress induced hypertension - A randomized controlled study. American Journal of Hypertension 2005; 18(5):89A-90A.

Manocha R. Sahaja yoga in asthma [2]. 2003; 58(9):825-6.

Mansky P, Sannes T, Wallerstedt D et al. Tai chi chuan: mind-body practice or exercise intervention? Studying the benefit for cancer survivors (Structured abstract). Integrative Cancer Therapies 2006; 5(3):192-201.

Manyam BV. Diabetes mellitus, Ayurveda, and yoga. J Altern Complement Med 2004; 10(2):223-5.

Marc I. Integrative approach for tinnitus: Potential for qigong. Focus on Alternative and Complementary Therapies 2011; (16 1):58.

Mariano C. A 16-week tai chi programme prevented falls in healthy older adults. Evid Based Nurs 2008; 11(2):60.

Marks I, Dar R. Fear reduction by psychotherapies. Recent findings, future directions. 2000; 176(JUN.):507-11.

Martiny PJ. Research on the physiological effects of transcendential meditation: studies show wholesome and good effects in meditators: Forskningen af de fysiologiske virkninger af Transcendental Meditation: forskningen viser sund og god virkning hos de mediterende. 1978; 78(17):4-7, 28.

Mathuna D. Tai chi for fall prevention among the elderly. Alternative Therapies in Women's Health 2005; 7(5):33-6.

Matsuda S, Martin D, Yu T. Ancient exercise for modern rehab. Rehab Manag 2005; 18(2):24-7.

McCown D. Cognitive and perceptual benefits of meditation. 2004; 2(4):148-51.

Meares A. A form of intensive meditation associated with the regression of cancer. Am J Clin Hypn 1982-1983; 25(2-3):114-21.

Miller JB. Yoga, visualisation and affirmation in YogaBirth. Pract Midwife 2010; 13(5):14-5.

Morse DR, Martin JS, Furst ML, Dubin LL. A physiological and subjective evaluation of neutral and emotionally-charged words for meditation. Part III. J Am Soc Psychosom Dent Med 1979; 26(3):106-12.

Morse DR, Martin JS, Furst ML, Dubin LL. A physiological and subjective evaluation of neutral and emotionally-charged words for meditation. Part II. J Am Soc Psychosom Dent Med 1979; 26(2):56-62.

Murphy L, Riley D, Rodgers J, Plank S, Lehman S, Duryea B. Effects of Tai Chi on balance, mobility, and strength among older persons participating in an osteoporosis prevention and education program. Explore (NY) 2005; 1(3):192-3.

Mustian KM, Katula JA, Roscoe J, Morrow G. The influence of Tai Chi (TC) and support therapy (ST) on fatigue and quality of life (QOL) in women with breast cancer (BC) [abstract]. Annual Meeting Proceedings of the American Society of Clinical Oncology 2004; 760.

NCT00558402 (2007). Meditation or Education for Alzheimer Caregivers Or Meditation for Alzheimer Caregivers: Stress & Physiology. Http://Www.Clinicaltrials.Gov 2007.

Nespor K. The combination of psychiatric treatment and yoga. Int J Psychosom 1985; 32(2):24-7.

Nichol G, Ding L, Mathias S, Lovell-Smith D, Low W. Transcendental meditation. N Z Med J 1983; 96(742):814.

Nolfe G. EEG and meditation. Clin Neurophysiol 2011.

Oh B, Butow P, Mullan B, Clarke SJ, Beale P, Rosenthal D. Randomized clinical trial: The Impact of Medical Qigong (traditional Chinese medicine) on fatique, quality of life, side effects, mood status and inlfammation of cancer patients [abstarct no. 9565]. Journal of Clinical Oncology: ASCO Annual Meeting Proceedings 2008; 26(15S part I):518.

Orme-Johnson DW. Transcendental meditation does not predispose to epilepsy. Med Hypotheses 2005; 65(1):201-2.

Osteras N, Fongen C. Tai Chi reduces pain and improves physical function for people with knee OA. J Physiother 2010; 56(1):57.

Parati G, Steptoe A. Stress reduction and blood pressure control in hypertension: a role for transcendental meditation? J Hypertens 2004; 22(11):2057-60.

Pierce S, Rakel D. Is therapeutic yoga helpful for chronic low back pain? Evidence-Based Practice 2010; 13(8):4.

Porter N. Yoga & Tai Chi: stress management and low impact fitness from the East. Pa Health You 2002; 105(2):6-8.

Rakel D, Fortney L, Sierpina VS, Kreitzer MJ. Mindfulness in medicine. Explore (NY) 2011; 7(2):124-6.

Rasmussen LB. Transcendental meditation and mild hypertension: Transcendental meditasjon og mild hypertensjon. 1998; 118(5):775.

Rediger JD, Summers L. Mindfulness training and meditation for mental health. Adv Mind Body Med 2007; 22(1):16-26.

Riley D. Hatha yoga and the treatment of illness. Altern Ther Health Med 2004; 10(2):20-1.

Robertshawe P. Effects of yoga on maternal comfort, labour pain and birth outcomes. Journal of the Australian Traditional-Medicine Society 2009; 15(2):81.

Rogers C, Keller C, Larkey LK. Perceived benefits of meditative movement in older adults (Structured abstract). Geriatric Nursing 2010; 31(1):37-51.

Rosdahl D R L. The effect of mindfulness meditation on tension headaches and secretory immunoglobulin A in saliva [dissertation]. 2003.

Rosdahl D. The effect of mindfulness meditation on tension headaches and secretory immunoglobulin A in saliva. University of Arizona, 2003.

Roth B. Mindfulness-based stress reduction at the Yale School of Nursing. 2001; 74(4):249-58.

Roy DJ. The thistle is a flower? A meditation on seeing the unseen. J Palliat Care 2011; 27(2):67-8.

Rubenfire M. [Commentary on] Effects of tai chi mind-body movement therapy on functional status and exercise capacity in patients with chronic heart failure: a randomized controlled trial. ACC Current Journal Review 2005; 14(2):35.

Sagula D A. Varying treatment duration in a mindfulness meditation stress reduction program for chronic pain patients [dissertation]. 1999.

Salomons TV, Kucyi A. Does Meditation Reduce Pain through a Unique Neural Mechanism? J Neurosci 2011; 31(36):12705-7.

Sarukkai S. Inside/outside: Merleau-ponty/yoga. 2002; 52(4):459-78.

Schmidt S. Mindfulness meditation for the treatment of chronic low back pain in older adults: A randomized controlled pilot study - Commentary: Achtsamkeit hilft bei chronischen schmerzen: Kommentar. Forsch. Komplementarmed. 2008; 15(2):106-8.

Schneider R, Alexander C, Myers H et al. Lifestyle modification in the prevention of left ventricular hypertrophy: A randomized controlled trial of stress reduction and health education in hypertensive African Americans. Journal of Hypertension 2006; 24(Suppl. 6):90.

Schneider RH, Alexander CN, Staggers F et al. Long-term effects of stress reduction on mortality in persons > or = 55 years of age with systemic hypertension. Am J Cardiol 2005; 95(9):1060-4.

Schneider RH, Cavanaugh KL, Kasture HS, Rothenberg S. Health promotion with a traditional system of natural health care: Maharishi Ayur-Veda. Journal of Social Behavior & Personality 1990; 5(3):1-27.

Sengoku M, Murata H, Kawahara T, Nakagome K. 'Does daily Naikan therapy maintain the efficacy of intensive Naikan therapy against depression?': Erratum. Psychiatry and Clinical Neurosciences 2010; 64(2).

Shannahoff-Khalsa D. Kundalini yoga meditation techniques for psychiatric disorders. 157th Annual Meeting of the American Psychiatric Association; 2004 May 1-6; New York, NY 2004.

Steptoe A. New approaches to the management of essential hypertension with psychological techniques. 1978; 22(4):339-54.

Stevinson C. Preliminary results suggest that yoga can alleviate depression. Focus on Alternative & Complementary Therapies 2001; 6(1):27-8.

Stevinson C. Inconclusive trial on yoga for anxiety among breast cancer patients: Commentary. Focus Altern. Complement. Ther. 2009; 14(2):123-4.

Straus S. A 16-week tai chi programme prevented falls in healthy older adults. Evid Based Med 2008; 13(2):54.

Tavee J, Stone L. Healing the mind: meditation and multiple sclerosis. Neurology 2010; 75(13):1130-1.

Teasdale JD. Emotional processing, three modes of mind and the prevention of relapse in depression. Behav Res Ther 1999; 37 Suppl 1:S53-77.

Teerlink JR. Mind or body: evaluating mind-body therapy efficacy in heart failure trials. Arch Intern Med 2011; 171(8):758-9.

Telles S, Naveen KV. Changes in middle latency auditory evoked potentials during meditation. Psychol Rep 2004; 94(2):398-400.

Telles S, Naveen KV. Effect of yoga on somatic indicators of distress in professional computer users. Med Sci Monit 2006; 12(10):LE21-2.

Telles S, Singh N. High frequency yoga breathing increases energy -expenditure from carbohydrates. Comment to: Assessment of sleep patterns, energy expenditure and circadian rhythms of skin temperature in patients with acute coronary syndrome Hadil Al Otair, Mustafa Al-shamiri, Mohammed Bahobail, Munir M. Sharif, Ahmed S. BaHammam Med Sci Monit, 2011; 17(7): CR397-403. Med Sci Monit 2011; 17(9):LE7-8.

Theadom A, Cropley M, Hankins M, Smith HE. Mind and body therapy for fibromyalgia. 2009; (4).

Tsai P, Chang JY, Chowdhury N, Beck C, Roberson PK, Rosengren K. Enrolling older adults with cognitive impairment in research: lessons from a study of Tai Chi for osteoarthritis knee pain. Research in Gerontological Nursing 2009; 2(4):228-34.

Van Eijk-Hustings Y, Boonen A, Landew R. A randomized trial of tai chi for fibromyalgia [7]. 2010; 363(23):2266.

Vanfraechem-Raway R. [Fatigue. Relaxation therapy]. Arch Belg 1985; 43(11-12):511-7.

von Durckheim K. The use of meditative practices in psychotherapy. Praxis Der Psychotherapie 1973; 18(2):63-74.

Wang C, Xu D, Qian Y. Medical and health care Qigong (Qu Bing Yang Sheng Gong). J Tradit Chin Med 1991; 11(4):296-301, contd.

Wang YT. Effects of long term Tai Chi practice and jogging exercise on muscle strength and endurance in older people: Commentary. Br. J. Sports Med. 2006; 40(1):54.

Wayne P M, Krebs D E, Wolf S L et al. Can Tai Chi improve vestibulopathic postural control? (Structured abstract). Archives of Physical Medicine and Rehabilitation 2004; 85(1):142-52.

Wayne P, McGibbon C, Scarborough D et al. Tai chi improves dynamic postural stability in patients with vestibular disease: results of a randomized trial. Journal of Alternative & Complementary Medicine 2006; 12(2):214.

Whitebird RR, Kreitzer MJ, O'Connor PJ. Mindfulness-Based Stress Reduction and Diabetes. Diabetes Spectr 2009; 22(4):226-30.

Williams A, Selwyn P, McCorkle R, Molde S, Liberti L, Katz D. Application of community-based participatory research methods to a study of complementary medicine interventions at end of life. Complementary Health Practice Review 2005; 10(2):91-104.

Wolf DB. Effects of the hare krsna maha mantra on stress, depression, and the three gunas. (spirituality, yoga) [dissertation]. Dissertation Abstracts International 2000; 60(7-B).

Yalta K, Sivri N, Yetkin E. Sahaja yoga: A unique adjunctive approach for the management of cardiac arrhythmias? Int J Cardiol 2011; 152(1):99-100.

Yount G, Solfvin J, Moore D et al. In vitro test of external Qigong. BMC Complement Altern Med 2004; 4:5.

Zeeuwe PEM, Verhagen AP, Bierma-Zeinstra SMA, Van Rossum E, Faber MJ, Koes BW. The effect of Tai Chi Chuan in reducing falls among elderly people: Design of a randomized clinical trial in the Netherlands [ISRCTN98840266]. 2006; 6.

Zhang F, Wu Y. A randomized trial of tai chi for fibromyalgia [6]. 2010; 363(23):2265-6.

Zhou M, Zhou D, He L. A randomized trial of tai chi for fibromyalgia [5]. 2010; 363(23):2265.

Zwick D. Integrating Iyengar yoga into rehab for spinal cord injury. Nursing 2006; 36 Suppl P T:18-22.

Meeting Abstracts

Biofeedback and meditation have little effect on high blood pressure. AHRQ Research Activities 1993; (171):4-5.

Abstracts: archives journals. JAMA: Journal of the American Medical Association 2006; 296(6):633-5.

Anderson VL. The effects of meditation on teacher perceived occupational stress and trait anxiety. Dissertation Abstracts International 1996; 57(3-A):934.

Anon. The effects of meditation on selected measures of human potential. Dissertation Abstracts International 1982; 42((11-A)):4717.

Anthony Jr W. An evaluation of meditation as a stress reduction technique for persons with spinal cord injury. Dissertation Abstracts International 1986; 46(11):3251.

Arana D. The practice of mindfulness meditation to alleviate the symptoms of chronic shyness and social anxiety. Dissertation Abstracts International 2006; 67(5-B):2822.

Brach AW. Clinical applications of meditation: A treatment outcome evaluation study of an intervention for binge eating among the obese that combines formal meditation and contingent formal and informal meditation. Dissertation Abstracts International 1992; 52(7-B):3898.

Britton Willoughby B. Meditation and depression. Dissertation Abstracts International 2007; 68(5-B):3387.

Carlisle TW. Effects of the transcendental meditation program on Psychological, health, social, and behavioral indicators of stress reduction and Human Resource development in the indian workplace. Dissertation Abstracts International 2005; 65(12-A):4629.

Chang J, Chiung W. Effect of meditation on music performance anxiety. Dissertation Abstracts International 2001; 62(5-A):1765.

Chhabra AK. The effect of self-aware meditation on stress in Indian immigrants living in the United States. Dissertation Abstracts International: Section B: The Sciences and Engineering 2011; 71(10-B):6435.

Clark P, Cortese-Jimenez G, Cohen E. Using Reiki, Yoga, meditation or patient education to address physical and psychological symptoms related to chemotherapy-induced peripheral neuropathy: A pilot study [conference abstract]. Psycho-Oncology [Abstracts From the 8th Annual Conference of the American Psychosocial Oncology Society Anaheim, CA United States. Feb 17-19 2011] 2011.

Cole B, Broer K, Hopkins C et al. A randomized controlled trial of spiritually-focused meditation in patients newly diagnosed with acute leukemia [Abstract No. 1519]. Blood 2010; 116(21).

Collins LA. Stress management and yoga. Dissertation Abstracts International 1984; 45(1-A):0116.

Comer James F. Meditation and progressive relaxation in the treatment of test anxiety. Dissertation Abstracts International 1978; 38(12-B):6142-3.

DeBlassie PA. Christian meditation: A clinical investigation. Dissertation Abstracts International 1981; 42(3-B):1167.

Diner MD. The differential effects of meditation and systematic desensitization on specific and general anxiety. Dissertation Abstracts International 1978; 39(4-B):1950.

Donesky-Cuenco D, Carrieri-Kohlman V, Park SK, Jacobs B. Safety and feasibility of yoga in patients with COPD [Abstract]. Proceedings of the American Thoracic Society 2006; A221.

Dua JK. Effect of meditation and progressive relaxation training on reported relaxation and on blood pressure [abstract]. Aust Psychol 1984; 19(1):71.

Dudani U, Gupta HL, Singh SH, Selvamurthy W, and Surange SG. Effect of Sahaja yoga on the frequency of seizures in epileptics. 18th International Epilepsy Congress 1989; 161.

Frisvold MH. The "midlife study": Mindfulness as an intervention to change health behaviors in midlife women. University of Minnesota, 2009.

Gilmore JV. Relative effectiveness of meditation and autogenic training for the self-regulation of anxiety. Dissertation Abstracts International 1985; 45(8-B):2686.

Humphrey CW. A stress management intervention with forgiveness as the goal (Meditation, mind-body medicine). Dissertation Abstracts International : Section B: the Sciences and Engineering 1999; 60(4-B):1855.

Immink M. A pilot study on yoga and meditation as an adjunct to fitness rehabilitation programs for stroke patients with chronic hemiparesis. Australian New Zealand Clinical Trials Registry (ANZCTR) Http://Www.Anzctr.Org.Au/ 2009.

Jones Roger C. A comparison of aerobic exercise, anaerobic exercise and meditation on multidimensional stress measures. Dissertation Abstracts International 1981; 42(6-B):2504-5.

Katiyar SK, Singh L, Bihari S. Role of yogic exercises in rehabilitation of patients with chronic obstructive pulmonary disease [Abstract]. Indian Journal of Allergy Asthma and Immunology 2005; 19(2):123.

Klein P T, Adams W. Cardiopulmonary physiotherapeutic applications of taiji (Structured abstract). Cardiopulmonary Physical Therapy 2004; 15(4):5-11.

Kondwani KA, Kelley ME, Meng YX, Quyyumi AA, Gibbons GH, Vaccarino V. Effects of a meditation intervention on endothelial function in African americans with metabolic syndrome: A randomized trial [conference abstract]. Psychosomatic Medicine [Abstracts From the 69th Annual Meeting of the American Psychosomatic Society San Antonio, TX United States. Mar 9-12, 2011] 2011; 73(3).

Krueger RC. The comparative effects of Zen focusing and muscle relaxation training on selected experiential variables. Dissertation Abstracts International 1980; 41(4-A):1405.

Kulshreshtha A, Norton C, Veledar E, Eubanks G, Sheps D. Mindfulness based meditation results in improved subjective emotional assessment among patients with coronary artery disease: Results from the mindfulness based stress reduction study [conference abstract]. Psychosomatic Medicine [Abstracts From the 69th Annual Meeting of the American Psychosomatic Society San Antonio, TX United States. Mar 9-12, 2011] 2011; 73(3).

Lavretsky H, Irwin M. Meditation improves depressive symptoms, coping, cognition, and inflammation in family dementia caregivers in a randomized 8-week pilot study [conference abstract]. American Journal of Geriatric Psychiatry [Abstracts of the American Association for Geriatric Psychiatry, AAGP Annual Meeting, 2011 Mar 18-21. San Antonio, TX United States.] 2011.

Malphurs JE, Asebey-Birkholm MA, Petisco I, David D. A Randomized Clinical Trial of Meditation for Veterans with Post-Traumatic Stress Disorder. Military Health Research Forum, Kansas City, MO. August 31- September 3, 2009 [Conference Abstracts] 2009.

Manikonda P, Stoerk S, Toegel S et al. Influence of non-pharmacological treatment (contemplative meditation and breathing technique) on stress induced hypertension - A randomized controlled study. American Journal of Hypertension 2005; 18(5):89A-90A.

Marcel A de Dios, Herman D, Hagerty C, Anderson BJ, Britton W, Stein M. Motivational enhancment and mindfulness meditation for young adult female marijuana users. Proceedings of the 73rd Annual Scientific Meeting of the College on Problems of Drug Dependence; 2011 June 18-23, Hollywood, Florida 2011; 203 , Abstract no: 811.

Miro DJ. A comparative evaluation of relaxation training strategies utilizing EMG biofeedback. Dissertation Abstracts International 1981; 42(3-B):1183-4.

Oh B, Butow P, Mullan B, Clarke SJ, Beale P, Rosenthal D. Randomized clinical trial: The Impact of Medical Qigong (traditional Chinese medicine) on fatique, quality of life, side effects, mood status and inlfammation of cancer patients [abstarct no. 9565]. Journal of Clinical Oncology: ASCO Annual Meeting Proceedings 2008; 26(15S part I):518.

Price A, Meah M, O'Shaughnessy T. A pilot study to compare qigong exercises with conventional exercises in pulmonary rehabilitation [Abstract]. Thorax 2006; 61(Suppl 2):ii67 [P032].

Rosdahl D R L. The effect of mindfulness meditation on tension headaches and secretory immunoglobulin A in saliva [dissertation]. 2003.

Sagula D A. Varying treatment duration in a mindfulness meditation stress reduction program for chronic pain patients [dissertation]. 1999.

Schneider R, Alexander C, Myers H et al. Lifestyle modification in the prevention of left ventricular hypertrophy: A randomized controlled trial of stress reduction and health education in hypertensive African Americans. Journal of Hypertension 2006; 24(Suppl. 6):90.

Smith JC. Meditation as psychotherapy. Dissertation Abstracts International 1975; 36(6-B):3073.

Straus S. A 16-week tai chi programme prevented falls in healthy older adults. Evid Based Med 2008; 13(2):54.

Toomey M. The effects of the transcendental meditation program on carotid atherosclerosis and cardiovascular disease risk factors in Native Hawaiians. Dissertation Abstracts International: Section B: The Sciences and Engineering 2007; 68(6):4169.

Weiner Donald E. The effects of mantra meditation and progressive relaxation on self-actualization, state and trait anxiety, and frontalis muscle tension. Dissertation Abstracts International 1977; 37(8-B):4174.

Wilson HB. The specific effects model: Relaxation and meditation effects on cognitive and somatic anxiety. Dissertation Abstracts International 2001; 61(9-b):5013.

Wolf DB. Effects of the hare krsna maha mantra on stress, depression, and the three gunas. (spirituality, yoga) [dissertation]. Dissertation Abstracts International 2000; 60(7-B).

Wood DT. The effects of progressive relaxation, heart rate feedback, and content-specific meditation on anxiety and performance in a class situation. Dissertation Abstracts International 1978; 39(6-A):3458.

Young EC, Brown ND, Brammar C, Owen E, Lowe J, Johnson C et al. Effect of mindfulness meditation as a psychological intervention for chronic cough [Abstract]. American Thoracic Society International Conference, May 15-20, 2009, San Diego 2009; A5760 [Poster #F8].

Other Meditation

Alberts HJ, Thewissen R. The Effect of a Brief Mindfulness Intervention on Memory for Positively and Negatively Valenced Stimuli. Mindfulness (N Y) 2011; 2(2):73-7.

Dahl JC, Lundgren TL, and Yardi N. Evaluation of short term ACT psychotherapy and yoga in a RCT trial for refractory seizures in India. Epilepsia 2005; 46 Suppl 6:196.

Deberry S, Davis S, Reinhard KE. A comparison of meditation - Relaxtion and cognitive/behavioral techniques for reducing anxiety and depression in geriatric population. 1989; 22(2):231-47.

DeBerry S. The effects of meditation-relaxation on anxiety and depression in a geriatric population. Psychotherapy: Theory, Research & Practice 1982; 19(4):512-21.

Fledderus M, Bohlmeijer ET, Smit F, Westerhof GJ. Mental health promotion as a new goal in public mental health care: a randomized controlled trial of an intervention enhancing psychological flexibility. Am J Public Health 2010; 100(12):2372.

Gaudiano BA, Herbert JD. Acute treatment of inpatients with psychotic symptoms using Acceptance and Commitment Therapy: pilot results. Behav Res Ther 2006; 44(3):415-37.

Khumar SS, Kaur P, Kaur S. Effectiveness of Shavasana on depression among university students. Indian Journal of Clinical Psychology 1993; 20(2):82-7.

Lillis J, Hayes SC, Bunting K, Masuda A. Teaching acceptance and mindfulness to improve the lives of the obese: a preliminary test of a theoretical model. Ann Behav Med 2009; 37(1):58-69.

Lundgren T, Dahl J, Yardi N, Melin L. Acceptance and Commitment Therapy and yoga for drug-refractory epilepsy: a randomized controlled trial. Epilepsy Behav 2008; 13(1):102-8.

Margolin A, Schuman-Olivier Z, Beitel M, Arnold RM, Fulwiler CE, Avants SK. A preliminary study of spiritual self-schema (3-S) therapy for reducing impulsivity in HIV positive drug users. 2007; 63(10):979-99.

McMillan TM, Robertson IH, Brock D, Chorlton L. Brief mindfulness training for attentional problems after traumatic brain injury: A randomised control treatment trial. Neuropsychological Rehabilitation 2002; 12(2):117-25.

Sengoku M, Murata H, Kawahara T, Imamura K, Nakagome K. Does daily Naikan therapy maintain the efficacy of intensive Naikan therapy against depression? Psychiatry and Clinical Neurosciences 2010; 64(1):44-51.

Smith WP, Compton WC, West WB. Meditation as an adjunct to a happiness enhancement program. J Clin Psychol 1995; 51(2):269-73.

Targ EF, Levine EG. The efficacy of a mind-body-spirit group for women with breast cancer: a randomized controlled trial. Gen Hosp Psychiatry 2002; 24(4):238-48.

Other Population

Carei TR, Fyfe-Johnson AL, Breuner CC, Brown MA. Randomized controlled clinical trial of yoga in the treatment of eating disorders. J Adolesc Health 2010; 46(4):346-51.

Franco Justo C, de la Fuente Arias M, Salvador Granados M. [Impact of a training program in full consciousness (mindfulness) in the measure of growth and personal self-realization]. Psicothema 2011; 23(1):58-65.

Kratter J. The use of meditation in the treatment of attention deficit disorder with hyperactivity [dissertation]. 1983.

Madanmohan, Udupa K, Bhavanani AB, Vijayalakshmi P, Surendiran A. Effect of slow and fast pranayams on reaction time and cardiorespiratory variables. Indian J Physiol Pharmacol 2005; 49(3):313-8.

Moretti-Altuna G. The effects of meditation versus medication in the treatment of Attention Deficit Disorder with Hyperactivity [dissertation]. 1987.

Verma IC, Jayashankarappa BS, Palani M. Effect of transcendental meditation on the performance of some cognitive psychological tests. Indian J Med Res 1982; 76 Suppl:136-43.

No Control Group

Agarwal BL, Kharbanda A. Effect of transcendental meditation on mild and moderate hypertension. J Assoc Physicians India 1981; 29(8):591-6.

Allison J. Respiratory changes during transcendental meditation. Lancet 1970; 1(7651):833-4.

An H, Kulkarni R, Nagarathna R, Nagendra H. Measures of heart rate variability in women following a meditation technique. Int J Yoga 2010; 3(1):6-9.

Andrade C, Andrade AC. Meditation versus medication. Indian J Psychiatry 1991; 33(1):39-43.

Astin J. Effects of transcendental meditation on patients with cardiac syndrome X. Focus on Alternative & Complementary Therapies 2000; 5(3):216-7.

Beauregard M, Courtemanche J, Paquette V. Brain activity in near-death experiencers during a meditative state. Resuscitation 2009; 80(9):1006-10.

Benson H, Lehmann JW, Malhotra MS, Goldman RF, Hopkins J, Epstein MD. Body temperature changes during the practice of g Tum-mo yoga. Nature 1982; 295(5846):234-6.

Benson H, Malvea BP, Graham JR. Physiologic correlates of meditation and their clinical effects in headache: an ongoing investigation. Headache 1973; 13(1):23-4.

Bera TK, Gore MM, Oak JP. Recovery from stress in two different postures and in Shavasana--a yogic relaxation posture. Indian J Physiol Pharmacol 1998; 42(4):473-8.

Carlson LE, Garland SN. Impact of mindfulness-based stress reduction (MBSR) on sleep, mood, stress and fatigue symptoms in cancer outpatients. Int J Behav Med 2005; 12(4):278-85.

Chalmers R. Transcendental meditation does not predispose to epilepsy. Med Hypotheses 2005; 65(3):624-5.

Chambers SK, Foley E, Galt E, Ferguson M, Clutton S. Mindfulness groups for men with advanced prostate cancer: a pilot study to assess feasibility and effectiveness and the role of peer support. Support Care Cancer 2011.

Chang J, Midlarsky E, Lin P. Effects of meditation on music performance anxiety. Medical Problems of Performing Artists 2003; 18(3):126-30.

Chen K, He B, Rihacek G, Sigal LH. A pilot trial of external Qigong therapy for arthritis. J Clin Rheumatol 2003; 9(5):332-5.

Chen KM, Hsu YC, Chen WT, Tseng HF. Well-being of institutionalized elders after Yang-style Tai Chi practice. J Clin Nurs 2007; 16(5):845-52.

Chen KW, Marbach JJ. External qigong therapy for chronic orofacial pain [2]. 2002; 8(5):532-4.

Cohen-Katz J, Wiley S, Capuano T, Baker DM, Deitrick L, Shapiro S. The effects of mindfulness-based stress reduction on nurse stress and burnout: a qualitative and quantitative study, part III. Holist Nurs Pract 2005; 19(2):78-86.

Duncan L, Weissenburger D. Effects of a Brief Meditation Program on Well-being and Loneliness. TCA Journal 2003; 31(1):4-14.

Dunn BR, Hartigan JA, Mikulas WL. Concentration and mindfulness meditations: unique forms of consciousness? Appl Psychophysiol Biofeedback 1999; 24(3):147-65.

Galantino ML, Desai K, Greene L, Demichele A, Stricker CT, Mao JJ. Impact of Yoga on Functional Outcomes in Breast Cancer Survivors With Aromatase Inhibitor-Associated Arthralgias. Integr Cancer Ther 2011.

Ghista DN, Nandagopal D, Ramamurthi B, Das A, Mukherju A, Krinivasan TM. Physiological characterisation of the 'meditative state' during intutional practice (the Ananda Marga system of meditation) and its therapeutic value. Med Biol Eng 1976; 14(2):209-13.

Gonzalez A, Solomon SE, Zvolensky MJ, Miller CT. The interaction of mindful-based attention and awareness and disengagement coping with HIV/AIDS-related stigma in regard to concurrent anxiety and depressive symptoms among adults with HIV/AIDS. J Health Psychol 2009; 14(3):403-13.

Greendale GA, McDivit A, Carpenter A, Seeger L, Huang MH. Yoga for women with hyperkyphosis: results of a pilot study. Am J Public Health 2002; 92(10):1611-4.

Gururaja D, Harano K, Toyotake I, Kobayashi H. Effect of yoga on mental health: Comparative study between young and senior subjects in Japan. Int J Yoga 2011; 4(1):7-12.

Haas M. Economic analysis of tai chi as a means of preventing falls and falls related injuries among older adults (Structured abstract). 2006; 1-14.

Heidenreich T, Tuin I, Pflug B, Michal M, Michalak J. Mindfulness-based cognitive therapy for persistent insomnia: a pilot study. Psychother Psychosom 2006; 75(3):188-9.

Hyeong-Dong Kim, Tae-You Kim, Hyun Dong J, Seon-Tae Son. The Effects of Tai Chi Based Exercise on Dynamic Postural Control of Parkinson's Disease Patients while Initiating Gait. Journal of Physical Therapy Science 2011; 23(2):265-9.

Johnson DP, Penn DL, Fredrickson BL et al. A pilot study of loving-kindness meditation for the negative symptoms of schizophrenia. Schizophr Res 2011; 129(2-3):137-40.

Joseph S, Sridharan K, Patil SK et al. Study of some physiological and biochemical parameters in subjects undergoing yogic training. Indian J Med Res 1981; 74:120-4.

Kaul P, Passafiume J, Sargent CR, O'Hara BF. Meditation acutely improves psychomotor vigilance, and may decrease sleep need. Behav Brain Funct 2010; 6:47.

Kinoshita K. [A study on response of EEG during Zen meditation--alpha-blocking to name calling (author's transl)]. Seishin Shinkeigaku Zasshi 1975; 77(9):623-58.

Kjaer TW, Bertelsen C, Piccini P, Brooks D, Alving J, Lou HC. Increased dopamine tone during meditation-induced change of consciousness. Brain Res Cogn Brain Res 2002; 13(2):255-9.

Lee KYT, Jones AYM, Hui-Chan CWY, Tsang WWN. Kinematics and energy expenditure of sitting T'ai Chi. 2011; 17(8):665-8.

Lee MS, Kang C-W, Ryu H, Moon S-R. Endocrine and immune effects of Qi-training. International Journal of Neuroscience 2004; 114(4):529-37.

Li J, Sharma K, Finkelstein J. Feasibility of computer-assisted Tai Chi education. AMIA Annu Symp Proc 2005; 1027.

Madhavi S, Raju PS, Reddy MV et al. Effect of yogic exercises on lean body mass. J Assoc Physicians India 1985; 33(7):465-6.

Maras ML, Rinke WJ, Stephens CR, Boehm TM. Effect of meditation on insulin dependent diabetes mellitus. Diabetes Educ 1984; 10(1):22-5.

McIver S, O'Halloran P, McGartland M. The impact of Hatha yoga on smoking behavior. Altern Ther Health Med 2004; 10(2):22-3.

McManus F, Muse K, Surawy C. Mindfulness-based cognitive therapy (MBCT) for severe health anxiety. Healthcare Counselling & Psychotherapy Journal 2011; 11(1):19-23.

Morse DR. An exploratory study of the use of meditation alone and in combination with hypnosis in clinical dentistry. J Am Soc Psychosom Dent Med 1977; 24(4):113-20.

Morse DR, Cohen L, Furst ML, Martin JS. A physiological evaluation of the yoga concept of respiratory control of autonomic nervous system activity. Int J Psychosom 1984; 31(1):3-19.

Morse DR, Schacterle GR, Esposito JV et al. Stress, meditation and saliva: a study of separate salivary gland secretions in endodontic patients. J Oral Med 1983; 38(4):150-60.

Morse DR, Schacterle GR, Furst ML et al. The effect of stress and meditation on salivary protein and bacteria: a review and pilot study. J Human Stress 1982; 8(4):31-9.

Moustgaard A, Bedard M, Felteau M. Mindfulness-based cognitive therapy (MBCT) for individuals who had a stroke: results from a pilot study. Journal of Cognitive Rehabilitation 2007; 25(4):4-10.

Murphy L, Riley D, Rodgers J, Plank S, Lehman S, Duryea B. Effects of Tai Chi on balance, mobility, and strength among older persons participating in an osteoporosis prevention and education program. Explore (NY) 2005; 1(3):192-3.

Mustata S, Cooper L, Langrick N, Simon N, Jassal SV, Oreopoulos DG. The effect of a Tai Chi exercise program on quality of life in patients on peritoneal dialysis: a pilot study. Perit Dial Int 2005; 25(3):291-4.

Narahari SR, Aggithaya MG, Prasanna KS, Bose KS. An integrative treatment for lower limb lymphedema (elephantiasis). J Altern Complement Med 2010; 16(2):145-9.

Orme-Johnson DW. Transcendental meditation does not predispose to epilepsy. Med Hypotheses 2005; 65(1):201-2.

Patra S, Telles S. Positive impact of cyclic meditation on subsequent sleep. Med Sci Monit 2009; 15(7):CR375-81.

Patra S, Telles S. Heart rate variability during sleep following the practice of cyclic meditation and supine rest. Appl Psychophysiol Biofeedback 2010; 35(2):135-40.

Robins JL, McCain NL, Gray DP, Elswick RK Jr, Walter JM, McDade E. Research on psychoneuroimmunology: tai chi as a stress management approach for individuals with HIV disease. Appl Nurs Res 2006; 19(1):2-9.

Sakata T, Li Q, Tanaka M, Tajima F. Positive effects of a qigong and aerobic exercise program on physical health in elderly Japanese women: an exploratory study. Environ Health Prev Med 2008; 13(3):162-8.

Satyanarayanamurthi GV, Sastry PB. A preliminary scientific investigation into some of the unusual physiological manifestations acquired as a result of yogic practices in India. Wien Z Nervenheilkd Grenzgeb 1958; 15(1-4):239-49.

Schneider B, Ercoli L, Siddarth P, Lavretsky H. Vascular Burden and Cognitive Functioning in Depressed Older Adults. Am J Geriatr Psychiatry 2011.

Shah AH, Joshi SV, Mehrotra PP, Potdar N, Dhar HL. Effect of Saral meditation on intelligence, performance and cardiopulmonary functions. Indian J Med Sci 2001; 55(11):604-8.

Singh N N, Lancioni G E, Winton A S, Singh A N, Adkins A D, Singh J. Clinical and benefit-cost outcomes of teaching a mindfulness-based procedure to adult offenders with intellectual disabilities (Provisional abstract). Behavior Modification 2008; 32(5):622-37.

Spanos NP, Rivers SM, Gottlieb J. Hypnotic responsivity, meditation, and laterality of eye movements. J Abnorm Psychol 1978; 87(5):566-9.

Subramanya P, Telles S. Effect of two yoga-based relaxation techniques on memory scores and state anxiety. Biopsychosoc Med 2009; 3:8.

Taggart HM. Effects of Tai Chi exercise on balance, functional mobility, and fear of falling among older women. Appl Nurs Res 2002; 15(4):235-42.

Telles S, Naveen KV. Changes in middle latency auditory evoked potentials during meditation. Psychol Rep 2004; 94(2):398-400.

Uhlig T, Larsson C, Hjorth AG, Odegard S, Kvien TK. No improvement in a pilot study of tai chi exercise in rheumatoid arthritis. Ann Rheum Dis 2005; 64(3):507-9.

Weissbecker I, Salmon P, Studts JL, Floyd AR, Dedert EA, Sephton SE. Mindfulness-based stress reduction and sense of coherence among women with fibromyalgia. Journal of Clinical Psychology in Medical Settings 2002; 9(4):297-307.

Wenger Ma, Bagchi Bk, Anand Bk. Experiments in India on "voluntary" control of the heart and pulse. Circulation 1961; 24:1319-25.

Yeh SH, Chuang H, Lin LW, Hsiao CY, Wang PW, Yang KD. Tai chi chuan exercise decreases A1C levels along with increase of regulatory T-cells and decrease of cytotoxic T-cell population in type 2 diabetic patients. Diabetes Care 2007; 30(3):716-8.

Oktedalen O, Solberg EE, Haugen AH, Opstad PK. The influence of physical and mental training on plasma beta-endorphin level and pain perception after intensive physical exercise. Stress and Health: Journal of the International Society for the Investigation of Stress 2001; 17(2):121-7.

Zeidan F, Martucci KT, Kraft RA, Gordon NS, McHaffie JG, Coghill RC. Brain mechanisms supporting the modulation of pain by mindfulness meditation. J Neurosci 2011; 31(14):5540-8.

Not Randomized

Acharya B, Upadhyay A, Upadhyay RT, Kumar A. Effect of Pranayama (voluntary regulated breathing) and Yogasana (yoga postures) on lipid profile in normal healthy junior footballers. Int J Yoga 2010; 3(2):70.

Aftanas LI, Golocheikine SA. Human anterior and frontal midline theta and lower alpha reflect emotionally positive state and internalized attention: high-resolution EEG investigation of meditation. Neurosci Lett 2001; 310(1):57-60.

Aftanas LI, Golosheikin SA. [Changes in cortical activity during altered state of consciousness: study of meditation by high resolution EEG]. Fiziol Cheloveka 2003; 29(2):18-27.

Agarwal BL, Kharbanda A. Effect of transcendental meditation on mild and moderate hypertension. J Assoc Physicians India 1981; 29(8):591-6.

Agte V, Tarwadi K. Sudarshan Kriya yoga for treating type 2 diabetes: a preliminary study. Alternative & Complementary Therapies 2004; 10(4):220-2.

Alexander CN, Swanson GC, Rainforth MV, Carlisle TW. Effects of the transcendental meditation program on stress reduction, health, and employee development: A prospective study in two occupational settings. Anxiety, Stress & Coping: An International Journal 1993; 6(3):245-62.

Allison J. Respiratory changes during transcendental meditation. Lancet 1970; 1(7651):833-4.

An H, Kulkarni R, Nagarathna R, Nagendra H. Measures of heart rate variability in women following a meditation technique. Int J Yoga 2010; 3(1):6-9.

Andrade C, Andrade AC. Meditation versus medication. Indian J Psychiatry 1991; 33(1):39-43.

Anon. Transcendental Meditation in the treatment of post-Vietnam adjustment. Journal of Counseling & Development 1985; 64(3):212-5.

Astin J. Effects of transcendental meditation on patients with cardiac syndrome X. Focus on Alternative & Complementary Therapies 2000; 5(3):216-7.

Badawi K, Wallace RK, Orme-Johnson D, Rouzere AM. Electrophysiologic characteristics of respiratory suspension periods occurring during the practice of the Transcendental Meditation Program. Psychosom Med 1984; 46(3):267-76.

Baijal S, Srinivasan N. Theta activity and meditative states: spectral changes during concentrative meditation. Cogn Process 2010; 11(1):31-8.

Banquet JP. Spectral analysis of the EEG in meditation. Electroencephalogr Clin Neurophysiol 1973; 35(2):143-51.

Barmark SM, Gaunitz SC. Transcendental meditation and heterohypnosis as altered states of consciousness. Int J Clin Exp Hypn 1979; 27(3):227-39.

Battle CL, Uebelacker LA, Howard M, Castaneda M. Prenatal yoga and depression during pregnancy. Birth 2010; 37(4):353-4.

Bay R, Bay F. Combined Therapy Using Acupressure Therapy, Hypnotherapy, and Transcendental Meditation versus Placebo in Type 2 Diabetes. J Acupunct Meridian Stud 2011; 4(3):183-6.

Beauregard M, Courtemanche J, Paquette V. Brain activity in near-death experiencers during a meditative state. Resuscitation 2009; 80(9):1006-10.

Bedard M, Felteau M, Gibbons C et al. A mindfulness-based intervention to improve quality of life among individuals who sustained traumatic brain injuries: one-year follow-up. Journal of Cognitive Rehabilitation 2005; 23(1):8-13.

Benson H, Lehmann JW, Malhotra MS, Goldman RF, Hopkins J, Epstein MD. Body temperature changes during the practice of g Tum-mo yoga. Nature 1982; 295(5846):234-6.

Benson H, Malvea BP, Graham JR. Physiologic correlates of meditation and their clinical effects in headache: an ongoing investigation. Headache 1973; 13(1):23-4.

Benson H, Rosner BA, Marzetta BR, Klemchuk HP. Decreased blood pressure in borderline hypertensive subjects who practiced meditation. J Chronic Dis 1974; 27(3):163-9.

Bera TK, Gore MM, Oak JP. Recovery from stress in two different postures and in Shavasana--a yogic relaxation posture. Indian J Physiol Pharmacol 1998; 42(4):473-8.

Berkovich-Ohana A, Glicksohn J, Goldstein A. Mindfulness-induced changes in gamma band activity - Implications for the default mode network, self-reference and attention. Clin Neurophysiol 2011.

Bernardi L, Passino C, Spadacini G et al. Reduced hypoxic ventilatory response with preserved blood oxygenation in yoga trainees and Himalayan Buddhist monks at altitude: evidence of a different adaptive strategy? Eur J Appl Physiol 2007; 99(5):511-8.

Bharshankar JR, Bharshankar RN, Deshpande VN, Kaore SB, Gosavi GB. Effect of yoga on cardiovascular system in subjects above 40 years. Indian J Physiol Pharmacol 2003; 47(2):202-6.

Bhatia M, Kumar A, Kumar N, Pandey RM, Kochupillai V. Electrophysiologic evaluation of Sudarshan Kriya: an EEG, BAER, P300 study. Indian J Physiol Pharmacol 2003; 47(2):157-63.

Bhatnagar OP, Anantharaman V. The effect of yoga training on neuromuscular excitability and muscular relaxation. Neurol India 1977; 25(4):230-2.

Bhattacharya S, Pandey US, Verma NS. Improvement in oxidative status with yogic breathing in young healthy males. Indian J Physiol Pharmacol 2002; 46(3):349-54.

Borker AS, Pednekar JR. Effect of pranayam on visual and auditory reaction time [2]. 2003; 47(2):229-30.

Bosch PR, Traustadottir T, Howard P, Matt KS. Functional and physiological effects of yoga in women with rheumatoid arthritis: a pilot study. Altern Ther Health Med 2009; 15(4):24-31.

Bowen S, Witkiewitz K, Dillworth TM et al. Mindfulness meditation and substance use in an incarcerated population. Psychol Addict Behav 2006; 20(3):343-7.

Bowen S, Witkiewitz K, Dillworth TM, Marlatt GA. The role of thought suppression in the relationship between mindfulness meditation and alcohol use. Addictive Behaviors 2007; 32(10):2324-8.

Brooks JS, Scarano T. Transcendental Meditation in the treatment of post-Vietnam adjustment. Journal of Counseling & Development 1985; 64(3):212-5.

Brown KD, Koziol JA, Lotz M. A yoga-based exercise program to reduce the risk of falls in seniors: a pilot and feasibility study. J Altern Complement Med 2008; 14(5):454-7.

Brown LL, Robinson SE. The relationship between meditation and/or exercise and three measures of self-actualization. Journal of Mental Health Counseling 1993; 15(1):85-93.

Caldwell K, Harrison M, Adams M, Triplett NT. Effect of Pilates and taiji quan training on self-efficacy, sleep quality, mood, and physical performance of college students. J Bodyw Mov Ther 2009; 13(2):155-63.

Campbell JF, Stenstrom RJ, Bertrand D. Systematic changes in perceptual reactance induced by physical fitness training. Percept Mot Skills 1985; 61(1):279-84.

Carlson CR, Bacaseta PE, Simanton DA. A controlled evaluation of devotional meditation and progressive relaxation. Journal of Psychology and Theology 1988; 16(4):362-8.

Carter OL, Presti DE, Callistemon C, Ungerer Y, Liu GB, Pettigrew JD. Meditation alters perceptual rivalry in Tibetan Buddhist monks. Curr Biol 2005; 15(11):R412-3.

Cazard P. Interhemispheric synchronism of parieto-occipital alpha rhythm. Attention and conscious experience: Synchronie interhemispherique des rythmes alpha parito-occipitaux. Attention et experience consciente. 1974; 74(1):7-22.

Chang RY, Koo M, Kan CB et al. Effects of Tai Chi rehabilitation on heart rate responses in patients with coronary artery disease. Am J Chin Med 2010; 38(3):461-72.

Chatzisarantis NL, Hagger MS. Mindfulness and the intention-behavior relationship within the theory of planned behavior. Pers Soc Psychol Bull 2007; 33(5):663-76.

Chaudhary AK, Bhatnagar HN, Bhatnagar LK, Chaudhary K. Comparative study of the effect of drugs and relaxation exercise (yoga shavasan) in hypertension. J Assoc Physicians India 1988; 36(12):721-3.

Chaya MS, Nagendra HR. Long-term effect of yogic practices on diurnal metabolic rates of healthy subjects. Int J Yoga 2008; 1(1):27-32.

Chen K, He B, Rihacek G, Sigal LH. A pilot trial of external Qigong therapy for arthritis pain [2]. 2003; 9(5):332-5.

Chen KM, Hsu YC, Chen WT, Tseng HF. Well-being of institutionalized elders after Yang-style Tai Chi practice. J Clin Nurs 2007; 16(5):845-52.

Chen KW, Marbach JJ. External qigong therapy for chronic orofacial pain [2]. 2002; 8(5):532-4.

Chen WW, Sun WY. Tai Chi Chuan, an alternative form of exercise for health promotion and disease prevention for older adults in the community. International Quarterly of Community Health Education 1997; 16(4):333-9.

Chen YS, Crowley Z, Zhou S, Cartwright C. Effects of 12-week Tai Chi training on soleus H-reflex and muscle strength in older adults: a pilot study. Eur J Appl Physiol 2011.

Chen YS, Zhou S, Cartwright C. Effect of 12 weeks of Tai Chi training on soleus Hoffmann reflex and control of static posture in older adults. Arch Phys Med Rehabil 2011; 92(6):886-91.

Cheung SY, Tsai E, Fung L, Ng J. Physical benefits of Tai Chi Chuan for individuals with lower-limb disabilities. Occup Ther Int 2007; 14(1):1-10.

Choi KE, Rampp T, Saha FJ, Dobos GJ, Musial F. Pain modulation by meditation and electroacupuncture in experimental submaximum effort tourniquet technique (SETT). Explore (NY) 2011; 7(4):239-45.

Coelho CM, Lessa TT, Coelho LAMC, da Silva Scari R, Junior JMN, de Carvalho RM. Ventilatory function in female practitionersof Hatha Yoga: Funcao ventilatoria em mulheres praticantes de Hatha Ioga. 2011; 13(4):279-84.

Colby F. An analogue study of the initial carryover effects of meditation, hypnosis, and relaxation using native college students. Biofeedback Self Regul 1991; 16(2):157-65.

Cooper MJ, Aygen MM. A relaxation technique in the management of hypercholesterolemia. J Human Stress 1979; 5(4):24-7.

Coubard OA, Duretz S, Lefebvre V, Lapalus P, Ferrufino L. Practice of contemporary dance improves cognitive flexibility in aging. Front Aging Neurosci 2011; 3:13.

Cowger EL, Torrance EP. Further examination of the quality of changes in creative functioning resulting from meditation (Zazen) training. Creative Child & Adult Quarterly 1982; 7(4):211-7.

Danhauer S, Rutherford C, McQuellon R et al. Restorative yoga as a supportive intervention for women with ovarian or breast cancer... American Psychosocial Oncology Society (APOS) Third Annual Conference, Amelia Island, Florida, 16th-19th February 2006. Psycho-Oncology 2006-; 15(1):S72-3.

Dash M, Telles S. Improvement in hand grip strength in normal volunteers and rheumatoid arthritis patients following yoga training. Indian J Physiol Pharmacol 2001; 45(3):355-60.

De La Arias JF, Justo CF, Manas I. Results of a program on mindfulness on the emotional situation of university students: Efectos de un programa de entrenamiento en conciencia plena (mindfulness) en el estado emocional de estudiantes universitarios. 2010; (19):31-52.

Deberry S, Davis S, Reinhard KE. A comparison of meditation - Relaxtion and cognitive/ behavioral techniques for reducing anxiety and depression in geriatric population. 1989; 22(2):231-47.

Delgado LC, Guerra P, Perakakis P, Viedma MI, Robles H, Vila J. Human values education and mindfulness meditation as a tool for emotional regulation and stress prevention for teachers: An efficiency study: Eficacia de un programa de entrenamiento en conciencia plena (mindfulness) y valores humanos como herramienta de regulacion emocional y prevencion del estres para profesores. 2010; 18(3):511-33.

Delmonte MM. Response to meditation in terms of physiological, behavioral and self-report measures. Int J Psychosom 1984; 31(2):3-17.

Delmonte MM. Effects of expectancy on physiological responsivity in novice meditators. Biol Psychol 1985; 21(2):107-21.

Delmonte MM. Expectancy and response to meditation. Int J Psychosom 1986; 33(2):28-34.

Dhikav V, Karmarkar G, Gupta M, Anand KS. Yoga in premature ejaculation: a comparative trial with fluoxetine. J Sex Med 2007; 4(6):1726-32.

Dunn BR, Hartigan JA, Mikulas WL. Concentration and mindfulness meditations: unique forms of consciousness? Appl Psychophysiol Biofeedback 1999; 24(3):147-65.

Eisendrath SJ, Delucchi K, Bitner R, Fenimore P, Smit M, McLane M. Mindfulness-based cognitive therapy for treatment-resistant depression: a pilot study. Psychother Psychosom 2008; 77(5):319-20.

Elson BD, Hauri P, Cunis D. Physiological changes in yoga meditation. Psychophysiology 1977; 14(1):52-7.

Emavardhana T, Tori CD. Changes in self-concept, ego defense mechanisms, and religiosity following seven-day Vipassana meditation retreats. Journal for the Scientific Study of Religion 1997; 36(2):194-206.

Fan J-T, Chen K-M. Using silver yoga exercises to promote physical and mental health of elders with dementia in long-term care facilities. 2011:1-9.

Ferguson JK, Willemsen EW, Castaneto MV. Centering prayer as a healing response to everyday stress: A psychological and spiritual process. Pastoral Psychology 2010; 59(3):305-29.

Fishman L. Yoga for osteoporosis: a pilot study. Topics in Geriatric Rehabilitation 2009; 25(3):244-50.

Fjellman-Wiklund A, Stenlund T, Steinholtz K, Ahlgren C. Take charge: Patients' experiences during participation in a rehabilitation programme for burnout. J Rehabil Med 2010; 42(5):475-81.

Franco C, Sola MadM, Justo E. Reduccion del malestar psicolgico y de la sobrecarga en familiares cuidadores de enfermos de Alzheimer mediante la aplicacion de un programa de entrenamiento en mindfulness (conciencia plena). Revista Espanola De Geriatria y Gerontologia 2010; 45(5):252-8.

Frumkin LR, Pagano RR. The effect of transcendental meditation on iconic memory. Biofeedback Self Regul 1979; 4(4):313-22.

Galantino ML, Desai K, Greene L, Demichele A, Stricker CT, Mao JJ. Impact of Yoga on Functional Outcomes in Breast Cancer Survivors With Aromatase Inhibitor-Associated Arthralgias. Integr Cancer Ther 2011.

Gallois P. [Neurophysiologic and respiratory changes during the practice of relaxation technics]. Encephale 1984; 10(3):139-44.

Gallois P, Forzy G, Dhont JL. [Hormonal changes during relaxation]. Encephale 1984; 10(2):79-82.

Gardner-Nix J, Backman S, Barbati J, Grummitt J. Evaluating distance education of a mindfulness-based meditation programme for chronic pain management. J Telemed Telecare 2008; 14(2):88-92.

Ghista DN, Nandagopal D, Ramamurthi B, Das A, Mukherju A, Krinivasan TM. Physiological characterisation of the 'meditative state' during intutional practice (the Ananda Marga system of meditation) and its therapeutic value. Med Biol Eng 1976; 14(2):209-13.

Gode JD, Singh RH, Settiwar RM, Gode KD, Udupa KN. Increased urinary excretion of testosterone following a course of yoga in normal young volunteers. Indian J Med Sci 1974; 28(4-5):212-5.

Gokal R, Shillito L, Maharaj SR. Positive impact of yoga and pranayam on obesity, hypertension, blood sugar, and cholesterol: a pilot assessment. J Altern Complement Med 2007; 13(10):1056-7.

Gokhan N, Meehan EF, Peters K. The value of mindfulness-based methods in teaching at a clinical field placement. Psychol Rep 2010; 106(2):455-66.

Goldenberg DL, Kaplan KH, Nadeau MG, Brodeur C, Smith S, Schmid CH. A controlled study of a stress-reduction, cognitive-behavioral treatment program in fibromyalgia. 1994; 2(2):53-66.

Goncalves LC, Vale RGDS, Barata NJF, Varejao RV, Dantas EHM. Flexibility, functional autonomy and quality of life (QoL) in elderly yoga practitioners. 2011; 53(2):158-62.

Gonzalez A, Solomon SE, Zvolensky MJ, Miller CT. The interaction of mindful-based attention and awareness and disengagement coping with HIV/AIDS-related stigma in regard to concurrent anxiety and depressive symptoms among adults with HIV/AIDS. J Health Psychol 2009; 14(3):403-13.

Gopal KS, Anantharaman V, Balachander S, Nishith SD. The cardiorespiratory adjustments in 'Pranayama', with and without 'Bandhas', in 'Vajrasana'. Indian J Med Sci 1973; 27(9):686-92.

Gopal KS, Anantharamn V, Nishith SD, Bhatnagar OP. The effect of yogasanas on muscular tone and cardio-respiratory adjustments. Indian J Med Sci 1974; 28(10):438-43.

Gopal KS, Bhatnagar OP, Subramanian N, Nishith SD. Effect of yogasanas and pranayamas on blood pressure, pulse rate and some respiratory functions. Indian J Physiol Pharmacol 1973; 17(3):273-6.

Greendale GA, McDivit A, Carpenter A, Seeger L, Huang MH. Yoga for women with hyperkyphosis: results of a pilot study. Am J Public Health 2002; 92(10):1611-4.

Greene YN, Hiebert B. A comparison of mindfulness meditation and cognitive self-observation. Canadian Journal of Counselling 1988; 22(1):25-34.

Grepmair L, Mitterlehner F, Rother W, Nickel M. Promotion of mindfulness in psychotherapists in training and treatment results of their patients. J Psychosom Res 2006; 60(6):649-50.

Grover P, Varma VK, Verma SK, Pershad D. Factors influencing treatment acceptance in neurotic patients referred for yoga therapy-;an exploratory study. Indian J Psychiatry 1989; 31(3):250-7.

Gururaja D, Harano K, Toyotake I, Kobayashi H. Effect of yoga on mental health: Comparative study between young and senior subjects in Japan. Int J Yoga 2011; 4(1):7-12.

Holzel BK, Carmody J, Vangel M et al. Mindfulness practice leads to increases in regional brain gray matter density. Psychiatry Research: Neuroimaging 2011; 191(1):36-43.

Haas M. Economic analysis of tai chi as a means of preventing falls and falls related injuries among older adults (Structured abstract). 2006; 1-14.

Hart CE, Tracy BL. Yoga as steadiness training: effects on motor variability in young adults. J Strength Cond Res 2008; 22(5):1659-69.

Harvey JR. The effect of yogic breathing exercises on mood. J Am Soc Psychosom Dent Med 1983; 30(2):39-48.

Hawkins MA, Alexander CN, Travis FT et al. Consciousness-Based rehabilitation of inmates in the Netherlands Antilles: Psychosocial and cognitive changes. Journal of Offender Rehabilitation 2003; 36(1-4):205-28.

He Q, Zhang JZ, Li JZ. The effects of long-term Qi Gong exercise on brain function as manifested by computer analysis. J Tradit Chin Med 1988; 8(3):177-82.

Hegde SV, Adhikari P, Kotian S, Pinto VJ, D'Souza S, D'Souza V. Effect of 3-Month Yoga on Oxidative Stress in Type 2 Diabetes With or Without Complications: A controlled clinical trial. Diabetes Care 2011; 34(10):2208-10.

Heide FJ. Psychophysiological responsiveness to auditory stimulation during transcendental meditation. Psychophysiology 1986; 23(1):71-5.

Heidenreich T, Tuin I, Pflug B, Michal M, Michalak J. Mindfulness-based cognitive therapy for persistent insomnia: A pilot study [2]. 2006; 75(3):188-9.

Heppner WL, Kernis MH, Lakey CE et al. Mindfulness as a means of reducing aggressive behavior: dispositional and situational evidence. Aggress Behav 2008; 34(5):486-96.

Hill JM, Vernig PM, Lee JK, Brown C, Orsillo SM. The development of a brief acceptance and mindfulness-based program aimed at reducing sexual revictimization among college women with a history of childhood sexual abuse. J Clin Psychol 2011; 67(9):969-80.

Hjelle LA. Transcendental meditation and psychological health. Percept Mot Skills 1974; 39(1 Pt 2):623-8.

Hui PN, Wan M, Chan WK, Yung PM. An evaluation of two behavioral rehabilitation programs, qigong versus progressive relaxation, in improving the quality of life in cardiac patients. J Altern Complement Med 2006; 12(4):373-8.

Jacobs B, Nagel L. The Impact of a Brief Mindfulness-Based Stress Reduction Program on Perceived Quality of Life. 2003; 2(2):155-68.

Jevning R, Wilson AF, VanderLaan EF. Plasma prolactin and growth hormone during meditation. Psychosom Med 1978; 40(4):329-33.

Johnson DP, Penn DL, Fredrickson BL et al. A pilot study of loving-kindness meditation for the negative symptoms of schizophrenia. Schizophr Res 2011; 129(2-3):137-40.

Jung YH, Kang DH, Byun MS et al. Influence of brain-derived neurotrophic factor and catechol O-methyl transferase polymorphisms on effects of meditation on plasma catecholamines and stress. Stress 2011.

Jung YH, Kang DH, Jang JH et al. The effects of mind-body training on stress reduction, positive affect, and plasma catecholamines. Neurosci Lett 2010; 479(2):138-42.

Kang HY, Yoo YS. Effects of a bereavement intervention program in middle-aged widows in Korea. Arch Psychiatr Nurs 2007; 21(3):132-40.

Karambelkar PV, Bhole MV, Gharote ML. Effect of Yogic asanas on uropepsin excretion. Indian J Med Res 1969; 57(5):944-7.

Kasamatsu A, Hirai T. An electroencephalographic study on the zen meditation (Zazen). Folia Psychiatr Neurol Jpn 1966; 20(4):315-36.

Kaul P, Passafiume J, Sargent CR, O'Hara BF. Meditation acutely improves psychomotor vigilance, and may decrease sleep need. Behav Brain Funct 2010; 6:47.

Khalsa SB, Cope S. Effects of a yoga lifestyle intervention on performance-related characteristics of musicians: a preliminary study. Med Sci Monit 2006; 12(8):CR325-31.

Khalsa SB, Shorter SM, Cope S, Wyshak G, Sklar E. Yoga ameliorates performance anxiety and mood disturbance in young professional musicians. Appl Psychophysiol Biofeedback 2009; 34(4):279-89.

Kim SJ, Lee CS. The Effects of Meditation on Stress and Self Efficacy of College Students. Chonnam Medical Journal 2000; 36(4):403-14.

Kim TS, Park JS, Kim MA. The relation of meditation to power and well-being. Nurs Sci Q 2008; 21(1):49-58.

Kingston T, Dooley B, Bates A, Lawlor E, Malone K. Mindfulness-based cognitive therapy for residual depressive symptoms. Psychol Psychother 2007; 80(Pt 2):193-203.

Kirk U, Downar J, Montague PR. Interoception drives increased rational decision-making in meditators playing the ultimatum game. Front Neurosci 2011; 5:49.

Kirsteins AE, Dietz F, Hwang SM. Evaluating the safety and potential use of a weight-bearing exercise, Tai-Chi Chuan, for rheumatoid arthritis patients. Am J Phys Med Rehabil 1991; 70(3):136-41.

Kjaer TW, Bertelsen C, Piccini P, Brooks D, Alving J, Lou HC. Increased dopamine tone during meditation-induced change of consciousness. Brain Res Cogn Brain Res 2002; 13(2):255-9.

Kjellgren A, Bood SA, Axelsson K, Norlander T, Saatcioglu F. Wellness through a comprehensive yogic breathing program - a controlled pilot trial. BMC Complement Altern Med 2007; 7:43.

Kligler B, Homel P, Harrison LB et al. Impact of the Urban Zen Initiative on patients' experience of admission to an inpatient oncology floor: a mixed-methods analysis. J Altern Complement Med 2011; 17(8):729-34.

Kline KS, Docherty EM, Farley FH. Transcendental Meditation, self/actualization, and global personality. Journal of General Psychology 1982; 106(1):3-8.

Kochupillai V, Kumar P, Singh D et al. Effect of rhythmic breathing (Sudarshan Kriya and Pranayam) on immune functions and tobacco addiction. Ann N Y Acad Sci 2005; 1056:242-52.

Kolsawalla MB. An experimental investigation into the effectiveness of some yogic variables as a mechanism of change in the value-attitude system. Journal of Indian Psychology 1978; 1(1):59-68.

Kozasa EH, Santos RF, Rueda AD, Benedito-Silva AA, De Ornellas FL, Leite JR. Evaluation of Siddha Samadhi Yoga for anxiety and depression symptoms: a preliminary study. Psychol Rep 2008; 103(1):271-4.

Kozasa EH, Sato JR, Lacerda SS et al. Meditation training increases brain efficiency in an attention task. Neuroimage 2011.

Kuan SC, Chen KM, Wang C. Effects of Qigong in Promoting Health of the Wheelchair-Bound Older Adults in Long-Term Care Facilities. Biol Res Nurs 2011.

Kuang AK, Wang CX, Zhao GS et al. Long-term observation on qigong in prevention of stroke--follow-up of 244 hypertensive patients for 18-22 years. J Tradit Chin Med 1986; 6(4):235-8.

Kulkarni R, Nagarathna R, Nagendra HR, An H. Measures of heart rate variability in women following a meditation technique. International Journal of Yoga 2010; 3(1):6-9.

Kyizom T, Singh S, Singh KP, Tandon OP, Kumar R. Effect of pranayama & yoga-asana on cognitive brain functions in type 2 diabetes-P3 event related evoked potential (ERP). Indian J Med Res 2010; 131:636-40.

Labelle LE, Campbell TS, Carlson LE. Mindfulness-based stress reduction in oncology: Evaluating mindfulness and rumination as mediators of change in depressive symptoms. Mindfulness 2010; 1(1):28-40.

Lakey CE, Berry DR, Sellers EW. Manipulating attention via mindfulness induction improves P300-based brain-computer interface performance. J Neural Eng 2011; 8(2):025019.

Lan C, Lai JS, Chen SY, Wong MK. 12-month Tai Chi training in the elderly: its effect on health fitness. Med Sci Sports Exerc 1998; 30(3):345-51.

Langer AI, Cangas AJ, Gallego J. Mindfulness-based intervention on distressing hallucination-like experiences in a nonclinical sample. Behav. Change 2010; 27(3):176-83.

Lavallee CF, Hunter MD, Persinger MA. Intracerebral source generators characterizing concentrative meditation. Cogn Process 2011; 12(2):141-50.

Lee EN, Kim YH, Chung WT, Lee MS. Tai chi for disease activity and flexibility in patients with ankylosing spondylitis--a controlled clinical trial. Evid Based Complement Alternat Med 2008; 5(4):457-62.

Lee KYT, Jones AYM, Hui-Chan CWY, Tsang WWN. Kinematics and energy expenditure of sitting T'ai Chi. 2011; 17(8):665-8.

Lee LY, Lee DT, Woo J. Effect of Tai Chi on state self-esteem and health-related quality of life in older Chinese residential care home residents J Clin Nurs. 2007 Sep;16(9):1592. Journal of Clinical Nursing 2007; 16(8):1580-2.

Lee LY, Lee DT, Woo J. Tai Chi and health-related quality of life in nursing home residents. J Nurs Scholarsh 2009; 41(1):35-43.

Lee MS, Lim HJ, Lee MS. Impact of qigong exercise on self-efficacy and other cognitive perceptual variables in patients with essential hypertension. J Altern Complement Med 2004; 10(4):675-80.

Lee MS, Rim YH, Kang C-W. Effects of external Qi-therapy on emotions, electroencephalograms, and plasma cortisol. 2004; 114(11):1493-502.

Lee MS, Kang C-W, Ryu H, Moon S-R. Endocrine and immune effects of Qi-training. International Journal of Neuroscience 2004; 114(4):529-37.

Lee TI, Chen HH, Yeh ML. Effects of chan-chuang qigong on improving symptom and psychological distress in chemotherapy patients. Am J Chin Med 2006; 34(1):37-46.

Lehrer PM, Schoicket S, Carrington P, Woolfolk RL. Psychophysiological and cognitive responses to stressful stimuli in subjects practicing progressive relaxation and clinically standardized meditation. Behaviour Research and Therapy 1980; 18(4):293-303.

Lesh TV. Zen meditation and the development of empathy in counselors. Journal of Humanistic Psychology 1970; 10(1):39-74.

Li M, Chen K, Mo Z. Use of qigong therapy in the detoxification of heroin addicts. Altern Ther Health Med 2002; 8(1):50-4, 56-9.

Li Y, Devault CN, Van Oteghen S. Effects of extended Tai Chi intervention on balance and selected motor functions of the elderly. Am J Chin Med 2007; 35(3):383-91.

Lin MR, Hwang HF, Wang YW, Chang SH, Wolf SL. Community-based tai chi and its effect on injurious falls, balance, gait, and fear of falling in older people. Phys Ther 2006; 86(9):1189-201.

Little SA, Kligler B, Homel P, Belisle SS, Merrell W. Multimodal mind/body group therapy for chronic depression: a pilot study. Explore (NY) 2009; 5(6):330-7.

Liu CY, Wei CC, Lo PC. Variation Analysis of Sphygmogram to Assess Cardiovascular System under Meditation. Evid Based Complement Alternat Med 2009; 6(1):107-12.

Logghe IH, Verhagen AP, Rademaker AC et al. Explaining the ineffectiveness of a Tai Chi fall prevention training for community-living older people: a process evaluation alongside a randomized clinical trial (RCT). Arch Gerontol Geriatr 2011; 52(3):357-62.

Lu WA, Kuo CD. Comparison of the effects of Tai Chi Chuan and Wai Tan Kung exercises on autonomic nervous system modulation and on hemodynamics in elder adults. Am J Chin Med 2006; 34(6):959-68.

Madanmohan, Bhavanani AB, Prakash ES, Kamath MG, Amudhan J. Effect of six weeks of shavasan training on spectral measures of short-term heart rate variability in young healthy volunteers. Indian J Physiol Pharmacol 2004; 48(3):370-3.

Madanmohan, Mahadevan SK, Balakrishnan S, Gopalakrishnan M, Prakash ES. Effect of six weeks yoga training on weight loss following step test, respiratory pressures, handgrip strength and handgrip endurance in young healthy subjects. Indian J Physiol Pharmacol 2008; 52(2):164-70.

Madanmohan, Udupa K, Bhavanani AB, Vijayalakshmi P, Surendiran A. Effect of slow and fast pranayams on reaction time and cardiorespiratory variables. Indian J Physiol Pharmacol 2005; 49(3):313-8.

Mahapure HH, Shete SU, Bera TK. Effect of yogic exercise on super oxide dismutase levels in diabetics. Int J Yoga 2008; 1(1):21-6.

Malhotra V, Singh S, Tandon OP, Madhu SV, Prasad A, Sharma SB. Effect of Yoga asanas on nerve conduction in type 2 diabetes. Indian J Physiol Pharmacol 2002; 46(3):298-306.

Maloney R, Altmaier E. An initial evaluation of a mindful parenting program. J Clin Psychol 2007; 63(12):1231-8.

Manjunath NK, Telles S. Factors influencing changes in tweezer dexterity scores following yoga training. Indian J Physiol Pharmacol 1999; 43(2):225-9.

Maras ML, Rinke WJ, Stephens CR, Boehm TM. Effect of meditation on insulin dependent diabetes mellitus. Diabetes Educ 1984; 10(1):22-5.

Marc I, Langguth B, Biesinger E. Integrative approach for tinnitus: potential for qigong. Focus on Alternative & Complementary Therapies 2011; 16(1):58-9.

Marcus MT, Schmitz J, Moeller G et al. Mindfulness-based stress reduction in therapeutic community treatment: a stage 1 trial. Am J Drug Alcohol Abuse 2009; 35(2):103-8.

Marcus M, Fine M, Kouzekanani K. Mindfulness-based meditation in a therapeutic community. Journal of Substance Use 2001; 5(4):305-11.

Margolin A, Schuman-Olivier Z, Beitel M, Arnold RM, Fulwiler CE, Avants SK. A preliminary study of spiritual self-schema (3-S+) therapy for reducing impulsivity in HIV positive drug users. 2007; 63(10):979-99.

Maupin Ew. Individual Differences In Response To A Zen Meditation Exercise. J Consult Psychol 1965; 29:139-45.

McIver S, O'Halloran P, McGartland M. The impact of Hatha yoga on smoking behavior. Altern Ther Health Med 2004; 10(2):22-3.

Meares A. A form of intensive meditation associated with the regression of cancer. Am J Clin Hypn 1982-1983; 25(2-3):114-21.

Mills PJ, Schneider RH, Hill D, Walton KG, Wallace RK. Beta-adrenergic receptor sensitivity in subjects practicing transcendental meditation. J Psychosom Res 1990; 34(1):29-33.

Mirabel-Sarron C, Dorocant ES, Sala L, Bachelart M, Guelfi J-D, Rouillon F. Mindfulness based cognitive therapy (MBCT): A pilot study in bipolar patients: Mindfulness based cognitive therapy (MBCT) dans la prevention des rechutes thymiques chez le patient bipolaire I : une etude pilote. Ann. Med.-Psychol. 2009; 167(9):686-92.

Mohan A, Sharma R, Bijlani RL. Effect of meditation on stress-induced changes in cognitive functions. J Altern Complement Med 2011; 17(3):207-12.

Monk-Turner E, Turner C. Does yoga shape body, mind and spiritual health and happiness: Differences between yoga practitioners and college students. Int J Yoga 2010; 3(2):48-54.

Monk-Turner E. The benefits of meditation: Experimental findings. The Social Science Journal 2003; 40(3):465-70.

Morse DR. An exploratory study of the use of meditation alone and in combination with hypnosis in clinical dentistry. J Am Soc Psychosom Dent Med 1977; 24(4):113-20.

Morse DR, Cohen L, Furst ML, Martin JS. A physiological evaluation of the yoga concept of respiratory control of autonomic nervous system activity. Int J Psychosom 1984; 31(1):3-19.

Morse DR, Furst ML. Meditation: an in depth study. J Am Soc Psychosom Dent Med 1982; 29(5):1-96.

Morse DR, Martin JS, Furst ML, Dubin LL. A physiological and subjective evaluation of neutral and emotionally-charged words for meditation. Part III. J Am Soc Psychosom Dent Med 1979; 26(3):106-12.

Morse DR, Martin JS, Furst ML, Dubin LL. A physiological and subjective evaluation of neutral and emotionally-charged words for meditation. Part I. J Am Soc Psychosom Dent Med 1979; 26(1):31-8.

Morse DR, Schacterle GR, Esposito JV et al. Stress, meditation and saliva: a study of separate salivary gland secretions in endodontic patients. J Oral Med 1983; 38(4):150-60.

Morse DR, Schacterle GR, Furst ML et al. The effect of stress and meditation on salivary protein and bacteria: a review and pilot study. J Human Stress 1982; 8(4):31-9.

Motivala SJ, Sollers J, Thayer J, Irwin MR. Tai Chi Chih acutely decreases sympathetic nervous system activity in older adults. J Gerontol A Biol Sci Med Sci 2006; 61(11):1177-80.

Mourya M, Mahajan AS, Singh NP, Jain AK. Effect of slow- and fast-breathing exercises on autonomic functions in patients with essential hypertension. J Altern Complement Med 2009; 15(7):711-7.

Moustgaard A, Bedard M, Felteau M. Mindfulness-based cognitive therapy (MBCT) for individuals who had a stroke: results from a pilot study. Journal of Cognitive Rehabilitation 2007; 25(4):4-10.

Myint K, Choy KL, Su TT, Lam SK. The effect of short-term practice of mindfulness meditation in alleviating stress in university students. 2011; 22(2):165-71.

Nagarathna R, Nagendra HR. Yoga for bronchial asthma: a controlled study. Br Med J (Clin Res Ed) 1985; 291(6502):1077-9.

Narahari SR, Aggithaya MG, Prasanna KS, Bose KS. An integrative treatment for lower limb lymphedema (elephantiasis). J Altern Complement Med 2010; 16(2):145-9.

Narendran S, Nagarathna R, Narendran V, Gunasheela S, Nagendra HR. Efficacy of yoga on pregnancy outcome. J Altern Complement Med 2005; 11(2):237-44.

Naruka JS, Mathur R, Mathur A. Effect of pranayama practices on fasting blood glucose and serum cholesterol. Indian J Med Sci 1986; 40(6):149-52.

Neumark-Sztainer D, Eisenberg ME, Wall M, Loth KA. Yoga and Pilates: associations with body image and disordered-eating behaviors in a population-based sample of young adults. Int J Eat Disord 2011; 44(3):276-80.

Newberg AB, Wintering N, Waldman MR, Amen D, Khalsa DS, Alavi A. Cerebral blood flow differences between long-term meditators and non-meditators. Conscious Cogn 2010; 19(4):899-905.

Nidich S, Seeman W, Dreskin T. Influence of transcendental meditation: A replication. Journal of Counseling Psychology 1973; 20(6):565-6.

Nomura T, Nagano K, Takato J, Ueki S, Matsuzaki Y, Yasumura S. The development of a Tai Chi exercise regimen for the prevention of conditions requiring long-term care in Japan. Arch Gerontol Geriatr 2011; 52(3):e198-203.

Norton GR, Rhodes L, Hauch J, Kaprowy EA. Characteristics of subjects experiencing relaxation and relaxation-induced anxiety. J Behav Ther Exp Psychiatry 1985; 16(3):211-6.

Nowakowska C, Fellmann B, Pasek T, Hauser J, Sluzewska A. [Evaluation of the effect of relaxation and concentration exercises based on yoga on patients with psychogenic mental disorders]. Psychiatr Pol 1982; 16(5-6):365-70.

Orme-Johnson D, Dillbeck MC, Wallace RK, Landrith GS 3rd. Intersubject EEG coherence: is consciousness a field? Int J Neurosci 1982; 16(3-4):203-9.

Orme-Johnson DW. Autonomic stability and Transcendental Meditation. Psychosom Med 1973; 35(4):341-9.

Orme-Johnson DW, Schneider RH, Son YD, Nidich S, Cho ZH. Neuroimaging of meditation's effect on brain reactivity to pain. Neuroreport 2006; 17(12):1359-63.

Orzech KM, Shapiro SL, Brown KW, McKay M. Intensive mindfulness training-related changes in cognitive and emotional experience. The Journal of Positive Psychology 2009; 4(3):212-22.

Ospina-Kammerer V, Figley CR. An evaluation of the Respiratory One Method (ROM) in reducing emotional exhaustion among family physician residents. International Journal of Emergency Mental Health 2003; 5(1):29-32.

Overbeck KD. [Effects of the transcendental meditation technic on the psychological and psychosomatic state]. Psychother Psychosom Med Psychol 1982; 32(6):188-92.

Palta A. Sahajayoga and quality of life: An empirical study. Journal of Indian Psychology 2009; 27(1-2):21-34.

Pandey S, Mahato NK, Navale R. Role of self-induced sound therapy: Bhramari Pranayama in tinnitus. Audiological Medicine 2010; 8(3):137-41.

Pattanashetty R, Sathiamma S, Talakkad S, Nityananda P, Trichur R, Kutty BM. Practitioners of vipassana meditation exhibit enhanced slow wave sleep and REM sleep states across different age groups. Sleep and Biological Rhythms 2010; 8(1):34-41.

Paty J, Brenot P, Tignol J, Bourgeois M. [Evoked cerebral activity (contingent negative variation and evoked potentials) and modified states of consciousness (sleeplike relaxation, transcendential meditation)]. Ann Med Psychol (Paris) 1978; 136(1):143-69.

Peng CK, Mietus JE, Liu Y et al. Exaggerated heart rate oscillations during two meditation techniques. Int J Cardiol 1999; 70(2):101-7.

Poulin P, Mackenzie C, Soloway G, Karayolas E. Mindfulness training as an evidenced-based approach to reducing stress and promoting well-being among human services professionals. International Journal of Health Promotion & Education 2008; 46(2):72-80.

Radin DI, Vieten C, Michel L, Delorme A. Electrocortical activity prior to unpredictable stimuli in meditators and nonmeditators. Explore (NY) 2011; 7(5):286-99.

Rakoviç D, Tomaíeviç M, Jovanov E et al. Electroencephalographic (EEG) correlates of some activities which may alter consciousness: The transcendental meditation technique, musicogenic states, microwave resonance relaxation, healer/healee interaction, and alertness/drowsiness. 1999; 23(3):399-412.

Ramachandran AK, Rosengren KS, Yang Y, Hsiao-Wecksler ET. Effect of Tai Chi on gait and obstacle crossing behaviors in middle-aged adults. Gait Posture 2007; 26(2):248-55.

Ramos NS, Hernandez SM, Bianca MaJ. Efecto de un programa integrado de mindfulness e inteligencia emocional sobre las estrategias cognitivas de regulacion emocional. Ansiedad y Estres 2009; 15(2-3):207-16.

Randolph PD, Caldera YM, Tacone AM, Greak BL. The long-term combined effects of medical treatment and a mindfulness-based behavioral program for the multidisciplinary management of chronic pain in west Texas. 1999; 9(2):103-12.

Robertshawe P. Glutathione and total antioxidant status improved with yoga. Journal of the Australian Traditional-Medicine Society 2008; 14(1):29.

Robertson DW. The short and long range effects of the Transcendental Meditation technique on fractionated reaction time. J Sports Med Phys Fitness 1983; 23(1):113-20.

Roth B, Robbins D. Mindfulness-based stress reduction and health-related quality of life: findings from a bilingual inner-city patient population. Psychosom Med 2004; 66(1):113-23.

Rubik B. Neurofeedback-enhanced gamma brainwaves from the prefrontal cortical region of meditators and non-meditators and associated subjective experiences. J Altern Complement Med 2011; 17(2):109-15.

Rungreangkulkij S, Wongtakee W, Thongyot S. Buddhist group therapy for diabetes patients with depressive symptoms. Arch Psychiatr Nurs 2011; 25(3):195-205.

Sahay BK, Sadasivudu B, Yogi R et al. Biochemical parameters in normal volunteers before and after yogic practices. Indian J Med Res 1982; 76 Suppl:144-8.

Sahdra BK, MacLean KA, Ferrer E et al. Enhanced response inhibition during intensive meditation training predicts improvements in self-reported adaptive socioemotional functioning. Emotion 2011; 11(2):299-312.

Saito Y, Sasaki Y. The effect of transcendental meditation training on psychophysiological reactivity to stressful situations. Japanese Journal of Hypnosis 1993; 38(1):20-6.

Sakata T, Li Q, Tanaka M, Tajima F. Positive effects of a qigong and aerobic exercise program on physical health in elderly Japanese women: an exploratory study. Environ Health Prev Med 2008; 13(3):162-8.

Sampalli T, Berlasso E, Fox R, Petter M. A controlled study of the effect of a mindfulness-based stress reduction technique in women with multiple chemical sensitivity, chronic fatigue syndrome, and fibromyalgia. J Multidiscip Healthc 2009; 2:53-9.

Sarang SP, Telles S. Immediate effect of two yoga-based relaxation techniques on performance in a letter-cancellation task. Percept Mot Skills 2007; 105(2):379-85.

Sathyaprabha TN, Satishchandra P, Netravati K et al. Effect of yoga on autonomic dysfunction associated with refractory epilepsy. Epilepsia 2005; 46 Suppl 6:353.

Schejbal P, Kroner B, Niesel W. [An attempt to determine the effects of autogenic training and transcendental meditation on the variables of a personality inventory (author's transl)]. Psychother Med Psychol (Stuttg) 1978; 28(5):158-64.

Seeman W, Nidich S, Banta T. Influence of transcendental meditation on a measure of self-actualization. Journal of Counseling Psychology 1972; 19(3):184-7.

Seiler G, Seiler V. The effects of transcendental meditation on periodontal tissue. J Am Soc Psychosom Dent Med 1979; 26(1):8-12.

Sengoku M, Murata H, Kawahara T, Imamura K, Nakagome K. Does daily Naikan therapy maintain the efficacy of intensive Naikan therapy against depression? Psychiatry and Clinical Neurosciences 2010; 64(1):44-51.

Sengoku M, Murata H, Kawahara T, Nakagome K. 'Does daily Naikan therapy maintain the efficacy of intensive Naikan therapy against depression?': Erratum. Psychiatry and Clinical Neurosciences 2010; 64(2).

Shah AH, Joshi SV, Mehrotra PP, Potdar N, Dhar HL. Effect of Saral meditation on intelligence, performance and cardiopulmonary functions. Indian J Med Sci 2001; 55(11):604-8.

Shapiro SL, Figueredo AJ, Caspi O et al. Going Quasi: The Premature Disclosure Effect in a Randomized Clinical Trial. 2002; 25(6):605-21.

Singh N N, Lancioni G E, Winton A S, Singh A N, Adkins A D, Singh J. Clinical and benefit-cost outcomes of teaching a mindfulness-based procedure to adult offenders with intellectual disabilities (Provisional abstract). Behavior Modification 2008; 32(5):622-37.

Sinha S, Singh SN, Monga YP, Ray US. Improvement of glutathione and total antioxidant status with yoga. J Altern Complement Med 2007; 13(10):1085-90.

Skoglund L, Jansson E. Qigong reduces stress in computer operators. Complement Ther Clin Pract 2007; 13(2):78-84.

Slagter HA, Lutz A, Greischar LL et al. Mental training affects distribution of limited brain resources. PLoS Biol 2007; 5(6):e138.

Son'kin VD, Zaitseva VV, Ivanov SA. [The effect of a complex of meditation exercises on the psychophysiological state of young men]. Fiziol Cheloveka 2006; 32(5):128-31.

Soriano En, Franco C, Justo E. Reducing psychological distress in immigrants living in Spain through the practice of flow meditation. European Journal of Education and Psychology 2009; 2(3):223-33.

Spanos NP, Rivers SM, Gottlieb J. Hypnotic responsivity, meditation, and laterality of eye movements. J Abnorm Psychol 1978; 87(5):566-9.

Spanos NP, Steggles S, Radtke-Bodorik HL, Rivers SM. Nonanalytic attending, hypnotic susceptibility, and psychological well-being in trained meditators and nonmeditators. J Abnorm Psychol 1979; 88(1):85-7.

Spicuzza L, Gabutti A, Porta C, Montano N, Bernardi L. Yoga and chemoreflex response to hypoxia and hypercapnia. Lancet 2000; 356(92-40):1495-6.

Srivastava M, Talukdar U, Lahan V. Application of meditation training in managing the symptoms of adjustment disorder with mixed anxiety and depression.

Stek RJ, Bass BA. Personal adjustment and perceived locus of control among students interested in meditation. Psychol Rep 1973; 32(3):1019-22.

Steptoe A. New approaches to the management of essential hypertension with psychological techniques. 1978; 22(4):339-54.

Subrahmanyam S, Satyanarayana M, Rajeswari KR. Alcoholism: newer methods of management. Indian J Physiol Pharmacol 1986; 30(1):43-54.

Subramanya P, Telles S. Changes in midlatency auditory evoked potentials following two yoga-based relaxation techniques. Clin EEG Neurosci 2009; 40(3):190-5.

Sudheesh NN, Joseph KP. Investigation into the effects of music and meditation on galvanic skin response. 2000; 21(3):158-63.

Sulekha S, Thennarasu K, Vedamurthachar A, Raju TR, Kutty BM. Evaluation of sleep architecture in practitioners of Sudarshan Kriya yoga and Vipassana meditation. Sleep and Biological Rhythms 2006; 4(3):207-14.

Sundar S, Agrawal SK, Singh VP, Bhattacharya SK, Udupa KN, Vaish SK. Role of yoga in management of essential hypertension. Acta Cardiol 1984; 39(3):203-8.

Surwillo WW, Hobson DP. Brain electrical activity during prayer. Psychol Rep 1978; 43(1):135-43.

Taggart HM. Effects of Tai Chi exercise on balance, functional mobility, and fear of falling among older women. Appl Nurs Res 2002; 15(4):235-42.

Tebecis AK. A controlled study of the EEG during transcendental meditation: comparison with hypnosis. Folia Psychiatr Neurol Jpn 1975; 29(4):305-13.

Telles S, Gaur V, Balkrishna A. Effect of a yoga practice session and a yoga theory session on state anxiety. Percept Mot Skills 2009; 109(3):924-30.

Telles S, Joshi M, Dash M, Raghuraj P, Naveen KV, Nagendra HR. An evaluation of the ability to voluntarily reduce the heart rate after a month of yoga practice. Integr Physiol Behav Sci 2004; 39(2):119-25.

Telles S, Maharana K, Balrana B, Balkrishna A. Effects of high-frequency yoga breathing called kapalabhati compared with breath awareness on the degree of optical illusion perceived. Percept Mot Skills 2011; 112(3):981-90.

Telles S, Raghuraj P, Arankalle D, Naveen KV. Immediate effect of high-frequency yoga breathing on attention. Indian J Med Sci 2008; 62(1):20-2.

Thomas D, Abbas KA. Comparison of transcendental meditation and progressive relaxation in reducing anxiety. Br Med J 1978; 2(6154):1749.

Throll DA. Transcendental meditation and progressive relaxation: Their psychological effects. Journal of Clinical Psychology 1981; 37(4):776-81.

Throll DA. Transcendental meditation and progressive relaxation: their physiological effects. J Clin Psychol 1982; 38(3):522-30.

Tloczynski J, Tantriella M. A comparison of the effects of Zen breath meditation or relaxation on college adjustment. Psychologia: An International Journal of Psychology in the Orient 1998; 41(1):32-43.

Travis F, Arenander A. Cross-sectional and longitudinal study of effects of transcendental meditation practice on interhemispheric frontal asymmetry and frontal coherence. Int J Neurosci 2006; 116(12):1519-38.

Travis F, Olson T, Egenes T, Gupta HK. Physiological patterns during practice of the Transcendental Meditation technique compared with patterns while reading Sanskrit and a modern language. Int J Neurosci 2001; 109(1-2):71-80.

Travis F, Tecce J, Arenander A, Wallace RK. Patterns of EEG coherence, power, and contingent negative variation characterize the integration of transcendental and waking states. Biol Psychol 2002; 61(3):293-319.

Travis F, Tecce JJ, Guttman J. Cortical plasticity, contingent negative variation, and transcendent experiences during practice of the Transcendental Meditation technique. Biol Psychol 2000; 55(1):41-55.

Travis FT, Orme-Johnson DW. Field model of consciousness: EEG coherence changes as indicators of field effects. Int J Neurosci 1989; 49(3-4):203-11.

Travis FT, Orme-Johnson DW. EEG coherence and power during Yogic Flying. Int J Neurosci 1990; 54(1-2):1-12.

Turnbull MJ, Norris H. Effects of Transcendental Meditation on self-identity indices and personality. British Journal of Psychology 1982; 73(1):57-68.

Udupa KN, Singh RH, Dwivedi KN, Pandey HP, Rai V. Comparative biochemical studies on meditation. Indian J Med Res 1975; 63(12):1676-9.

van den Hout MA, Engelhard IM, Beetsma D et al. EMDR and mindfulness. Eye movements and attentional breathing tax working memory and reduce vividness and emotionality of aversive ideation. J Behav Ther Exp Psychiatry 2011; 42(4):423-31.

van den Hurk PA, Wingens T, Giommi F, Barendregt HP, Speckens AE, van Schie HT. On the Relationship Between the Practice of Mindfulness Meditation and Personality-an Exploratory Analysis of the Mediating Role of Mindfulness Skills. Mindfulness (N Y) 2011; 2(3):194-200.

van Vugt MK, Jha AP. Investigating the impact of mindfulness meditation training on working memory: a mathematical modeling approach. Cogn Affect Behav Neurosci 2011; 11(3):344-53.

Verma IC, Jayashankarappa BS, Palani M. Effect of transcendental meditation on the performance of some cognitive psychological tests. Indian J Med Res 1982; 76 Suppl:136-43.

Walach H, Nord E, Zier C, Dietz-Waschkowski B, Kersig S, Schpbach H. Mindfulness-based stress reduction as a method for personnel development: A pilot evaluation. International Journal of Stress Management 2007; 14(2):188-98.

Walia IJ, Mehra P, Grover P, Verma SK, Sanjeev. Health status of nurses and Yoga. II. Subjects with and without-health problems. Nurs J India 1989; 80(10):256-8, 278.

Wallace RK, Mills PJ, Orme-Johnson DW, Dillbeck MC, Jacobe E. Modification of the paired H reflex through the transcendental meditation and TM-Sidhi program. Exp Neurol 1983; 79(1):77-86.

Walrath LC, Hamilton DW. Autonomic correlates of meditation and hypnosis. Am J Clin Hypn 1975; 17(3):190-7.

Wandhofer A, Kobal G, Plattig KH. [Decrease of latency of auditory evoked potentials in humans practicing transcendental meditation (author's transl]. EEG EMG Z Elektroenzephalogr Elektromyogr Verwandte Geb 1976; 7(2):99-103.

Wang YT. Effects of long term Tai Chi practice and jogging exercise on muscle strength and endurance in older people: Commentary. Br. J. Sports Med. 2006; 40(1):54.

Watkins E, Teasdale JD. Adaptive and maladaptive self-focus in depression. J Affect Disord 2004; 82(1):1-8.

Weissbecker I, Salmon P, Studts JL, Floyd AR, Dedert EA, Sephton SE. Mindfulness-based stress reduction and sense of coherence among women with fibromyalgia. Journal of Clinical Psychology in Medical Settings 2002; 9(4):297-307.

Wenger Ma, Bagchi Bk, Anand Bk. Experiments in India on "voluntary" control of the heart and pulse. Circulation 1961; 24:1319-25.

Wenk-Sormaz H. Meditation can reduce habitual responding. Adv Mind Body Med 2005; 21(3-4):33-49.

West MA. Physiological effects of meditation: a longitudinal study. Br J Soc Clin Psychol 1979; 18(2):219-26.

Williams LR, Lodge B, Reddish PS. Effects of transcendental meditation on rotary pursuit skill. Res Q 1977; 48(1):196-201.

Wilson AF, Jevning R, Guich S. Marked reduction of forearm carbon dioxide production during states of decreased metabolism. Physiol Behav 1987; 41(4):347-52.

Wood CJ. Evaluation of meditation and relaxation on physiological response during the performance of fine motor and gross motor tasks. Percept Mot Skills 1986; 62(1):91-8.

Woolfolk RL, Lehrer PM, McCann BS, Rooney AJ. Effects of progressive relaxation and meditation on cognitive and somatic manifestations of daily stress. Behav Res Ther 1982; 20(5):461-7.

Woolfolk RL, Carr-Kaffashan L, McNulty TF, Lehrer PM. Meditation training as a treatment for insomnia. Behavior Therapy 1976; 7(3):359-65.

Xu D, Hong Y, Li J, Chan K. Effect of tai chi exercise on proprioception of ankle and knee joints in old people. Br J Sports Med 2004; 38(1):50-4.

Yan JH. Tai chi practice reduces movement force variability for seniors. J Gerontol A Biol Sci Med Sci 1999; 54(12):M629-34.

Yan X, Shen H, Jiang H et al. External Qi of Yan Xin Qigong induces G2/M arrest and apoptosis of androgen-independent prostate cancer cells by inhibiting Akt and NF-kappa B pathways. Mol Cell Biochem 2008; 310(1-2):227-34.

Yeh ML, Lee TI, Chen HH, Chao TY. The influences of Chan-Chuang qi-gong therapy on complete blood cell counts in breast cancer patients treated with chemotherapy. Cancer Nurs 2006; 29(2):149-55.

Yip VYB, Sit JWH, Wong DYS. A quasi-experimental study on improving arthritis self-management for residents of an aged people's home in Hong Kong. 2004; 9(2):235-46.

Yong WK, Lee S-H, Tae KC et al. Effectiveness of mindfulness-based cognitive therapy as an adjuvant to pharmacotherapy in patients with panic disorder or generalized anxiety disorder. 2009; 26(7):601-6.

Zamarra JW, Schneider RH, Besseghini I, Robinson DK, Salerno JW. Usefulness of the transcendental meditation program in the treatment of patients with coronary artery disease. Am J Cardiol 1996; 77(10):867-70.

Zeidan F, Martucci KT, Kraft RA, Gordon NS, McHaffie JG, Coghill RC. Brain mechanisms supporting the modulation of pain by mindfulness meditation. J Neurosci 2011; 31(14):5540-8.

Zettergren KK, Lubeski JM, Viverito JM. Effects of a yoga program on postural control, mobility, and gait speed in community-living older adults: a pilot study. J Geriatr Phys Ther 2011; 34(2):88-94.

Not Relevant to Key Questions

Aherne C, Moran AP, Lonsdale C. The effect of mindfulness training on athletes' flow: An initial investigation. The Sport Psychologist 2011; 25(2):177-89.

Alberts HJ, Mulkens S, Smeets M, Thewissen R. Coping with food cravings. Investigating the potential of a mindfulness-based intervention. Appetite 2010; 55(1):160-3.

Alexander CN, Schneider RH, Staggers F et al. Trial of stress reduction for hypertension in older African Americans. II. Sex and risk subgroup analysis. Hypertension 1996; 28(2):228-37.

Alpher VS, Blanton RL. Motivational processes and behavioral inhibition in breath holding. J Psychol 1991; 125(1):71-81.

Anon. Self-desensitization and meditation in the reduction of public speaking anxiety. Journal of Consulting and Clinical Psychology 1979; 47(3):536-41.

Arch JJ, Craske MG. Mechanisms of mindfulness: emotion regulation following a focused breathing induction. Behav Res Ther 2006; 44(12):1849-58.

Bagga OP, Gandhi A. A comparative study of the effect of Transcendental Meditation (T.M.) and Shavasana practice on cardiovascular system. Indian Heart J 1983; 35(1):39-45.

Bahrke MS, Morgan WP. Anxiety reduction following exercise and meditation. Cognitive Therapy and Research 1978; 2(4):323-33.

Banquet JP, Bourzeix JC, Lesevre N. [Evoked potentials and vigilance states induced during the course of choice reaction time tests]. Rev Electroencephalogr Neurophysiol Clin 1979; 9(3):221-7.

Barovick H. What's so funny? Laughter-yoga fans hail the health benefits of giggling for no reason. Time 2010; 176(11):54.

Bera TK, Gore MM, Oak JP. Recovery from stress in two different postures and in Shavasana--a yogic relaxation posture. Indian J Physiol Pharmacol 1998; 42(4):473-8.

Berghmans C, Tarquinio C, Kretsch M. Impact of the therapeutic approach of mindfulness-based stress reduction (MBSR) on psychic health (stress, anxiety, depression) in students: A controlled and randomized pilot study: Impact de l'approche therapeutique de pleine conscience mindfulness-based stress reduction (MBSR) sur la sant psychique (stress, anxiety, depression) chez des etudiants : une etude pilote controle et randomise. 2010; 20(1):11-5.

Blanchard EB, Appelbaum KA, Radnitz CL et al. A controlled evaluation of thermal biofeedback and thermal biofeedback combined with cognitive therapy in the treatment of vascular headache. J Consult Clin Psychol 1990; 58(2):216-24.

Bormann JE, Carrico AW. Increases in positive reappraisal coping during a group-based mantram intervention mediate sustained reductions in anger in HIV-positive persons. Int J Behav Med 2009; 16(1):74-80.

Boudette R. Integrating mindfulness into the therapy hour. Eat Disord 2011; 19(1):108-15.

Bradley BW, McCanne TR. Autonomic responses to stress: the effects of progressive relaxation, the relaxation response, and expectancy of relief. Biofeedback Self Regul 1981; 6(2):235-51.

Brandon, Jeffrey E. and Poppen, Roger. A Comparison of Behaviorial, Meditation, and Placebo Control Relaxation Training Procedures. Health-Education 1985; 16(5):42-6,33.

Broota A, Dhir R. Efficacy of two relaxation techniques in depression. Journal of Personality and Clinical Studies 1990; 6(1):83-90.

Broota A, Sanghvi C. Efficacy of two relaxation techniques in examination anxiety. Journal of Personality and Clinical Studies 1994; 10(1-2):29-35.

Bruning NS, Frew DR. Effects of exercise, relaxation, and management skills training on physiological stress indicators: A field experiment. Journal of Applied Psychology 1987; 72(4):515-21.

Campbell JF, Stenstrom RJ, Bertrand D. Systematic changes in perceptual reactance induced by physical fitness training. Percept Mot Skills 1985; 61(1):279-84.

Cardozo B, Thakar AB, Skandhan KP. A clinical study on psyco-somatic management of shukraavrlta vata (premature ejaculation) with rasayana yoga and shirodhara. AYU 2006; 27(4):94-8.

Carlson CR, Bacaseta PE, Simanton DA. A controlled evaluation of devotional meditation and progressive relaxation. Journal of Psychology and Theology 1988; 16(4):362-8.

Carmody J, Olendzki B, Reed G, Andersen V, Rosenzweig P. A dietary intervention for recurrent prostate cancer after definitive primary treatment: results of a randomized pilot trial. Urology 2008; 72(6):1324-8.

Carson JW, Carson KM, Gil KM, Baucom DH. Self-expansion as a mediator of relationship improvements in a mindfulness intervention. J Marital Fam Ther 2007; 33(4):517-28.

Carson JW. Mindfulness meditation-based treatment for relationship enhancement [dissertation]. Dissertation Abstracts International 2003; 63(8-B).

Carter OL, Presti DE, Callistemon C, Ungerer Y, Liu GB, Pettigrew JD. Meditation alters perceptual rivalry in Tibetan Buddhist monks. Curr Biol 2005; 15(11):R412-3.

Cazard P. Interhemispheric synchronism of parieto-occipital alpha rhythm. Attention and conscious experience: Synchronie interhemispherique des rythmes alpha parieto-occipitaux. Attention et experience consciente. 1974; 74(1):7-22.

Chan AS, Han YM, Cheung MC. Electroencephalographic (EEG) measurements of mindfulness-based Triarchic body-pathway relaxation technique: a pilot study. Appl Psychophysiol Biofeedback 2008; 33(1):39-47.

Chatzisarantis NL, Hagger MS. Mindfulness and the intention-behavior relationship within the theory of planned behavior. Pers Soc Psychol Bull 2007; 33(5):663-76.

Cheema BS, Marshall PW, Chang D, Colagiuri B, Machliss B. Effect of an office worksite-based yoga program on heart rate variability: a randomized controlled trial. BMC Public Health 2011; 11:578.

Chen K, He B, Rihacek G, Sigal LH. A pilot trial of external Qigong therapy for arthritis pain [2]. 2003; 9(5):332-5.

Chen K, He B, Rihacek G, Sigal LH. A pilot trial of external Qigong therapy for arthritis. J Clin Rheumatol 2003; 9(5):332-5.

Chen KW, Marbach JJ. External qigong therapy for chronic orofacial pain [2]. 2002; 8(5):532-4.

Chu L. The benefits of meditation vis-a-vis emotional intelligence, perceived stress and negative mental health. Stress & Health: Journal of the International Society for the Investigation of Stress 2010; 26(2):169-80.

Clark MM, Abrams DB, Niaura RS, Eaton CA, Rossi JS. Self-efficacy in weight management. 1991; 59(5):739-44.

Coatsworth JD, Duncan LG, Greenberg MT, Nix RL. Changing parent's mindfulness, child management skills and relationship quality with their youth: Results from a randomized pilot intervention trial. 2010; 19(2):203-17.

Colby F. An analogue study of the initial carryover effects of meditation, hypnosis, and relaxation using native college students. Biofeedback Self Regul 1991; 16(2):157-65.

Cooper S, Oborne J, Newton S et al. Do breathing exercises (buteyko and pranayama) help to control asthma: a randomised controlled trial [abstract]. European Respiratory Society Annual Congress 2002 2002; abstract P1929.

Cooper S, Oborne J, Newton S et al. Effect of two breathing exercises (Buteyko and pranayama) in asthma: a randomised controlled trial. Thorax 2003; 58(8):674-9.

Cooper SE, Oborne J, Newton S et al. The effect of two breathing exercises (Buteyko and Pranayama) on the ability to reduce inhaled corticosteroids in asthma: a randomised controlled trial [abstract]. American Thoracic Society 99th International Conference 2003; B023 Poster 924.

Cowger EL, Torrance EP. Further examination of the quality of changes in creative functioning resulting from meditation (Zazen) training. Creative Child & Adult Quarterly 1982; 7(4):211-7.

Crane C, Winder R, Hargus E, Amarasinghe M, Barnhofer T. Effects of Mindfulness-Based Cognitive Therapy on Specificity of Life Goals. 2011:1-8.

Credidio SG. Comparative effectiveness of patterned biofeedback vs meditation training on EMG and skin temperature changes. Behav Res Ther 1982; 20(3):233-41.

Curiati JA, Bocchi E, Freire JO et al. Meditation reduces sympathetic activation and improves the quality of life in elderly patients with optimally treated heart failure: a prospective randomized study. J Altern Complement Med 2005; 11(3):465-72.

Cuthbert B, Kristeller J, Simons R, Hodes R, Lang PJ. Strategies of arousal control: biofeedback, meditation, and motivation. J Exp Psychol Gen 1981; 110(4):518-46.

da Silva GD, Lorenzi-Filho G, Lage LV. Effects of yoga and the addition of Tui Na in patients with fibromyalgia. J Altern Complement Med 2007; 13(10):1107-13.

Danusantoso H, Heijnen L. Tai Chi Chuan for people with haemophilia [1]. 2001; 7(4):[d]437-9.

Dave HR, Srikrishna Ch, Vyas SN, Dave AR. A comparative study on the role of medhya rasayana yoga and dashamula kwathadhara in the management of vatika shirahshula (tension headache). AYU 2006; 27(2):36-40.

de la Fuente Arias M, Granados MS, Justo CF. Efectos de un programa de entrenamiento en conciencia plena (mindfulness) en la autoestima y la inteligencia emocional percibidas. Behavioral Psychology/Psicologia Conductual: Revista Internacional Clinica y De La Salud 2010; 18(2):297-315.

de la Fuente Arias M, Justo CF, Granados MS. Effects of a meditation program (mindfulness) on the measure of alexithymia and social skills: Efectos de un programa de meditacion (mindfulness) en la medida de la alexitimia y las habilidades sociales. 2010; 22(3):369-75.

de Santana JS, de Almeida APG, Brandúo PMC. The effect of Ai Chi method in fybromialgic patients: Os efeitos do mtodo Ai Chi em pacientes portadoras da syndrome fibromiílgica. 2010; 15(SUPPL. 1):1433-8.

Deberry S, Davis S, Reinhard KE. A comparison of meditation-relaxation and cognitive/behavioral techniques for reducing anxiety and depression in a geriatric population. J Geriatr Psychiatry 1989; 22(2):231-47.

Delinsky SS, Wilson GT. Mirror exposure for the treatment of body image disturbance. Int J Eat Disord 2006; 39(2):108-16.

Delmonte MM. Effects of expectancy on physiological responsivity in novice meditators. Biol Psychol 1985; 21(2):107-21.

Delmonte MM. Response to meditation in terms of physiological, behavioral and self-report measures. Int J Psychosom 1984; 31(2):3-17.

Dillbeck MC, Bronson EC. Short-term longitudinal effects of the transcendental meditation technique on EEG power and coherence. Int J Neurosci 1981; 14(3-4):147-51.

Dillbeck MC. The effect of the Transcendental Meditation technique on anxiety level. J Clin Psychol 1977; 33(4):1076-8.

Ditto B, Eclache M, Goldman N. Short-Term Autonomic and Cardiovascular Effects of Mindfulness Body Scan Meditation. Annals of Behavioral Medicine 2006; 32(3):227-34.

Domino G. Transcendental meditation and creativity: an empirical investigation. J Appl Psychol 1977; 62(3):358-62.

Dosh SA. The treatment of adults with essential hypertension. J. Fam. Pract. 2002; 51(1):74-80.

Downey N. Mindfulness training: The effect of process and outcome instructions on the experience of control and the level of mindfulness among older women. Educational Gerontology 1991; 17(2):97-109.

Dunn BR, Hartigan JA, Mikulas WL. Concentration and mindfulness meditations: unique forms of consciousness? Appl Psychophysiol Biofeedback 1999; 24(3):147-65.

Duraiswamy G, Thirthalli J, Nagendra HR, Gangadhar BN. Yoga therapy as an add-on treatment in the management of patients with schizophrenia--a randomized controlled trial. Acta Psychiatr Scand 2007; 116(3):226-32.

Eifert GH, Heffner M. The effects of acceptance versus control contexts on avoidance of panic-related symptoms. J Behav Ther Exp Psychiatry 2003; 34(3-4):293-312.

Elson BD, Hauri P, Cunis D. Physiological changes in yoga meditation. Psychophysiology 1977; 14(1):52-7.

Erisman SM, Roemer L. A preliminary investigation of the effects of experimentally induced mindfulness on emotional responding to film clips. Emotion 2010; 10(1):72-82.

Fan Y, Tang YY, Ma Y, Posner MI. Mucosal immunity modulated by integrative meditation in a dose-dependent fashion. J Altern Complement Med 2010; 16(2):151-5.

Fang W, Weidong W, Rongrui Z et al. Clinical observation on physiological and psychological effects of Eight-Section Brocade on type 2 diabetic patients. 2008; 28(2):101-5.

Fee RA, Girdano DA. The relative effectiveness of three techniques to induce the trophotropic response. Biofeedback Self Regul 1978; 3(2):145-57.

Feldman G, Greeson J, Senville J. Differential effects of mindful breathing, progressive muscle relaxation, and loving-kindness meditation on decentering and negative reactions to repetitive thoughts. Behav Res Ther 2010; 48(10):1002-11.

Fiebert MS, Mead TM. Meditation and academic performance. Perceptual and Motor Skills 1981; 53(2):447-50.

Fling S, Thomas A, Gallaher M. Participant characteristics and the effects of two types of meditation vs. quiet sitting. Journal of Clinical Psychology 1981; 37(4):784-90.

Fragoso CM, Grinberg-Zylberbaum J, Perez MAG, Ortiz CA, Loyo JR. Efectos de la meditacion sobre la actividad electrica cerebral. Revista Mexicana De Psicologia 1999; 16(1):101-15.

Franco C, Manas I, Cangas AJ, Moreno E, Gallego J. Reducing teachers' psychological distress through a mindfulness training program. Span J Psychol 2010; 13(2):655-66.

Franco C, Sola Mdel M, Justo E. [Reducing psychological discomfort and overload in Alzheimer's family caregivers through a mindfulness meditation program]. Rev Esp Geriatr Gerontol 2010; 45(5):252-8.

Franco Justo C, de la Fuente Arias M, Salvador Granados M. [Impact of a training program in full consciousness (mindfulness) in the measure of growth and personal self-realization]. Psicothema 2011; 23(1):58-65.

Franco Justo C. Reducing stress levels and anxiety in primary-care physicians through training and practice of a mindfulness meditation technique: Reduccion de los niveles de estres y ansiedad en medicos de Atencion Primaria mediante la aplicacion de un programa de entrenamiento en conciencia plena (mindfulness). 2010; 42(11):564-70.

Freret N, Ricci L, Murphy S. Recruiting and screening older, transitional to frail adults in congregate living facilities. Appl Nurs Res 2003; 16(2):118-25.

Fukushima M, Kataoka T, Hamada C, Matsumoto M. Evidence of Qi-gong energy and its biological effect on the enhancement of the phagocytic activity of human polymorphonuclear leukocytes. Am J Chin Med 2001; 29(1):1-16.

Gallois Ph, Forzy G, Dhont JL. Changements hormonaux durant la relaxation. L'Encéphale: Revue de psychiatrie clinique biologique et thérapeutique 1984; 10(2):79-82.

Gaston L, Crombez J-C, Joly J, Hodgins S. Efficacy of imagery and meditation techniques in treating psoriasis. Imagination, Cognition and Personality 1988; 8(1):25-38.

Gaylord SA, Whitehead WE, Coble RS et al. Mindfulness for irritable bowel syndrome: protocol development for a controlled clinical trial. BMC Complement Altern Med 2009; 9:24.

Geisler M. Transcendental meditation as a therapeutic tool for drug users. Zeitschrift Fr Klinische Psychologie 1978; 7(4):235-55.

Gilbert GS, Parker JC, Claiborn CD. Differential mood changes in alcoholics as a function of anxiety management strategies. J Clin Psychol 1978; 34(1):229-32.

Gokhan N, Meehan EF, Peters K. The value of mindfulness-based methods in teaching at a clinical field placement. Psychol Rep 2010; 106(2):455-66.

Goldman BL, Domitor PJ, Murray EJ. Effects of Zen meditation on anxiety reduction and perceptual functioning. J Consult Clin Psychol 1979; 47(3):551-6.

Grant AM, Langer EJ, Falk E, Capodilupo C. Mindful creativity: Drawing to draw distinctions. Creativity Research Journal 2004; 16(2-3):261-5.

Grepmair L, Mitterlehner F, Rother W, Nickel M. Promotion of mindfulness in psychotherapists in training and treatment results of their patients. J Psychosom Res 2006; 60(6):649-50.

Griffiths TJ, Steel DH, Vaccaro P, Karpman MB. The effects of relaxation techniques on anxiety and underwater performance. International Journal of Sport Psychology 1981; 12(3):176-82.

Gross CR, Kreitzer MJ, Reilly-Spong M, Winbush NY, Schomaker EK, Thomas W. Mindfulness meditation training to reduce symptom distress in transplant patients: rationale, design, and experience with a recycled waitlist. Clin Trials 2009; 6(1):76-89.

Hakim R, Segal J, Newton R, DuCette J. A fall risk reduction intervention for community-dwelling older adults. Journal of Geriatric Physical Therapy 2001; 24(3):21-2.

Hall EG, Hardy CJ. Ready, aim, fire
Perceptual and Motor Skills 1991; 72(3, Pt 1):775-86.

Hall PD. The effect of meditation on the academic performance of African American college students. Journal of Black Studies 1999; 29(3):408-15.

Hart DE, Means JR. Effects of meditation vs professional reading on students' perceptions of paraprofessional counselors' effectiveness. Psychol Rep 1982; 51(2):479-82.

Hart J, Kanner H, Gilboa-Mayo R, Haroeh-Peer O, Rozenthul-Sorokin N, Eldar R. Tai Chi Chuan practice in community-dwelling persons after stroke. Int J Rehabil Res 2004; 27(4):303-4.

Harvey JR. The effect of yogic breathing exercises on mood. J Am Soc Psychosom Dent Med 1983; 30(2):39-48.

Heppner WL, Kernis MH, Lakey CE et al. Mindfulness as a means of reducing aggressive behavior: dispositional and situational evidence. Aggress Behav 2008; 34(5):486-96.

Hillemeier MM, Downs DS, Feinberg ME et al. Improving women's preconceptional health: findings from a randomized trial of the Strong Healthy Women intervention in the Central Pennsylvania women's health study. Womens Health Issues 2008; 18(6 Suppl):S87-96.

Holt WR, Caruso JL, Riley JB. Transcendental meditation vs pseudo-meditation on visual choice reaction time. Perceptual and Motor Skills 1978; 46(3, Pt 1).

Hong PY, Lishner DA, Han KH, Huss EA. The positive impact of mindful eating on expectations of food liking. Mindfulness 2011; 2(2):103-13.

Hooper N, Villatte M, Neofotistou E, McHugh L. The effects of mindfulness versus thought suppression on implicit and explicit measures of experiential avoidance. International Journal of Behavioral Consultation and Therapy 2010; 6(3):233-44.

Innes KE, Selfe TK, Alexander GK, Taylor AG. A new educational film control for use in studies of active mind-body therapies: acceptability and feasibility. J Altern Complement Med 2011; 17(5):453-8.

Jain S, Jain M, Sharma CS. Effect of yoga and relaxation techniques on cardiovascular system. Indian J Physiol Pharmacol 2010; 54(2):183-5.

Jain S, Shapiro SL, Swanick S et al. A randomized controlled trial of mindfulness meditation versus relaxation training: effects on distress, positive states of mind, rumination, and distraction. Ann Behav Med 2007; 33(1):11-21.

Jang H-S, Lee MS, Kim M-J, Chong ES. Effects of Qi-therapy on premenstrual syndrome. 2004; 114(8):909-21.

Jang HS, Lee MS. Effects of qi therapy (external qigong) on premenstrual syndrome: a randomized placebo-controlled study. J Altern Complement Med 2004; 10(3):456-62.

Janowiak JJ, Hackman R. Meditation and college students' self-actualization and rated stress. Psychol Rep 1994; 75(2):1007-10.

Jensen CG, Vangkilde S, Frokjaer V, Hasselbalch SG. Mindfulness training affects attention-or is it attentional effort? J Exp Psychol Gen 2011.

Kabat-Zinn J, Wheeler E, Light T et al. Part II: Influence of a mindfulness meditation-based stress reduction intervention on rates of skin clearing in patients with moderate to severe psoriasis undergoing phototherapy (UVB) and photochemo-therapy (PUVA). [References]. Constructivism in the Human Sciences 2003; 8(2):85-106.

Katiyar SK, Bihari S. Role of pranayama in rehabilitation of copd patients - a randomized controlled study. Indian Journal of Allergy Asthma Immunology 2006; 20(2):98-104.

Kaviani A, Hatami N, ShafiAbadi A. The impact of mindfulness-based cognitive therapy on the quality of life in non-clinically depressed people. Advances in Cognitive Science 2008; 10(4).

Keller S, Seraganian P. Physical fitness level and autonomic reactivity to psychosocial stress. J Psychosom Res 1984; 28(4):279-87.

Kember P. The Transcendental Meditation technique and postgraduate academic performance. British Journal of Educational Psychology 1985; 55(2):164-6.

Kepner J. Yoga research and Richard Freeman. Altern Ther Health Med 2004; 10(4):14.

Kerr D, Gillam E, Ryder J, Trowbridge S, Cavan D, Thomas P. An Eastern art form for a Western disease: randomised controlled trial of yoga in patients with poorly controlled insulin-treated diabetes. Practical Diabetes International 2002; 19(6):164-6.

Khasky AD, Smith JC. Stress, relaxation states, and creativity. Percept Mot Skills 1999; 88(2):409-16.

Kiken LG, Shook NJ. Looking up: Mindfulness increases positive judgments and reduces negativity bias. Social Psychological and Personality Science 2011; 2(4):425-31.

Kingston J, Chadwick P, Meron D, Skinner TC. A pilot randomized control trial investigating the effect of mindfulness practice on pain tolerance, psychological well-being, and physiological activity. J Psychosom Res 2007; 62(3):297-300.

Kinoshita K. [A study on response of EEG during Zen meditation--alpha-blocking to name calling (author's transl)]. Seishin Shinkeigaku Zasshi 1975; 77(9):623-58.

Kirsch I, Henry D. Self-desensitization and meditation in the reduction of public speaking anxiety. J Consult Clin Psychol 1979; 47(3):536-41.

Knox SS. Effect of passive concentration as instructional set for training enhancement of EEG alpha. Percept Mot Skills 1980; 51(3 Pt 1):767-75.

Koole SL, Govorun O, Cheng CM, Gallucci M. Pulling yourself together: Meditation promotes congruence between implicit and explicit self-esteem. Journal of Experimental Social Psychology 2009; 45(6):1220-6.

Kova-ii-i T, Kova-ii-i M. Impact of relaxation training according to Yoga in Daily Life-« system on perceived stress after breast cancer surgery. 2011; 10(1):16-26.

Kuang AK, Jiang MD, Wang CX, Zhao GS, Xu DH. Research on the mechanism of "Qigong (breathing exercise)". A preliminary study on its effect in balancing "Yin" and "Yang", regulating circulation and promoting flow in the meridian system. J Tradit Chin Med 1981; 1(1):7-10.

Kubose SK. An experimental investigation of psychological aspects of meditation. Psychologia: An International Journal of Psychology in the Orient 1976; 19(1):1-10.

Kuehner C, Huffziger S, Liebsch K. Rumination, distraction and mindful self-focus: effects on mood, dysfunctional attitudes and cortisol stress response. Psychol Med 2009; 39(2):219-28.

Kugler JE. Meditation and the electroencephalogram. Electroencephalogr Clin Neurophysiol Suppl 1982; (35):391-8.

Kumari S, Nath NCB, Nagendra HR. Enhancing emotional competence among managers through SMET. Psychological Studies 2007; 52(2):171-3.

Lee EN. [The effects of tai chi exercise program on blood pressure, total cholesterol and cortisol level in patients with essential hypertension]. Taehan Kanho Hakhoe Chi 2004; 34(5):829-37.

Lee KY, Jeong OY. [The effect of Tai Chi movement in patients with rheumatoid arthritis]. Taehan Kanho Hakhoe Chi 2006; 36(2):278-85.

Lee MS, Jeong SM, Jang H-S, Ryu H, Moon S-R. Effects of in vitro and in vivo Qi-therapy on neutrophil superoxide generation in healthy male subjects. 2003; 31(4):623-8.

Lee MS, Kim MK, Lee YH. Effects of Qi-therapy (external Qigong) on cardiac autonomic tone: a randomized placebo controlled study. Int J Neurosci 2005; 115(9):1345-50.

Lee MS, Rim YH, Jeong DM, Kim MK, Joo MC, Shin SH. Nonlinear analysis of heart rate variability during Qi therapy (external Qigong). Am J Chin Med 2005; 33(4):579-88.

Lee MS, Rim YH, Kang C-W. Effects of external Qi-therapy on emotions, electroencephalograms, and plasma cortisol. 2004; 114(11):1493-502.

Lehrer PM, Schoicket S, Carrington P, Woolfolk RL. Psychophysiological and cognitive responses to stressful stimuli in subjects practicing progressive relaxation and clinically standardized meditation. Behav Res Ther 1980; 18(4):293-303.

Leung RW, Alison JA, McKeough ZJ, Peters MJ. A study design to investigate the effect of short-form Sun-style Tai Chi in improving functional exercise capacity, physical performance, balance and health related quality of life in people with Chronic Obstructive Pulmonary Disease (COPD). Contemp Clin Trials 2011; 32(2):267-72.

Li J, Sharma K, Finkelstein J. Feasibility of computer-assisted Tai Chi education. AMIA Annu Symp Proc 2005; 1027.

Liu X, Miller YD, Burton NW, Brown WJ. Changes in mechanical loading lead to tendonspecific alterations in MMP and TIMP expression: Influence of stress deprivation and intermittent cyclic hydrostatic compression on rat supraspinatus and Achilles tendons. 2010; 44(10):704-9.

Liu YS. Analysis of the curative effect of electroacupuncture plus qigong on ulcerative colonitis. J Acu Tuina Sci 2003; 1(2):23.

Liu YS. Analysis on the therapeutic effect of ulcerative colitis treated with electroacupuncture plus qigong. [World Journal of Acupuncture-Moxibustion]: World J Acup-Moxi: Shi Jie Zhen Jiu Za Zhi 1998; 8(1):3-8.

Liubimov NN. [Changes in the electroencephalogram and evoked potentials while using a special form of psychological training (meditation)]. Fiziol Cheloveka 1999; 25(2):56-66.

Lu CF, Liao JC, Liu CY, Liu HY, Chang YH. Meditation therapy in the treatment of anxiety disorders. Taiwanese Journal of Psychiatry 1998; 12(4):343-51.

MacLean CR, Walton KG, Wenneberg SR et al. Effects of the Transcendental Meditation program on adaptive mechanisms: changes in hormone levels and responses to stress after 4 months of practice. Psychoneuroendocrinology 1997; 22(4):277-95.

Mamatha SD, Gorkal AR. Comparative study of breath holding time in pranayama practitioners, suryanamaskara practitioners and in non-yogic individuals (Biomedicine). 2010; 30(3):403.

Maupin EW. Individual Differences In Response To A Zen Meditation Exercise. J Consult Psychol 1965; 29:139-45.

Maybery DJ, Graham D. The influence of physical and mental training on plasma beta-endorphin level and pain perception after intensive physical exercise. 2001; 17(2):121-7.

McGibbon CA, Krebs DE, Wolf SL, Wayne PM, Scarborough DM, Parker SW. Tai Chi and vestibular rehabilitation effects on gaze and whole-body stability. J Vestib Res 2004; 14(6):467-78.

Mehling WE. Breath therapy for chronic low back pain. 2006; 10(2):96-8.

Monk-Turner E, Turner C. Does yoga shape body, mind and spiritual health and happiness: Differences between yoga practitioners and college students. Int J Yoga 2010; 3(2):48-54.

Morrell EM, Hollandsworth JG Jr. Norepinephrine alterations under stress conditions following the regular practice of meditation. Psychosom Med 1986; 48(3-4):270-7.

Morse DR, Furst ML. Meditation: an in depth study. J Am Soc Psychosom Dent Med 1982; 29(5):1-96.

Morse DR, Martin JS, Furst ML, Dubin LL. A physiological and subjective evaluation of neutral and emotionally-charged words for meditation. Part I. J Am Soc Psychosom Dent Med 1979; 26(1):31-8.

Nakamura Y, Lipschitz DL, Landward R, Kuhn R, West G. Two sessions of sleep-focused mind-body bridging improve self-reported symptoms of sleep and PTSD in veterans: A pilot randomized controlled trial. J Psychosom Res 2011; 70(4):335-45.

Narahari SR, Aggithaya MG, Prasanna KS, Bose KS. An integrative treatment for lower limb lymphedema (elephantiasis). J Altern Complement Med 2010; 16(2):145-9.

Neumark-Sztainer D, Eisenberg ME, Wall M, Loth KA. Yoga and Pilates: associations with body image and disordered-eating behaviors in a population-based sample of young adults. Int J Eat Disord 2011; 44(3):276-80.

Oman D, Shapiro SL, Thoresen CE, Flinders T, Driskill JD, Plante TG. Learning from spiritual models and meditation: A randomized evaluation of a college course. Pastoral Psychology 2007; 55(4):473-93.

Oman D, Shapiro SL, Thoresen CE, Plante TG, Flinders T. Meditation lowers stress and supports forgiveness among college students: a randomized controlled trial. J Am Coll Health 2008; 56(5):569-78.

Ortner CNM, Kilner SJ, Zelazo PD. Mindfulness meditation and reduced emotional interference on a cognitive task. Motivation and Emotion 2007; 31(4):271-83.

Pace TW, Negi LT, Adame DD et al. Effect of compassion meditation on neuroendocrine, innate immune and behavioral responses to psychosocial stress. Psychoneuroendocrinology 2009; 34(1):87-98.

Pandey S, Mahato NK, Navale R. Role of self-induced sound therapy: Bhramari Pranayama in tinnitus. Audiological Medicine 2010; 8(3):137-41.

Paty J, Brenot P, Tignol J, Bourgeois M. [Evoked cerebral activity (contingent negative variation and evoked potentials) and modified states of consciousness (sleeplike relaxation, transcendential meditation)]. Ann Med Psychol (Paris) 1978; 136(1):143-69.

Paty J, Brenot Ph, Tignol J, Bourgeois M. Cerebral activity (contingent negative variation and evoked potentials) evoked during modified states of consciousness (deep relaxation, transcendental meditation). Annales Medico-Psychologiques 1978; 136(1):143-69.

Puente AE. Psychophysiological investigations on transcendental meditation. Biofeedback Self Regul 1981; 6(3):327-42.

Puryear HB, Cayce CT, Thurston MA. Anxiety reduction associated with meditation: home study. Percept Mot Skills 1976; 42(43):527-31.

Rakhshaee Z. Effect of three yoga poses (cobra, cat and fish poses) in women with primary dysmenorrhea: a randomized clinical trial. J Pediatr Adolesc Gynecol 2011; 24(4):192-6.

Rakoviç D, Tomaseviç M, Jovanov E et al. Electroencephalographic (EEG) correlates of some activities which may alter consciousness: The transcendental meditation technique, musicogenic states, microwave resonance relaxation, healer/healee interaction, and alertness/drowsiness. 1999; 23(3):399-412.

Rani NJ. Impact of yoga training on triguna and self-ideal disparity. Psychological Studies 2007; 52(2):174-7.

Rao AV, Krishna DR, Ramanakar TV, Prabhakar MC. Jala Neti' a yoga technique for nasal comfort and hygiene in leprosy patients. Lepr India 1982; 54(4):691-4.

Rausch SM, Gramling SE, Auerbach SM. Effects of a single session of large-group meditation and progressive muscle relaxation training on stress reduction, reactivity, and recovery. International Journal of Stress Management 2006; 13(3):273-90.

Ray US, Hegde KS, Selvamurthy W. Improvement in muscular efficiency as related to a standard task after yogic exercises in middle aged men. Indian J Med Res 1986; 83:343-8.

Rejeski WJ, Mihalko SL, Ambrosius WT, Bearon LB, McClelland JW. Weight loss and self-regulatory eating efficacy in older adults: The cooperative lifestyle intervention program. 2011; 66 B(3):279-86.

Rogojanski J, Vettese LC, Antony MM. Coping with cigarette cravings: Comparison of suppression versus mindfulness-based strategies. Mindfulness 2011; 2(1):14-26.

Roldan E, Los J, Dostalek C, Bohdanecky Z. Frequency characteristics, distribution and dominance of the EEG during rest and a yogic breathing exercise
Activitas Nervosa Superior 1983; 25(3).

Roy DJ. The thistle is a flower? A meditation on seeing the unseen. J Palliat Care 2011; 27(2):67-8.

Sabel BA. Transcendental Meditation and concentration ability. Perceptual and Motor Skills 1980; 50(3, Pt 1):799-802.

Sadeghi S, Sohrabi F, Delavar A, Borjaali A, Ghassemi GR. Combined effect of anti depressant and mindfulness based group cognitive therapy (MBCT) on psychological well being of divorced women. 2010; 28(112).

Sarang SP, Telles S. Immediate effect of two yoga-based relaxation techniques on performance in a letter-cancellation task. Percept Mot Skills 2007; 105(2):379-85.

Saxena T, Saxena M. The effect of various breathing exercises (pranayama) in patients with bronchial asthma of mild to moderate severity. Int J Yoga 2009; 2(1):22-5.

Schejbal P, Krner B, Niesel W. An attempt to determine the effects of autogenic training and Transcendental Meditation on the variables of a personality inventory. Psychotherapie Und Medizinische Psychologie 1978; 28(5):158-64.

Schneider B, Ercoli L, Siddarth P, Lavretsky H. Vascular Burden and Cognitive Functioning in Depressed Older Adults. Am J Geriatr Psychiatry 2011.

Schneider RH, Alexander CN, Staggers F et al. A randomized controlled trial of stress reduction in African Americans treated for hypertension for over one year. Am J Hypertens 2005; 18(1):88-98.

Schneider RH, Alexander CN, Staggers F et al. Long-term effects of stress reduction on mortality in persons

Schneider RH, Staggers F, Alexander CN et al. A randomized controlled trial of stress reduction for hypertension in older African Americans. 1995; 26(5):820-7.

Schoicket SL, Bertelson AD, Lacks P. Is sleep hygiene a sufficient treatment for sleep-maintenance insomnia? Behavior Therapy 1988; 19(2):183-90.

Selfridge N. Meditation for fibromyalgia: Yea or nay? 2011; 14(3):34-6.

Severtsen B, Bruya MA. Effects of meditation and aerobic exercise on EEG patterns. J Neurosci Nurs 1986; 18(4):206-10.

Shapiro SL, Figueredo AJ, Caspi O et al. Going Quasi: The Premature Disclosure Effect in a Randomized Clinical Trial. 2002; 25(6):605-21.

Shapiro SL, Oman D, Thoresen CE, Plante TG, Flinders T. Cultivating mindfulness: effects on well-being. J Clin Psychol 2008; 64(7):840-62.

Sharma VK, Das S, Mondal S, Goswami U. Comparative effect of Sahaj Yoga on EEG in patients of major depression and healthy subjects. 2007; 27(3):95-9.

Sharma VK, Das S, Mondal S, Goswami U. Effect of Sahaj yoga on autonomic functions in healthy subjects and patients of major depression. 2008; 28(2):139-41.

Shin T-B, Jin S-R. The qualitative study of "mindfulness group" toward the self-care and counseling practice of counselor interns. Bulletin of Educational Psychology 2010; 42(1):163-84.

Sime W. A comparison of exercise and meditation in reducing physiological responses to stress. Medicine in Sports and Science 1977; 9:55.

Smith WP, Compton WC, West WB. Meditation as an adjunct to a happiness enhancement program. J Clin Psychol 1995; 51(2):269-73.

Solberg EE, Ingjer F, Holen A, Sundgot-Borgen J, Nilsson S, Holme I. Stress reactivity to and recovery from a standardised exercise bout: a study of 31 runners practising relaxation techniques. Br J Sports Med 2000; 34(4):268-72.

Spanos NP, Stam HJ, Rivers SM, Radtke HL. Meditation, expectation and performance on indices of nonanalytic attending. Int J Clin Exp Hypn 1980; 28(3):244-51.

Spence GB, Cavanagh MJ, Grant AM. The integration of mindfulness training and health coaching: An exploratory study. Coaching: An International Journal of Theory, Research and Practice 2008; 1(2):145-63.

Sridevi K, Sitamma M, Krishna Rao PV. Perceptual organisation and yoga training. Journal of Indian Psychology 1995; 13(2):21-7.

Steinhauser KE, Alexander SC, Byock IR, George LK, Tulsky JA. Seriously ill patients' discussions of preparation and life completion: an intervention to assist with transition at the end of life. Palliat Support Care 2009; 7(4):393-404.

Stek RJ, Bass BA. Personal adjustment and perceived locus of control among students interested in meditation. Psychol Rep 1973; 32(3):1019-22.

Steptoe A. New approaches to the management of essential hypertension with psychological techniques. 1978; 22(4):339-54.

Stormer-Labonte M, Machemer P, Hardinghaus W. A Meditative Stress-Management-Programm For Psychosomatic Patients: Ein Meditatives Stressbewaltigungsprogramm Bei Psychosomatischen Patienten. 1992; 42(12):436-44.

Strijk JE, Proper KI, van der Beek AJ, van Mechelen W. A process evaluation of a worksite vitality intervention among ageing hospital workers. Int J Behav Nutr Phys Act 2011; 8:58.

Subramanya P, Telles S. Changes in midlatency auditory evoked potentials following two yoga-based relaxation techniques. Clin EEG Neurosci 2009; 40(3):190-5.

Sudheesh NN, Joseph KP. Investigation into the effects of music and meditation on galvanic skin response. 2000; 21(3):158-63.

Surwillo WW, Hobson DP. Brain electrical activity during prayer. Psychol Rep 1978; 43(1):135-43.

Surwit RS, Shapiro D, Good MI. Comparison of cardiovascular biofeedback, neuromuscular biofeedback, and meditation in the treatment of borderline essential hypertension. J Consult Clin Psychol 1978; 46(2):252-63.

Tang YY, Ma Y, Wang J et al. Short-term meditation training improves attention and self-regulation. Proc Natl Acad Sci U S A 2007; 104(43):17152-6.

Targ EF, Levine EG. The efficacy of a mind-body-spirit group for women with breast cancer: a randomized controlled trial. Gen Hosp Psychiatry 2002; 24(4):238-48.

Taylor DN. Effects of a behavioral stress-management program on anxiety, mood, self-esteem, and T-cell count in HIV positive men. Psychol Rep 1995; 76(2):451-7.

Telles S, Balkrishna A, Maharana K. Effect of yoga and ayurveda on duchenne muscular dystrophy. Indian J Palliat Care 2011; 17(2):169-70.

Telles S, Maharana K, Balrana B, Balkrishna A. Effects of high-frequency yoga breathing called kapalabhati compared with breath awareness on the degree of optical illusion perceived. Percept Mot Skills 2011; 112(3):981-90.

Thiede W. [Occultism in children and adolescents. Search movements by youth for an orienting world view and possible transcendence--theological observations and reflections]. Kinderkrankenschwester 2005; 24(12):510-3.

Thomas M, Sadlier M, Smith A. A multiconvergent approach to the rehabilitation of patients with chronic fatigue syndrome: a comparative study. Physiotherapy 2008; 94(1):35-42.

Tloczynski J, Malinowski A, Lamorte R. Rediscovering and reapplying contingent informal meditation. Psychologia: An International Journal of Psychology in the Orient 1997; 40(1):14-21.

Tloczynski J. A preliminary study of opening-up meditation college adjustment, and self-actualization. Psychol Rep 1994; 75(1 Pt 2):449-50.

Travis F, Olson T, Egenes T, Gupta HK. Physiological patterns during practice of the Transcendental Meditation technique compared with patterns while reading Sanskrit and a modern language. Int J Neurosci 2001; 109(1-2):71-80.

Travis F. Comparison of coherence, amplitude, and eLORETA patterns during Transcendental Meditation and TM-Sidhi practice. Int J Psychophysiol 2011.

Travis FT, Orme-Johnson DW. EEG coherence and power during Yogic Flying. Int J Neurosci 1990; 54(1-2):1-12.

Tsang WW, Hui-Chan CW. Effect of 4- and 8-wk intensive Tai Chi Training on balance control in the elderly. Med Sci Sports Exerc 2004; 36(4):648-57.

Ussher M, Cropley M, Playle S, Mohidin R, West R. Effect of isometric exercise and body scanning on cigarette cravings and withdrawal symptoms. 2009; 104(7):1251-7.

Vahia VN, Shetty HK, Motiwala S, Thakkar G, Fernandes L, Sharma JC. Efficacy of meditation in generalized anxiety disorder. Indian J Psychiatry 1993; 35(2):87-91.

van den Hout MA, Engelhard IM, Beetsma D et al. EMDR and mindfulness. Eye movements and attentional breathing tax working memory and reduce vividness and emotionality of aversive ideation. J Behav Ther Exp Psychiatry 2011; 42(4):423-31.

Vandana B, Vaidyanathan K, Saraswathy LA, Sundaram KR, Kumar H. Impact of integrated amrita meditation technique on adrenaline and cortisol levels in healthy volunteers. Evid Based Complement Alternat Med 2011; 2011:379645.

von Trott P, Wiedemann AM, Ludtke R, Reishauer A, Willich SN, Witt CM. Qigong and exercise therapy for elderly patients with chronic neck pain (QIBANE): a randomized controlled study. J Pain 2009; 10(5):501-8.

Wachholtz AB, Pargament KI. Migraines and meditation: does spirituality matter? J Behav Med 2008; 31(4):351-66.

Wang F, Wang W, Zhang R et al. Clinical observation on physiological and psychological effects of Eight-Section Brocade on type 2 diabetic patients. J Tradit Chin Med 2008; 28(2):101-5.

Warber SL, Ingerman S, Moura VL et al. Healing the heart: a randomized pilot study of a spiritual retreat for depression in acute coronary syndrome patients. Explore (NY) 2011; 7(4):222-33.

Watkins E, Teasdale JD. Adaptive and maladaptive self-focus in depression. J Affect Disord 2004; 82(1):1-8.

Wenk-Sormaz H. Meditation can reduce habitual responding. Altern Ther Health Med 2005; 11(2):42-58.

Williams JMG, Russell IT, Crane C et al. Staying well after depression: Trial design and protocol. BMC Psychiatry 2010; 10.

Wilson AF, Honsberger R, Chiu JT, Novey HS. Transcendental meditation and asthma. Respiration 1975; 32(1):74-80.

Winzelberg AJ, Luskin FM. The effect of a meditation training in stress levels in secondary school teachers. Stress Medicine 1999; 15(2):69-77.

Wirth DP, Cram JR. Multisite surface electromyography and complementary healing intervention: a comparative analysis. J Altern Complement Med 1997; 3(4):355-64.

Wolfson L, Whipple R, Derby C et al. Balance and strength training in older adults: intervention gains and Tai Chi maintenance. J Am Geriatr Soc 1996; 44(5):498-506.

Wood C. Mood change and perceptions of vitality: a comparison of the effects of relaxation, visualization and yoga. J R Soc Med 1993; 86(5):254-8.

Xu WS. [Meditating on the management of sepsis at early stage of burns]. Zhonghua Shao Shang Za Zhi 2005; 21(2):81-2.

Xu YH, Wang JH, Li HF, Zhu XH, Wang G. [Efficacy of integrative respiratory rehabilitation training in exercise ability and quality of life of patients with chronic obstructive pulmonary disease in stable phase: a randomized controlled trial]. Zhong Xi Yi Jie He Xue Bao 2010; 8(5):432-7.

Yan X, Shen H, Jiang H et al. External Qi of Yan Xin Qigong differentially regulates the Akt and extracellular signal-regulated kinase pathways and is cytotoxic to cancer cells but not to normal cells. Int J Biochem Cell Biol 2006; 38(12):2102-13.

Yan X, Shen H, Jiang H et al. External Qi of Yan Xin Qigong Induces apoptosis and inhibits migration and invasion of estrogen-independent breast cancer cells through suppression of Akt/NF-kB signaling. Cell Physiol Biochem 2010; 25(2-3):263-70.

Yan X, Shen H, Jiang H et al. External Qi of Yan Xin Qigong induces G2/M arrest and apoptosis of androgen-independent prostate cancer cells by inhibiting Akt and NF-kappa B pathways. Mol Cell Biochem 2008; 310(1-2):227-34.

Young EC, Brammer C, Owen E et al. The effect of mindfulness meditation on cough reflex sensitivity. Thorax 2009; 64(11):993-8.

Yount G, Solfvin J, Moore D et al. In vitro test of external Qigong. BMC Complement Altern Med 2004; 4:5.

Zaichkowsky LD, Kamen R. Biofeedback and meditation: effects on muscle tension and locus of control. Percept Mot Skills 1978; 46(3 Pt 1):955-8.

Zautra AJ, Fasman R, Davis MC, Craig AD. The effects of slow breathing on affective responses to pain stimuli: an experimental study. Pain 2010; 149(1):12-8.

Zeidan F, Johnson SK, Diamond BJ, David Z, Goolkasian P. Mindfulness meditation improves cognition: evidence of brief mental training. Conscious Cogn 2010; 19(2):597-605.

Zeidan F, Johnson SK, Gordon NS, Goolkasian P. Effects of brief and sham mindfulness meditation on mood and cardiovascular variables. J Altern Complement Med 2010; 16(8):867-73.

Zeier H. [Relaxation by biofeedback controlled respiratory meditation and autogenic training]. Z Exp Angew Psychol 1985; 32(4):682-95.

Zhuo D, Dighe J, Basmajian JV. EMG biofeedback and Chinese 'Chi Kung': relaxation effects in patients with low back pain. Physiother. Can. 1983; 35(1):13-7.

Zuroff DC, Schwarz JC. Effects of transcendental meditation and muscle relaxation on trait anxiety, maladjustment, locus of control, and drug use. J Consult Clin Psychol 1978; 46(2):264-71.

Zuroff DC, Schwarz JC. Transcendental meditation versus muscle relaxation: A two-year follow-up of a controlled experiment. The American Journal of Psychiatry 1980; 137(10):1229-31.

Movement-Based Meditation

Adjunctive T'ai Chi Chih with escitalopram for geriatric depression. Brown University Psychopharmacology Update 2011; 22(5):3-4.

Adler P. The effects of Tai Chi on pain and function in older adults with osteoarthritis. Case Western Reserve University, 2007.

Agte V, Tarwadi K. Sudarshan Kriya yoga for treating type 2 diabetes: a preliminary study. Alternative & Complementary Therapies 2004; 10(4):220-2.

Ahmadi A, Nikbakh M, Arastoo A, Habibi A-H. The Effects of a yoga intervention on balance, speed and endurance of walking, fatigue and quality of life in people with multiple sclerosis. 2010; 23(1):71-8.

Alp A, Cansever S, Gorgec N, Yurtkuran M, Topsac T. Effects of Tai Chi exercise on functional and life quality assessments in senile osteoporosis. 2009; 29(3):687-95.

Amita S, Prabhakar S, Manoj I, Harminder S, Pavan T. Effect of yoga-nidra on blood glucose level in diabetic patients. Indian J Physiol Pharmacol 2009; 53(1):97-101.

Annapoorna K, Latha KS, Bhat SM, Bhandary PV. Effectiveness of the practice of yoga therapy in anxiety disorders: A randomized controlled trial. Asian J. Psychiatry 2011; 4:S45.

Anon. [The effect of 'QiGong' training on the rheoencephalogram]. Chinese Journal of Sports Medicine 1993; 12(1):55-6.

Armstrong W, Smedley J. Effects of a home-based yoga exercise program on flexibility in older women. Clinical Kinesiology: Journal of the American Kinesiotherapy Association 2003; 57(1):1-6.

Aslan U, Livanelioglu A. The effects of Hatha yoga on flexibility [Turkish]. Fizyoterapi Rehabilitasyon 2001; 12(1):25-30.

Attanayake AMP, Somarathna KIWK, Vyas GH, Dash SC. Clinical evaluation of selected yogic procedures in individuals with low back pain. AYU 2010; 31(2):245-50.

Audette JF, Jin YS, Newcomer R, Stein L, Duncan G, Frontera WR. Tai Chi versus brisk walking in elderly women. Age Ageing 2006; 35(4):388-93.

Baker MA. The effects of Hatha Yoga and self-recording on trait anxiety and locus of control. Dissertation Abstracts International 1980; 41(2-B):680.

Balk JL. Does yoga untie the pretzel of anxiety and depression? 2009; 12(9):100-2.

Balzano J, Burke J, Hoy T, Roberts E, Hakim R. A comparative study of balance measures among elderly persons participating in Tai Chi or structured exercise programs. Journal of Geriatric Physical Therapy 2002; 25(3):44.

Barovick H. What's so funny? Laughter-yoga fans hail the health benefits of giggling for no reason. Time 2010; 176(11):54.

Barrow DE, Bedford A, Ives G, O'Toole L, Channer KS. An evaluation of the effects of Tai Chi Chuan and Chi Kung training in patients with symptomatic heart failure: a randomised controlled pilot study. Postgrad Med J 2007; 83(985):717-21.

Belaia NA, Zhuravleva AI, Andreeva VM. Effect of certain asanas used in the system of yoga on the central nervous and cardiovascular systems: Vliiani nekotorykh asan, primeniaemykh po sisteme ¦Éogov, na tsentral'nuiu nervnuiu i serdechno-cosudistuiu sistemy. 1976; 0(3):13-8.

Bezerra L, Bottaro M, Reis VM et al. Effects of yoga on bone metabolism in postmenopausal women. 2010; 13(4):58-65.

Bhat R, Ganaraja B, Bhagylakshmi K. Yoga and exercise show beneficial effects on heart rate variability and blood pressure in geriatric hypertensivepatients. J. Gen. Intern. Med. 2010; 25:S434.

Bhatnagar OP, Anantharaman V. The effect of yoga training on neuromuscular excitability and muscular relaxation. Neurol India 1977; 25(4):230-2.

Bhatti TI, Gillin JC, Atkinson JH et al. T'ai chi chih as a treatment for chronic low back pain: a randomized, controlled study (abstract). Alternative Therapies in Health and Medicine 1998; 4(2):90-1.

Bijlani RL. Influence of yoga on brain and behaviour: facts and speculations. Indian J Physiol Pharmacol 2004; 48(1):1-5.

Blom KC, Baker B, Irvine J et al. The harmony study: Hypertension analysis of stress reduction using mindfulness meditation and yoga. J. Clin. Hypertens. 2011; 13(4):A141.

Blumenthal JA, Emery CF, Madden DJ et al. Effects of exercise training on bone density in older men and women. J Am Geriatr Soc 1991; 39(11):1065-70.

Bobby. Effect of Qigong on physical and psychosocial status of Chinese COPD patients: a randomized controlled trial. Hong Kong Polytechnic University (Hong Kong), 2010.

Bosch P. Stress responsiveness and adaptations of the neuroendocrine system in women with rheumatoid arthritis. Arizona State University, 2003.

Boylan M. External Qigong therapy and fibromyalgia -- a pilot study. Journal of the Australian Traditional-Medicine Society 2007; 13(2):105.

Brady Michele Ruggiero. The effects of Hatha yoga and weight training on trait and state anxiety. Dissertation Abstracts International 2007; 67(8-B):4699.

Broota A, Varma R, Singh A. Role of relaxation in hypertension. Journal of the Indian Academy of Applied Psychology 1995; 21(1):29-36.

Bulavin VV, Kliuzhev VM, Kliachkin LM, Lakshmankumar, Zuikhin ND, Vlasova TN. [Elements of yoga therapy in the combined rehabilitation of myocardial infarct patients in the functional recovery period]. Vopr Kurortol Fizioter Lech Fiz Kult 1993; (4):7-9.

Cespedes EM, Riveron G, Alonso CA, Gordon L. Evolucion metabolica de pacientes diabeticos tipo 2 sometidos a un tratamiento combinado de dieta y ejercicios yoga. 2002; 21(2):98-101.

Caldwell K, Harrison M, Adams M, Triplett NT. Effect of Pilates and taiji quan training on self-efficacy, sleep quality, mood, and physical performance of college students. J Bodyw Mov Ther 2009; 13(2):155-63.

Canter P, Brazier A. Inconclusive study of yoga and meditation in HIV/AIDS. Focus on Alternative & Complementary Therapies 2006; 11(3):227-8.

Canter P, Gangadhar B. Possible antidepressant effects of yogic breathing during early stage alcohol detoxification. Focus on Alternative & Complementary Therapies 2006; 11(4):318-9.

Cardozo B, Thakar AB, Skandhan KP. A clinical study on psyco-somatic management of shukraavrlta vata (premature ejaculation) with rasayana yoga and shirodhara. AYU 2006; 27(4):94-8.

Carei TR, Fyfe-Johnson AL, Breuner CC, Brown MA. Randomized controlled clinical trial of yoga in the treatment of eating disorders. J Adolesc Health 2010; 46(4):346-51.

Carei Tiffany Rain. Randomized controlled clinical trial of yoga in the treatment of eating disorders. Dissertation Abstracts International 2008; 68(8-B):5560.

Carrieri-Kohlmann V, Stulbarg S. Yoga for treating shortness of breath in chronic obstructive pulmonary disease (COPD). ClinicalTrials.Gov 2003.

Carter JJ. Evaluation of a multi-component yoga intervention as adjunct to psychiatric treatment for Vietnam veterans with posttraumatic stress disorder (PTSD): A randomized controlled trial (RCT). Controlled-Trials.Com 2006.

Chandwani KD, Thornton B, Perkins GH et al. Yoga improves quality of life and benefit finding in women undergoing radiotherapy for breast cancer. J Soc Integr Oncol 2010; 8(2):43-55.

Chaudhary AK, Bhatnagar HN, Bhatnagar LK, Chaudhary K. Comparative study of the effect of drugs and relaxation exercise (yoga shavasan) in hypertension. J Assoc Physicians India 1988; 36(12):721-3.

Cheema BS, Marshall PW, Chang D, Colagiuri B, Machliss B. Effect of an office worksite-based yoga program on heart rate variability: a randomized controlled trial. BMC Public Health 2011; 11:578.

Chen HH, Yeh ML, Lee FY. The effects of Baduanjin qigong in the prevention of bone loss for middle-aged women. Am J Chin Med 2006; 34(5):741-7.

Chen KM, Fan JT, Wang HH, Wu SJ, Li CH, Lin HS. Silver yoga exercises improved physical fitness of transitional frail elders. Nurs Res 2010; 59(5):364-70.

Chen L-X. Curative effect of yoga exercise prescription in treating menstrual disorders. 2005; 9(4):164-5.

Chen WW, Sun WY. Tai chi chuan, an alternative form of exercise for health promotion and disease prevention for older adults in the community. Int Q Community Health Educ 1996; 16(4):333-9.

Chen ZX, Lin BL, Chen JY et al. Effect of Qigong exercise on the contentration of plasma fibronectin. Journal of Guangzhou University of Traditional Chinese Medicine [Guang Zhou Zhong Yi Xue Yuan Xue Bao] 1989; 6(1):46-, 48.

Chi I, Jordan-Marsh M, Guo M, Xie B, Zhang M. Tai Chi for depression. 2008; (2).

Cho HS. The Effects of Yoga Exercise on Stress and Health status in Clinical Nurses. Korean J Rehabil Nurs 2004; 7(1):15-23.

Cho KL. Effect of Tai Chi on depressive symptoms amongst Chinese older patients with major depression: the role of social support. Med Sport Sci 2008; 52:146-54.

Christou EA, Yang Y, Rosengren KS. Taiji training improves knee extensor strength and force control in older adults. J Gerontol A Biol Sci Med Sci 2003; 58(8):763-6.

Chyu MC, James CR, Sawyer SF et al. Effects of tai chi exercise on posturography, gait, physical function and quality of life in postmenopausal women with osteopaenia: a randomized clinical study. Clin Rehabil 2010; 24(12):1080-90.

Clark P, Cortese-Jimenez G, Cohen E. Using Reiki, Yoga, meditation or patient education to address physical and psychological symptoms related to chemotherapy-induced peripheral neuropathy: A pilot study [conference abstract]. Psycho-Oncology [Abstracts From the 8th Annual Conference of the American Psychosocial Oncology Society Anaheim, CA United States. Feb 17-19 2011] 2011.

Coelho CM, Lessa TT, Coelho LAMC, da Silva Scari R, Junior JMN, de Carvalho RM. Ventilatory function in female practitionersof Hatha Yoga: Funcao ventilatoria em mulheres praticantes de Hatha Ioga. 2011; 13(4):279-84.

Cohen L. Randomized Controlled Trial of Yoga Among a Multiethnic Sample of Breast Cancer Patients: Effects on Quality of Life. 2008; 19(2):129.

Cohen L, Chandwani K, Thornton B, Perkins G, et al. Randomized trial of yoga in women with breast cancer undergoing radiation treatment. Journal of Clinical Oncology 2006; 24(18 Suppl):469s.

Collins LA. Stress management and yoga. Dissertation Abstracts International 1984; 45(1-A):0116.

Cowen V, Adams T. Physical and perceptual benefits of yoga asana practice: results of a pilot study. Journal of Bodywork & Movement Therapies 2005; 9(3):211-9.

Cromwell S. Benefits of Tai Chi for sedentary Mexican-American women. Communicating Nursing Research 2005; 38:259.

Culos-Reed SN, Carlson LE, Daroux LM, Hately-Aldous S. A pilot study of yoga for breast cancer survivors: physical and psychological benefits. Psychooncology 2006; 15(10):891-7.

Cusumano JA. The short-term psychophysiological effects of Hatha Yoga and progressive relaxation on female Japanese students. Dissertation Abstracts International 1991; 51(10):3333.

Cusumano JA, Robinson SE. The short-term psychophysiological effects of hatha yoga and progressive relaxation on female Japanese students. Applied Psychology: An International Review 1993; 42(1):77-90.

Dahl JC, Lundgren TL, and Yardi N. Evaluation of short term ACT psychotherapy and yoga in a RCT trial for refractory seizures in India. Epilepsia 2005; 46 Suppl 6:196.

Danhauer S, Rutherford C, McQuellon R et al. Restorative yoga as a supportive intervention for women with ovarian or breast cancer... American Psychosocial Oncology Society (APOS) Third Annual Conference, Amelia Island, Florida, 16th-19th February 2006. Psycho-Oncology 2006-; 15(1):S72-3.

Dave HR, Srikrishna Ch, Vyas SN, Dave AR. A comparative study on the role of medhya rasayana yoga and dashamula kwathadhara in the management of vatika shirahshula (tension headache). AYU 2006; 27(2):36-40.

de Godoy DV, Bringhenti RL, Severa A, de Gasperi R, Poli LV. Yoga versus aerobic activity: effects on spirometry results and maximal inspiratory pressure. J Bras Pneumol 2006; 32(2):130-5.

Dechamps A, Onifade C, Decamps A, Bourdel-Marchasson I. Health-related quality of life in frail institutionalized elderly: effects of a cognition-action intervention and Tai Chi. Journal of Aging & Physical Activity 2009; 17(2):236-48.

Dechamps A, Quintard B, Lafont L. Effects of a short-term tai-chi-chuan mind-body approach on self-efficacy, anxiety and mood among sedentary lifestyle students. [French]. [References]. European Review of Applied Psychology/Revue Europeenne De Psychologie Appliquee 2008; 58(2):125-32.

Deuskar M, Poonawala N, Bhatewara SA. Effect of Yoga Nidra and Applied Relaxation Technique on Steadiness and Performance of Archers. Psychological Studies 2006; 51(1):64-8.

Djelic M, Nesic D, Ilic V et al. Positive impact of yoga exercise program for female seniors on risk profiles of cardiovascular diseases. Eur. J. Cardiovasc. Prev. Rehabil. 2011; 18(1):S31.

Donesky-Cuenco D, Carrieri-Kohlman V, Park SK, Jacobs B. Safety and feasibility of yoga in patients with COPD [Abstract]. Proceedings of the American Thoracic Society 2006; A221.

Du ZY, Zhang JZ Li XG Di XM. [Cardiovascular effect of different 'QiGong']. Chinese Journal of Sports Medicine 1992; 11(1):32-5.

Dudani U, Gupta HL, Singh SH, Selvamurthy W, and Surange SG. Effect of Sahaja yoga on the frequency of seizures in epileptics. 18th International Epilepsy Congress 1989; 161.

Dvivedi J, Dvivedi S, Mahajan KK, Mittal S, Singhal A. Effect of '61-points relaxation technique' on stress parameters in premenstrual syndrome. Indian J Physiol Pharmacol 2008; 52(1):69-76.

Engelman SR, Clance PR, Imes S. Self and body-cathexis change in therapy and yoga groups. J Am Soc Psychosom Dent Med 1982; 29(3):77-88.

Evans AT, Hadler NM. Yoga improved function and reduced symptoms of chronic low-back pain more than a self-care book. ACP J Club 2006; 145(1):16.

Faber MJ, Bosscher RJ, Chin A Paw MJ, van Wieringen PC. Effects of exercise programs on falls and mobility in frail and pre-frail older adults: A multicenter randomized controlled trial. Arch Phys Med Rehabil 2006; 87(7):885-96.

Field T, Diego M, Hernandez-Reif M, Medina L, Delgado J, Hernandez A. Yoga and massage therapy reduce prenatal depression and prematurity.

Flegal KE, Kishiyama S, Zajdel D, Haas M, Oken BS. Adherence to yoga and exercise interventions in a 6-month clinical trial. BMC Complement Altern Med 2007; 7:37.

Fluge T, Richter J, Fabel H, Zysno E, Weller E, Wagner TO. [Long-term effects of breathing exercises and yoga in patients with bronchial asthma]. Pneumologie 1994; 48(7):484-90.

Friedman S. A qigong approach to treating breast cancer. California Journal of Oriental Medicine (CJOM) 2007; 18(1):18-9.

Frye B, Scheinthal S, Kemarskaya T, Pruchno R. Tai chi and low impact exercise: effects on the physical functioning and psychological well-being of older people. Journal of Applied Gerontology 2007; 26(5):433-53.

Furian TC, Wagner D, Ritthaler F. [Effect of tai chi training equipment on physical performance, ventilatory parameters and balance]. Deutsche Zeitschrift Fur Sportmedizin 1999; 50(S1):64.

Galani K, Vyas SN, Dave AR. A clinical study on role of of "Saptasamo yoga and darvyadi yamak malahara" In the management of ekakushtha (psoriasis). AYU 2009; 30(4):415-20.

Galantino M, Capito L, Kane R, Ottey N, Switzer S, Packel L. The effects of Tai Chi and walking on fatigue and body mass index in women living with breast cancer: a pilot study. Rehabilitation Oncology 2003; 21(1):17-22.

Galantino M. Blending traditional and alternative strategies for rehabilitation: measuring functional outcomes and quality of life issues in an AIDS population. Temple University, 1997.

Garfinkel MS, Schumacher HR Jr, Husain A, Levy M, Reshetar RA. Evaluation of a yoga based regimen for treatment of osteoarthritis of the hands. J Rheumatol 1994; 21(12):2341-3.

Gatts S. Neural mechanisms underlying balance control in Tai Chi. Med Sport Sci 2008; 52:87-103.

Gatts SK, Woollacott MH. How Tai Chi improves balance: biomechanics of recovery to a walking slip in impaired seniors. Gait Posture 2007; 25(2):205-14.

Gatts S. Neural and biomechanical mechanisms underlying balance improvement with short term Tai Chi training in balance impaired older adults. University of Oregon, 2005.

Gemmell C, Leathem JM. A study investigating the effects of Tai Chi Chuan: individuals with traumatic brain injury compared to controls. Brain Inj 2006; 20(2):151-6.

Gharote ML, Ganguly SK. Effects of a nine-week yogic training programme on some aspects of physical fitness of physically conditioned young males. Indian J Med Sci 1979; 33(10):258-63.

Gode JD, Singh RH, Settiwar RM, Gode KD, Udupa KN. Increased urinary excretion of testosterone following a course of yoga in normal young volunteers. Indian J Med Sci 1974; 28(4-5):212-5.

Gokal R, Shillito L, Maharaj SR. Positive impact of yoga and pranayam on obesity, hypertension, blood sugar, and cholesterol: A pilot assessment [3]. 2007; 13(10):1056-7.

Goncalves LC, Vale RGDS, Barata NJF, Varejao RV, Dantas EHM. Flexibility, functional autonomy and quality of life (QoL) in elderly yoga practitioners. 2011; 53(2):158-62.

Gopal A, Mondal S, Gandhi A, Arora S, Bhattacharjee J. Effect of integrated yoga practices on immune responses in examination stress - A preliminary study. Int J Yoga 2011; 4(1):26-32.

Gopal KS, Anantharaman V, Balachander S, Nishith SD. The cardiorespiratory adjustments in 'Pranayama', with and without 'Bandhas', in 'Vajrasana'. Indian J Med Sci 1973; 27(9):686-92.

Gopal KS, Anantharamn V, Nishith SD, Bhatnagar OP. The effect of yogasanas on muscular tone and cardio-respiratory adjustments. Indian J Med Sci 1974; 28(10):438-43.

Gopal KS, Bhatnagar OP, Subramanian N, Nishith SD. Effect of yogasanas and pranayamas on blood pressure, pulse rate and some respiratory functions. Indian J Physiol Pharmacol 1973; 17(3):273-6.

Gopinath KS, Rao R, Raghuram N et al. Evaluation of yoga therapy as a psychotherapeutic intervention in breast cancer patients on conventional combined modality of treatment. Proceedings of American Society of Clinical Oncology 2003; 22:26.

Gordon L, Morrison EY, McGrowder D et al. Effect of yoga and traditional physical exercise on hormones and percentage insulin binding receptor in patients with type 2 diabetes. 2008; 4(1):35-42.

Gordon L, Morrison EY, McGrowder DA et al. Changes in clinical and metabolic parameters after exercise therapy in patents with type 2 diabetes. 2008; 4(4):427-37.

Gordon LA, Morrison EY, McGrowder DA et al. Effect of exercise therapy on lipid profile and oxidative stress indicators in patients with type 2 diabetes. 2008; 8.

Grover P, Varma VK, Verma SK, Pershad D. Factors influencing treatment acceptance in neurotic patients referred for yoga therapy-;an exploratory study. Indian J Psychiatry 1989; 31(3):250-7.

Gundling K. A randomised trial of medical Qigong for cancer patients. Focus on Alternative and Complementary Therapies 2010; 15(4):299-300.

Haber D. Yoga as a preventive health care program for white and black elders: an exploratory study. Int J Aging Hum Dev 1983; 17(3):169-76.

Hackney ME, Earhart GM. Tai Chi improves balance and mobility in people with Parkinson disease. Gait Posture 2008; 28(3):456-60.

Hakim R, Segal J, Newton R, DuCette J. A fall risk reduction intervention for community-dwelling older adults. Journal of Geriatric Physical Therapy 2001; 24(3):21-2.

Halpern J, Cohen M, Kennedy G. Yoga for improving sleep and life quality in the elderly population. Sleep Biol. Rhythms 2010; 8:A41.

Halpern J, Cohen M, Kennedy G. Yoga for improving sleep and life quality in the elderly population [Abstract]. Sleep and Biological Rhythms 2010; 8(Suppl 1):A41 [P037].

Hart J, Kanner H, Gilboa-Mayo R, Haroeh-Peer O, Rozenthul-Sorokin N, Eldar R. Tai Chi Chuan practice in community-dwelling persons after stroke. Int J Rehabil Res 2004; 27(4):303-4.

Hartfiel N, Havenhand J, Khalsa SB, Clarke G, Krayer A. The effectiveness of yoga for the improvement of well-being and resilience to stress in the workplace. Scand J Work Environ Health 2011; 37(1):70-6.

Haslock I, Monro R, Nagarathna R, Nagendra HR, Raghuram NV. Measuring the effects of yoga in rheumatoid arthritis [3]. BR. J. Rheumatol. 1994; 33(8):787-8.

He Q, Zhang JZ, Li JZ. The effects of long-term Qi Gong exercise on brain function as manifested by computer analysis. J Tradit Chin Med 1988; 8(3):177-82.

Hipp A, Heitkamp HC, Rocker K, Schuller H, Dickhuth HH. Effects of yoga on lipid metabolism in patients with coronary artery disease. International Journal of Sports Medicine 1998; 19:S.

Hiraoka A, Kobayashi H, Shimono F, Ohsuga M. Effects of Kai-Gou (air-ball handling), a Qi-Gong strategy, on the biofeedback training for enhancement of the electroencephalographic activity. Japanese Journal of Biofeedback Research 1997; 24:74-8.

Hu X. Effects of Tai Chi on functional fitness and subjective health status in older Japanese returnees from China: A randomized controlled trial. 2007; 56(4):409-17.

Huang HC, Liu CY, Huang YT, Kernohan WG. Health education and Tai Chi reduce falls - a one-year follow-up RCT [abstract]. Irish Journal of Medical Science 2009; 178(Suppl 8):S289.

Huang T, Yang L, Liu C. Reducing the fear of falling among community adults through cognitive controlled trial. Journal of Advanced Nursing 2011; 67(5):961-71.

Hui G, Kaijun N, Yano H et al. The effect of a new exercise program including Tai Chi Chuan and Kung Fu gymnastics elements for the physical fitness of older subjects who have lower physical fitness - Compared to a well-accepted exercise program. 2007; 56(2):241-56.

Hung H, Chen K. Effects of the simplified Tai-Chi exercise program in promoting the health of the urban elderly [Chinese]. Journal of Evidence-Based Nursing 2007; 3(3):225-35.

Hyeong-Dong Kim, Tae-You Kim, Hyun Dong J, Seon-Tae Son. The Effects of Tai Chi Based Exercise on Dynamic Postural Control of Parkinson's Disease Patients while Initiating Gait. Journal of Physical Therapy Science 2011; 23(2):265-9.

Immink M. A pilot study on yoga and meditation as an adjunct to fitness rehabilitation programs for stroke patients with chronic hemiparesis. Australian New Zealand Clinical Trials Registry (ANZCTR) Http://Www.Anzctr.Org.Au/ 2009.

Immink M. A yoga and meditation program to improve physical function, mood and quality of life in individuals with chronic stroke hemiparesis. Australian New Zealand Clinical Trials Registry (ANZCTR) Http://Www.Anzctr.Org.Au/ 2009.

Innes KE, Selfe TK, Alexander GK, Taylor AG. A new educational film control for use in studies of active mind-body therapies: acceptability and feasibility. J Altern Complement Med 2011; 17(5):453-8.

Innes KE, Selfe TK, Vishnu A. Association of fructosamine to indices of dyslipidemia in older adults with type 2 diabetes. Diabetes Metab. Syndr. Clin. Res. Rev. 2010.

Irwin MR, Olmstead R. Mitigating Cellular Inflammation in Older Adults: A Randomized Controlled Trial of Tai Chi Chih. Am J Geriatr Psychiatry 2011.

Jaffe R. Tai Chi retards bone loss and improves muscle strenght. Phys. Sportsmed. 2003; 31(4):16-7.

Janelsins MC, Davis PG, Wideman L et al. Effects of Tai Chi Chuan on insulin and cytokine levels in a randomized controlled pilot study on breast cancer survivors. Clin Breast Cancer 2011; 11(3):161-70.

Jang HS, Lee MS. Effects of qi therapy (external qigong) on premenstrual syndrome: a randomized placebo-controlled study. J Altern Complement Med 2004; 10(3):456-62.

Jatuporn S, Sangwatanaroj S, Saengsiri AO et al. Short-term effects of an intensive lifestyle modification program on lipid peroxidation and antioxidant systems in patients with coronary artery disease. Clin Hemorheol Microcirc 2003; 29(3-4):429-36.

Jhansi Rani N. Impact of yoga training on cognitive style and body awareness. Journal of Indian Psychology 2008; 26(1-2):69-78.

Johansson M, Hassmen P, Jouper J. Acute effects of qigong exercise on mood and anxiety. International Journal of Stress Management 2008; 15(2):199-207.

Joseph S, Sridharan K, Patil SK et al. Study of some physiological and biochemical parameters in subjects undergoing yogic training. Indian J Med Res 1981; 74:120-4.

Karambelkar PV, Bhole MV, Gharote ML. Effect of Yogic asanas on uropepsin excretion. Indian J Med Res 1969; 57(5):944-7.

Katiyar SK, Bihari S. Role of pranayama in rehabilitation of copd patients - a randomized controlled study. Indian Journal of Allergy Asthma Immunology 2006; 20(2):98-104.

Kepner J. Yoga research and Richard Freeman. Altern Ther Health Med 2004; 10(4):14.

Kerr D, Gillam E, Ryder J, Trowbridge S, Cavan D, Thomas P. An Eastern art form for a Western disease: randomised controlled trial of yoga in patients with poorly controlled insulin-treated diabetes. Practical Diabetes International 2002; 19(6):164-6.

Khalsa SB. Evaluation of a yoga breathing meditation as a treatment for chronic insomnia. Biological Psychology 2006; 72(3):232.

Khalsa SB, Cope S. Effects of a yoga lifestyle intervention on performance-related characteristics of musicians: a preliminary study. Med Sci Monit 2006; 12(8):CR325-31.

Khalsa SB, Shorter SM, Cope S, Wyshak G, Sklar E. Yoga ameliorates performance anxiety and mood disturbance in young professional musicians. Appl Psychophysiol Biofeedback 2009; 34(4):279-89.

Khare KC, Sanghvi VC, Bhatnagar AD, Khare R. Effect of Yoga in treatment of bronchial asthma. Indian Practitioner 1991; 44(1):23-7.

Khemka SS, Rao NH, Nagarathna R. Immediate effects of two relaxation techniques on healthy volunteers. Indian J Physiol Pharmacol 2009; 53(1):67-72.

Khumar SS, Kaur P, Kaur S. Effectiveness of Shavasana on depression among university students. Indian Journal of Clinical Psychology 1993; 20(2):82-7.

Kim H. Effects of Tai Chi exercise on the center of pressure trace during obstacle crossing in older adults who are at a risk of falling. Journal of Physical Therapy Science 2009; 21(1):49-54.

Kim H, Han J, Cho Y. The effectiveness of community-based Tai Chi training on balance control during stair descent by older adults. Journal of Physical Therapy Science 2009; 21(4):317-23.

Kimbrough S, Balkin R, Rancich A. The effect of inverted yoga positions on short-term memory. Athletic Insight: The Online Journal of Sport Psychology 2007; 9(2).

Kin SK, Kurosawa K. Effect of Tai Chi on improving physical performance and preventing falling in community-dwelling old women. 2006; 21(3):275-9.

Kinney A, Campo R, O'Connor K et al. Feasibility and acceptability of a randomized trial of tai chi chih in senior female cancer survivors. Psycho-Oncology 2011; 20:235-6.

Klein P T, Adams W. Cardiopulmonary physiotherapeutic applications of taiji (Structured abstract). Cardiopulmonary Physical Therapy 2004; 15(4):5-11.

Kligler B, Homel P, Blank AE, Kenney J, Levenson H, Merrell W. Randomized trial of the effect of an integrative medicine approach to the management of asthma in adults on disease-related quality of life and pulmonary function. Altern Ther Health Med 2011; 17(1):10-5.

Kolsawalla MB. An experimental investigation into the effectiveness of some yogic variables as a mechanism of change in the value-attitude system. Journal of Indian Psychology 1978; 1(1):59-68.

Kova-ii-ì T, Kova-ii-ì M. Impact of relaxation training according to Yoga in Daily Life-« system on perceived stress after breast cancer surgery. 2011; 10(1):16-26.

Kovacic T, Kovacic M. Impact of relaxation training according to Yoga In Daily Life(R) system on perceived stress after breast cancer surgery. Integr Cancer Ther 2011; 10(1):16-26.

Kroner-Herwig B, Hebing G, Van Rijn-Kalkmann U, Frenzel A. The management of chronic tinnitus: Comparison of a cognitive-behavioural group training with yoga. Journal of Psychosomatic Research 1995; 39(2):153-65.

Krishnamurthy M, Telles S. Effects of Yoga and an Ayurveda preparation on gait, balance and mobility in older persons. Med Sci Monit 2007; 13(12):LE19-20.

Kuang A, Wang C, Xu D, Qian Y. Research on "anti-aging" effect of qigong. J Tradit Chin Med 1991; 11(2):153-8.

Kuang AK. [Treatment of hypertensive patients with Chi-kung and regular antihypertensive therapy--a comparative study of 4-year treatment results of 135 cases (author's transl)]. Zhonghua Nei Ke Za Zhi 1979; 18(3):187-91.

Kuang AK, Chen JL, Lu YR. [Changes of the sex hormones in female type II diabetics, coronary heart disease, essential hypertension and its relations with kidney deficiency, cardiovascular complications and efficacy of traditional Chinese medicine or qigong treatment]. Zhong Xi Yi Jie He Za Zhi 1989; 9(6):331-4, 323.

Kuang AK, Jiang MD, Wang CX, Zhao GS, Xu DH. Research on the mechanism of "Qigong (breathing exercise)". A preliminary study on its effect in balancing "Yin" and "Yang", regulating circulation and promoting flow in the meridian system. J Tradit Chin Med 1981; 1(1):7-10.

Kuang AK, Wang CX, Zhao GS et al. Long-term observation on qigong in prevention of stroke--follow-up of 244 hypertensive patients for 18-22 years. J Tradit Chin Med 1986; 6(4):235-8.

Kuang AX, Wang CX, Xu DH, Qian YC, Huang ML. [Study of the anti-aging effect of Qigong]. Zhong Xi Yi Jie He Za Zhi = Chinese Journal of Modern Developments in Traditional Medicine / Zhongguo Zhong Xi Yi Jie He Yan Jiu Hui (Chou), Zhong Yi Yan Jiu Yuan, Zhu Ban 1987; 7(8):455-8.

Kuang Anbi, Wang Chongxing, Xu Dinghai, Qian Yuecheng, Huang Meiling. The washback study of Qigong in anti-aging. Zhong Xi Yi Jie He Za Zhi = Chinese Journal of Modern Developments in Traditional Medicine / Zhongguo Zhong Xi Yi Jie He Yan Jiu Hui (Chou), Zhong Yi Yan Jiu Yuan, Zhu Ban 1987; 7(8):455-8.

Kulmatycki L, Burzäski Z. Yoga nidra and Benson's meditative relaxation and anxiety level, anger and depression emotions: Relaksacja joga nidry i medytacji Bensona a poziom leku oraz emocje gniewu i depresji. 2007; 21(3):23-8.

Kulpati DD, Kamath RK, Chauhan MR. The influence of physical conditioning by yogasanas and breathing exercises in patients of chronic obstructive lung disease. J Assoc Physicians India 1982; 30(12):865-8.

Kumari S, Nath NCB, Nagendra HR. Enhancing emotional competence among managers through SMET. Psychological Studies 2007; 52(2):171-3.

Kutner NG, Barnhart H, Wolf SL, McNeely E, Xu T. Self-report benefits of Tai Chi practice by older adults. J Gerontol B Psychol Sci Soc Sci 1997; 52(5):P242-6.

Kyizom T, Singh S, Singh KP, Tandon OP, Kumar R. Effect of pranayama & yoga-asana on cognitive brain functions in type 2 diabetes-P3 event related evoked potential (ERP). Indian J Med Res 2010; 131:636-40.

LaDue L. A quantitative study comparing tai chi and traditional balance exercises on emotional well-being, balance control and mobility efficacy in older adults. Walden University, 2009.

Lakshmikanthan C, Alagesan R, Thanikachalam S et al. Long term effects of yoga on hypertension and/or coronary artery disease. J Assoc Physicians India 1979; 27(12):1055-8.

Lam LC, Chau RC, Wong BM et al. Interim follow-up of a randomized controlled trial comparing Chinese style mind body (Tai Chi) and stretching exercises on cognitive function in subjects at risk of progressive cognitive decline. Int J Geriatr Psychiatry 2011; 26(7):733-40.

Latha, Kaliappan KV. Yoga, pranayama, thermal biofeedback techniques in the management of stress and high blood pressure. Journal of Indian Psychology 1991; 9(1-2):36-46.

Latha Dr, Kaliappan KV. Efficacy of yoga therapy in the management of headaches. Journal of Indian Psychology 1992; 10(1-2):41-7.

Latha M, Kaliappan KV. The efficacy of yoga therapy in the treatment of migraine and tension headaches. Journal of the Indian Academy of Applied Psychology 1987; 13(2):95-100.

Lavretsky H, Irwin M. Complementary use of tai chi improves resilience, quality of life, and cognitive function in depressed older adults. 163rd Annual Meeting of the American Psychiatric Association; 2010 May 22-26; New Orleans, LA 2010; NR3-70.

Lavretsky H, Irwin M. Complementary use of Tai Chi improves resilience, quality of life, and cognitive function in depressed older adults. Biol. Psychiatry 2010; 67(9):58S-9S.

Lee KO, Kim KR, Ahn SH. Effects of a Qigong prenatal education program on anxiety, depression and physical symptoms in pregnant women. Korean Journal of Women Health Nursing 2006; 12(3):240-8.

Lee KY, Jeong OY. [The effect of Tai Chi movement in patients with rheumatoid arthritis]. Taehan Kanho Hakhoe Chi 2006; 36(2):278-85.

Lee KYT, Jones AYM, Hui-Chan CWY, Tsang WWN. Kinematics and energy expenditure of sitting T'ai Chi. 2011; 17(8):665-8.

Lee LKY, Tim HM, Lee DTF, Woo J. Tai chi and health-related quality of life among Chinese nursing home residents [abstract]. Quality of Life Research : an International Journal of Quality of Life Aspects of Treatment, Care and Rehabilitation 2005; 14(9):2049.

Lee LY, Lee DT, Woo J. Effect of Tai Chi on state self-esteem and health-related quality of life in older Chinese residential care home residents J Clin Nurs. 2007 Sep;16(9):1592. Journal of Clinical Nursing 2007; 16(8):1580-2.

Lee LY, Lee DT, Woo J. Tai Chi and health-related quality of life in nursing home residents. J Nurs Scholarsh 2009; 41(1):35-43.

Lee MS, Kang C-W, Lim H-J, Lee M-S. Effects of Qi-training on anxiety and plasma concentrations of cortisol, ACTH, and aldosterone: A randomized placebo-controlled pilot study. 2004; 20(5):243-8.

Lee MS, Lee MS, Kim HJ, Moon SR. Qigong reduced blood pressure and catecholamine levels of patients with essential hypertension. Int J Neurosci 2003; 113(12):1691-701.

Lee MS, Lim HJ, Lee MS. Impact of qigong exercise on self-efficacy and other cognitive perceptual variables in patients with essential hypertension. J Altern Complement Med 2004; 10(4):675-80.

Lee MS, Rim YH, Jeong DM, Kim MK, Joo MC, Shin SH. Nonlinear analysis of heart rate variability during Qi therapy (external Qigong). Am J Chin Med 2005; 33(4):579-88.

Lee M, Koo M. Is tai chi exercise programme beneficial for patients with coronary artery disease? Focus on Alternative & Complementary Therapies 2011; 16(1):60-1.

Leininger P. Physical and psychological effects of yoga exercise on healthy community-dwelling older adult women. Temple University, 2006.

Leung RW, Alison JA, McKeough ZJ, Peters MJ. A study design to investigate the effect of short-form Sun-style Tai Chi in improving functional exercise capacity, physical performance, balance and health related quality of life in people with Chronic Obstructive Pulmonary Disease (COPD). Contemp Clin Trials 2011; 32(2):267-72.

Li F, Duncan TE, Duncan SC, McAuley E, Chaumeton NR, Harmer P. Enhancing the psychological well-being of elderly individuals through Tai Chi exercise: A latent growth curve analysis. [References]. Structural Equation Modeling 2001; 8(1):53-83.

Li F, Harmer P, Chaumeton N, Duncan T, Duncan S. Tai Chi as a means to enhance self-esteem: a randomized controlled trial. Journal of Applied Gerontology 2002; 21(1):70-89.

Li F, Harmer P, Fisher KJ et al. Tai Chi and fall reductions in older adults: a randomized controlled trial. J Gerontol A Biol Sci Med Sci 2005; 60(2):187-94.

Li JP. [Effect of 'QiGong' on plasma norepinephrine and serotonin in patients with essential hypertension]. Chinese Journal of Sports Medicine 1993; 12(3):152-6.

Li JX, Xu DQ, Hong Y. Effects of 16-week Tai Chi intervention on postural stability and proprioception of knee and ankle in older people. Age Ageing 2008; 37(5):575-8.

Li M, Chen K, Mo Z. Use of qigong therapy in the detoxification of heroin addicts. Altern Ther Health Med 2002; 8(1):50-4, 56-9.

Li W, Pi DR, Xing ZH et al . The clinical observation on the effect of Qigong in treating patients with hypertension caused by liver-yang hyperactivity and Yang hyperactivity-Yin deficiency. Zhong Xi Yi Jie He Za Zhi = Chinese Journal of Modern Developments in Traditional Medicine/Zhongguo Zhong Xi Yi Jie Yan Jiu Hui (Chou), Zhong Yi Yan Jiu Yuan, Zhu Ban 1989; 9(1):34-5.

Li W, Xin Z, Pi D. [Effect of qigong on sympathetico-adrenomedullary function in patients with liver yang exuberance hypertension]. Zhong Xi Yi Jie He Za Zhi 1990; 10(5):283-5, 261.

Li W, Xing Z, Pi D, Li X. [Influence of qi-gong on plasma TXB2 and 6-keto-PGF1 alpha in two TCM types of essential hypertension]. Hunan Yi Ke Da Xue Xue Bao 1997; 22(6):497-9.

Li W, Xing Z, Pi D, Wu Y. The efficacy of Qigong training in patients with various TCM types of hypertension. 1996; 21(2):123-6.

Liem T. Osteopathy and Hatha Yoga: Osteopathie und (Hatha-)Yoga. 2009; 10(1):21-7.

Lin YG. [Effects of the skin potential activity and respiratory movement in the practice of Qi-Gong in different postures]. Zhong Xi Yi Jie He Za Zhi 1983; 3(5):304-6.

Linder K, Svardsudd K. [Qigong has a relieving effect on stress]. Lakartidningen 2006; 103(24-25):1942-5.

Liu C, Yang K-Y, Chen W-C, Shiang T-Y, Chuang L-R. Effects of Tai Chi Chuan combined with vibration training on the reflex activity of peripheral neuron. 2011; 26(4):329-34.

Liu J, Li B, Shnider R. Effects of Tai Chi Training on Improving Physical Function in Patients With Coronary Heart Diseases. 2010; 8(2):78-84.

Liu X, Miller YD, Burton NW, Brown WJ. Changes in mechanical loading lead to tendonspecific alterations in MMP and TIMP expression: Influence of stress deprivation and intermittent cyclic hydrostatic compression on rat supraspinatus and Achilles tendons. 2010; 44(10):704-9.

Liu X-D. Effect of 8-week Tai Chi Chuan on immune function of older people. 2006; 10(27):10-2.

Liu YS. Analysis on the therapeutic effect of ulcerative colitis treated with electroacupuncture plus qigong. [World Journal of Acupuncture-Moxibustion]: World J Acup-Moxi: Shi Jie Zhen Jiu Za Zhi 1998; 8(1):3-8.

Liu YS. Analysis of the curative effect of electroacupuncture plus qigong on ulcerative colonitis. J Acu Tuina Sci 2003; 1(2):23.

Lo RSK, Hui EST, Cheng JOY, Cheng HKT. Benefits of Tai Chi in palliative care for advanced cancer patients [3]. 2008; 22(1):93-4.

Logghe IH, Verhagen AP, Rademaker AC et al. Explaining the ineffectiveness of a Tai Chi fall prevention training for community-living older people: a process evaluation alongside a randomized clinical trial (RCT). Arch Gerontol Geriatr 2011; 52(3):357-62.

Lu C, Wang B. A study on effects of aerobics combined with yoga exercise on physical training. 2007; 22(10):885-7.

Lu WA, Kuo CD. Comparison of the effects of Tai Chi Chuan and Wai Tan Kung exercises on autonomic nervous system modulation and on hemodynamics in elder adults. Am J Chin Med 2006; 34(6):959-68.

Lu X, Wang B, Lee Y, Hui-Chan CWY. The effect of sitting Tai Chi on eye-hand coordination in frail older adults|. 2009; 24(3):236-9.

Lu ZC. [Comparative study on the therapeutic effects of a breathing exercise (qigong), jogging and drug therapy on essential hypertension]. Zhong Xi Yi Jie He Za Zhi 1987; 7(8):462-4, 452.

Lundgren T, Dahl J, Yardi N, Melin L. Acceptance and Commitment Therapy and yoga for drug-refractory epilepsy: a randomized controlled trial. Epilepsy Behav 2008; 13(1):102-8.

Lv ZC, Yu HP, Liu JW, Mo GM, Zhang YW. [Controlled study of qigong, jogging and drug therapy on essential hypertension]. Zhong Xi Yi Jie He Za Zhi = Chinese Journal of Modern Developments in Traditional Medicine / Zhongguo Zhong Xi Yi Jie He Yan Jiu Hui (Chou), Zhong Yi Yan Jiu Yuan, Zhu Ban 1987; 7(8):462-4.

Lv Zengchun, Yu Huapei, Liu Jingwen, Mo Guomeng, Zhang Yuwen. The comparative analysis of Qigong, jogging and medical therapy. Zhong Xi Yi Jie He Za Zhi = Chinese Journal of Modern Developments in Traditional Medicine / Zhongguo Zhong Xi Yi Jie He Yan Jiu Hui (Chou), Zhong Yi Yan Jiu Yuan, Zhu Ban 1987; 7(8):462-4.

Macfarlane D, Chou K, Cheng W. Effects of Tai Chi on the physical and psychological well-being of Chinese older women. Journal of Exercise Science & Fitness 2005; 3(2):87-94.

Madhavi S, Raju PS, Reddy MV et al. Effect of yogic exercises on lean body mass. J Assoc Physicians India 1985; 33(7):465-6.

Malathi A, Damodaran A, Shah N, Krishnamurthy G, Namjoshi P, Ghodke S. Psychophysiological changes at the time of examination in medical students before and after the practice of yoga and relaxation. Indian J Psychiatry 1998; 40(1):35-40.

Manjunath NK, Telles S. Influence of yoga & ayurveda on self-rated sleep in a geriatric population. Indian Journal of Medical Research 2005; 121:683-90.

Manjunath NK, Telles S. Effects of Yoga and an Ayurveda preparation on gait, balance and mobility in older persons. 2007; 13(12):LE19-LE20.

Manjunath NK, Telles S. Pulmonary functions following yoga in a community dwelling geriatric population in India. Journal of Indian Psychology 2006; 24(1-2):44-51.

Manocha R. Sahaja yoga in asthma [2]. 2003; 58(9):825-6.

Mao H-N, Sha P. Effect of Tai Chi exercise on blood pressure, plasma nitrogen monoxidum and endothelin in hypertensive patients. 2006; 10(48):65-7.

Marc I. Integrative approach for tinnitus: Potential for qigong. Focus on Alternative and Complementary Therapies 2011; (16 1):58.

Marc I, Langguth B, Biesinger E. Integrative approach for tinnitus: potential for qigong. Focus on Alternative & Complementary Therapies 2011; 16(1):58-9.

Mathuna D. Tai chi for fall prevention among the elderly. Alternative Therapies in Women's Health 2005; 7(5):33-6.

McGibbon CA, Krebs DE, Parker SW, Scarborough DM, Wayne PM, Wolf SL. Tai Chi and vestibular rehabilitation improve vestibulopathic gait via different neuromuscular mechanisms: preliminary report. BMC Neurol 2005; 5(1):3.

McGibbon CA, Krebs DE, Wolf SL, Wayne PM, Scarborough DM, Parker SW. Tai Chi and vestibular rehabilitation effects on gaze and whole-body stability. J Vestib Res 2004; 14(6):467-78.

McIver S. Yoga may help manage binge eating disorder. Focus on Alternative and Complementary Therapies 2010; 15(1):43-4.

Mihay L, Iltzsche E, Tribby A et al. Balance and perceived confidence with performance of instrumental activities of daily living: a pilot study of Tai Chi inspired exercise with elderly retirement-community dwellers. Physical & Occupational Therapy in Geriatrics 2003; 21(3):75-86.

Mihay L, Boggs K, Breck A, Dokken E, NaThalang G. The effect of Tai Chi inspired exercise compared to strength training: a pilot study. Physical & Occupational Therapy in Geriatrics 2006; 24(3):13-26.

Miles Wr. Oxygen Consumption During Three Yoga-Type Breathing Patterns. J Appl Physiol 1964; 19:75-82.

Mitchell KS, Mazzeo SE, Rausch SM, Cooke KL. Innovative interventions for disordered eating: evaluating dissonance-based and yoga interventions. Int J Eat Disord 2007; 40(2):120-8.

Mo FF, Yan RF. [A study of QiGong on aged microcirculation disability]. Chinese Journal of Geriatrics 1990; 9(2):108-.

Moadel A B, Shah C, Patel S et al. Randomized controlled trial of yoga for symptom management during breast cancer treatment [abstract]. Proceedings of the American Society of Clinical Oncology 2003; 726.

Moegling K. How Tai Chi Chuan influences health: some observations and results [German]. Krankengymnastik 1997; 49(6):950-8.

Mollo K, Schaaf R, Benevides T. The use of kripalu yoga to decrease sensory overresponsivity: a pilot study. Sensory Integration Special Interest Section Quarterly 2008; 31(3):1-4.

Monro R, Power J, Coumar A, Nagarathna R, Dandona P. Yoga therapy for NIDDM: A controlled trial. 1992; 6(2):66-8.

Morris DM. An evaluation of yoga for the reduction of fall risk factors in older adults. 2008.

Motajova J, Vicenik K. Effect of hatha yoga on heart activity in exercising women. ACT. NERV. SUPER. 1980; 22(2):125-6.

Mourya M, Mahajan AS, Singh NP, Jain AK. Effect of slow- and fast-breathing exercises on autonomic functions in patients with essential hypertension. J Altern Complement Med 2009; 15(7):711-7.

Muralidhara DV, Ranganathan KV. Effect of yoga practice on Cardiac Recovery Index. Indian J Physiol Pharmacol 1982; 26(4):279-83.

Mustian KM, Katula JA, Roscoe J, Morrow G. The influence of Tai Chi (TC) and support therapy (ST) on fatigue and quality of life (QOL) in women with breast cancer (BC) [abstract]. Annual Meeting Proceedings of the American Society of Clinical Oncology 2004; 760.

Mustian KM, Katula JA, Zhao H. A pilot study to assess the influence of tai chi chuan on functional capacity among breast cancer survivors. J Support Oncol 2006; 4(3):139-45.

Mustian KM, Palesh OG, Flecksteiner SA. Tai Chi Chuan for breast cancer survivors. Med Sport Sci 2008; 52:209-17.

Naruka JS, Mathur R, Mathur A. Effect of pranayama practices on fasting blood glucose and serum cholesterol. Indian J Med Sci 1986; 40(6):149-52.

Nau JY. [Heart and tai chi; Viagra and mountaineering]. Rev Med Suisse 2011; 7(294):1058-9.

Naveen KV, Telles S. Yoga and psychosis: Risks and therapeutic potential. Journal of Indian Psychology 2003; 21(1):34-7.

Nespor K. The combination of psychiatric treatment and yoga. Int J Psychosom 1985; 32(2):24-7.

Ng BHP. Effect of Qigong on physical and psychosocial status of Chinese COPD patients: a randomized controlled trial [Dissertation]. Hong Kong Polytechnic University (Hong Kong) 2010; 135 p.

Niranjan M, Bhagyalakshmi K, Ganaraja B, Adhikari P, Bhat R. Effects of yoga and supervised integrated exercise on heart rate variability and blood pressure in hypertensive patients. 2009; 4(3):139-43.

Nnodim JO, Strasburg D, Nabozny M et al. Dynamic balance and stepping versus tai chi training to improve balance and stepping in at-risk older adults. J Am Geriatr Soc 2006; 54(12):1825-31.

Nowakowska C, Fellmann B, Pasek T, Hauser J, Sluzewska A. [Evaluation of the effect of relaxation and concentration exercises based on yoga on patients with psychogenic mental disorders]. Psychiatr Pol 1982; 16(5-6):365-70.

O'Grady M, Wolf SL, Barnhart HX, Kutner N, McNeely E. Tai Chi effect on falls in frail older adults [abstract]. Archives of Physical Medicine and Rehabilitation 1997; 78:1028.

Oh B, Butow P, Mullan B, Clarke SJ, Beale P, Rosenthal D. Randomized clinical trial: The Impact of Medical Qigong (traditional Chinese medicine) on fatique, quality of life, side effects, mood status and inlfammation of cancer patients [abstarct no. 9565]. Journal of Clinical Oncology: ASCO Annual Meeting Proceedings 2008; 26(15S part I):518.

Oh B, Butow PN, Mullan BA et al. Effect of medical Qigong on cognitive function, quality of life, and a biomarker of inflammation in cancer patients: a randomized controlled trial. 2011:1-8.

Okoli U, Dehaney M, Hillman A, Robinson M. Can we get away with anything less? Evaluating health promotion interventions: A Tai Chi exercise programme for older people. 2002; 4(1):10-3.

Orr R, Tsang T, Lam P, Comino E, Singh MF. Mobility impairment in type 2 diabetes: association with muscle power and effect of Tai Chi intervention. Diabetes Care 2006; 29(9):2120-2.

Osteras N, Fongen C. Tai Chi reduces pain and improves physical function for people with knee OA. J Physiother 2010; 56(1):57.

Pages Bolibar E, Climent Barbera J, Iborra Urios J, Rodriguez-Pinero Duran M, Pena Arrebola A. Tai Chi, falls and osteoporosis [Spanish]. Rehabilitacion 2005; 39(5):230-45.

Pal A, Srivastava N, Tiwari S et al. Effect of yogic practices on lipid profile and body fat composition in patients of coronary artery disease. Complement Ther Med 2011; 19(3):122-7.

Palta A. Sahajayoga and quality of life: An empirical study. Journal of Indian Psychology 2009; 27(1-2):21-34.

Panjwani U, Gupta HL, Singh SH, Selvamurthy W, Rai UC. Effect of Sahaja yoga practice on stress management in patients of epilepsy. Indian J Physiol Pharmacol 1995; 39(2):111-6.

Panjwani U, Selvamurthy W, Singh SH, Gupta HL, Thakur L, Rai UC. Effect of Sahaja yoga practice on seizure control & EEG changes in patients of epilepsy. Indian J Med Res 1996; 103:165-72.

Patel C. Yoga and biofeedback in the management of 'stress' in hypertensive patients. Clin Sci Mol Med Suppl 1975; 2:171s-4s.

Paterna AA. The effectiveness of a recreational modality (Tai Chi Chuan) in enhancing health status in an older adult population. 2003; 124.

Patra S, Telles S. Positive impact of cyclic meditation on subsequent sleep. Med Sci Monit 2009; 15(7):CR375-81.

Peng Y, He S, Zhang X, Liu G, Xie J. [Effects of hypoxia and qigong on urine malondialdehyde, superoxide dismutase and circulating endothelial cell in humans during simulated weightlessness]. Space Med Med Eng (Beijing) 1998; 11(2):136-8.

Pereira MM, de Oliveira RJ, Silva MAF, Souza LHR, Vianna LG. Effects of Tai Chi Chuan on knee extensor muscle strength and balance in elderly women. 2008; 12(2):121-6.

Phoosuwan M, Kritpet T, Yuktanandana P. The effects of weight bearing yoga training on the bone resorption markers of the postmenopausal women. J Med Assoc Thai 2009; 92 Suppl5:S102-8.

Pierce S, Rakel D. Is therapeutic yoga helpful for chronic low back pain? Evidence-Based Practice 2010; 13(8):4.

Posadzki P. Tai chi/qigong improves selected indicators of metabolic syndrome, QoL, depression and perceived stress. Focus Altern. Complement. Ther. 2011; 16(2):161-2.

Price A, Meah M, O'Shaughnessy T. A pilot study to compare qiqong exercises with conventional exercises in pulmonary rehabilitation [Abstract]. Thorax 2006; 61(Suppl 2):ii67 [P032].

Pullen PR, Nagamia SH, Mehta PK et al. Effects of yoga on inflammation and exercise capacity in patients with chronic heart failure. J Card Fail 2008; 14(5):407-13.

Pullen PR. The benefits of yoga therapy for heart failure patients. Georgia State University, 2009.

Raghavendra RM, Ajaikumar BS, Patil S et al. Effects of pretreatment, pharmacologic factors, and yoga intervention on CINV outcomes in breast cancer [abstract no. 9599]. Journal of Clinical Oncology: ASCO Annual Meeting Proceedings 2008; 26:526.

Raghuraj P, Telles S. Improvement in spatial and temporal measures of visual perception following yoga training. Journal of Indian Psychology 2002; 20(1):23-31.

Rahnama N, Namazizadeh M, Etemadifar M, Bambaeichi E, Arbabzadeh S, Sadeghipour HR. Effects of yoga on depression in women with multiple sclerosis. 2011; 29(136).

Raina N, Chakraborty PK, Basit MA, Samarth SN, Singh H. Evaluation of yoga therapy in alcohol dependence syndrome. Indian Journal of Psychiatry 2001; 43(2).

Raju PS, Madhavi S, Prasad KV et al. Comparison of effects of yoga & physical exercise in athletes. Indian J Med Res 1994; 100:81-6.

Rakhshaee Z. Effect of Three Yoga Poses (Cobra, Cat and Fish Poses) in Women with Primary Dysmenorrhea: A Randomized Clinical Trial.

Rakhshani A, Maharana S, Raghuram N, Nagendra HR, Venkatram P. Effects of integrated yoga on quality of life and interpersonal relationship of pregnant women. Qual Life Res 2010; 19(10):1447-55.

Rani K, Tiwari S, Singh U, Agrawal G, Ghildiyal A, Srivastava N. Impact of Yoga Nidra on psychological general wellbeing in patients with menstrual irregularities: A randomized controlled trial. Int J Yoga 2011; 4(1):20-5.

Rani NJ. Impact of yoga training on triguna and self-ideal disparity. Psychological Studies 2007; 52(2):174-7.

Rani NJ, Rao PVK. Body awareness and yoga training. Perceptual and Motor Skills 1994; 79(3, Pt 1):1103-6.

Ranjbar F, Hemmati L, Rezaei S. The effects of yoga in women with generalized anxiety disorder [conference abstract]. European Psychiatry [Abstracts of the 19th European Congress of Psychiatry, EPA 2011 Vienna Austria. Conference Start: 20110312 Conference End: 20110315] 2011.

Rao AV, Krishna DR, Ramanakar TV, Prabhakar MC. Jala Neti' a yoga technique for nasal comfort and hygiene in leprosy patients. Lepr India 1982; 54(4):691-4.

Rao RM, Nagendra HR, Raghuram N et al. Influence of yoga on postoperative outcomes and wound healing in early operable breast cancer patients undergoing surgery. Int J Yoga 2008; 1(1):33-41.

Rao RM, Telles S, Nagendra HR et al. Effects of yoga on natural killer cell counts in early breast cancer patients undergoing conventional treatment. 2008; 14(2):LE3-LE4.

Ray US, Hegde KS, Selvamurthy W. Improvement in muscular efficiency as related to a standard task after yogic exercises in middle aged men. Indian J Med Res 1986; 83:343-8.

Ray US, Mukhopadhyaya S, Purkayastha SS et al. Effect of yogic exercises on physical and mental health of young fellowship course trainees. Indian J Physiol Pharmacol 2001; 45(1):37-53.

Razumov AN, Namsaraeva GT, Frolkov VK. [Some physiological aspects of the mechanism of action of traditional health-improving methods (Cigun, Indian, and Tibetan Yoga)]. Vopr Kurortol Fizioter Lech Fiz Kult 2008; (4):55-9.

Rendant D, Pach D, Ludtke R, Reisshauer A, Willich S, Witt CM. Qigong versus exercise versus no therapy for patients with chronic neck pain - a randomized controlled trial. Spine 2010; 36(6):419-27.

Ritter C, Aldridge D. Qigong Yangsheng as a therapeutic approach for the treatment of essential hypertension in comparison with a western muscle relaxation therapy: A randomised, controlled pilot study: Qigong Yangsheng in der anwendung bei essentieller hypertonie im vergleich mit einer westlichen muskelentspannungstherapie: Eine randomisierte, kontrollierte pilotstudie. 2001; 16(2):48-63.

Ritter C, Aldridge D. Qigong Yangsheng as a therapeutic approach for the treatment of essential hypertension in comparison with a western muscle relaxation therapy: A randomised, controlled pilot study. Chinesische Medizin 2001; 16(2):48-63.

Robertshawe P. A comparative trial of yoga and relaxation to reduce stress and anxiety. Journal of the Australian Traditional-Medicine Society 2007; 13(4):225.

Robertshawe P. Glutathione and total antioxidant status improved with yoga. Journal of the Australian Traditional-Medicine Society 2008; 14(1):29.

Robertshawe P. Effects of yoga on maternal comfort, labour pain and birth outcomes. Journal of the Australian Traditional-Medicine Society 2009; 15(2):81.

Rogers CE, Keller C, Larkey LK, Ainsworth BE. A Randomized Controlled Trial to Determine the Efficacy of Sign Chi Do Exercise on Adaptation to Aging. Res Gerontol Nurs 2011; 1-13.

Rohini V, Pandey RS, Janakiramaiah N, Gangadhar BN, Vedamurthachar A. A comparative study of full and partial Sudarshan Kriya Yoga (SKY) in major depressive disorder. NIMHANS Journal 2000; 18(1-2):53-7.

Rubenfire M. [Commentary on] Effects of tai chi mind-body movement therapy on functional status and exercise capacity in patients with chronic heart failure: a randomized controlled trial. ACC Current Journal Review 2005; 14(2):35.

Ryu H, Jun CD, Lee BS, Choi BM, Kim HM, Chung HT. Effect of qigong training on proportions of T lymphocyte subsets in human peripheral blood. Am J Chin Med 1995; 23(1):27-36.

Ryu H, Mo HY, Mo GD et al. Delayed cutaneous hypersensitivity reactions in Qigong (chun do sun bup) trainees by multitest cell mediated immunity. Am J Chin Med 1995; 23(2):139-44.

Sahasi G, Mohan D, Kacker C. Effectiveness of yogic techniques in the management of anxiety. Journal of Personality and Clinical Studies 1989; 5(1):51-5.

Sahay BK, Sadasivudu B, Yogi R et al. Biochemical parameters in normal volunteers before and after yogic practices. Indian J Med Res 1982; 76 Suppl:144-8.

Sanglier I, Sarazin M, Zinetti J. [Tai Chi, body and cognitive rehabilitation of Alzheimer's and related diseases]. Soins 2004; (685):42-3.

Santana JS, Almeida AP, Brandao PM. [The effect of Ai Chi method in fibromyalgic patients]. Cien Saude Colet 2010; 15 Suppl 1:1433-8.

Sareen S, Kumari V, Gajebasia KS, Gajebasia NK. Yoga: a tool for improving the quality of life in chronic pancreatitis. World J Gastroenterol 2007; 13(3):391-7.

Sathyaprabha TN, Satishchandra P, Pradhan C et al. Modulation of cardiac autonomic balance with adjuvant yoga therapy in patients with refractory epilepsy. Epilepsy Behav 2008; 12(2):245-52.

Sattin RW, Easley KA, Wolf SL, Chen Y, Kutner MH. Reduction in fear of falling through intense tai chi exercise training in older, transitionally frail adults. J Am Geriatr Soc 2005; 53(7):1168-78.

Satyanarayanamurthi Gv, Sastry Pb. A preliminary scientific investigation into some of the unusual physiological manifestations acquired as a result of yogic practices in India. Wien Z Nervenheilkd Grenzgeb 1958; 15(1-4):239-49.

Schell EJ, Allolio B, Schonecke OW. Physiological and psychological effects of Hatha-yoga exercise in health women. 1994; 41(1-4):46-52.

Selfridge N. From padasana to pain relief: Iyengar yoga for chronic low back pain. 2010; 13(1):9-11.

Selvamurthy W, Sridharan K, Ray US et al. A new physiological approach to control essential hypertension. Indian J Physiol Pharmacol 1998; 42(2):205-13.

Shaffer HJ, LaSalvia TA, Stein JP. Comparing Hatha yoga with dynamic group psychotherapy for enhancing methadone maintenance treatment: a randomized clinical trial. Altern Ther Health Med 1997; 3(4):57-66.

Shannahoff-Khalsa D. Kundalini yoga meditation for the treatment of OCD. 156th Annual Meeting of the American Psychiatric Association, May 17-22, San Francisco CA 2003.

Shannahoff-Khalsa D. Kundalini yoga meditation techniques for psychiatric disorders. 157th Annual Meeting of the American Psychiatric Association; 2004 May 1-6; New York, NY 2004.

Sharma I, Azmi SA, Settiwar RM. Evaluation of the effect of pranayama in anxiety state. Alternative Medicine 1991; 3(4):227-35.

Sharma VK, Das S, Mondal S, Goswami U. Comparative effect of Sahaj Yoga on EEG in patients of major depression and healthy subjects. 2007; 27(3):95-9.

Sharma VK, Das S, Mondal S, Goswampi U, Gandhi A. Effect of Sahaj Yoga on depressive disorders. Indian J Physiol Pharmacol 2005; 49(4):462-8.

Shen C-L, Chyu M-C, Yeh JK et al. Effect of green tea and Tai Chi on bone health in postmenopausal osteopenic women: a 6-month randomized placebo-controlled trial. 2011:1-12.

Sherman KJ, Cherkin DC, Erro J, Miglioretti DL, Deyo RA. Comparing yoga, exercise, and a self-care book for chronic low back pain: a randomized, controlled trial. Ann Intern Med 2005; 143(12):849-56.

Sherman K. Does tai chi chuan improve balance in less robust elderly? Focus on Alternative & Complementary Therapies 2006; 11(1):54-5.

Spicuzza L, Gabutti A, Porta C, Montano N, Bernardi L. Yoga and chemoreflex response to hypoxia and hypercapnia Lancet 2000 Nov 4;356(9241):1612. Lancet 2000; 356(9240):1495-6.

Sridevi K, Krishna Rao PV. Yoga practice and menstrual distress. Journal of the Indian Academy of Applied Psychology 1996; 22(1-2):47-54.

Sridevi K, Sitamma M, Krishna Rao PV. Perceptual organisation and yoga training. Journal of Indian Psychology 1995; 13(2):21-7.

Stenlund T, Ahlgren C, Lindahl B et al. Cognitively oriented behavioral rehabilitation in combination with Qigong for patients on long-term sick leave because of burnout: REST randomized clinical trial. International Journal of Behavioral Medicine 2009; 16(3):294-303.

Stevinson C. Preliminary results suggest that yoga can alleviate depression. Focus on Alternative & Complementary Therapies 2001; 6(1):27-8.

Stevinson C. Inconclusive trial on yoga for anxiety among breast cancer patients: Commentary. Focus Altern. Complement. Ther. 2009; 14(2):123-4.

Straus S. A 16-week tai chi programme prevented falls in healthy older adults. Evid Based Med 2008; 13(2):54.

Streeter CC, Whitfield TH, Owen L et al. Effects of yoga versus walking on mood, anxiety, and brain GABA levels: a randomized controlled MRS study. J Altern Complement Med 2010; 16(11):1145-52.

Streeter CC, Whitfield TH, Rein T, Ciraulo DA, Renshaw PF, Jensen E. Correlations between mood and brain gaba levels after yoga and walking. 163rd Annual Meeting of the American Psychiatric Association; 2010 May 22-26; New Orleans, LA 2010.

Suksom D, Siripatt A, Lapo P, Patumraj S. Effects of two modes of exercise on physical fitness and endothelial function in the elderly: exercise with a flexible stick versus Tai Chi. J Med Assoc Thai 2011; 94(1):123-32.

Sun G-C, Lovejoy J, Bradley R, Putiri A, Gillham S. Qigong therapy vs progressive resistance exercise in patients with type 2 diabetes: A pilot study. FASEB J. 2009; 23(S1).

Sun WY, Dosch M, Gilmore GD, Pemberton W, Scarseth T. Effects of a Tai Chi Chuan program on Hmong American older adults. Educational Gerontology 1996; 22(2):161-7.

Sundar S, Agrawal SK, Singh VP, Bhattacharya SK, Udupa KN, Vaish SK. Role of yoga in management of essential hypertension. Acta Cardiol 1984; 39(3):203-8.

Szabo A, Mesko A, Caputo A, Gill T. Examination of exercise-induced feeling states in four modes of exercise. International Journal of Sport Psychology 1998; 29(4):376-90.

Taboonpong S, Puthsri N, Kong-In W, Saejew A. The effects of Tai Chi on sleep quality, well-being and physical performances among older adults. Thai Journal of Nursing Research 2008; 12(1):1-13.

Taylor-Piliae RE, Newell KA, Cherin R, Lee MJ, King AC, Haskell WL. Effects of Tai Chi and Western exercise on physical and cognitive functioning in healthy community-dwelling older adults. J Aging Phys Act 2010; 18(3):261-79.

Telles S, Balkrishna A. Yoga and diet change influence renal functions in the obese. Med Sci Monit 2010; 16(10):LE15.

Telles S, Balkrishna A, Maharana K. Effect of yoga and ayurveda on duchenne muscular dystrophy. Indian J Palliat Care 2011; 17(2):169-70.

Telles S, Hanumanthaiah BH, Nagarathna R, Nagendra HR. Plasticity of motor control systems demonstrated by yoga training. Indian J Physiol Pharmacol 1994; 38(2):143-4.

Telles S, Joshi M, Dash M, Raghuraj P, Naveen KV, Nagendra HR. An evaluation of the ability to voluntarily reduce the heart rate after a month of yoga practice. Integr Physiol Behav Sci 2004; 39(2):119-25.

Telles S, Maharana K, Balrana B, Balkrishna A. Effects of high-frequency yoga breathing called kapalabhati compared with breath awareness on the degree of optical illusion perceived. Percept Mot Skills 2011; 112(3):981-90.

Telles S, Nagarathna R, Vani PR, Nagendra HR. A combination of focusing and defocusing through yoga reduces optical illusion more than focusing alone. Indian J Physiol Pharmacol 1997; 41(2):179-82.

Telles S, Praghuraj P, Ghosh A, Nagendra HR. Effect of a one-month yoga training program on performance in a mirror-tracing task. Indian J Physiol Pharmacol 2006; 50(2):187-90.

Telles S, Singh N. High frequency yoga breathing increases energy -expenditure from carbohydrates. Comment to: Assessment of sleep patterns, energy expenditure and circadian rhythms of skin temperature in patients with acute coronary syndrome Hadil Al Otair, Mustafa Al-shamiri, Mohammed Bahobail, Munir M. Sharif, Ahmed S. BaHammam Med Sci Monit, 2011; 17(7): CR397-403. Med Sci Monit 2011; 17(9):LE7-8.

Telles S, Nagarathna R, Nagendra HR. Improvement in visual perception following yoga training. Journal of Indian Psychology 1995; 13(1):30-2.

Thomas GN, Hong AW, Tomlinson B et al. Effects of Tai Chi and resistance training on cardiovascular risk factors in elderly Chinese subjects: a 12-month longitudinal, randomized, controlled intervention study. Clin Endocrinol (Oxf) 2005; 63(6):663-9.

Thomas M, Sadlier M, Smith A. A multiconvergent approach to the rehabilitation of patients with chronic fatigue syndrome: a comparative study. Physiotherapy 2008; 94(1):35-42.

Toise S, Sears SF, Schoenfeld MH et al. The efficacy of adapted yoga in managing anxiety and depression in implantable cardioverter defibrillator (ICD) patients [conference abstract]. Heart Rhythm [Abstracts From the 32nd Annual Scientific Sessions of the Heart Rhythm Society, Heart Rhythm San Francisco, CA United States. May 4-7 2011] 2011.

Tsai P. RIG sponsored biobehavioral symposium: use of Tai Chi to reduce cognitive deficits in elders -- a pilot study. Southern Online Journal of Nursing Research 2008; 8(2):2p.

Tsang T, Orr R, Lam P, Comino E, Singh MF. Effects of Tai Chi on glucose homeostasis and insulin sensitivity in older adults with type 2 diabetes: a randomised double-blind sham-exercise-controlled trial. Age Ageing 2008; 37(1):64-71.

Tsang WW, Hui-Chan CW. Effect of 4- and 8-wk intensive Tai Chi Training on balance control in the elderly. Med Sci Sports Exerc 2004; 36(4):648-57.

Udani JK, Ofman JJ. Tai Chi for the prevention of falls in the elderly. 1998; 1(4):167-9.

Udupa KN, Singh RH, Settiwar RM. A comparative study on the effect of some individual yogic practices in normal persons. Indian J Med Res 1975; 63(8):1066-71.

Udupa KN, Singh RH, Settiwar RM. Studies on the effect of some yogic breathing exercises (Pranayams) in normal persons. Indian J Med Res 1975; 63(8):1062-5.

Vadiraja HS, Raghavendra RM. Effects of a yoga program on cortisol rhythm and mood states in early breast cancer patients undergoing adjuvant radiotherapy: A randomized controlled trial (Integrative Cancer Therapies (2009) 8, 1, (37-46) DOI: 10.1177/1534735409331456). 2009; 8(2):195.

van Montfrans GA, Karemaker JM, Wieling W, Dunning AJ. Relaxation therapy and continuous ambulatory blood pressure in mild hypertension: a controlled study. BMJ 1990; 300(6736):1368-72.

Van Puymbroeck M, Payne LL, Hsieh PC. A phase I feasibility study of yoga on the physical health and coping of informal caregivers. Evid Based Complement Alternat Med 2007; 4(4):519-29.

Vancampfort D, De Hert M, Knapen J et al. State anxiety, psychological stress and positive well-being responses to yoga and aerobic exercise in people with schizophrenia: a pilot study. Disabil Rehabil 2011; 33(8):684-9.

Vedamurthachar A, Janakiramaiah N, Hegde JM et al. Antidepressant efficacy and hormonal effects of Sudarshana Kriya Yoga (SKY) in alcohol dependent individuals. J Affect Disord 2006; 94(1-3):249-53.

Vedanthan PK. Clinical study of yoga techniques in university students with asthma: A controlled study. 1998; 19(1):3-9.

Verma K K, Varstala V, Kytokorpi L, Telama R. The effects of a three-week hatha yoga programme on the reduction of anxiety level and neck and shoulder pain. Liikunnan Ja Kansanterveyden Julkaisuja 1990; (67):229.

Vijayalakshmi S, Satyanarayana M, Krishna Rao PV, Prakash V. Combined effect of yoga and psychotherapy on management of asthma: A preliminary study. Journal of Indian Psychology 1988; 7(2):32-9.

Visceglia E, Lewis S. Yoga therapy as an adjunctive treatment for schizophrenia: a randomized, controlled pilot study. J Altern Complement Med 2011; 17(7):601-7.

von Trott P, Wiedemann AM, Ludtke R, Reishauer A, Willich SN, Witt CM. Qigong and exercise therapy for elderly patients with chronic neck pain (QIBANE): a randomized controlled study. J Pain 2009; 10(5):501-8.

Voukelatos A, Cumming RG, Lord SR, Rissel C. A randomized, controlled trial of tai chi for the prevention of falls: the Central Sydney tai chi trial. J Am Geriatr Soc 2007; 55(8):1185-91.

Wallsten S, Bintrim K, Denman D, Parrish J, Hughes G. The effect of Tai Chi Chuan on confidence and lower extremity strength and balance in residents living independently at a continuing care retirement community. Journal of Applied Gerontology 2006; 25(1):82-95.

Wang C. Tai Chi improves pain and functional status in adults with rheumatoid arthritis: results of a pilot single-blinded randomized controlled trial. Med Sport Sci 2008; 52:218-29.

Wang C, Xu D, Qian Y. Medical and health care Qigong (Qu Bing Yang Sheng Gong). J Tradit Chin Med 1991; 11(4):296-301, contd.

Wang CX, Xu DH. [Influence of qigong therapy upon serum HDL-C in hypertensive patients]. Zhong Xi Yi Jie He Za Zhi 1989; 9(9):543-4, 516.

Wang CX, Xu DH. [The beneficial effect of qigong on the ventricular function and microcirculation in deficiency of heart-energy hypertensive patients]. Zhong Xi Yi Jie He Za Zhi 1991; 11(11):659-60, 644.

Wang CX, Xu DH, Qian YS, Zhao GS, Kuang AK. The influence of qigong therapy upon serum HDL-C of hypertensive patients. Zhong Xi Yi Jie He Za Zhi = Chinese Journal of Modern Developments in Traditional Medicine / Zhongguo Zhong Xi Yi Jie He Yan Jiu Hui (Chou), Zhong Yi Yan Jiu Yuan, Zhu Ban 1989; 9(9):543-4.

Wang CX, You CY. [The efficacy of qigong (breathing exercise) and antihypertensive drug therapy in 426 hypertensive patients and changes in plasma dopamine-beta-hydroxylase activity]. Zhong Xi Yi Jie He Za Zhi 1982; 2(4):195, 218-9.

Wang CX XDQYSW. Observation on the effect of QiGong on Serum Apolipoprotein in patients with Hypertension. Shanghai Journal of Traditional Chinese Medicine (Shang Hai Zhong Yi Yao Za Zhi) 1993; 39(5):22-3.

Wang M-Y, An L-G. Effects of 12 weeks' tai chi chuan practice on the immune function of female college students who lack physical exercise. 2011; 28(1):45-9.

Wang W, Sawada M, Noriyama Y, Arita K, Ota T, Kishimoto T. Effects of Qigong in Tai Chi in the elderly using General Health Questionnaire (GHQ). 2009; 60(5-6):159-65.

Wayne P, McGibbon C, Scarborough D et al. Tai chi improves dynamic postural stability in patients with vestibular disease: results of a randomized trial. Journal of Alternative & Complementary Medicine 2006; 12(2):214.

Wiholm C, Arnetz B. Stress management and musculoskeletal disorders in knowledge workers: The possible mediating effects of stress hormones. 2006; 8(1):5-14.

Williams KA, Petronis J, Smith D et al. Effect of Iyengar yoga therapy for chronic low back pain. Pain 2005; 115(1-2):107-17.

Wolf SL, Barnhart HX, Ellison GL, Coogler CE. The effect of Tai Chi Quan and computerized balance training on postural stability in older subjects. Atlanta FICSIT Group. Frailty and Injuries: Cooperative Studies on Intervention Techniques. Phys Ther 1997; 77(4):371-81; discussion 382-4.

Wolf SL, Barnhart HX, Kutner NG, McNeely E, Coogler C, Xu T. Reducing frailty and falls in older persons: An investigation of Tai Chi and computerized balance training. 1996; 44(5):489-97.

Wolf SL, O'Grady M, Easley KA, Guo Y, Kressig RW, Kutner M. The influence of intense Tai Chi training on physical performance and hemodynamic outcomes in transitionally frail, older adults. J Gerontol A Biol Sci Med Sci 2006; 61(2):184-9.

Wolf SL, Sattin RW, Kutner M, O'Grady M, Greenspan AI, Gregor RJ. Intense tai chi exercise training and fall occurrences in older, transitionally frail adults: a randomized, controlled trial. J Am Geriatr Soc 2003; 51(12):1693-701.

Wolfgang WJ, Mayer-Berger J, Kettner C et al. Randomized controlled trial of long-term use of yoga and progressive relaxation in cardiovascular rehabilitation. European Journal of Cardiovascular Prevention and Rehabilitation 2010; 17:S58.

Wood C. Mood change and perceptions of vitality: a comparison of the effects of relaxation, visualization and yoga. J R Soc Med 1993; 86(5):254-8.

Wu G, Keyes L, Callas P, Ren X, Bookchin B. Comparison of telecommunication, community, and home-based Tai Chi exercise programs on compliance and effectiveness in elders at risk for falls. Arch Phys Med Rehabil 2010; 91(6):849-56.

Xie J, Lin YH, Guo CR, Chen F. Study on influences of yoga on quailty of life of schizophrenic inpatients. Nanfang Journal of Nursing 2006; 13(1):9-10.

Xiong HF, Long YD Xu SM Liu PF Xiong Zh Wang KY. [A study on the mechanism of QiGong(breathing exercise) in the treatment of coronary heart disease]. Chinese Journal of Sports Medicine 1983; 2(3):29-34.

Xu H, Lawson D, Kras A. A study on Tai Ji exercise and traditional Chinese medical modalities in relation to bone structure, bone function and menopausal symptoms. J. Chin. Med. 2004; (74):10-4.

Xu H, Lawson D, Kras A. A study on Tai Ji exercise and traditional Chinese medical modalities in relation to bone structure, bone function and menopausal symptoms. Journal of Chinese Medicine 2004; (74):3-7.

Yang Y, Verkuilen J, Rosengren KS et al. Effects of a traditional Taiji/Qigong curriculum on older adults' immune response to influenza vaccine. Med Sport Sci 2008; 52:64-76.

Yao Q, Yujun T, Cunzhe Q. Effect of short wave infrared qigong information therapy on chronic active hepatitis. Chinese Journal of Infectious Diseases 1986; 4(Suppl 2):64-7.

Yeh GY, Mietus JE, Peng CK et al. Enhancement of sleep stability with Tai Chi exercise in chronic heart failure: preliminary findings using an ECG-based spectrogram method. Sleep Med 2008; 9(5):527-36.

Yeh GY, Wayne PM, Phillips RS. T'ai Chi exercise in patients with chronic heart failure. Med Sport Sci 2008; 52:195-208.

Yeh GY, Wood MJ, Lorell BH, Jha AK. Benefits of Tai Chi for elderly patients with congestive heart failure. J. Clin. Outcomes Manage. 2004; 11(11):690-1.

Yeh GY, Wood MJ, Lorell BH et al. Heart failure patients improve quality of life and exercise capacity with tai chi. 2005; 10(1):50-1.

Yogendra J, Yogendra HJ, Ambardekar S et al. Beneficial effects of yoga lifestyle on reversibility of ischaemic heart disease: caring heart project of International Board of Yoga. J Assoc Physicians India 2004; 52:283-9.

Youshan W, Wei L, Deren P, Zhihua X, Jinhui X. Laboratory study of Qigong therapy for patients with essential hypertension. 1993; 18(3):269-71.

Yurtkuran M, Alp A, Yurtkuran M, Dilek K. A modified yoga-based exercise program in hemodialysis patients: a randomized controlled study. Complement Ther Med 2007; 15(3):164-71.

Zeeuwe PEM, Verhagen AP, Bierma-Zeinstra SMA, Van Rossum E, Faber MJ, Koes BW. The effect of Tai Chi Chuan in reducing falls among elderly people: Design of a randomized clinical trial in the Netherlands [ISRCTN98840266]. 2006; 6.

Zhang BL, Song KZ, Zhang JX, Xie JS, Wang CM. [Counteracting effect of hypoxia and Qigong on cardiac rhythm during orthostatic test post simulated weightlessness]. Space Med Med Eng (Beijing) 1999; 12(1):59-61.

Zhang LT, Shen FD, Ji ZH, Luo XL, Qi FJ, Fan JY et al. [Clinical study on Yigan qigong in the treatment of chronic hepatitis B]. Chinese Journal of Integrated Traditional & Western Medicine on Liver Diseases 1993; 3(1):7-9.

Zhao J, Zhang L, Tian Y. Effect of 6 months of Tai Chi Chuan and calcium supplementation on bone health in females aged 50-59 years. Journal of Exercise Science & Fitness 2007; 5(2):88-94.

Zhou MR, Lian MR. [Observation of qi-gong treatment in 60 cases of pregnancy-induced hypertension]. Zhong Xi Yi Jie He Za Zhi 1989; 9(1):16-8, 4-5.

Zhuo D, Dighe J, Basmajian JV. EMG biofeedback and Chinese 'Chi Kung': relaxation effects in patients with low back pain. Physiother. Can. 1983; 35(1):13-7.

Zhuo D, Dighe J, Basmajian J. EMG biofeedback and Chinese "Chi Kung": relaxation effects in patients with low back pain. Physiotherapy Canada 1983; 35(1):13-8.

Other

Abstracts: archives journals. JAMA: Journal of the American Medical Association 2006; 296(6):633-5.

Retraction. Preliminary study of the effects of Tai Chi and Qigong medical exercise on indicators of metabolic syndrome and glycaemic control in adults with raised blood glucose levels. Br J Sports Med 2010; 44(8):608.

Abrams AI, Siegel LM. The Transcendental Meditation program and rehabilitation at Folsom State Prison: A cross-validation study. Criminal Justice and Behavior 1978; 5(1):3-20.

Agte V, Tarwadi K. Sudarshan Kriya yoga for treating type 2 diabetes: a preliminary study. Alternative & Complementary Therapies 2004; 10(4):220-2.

Alberts HJ, Thewissen R. The Effect of a Brief Mindfulness Intervention on Memory for Positively and Negatively Valenced Stimuli. Mindfulness (N Y) 2011; 2(2):73-7.

Alexander CN, Swanson GC, Rainforth MV, Carlisle TW. Effects of the transcendental meditation program on stress reduction, health, and employee development: A prospective study in two occupational settings. Anxiety, Stress & Coping: An International Journal 1993; 6(3):245-62.

Anderson VL. The effects of meditation on teacher perceived occupational stress and trait anxiety. Dissertation Abstracts International 1996; 57(3-A):934.

Anderson VL, Levinson EM, Barker W, Kiewra KR. The Effects of Meditation on Teacher Perceived Occupational Stress, State and Trait Anxiety, and Burnout 1. 1999; 14(1):3-25.

Andrew J, Winzelberg Ma, Frederic M, Luskin MS. The effect of a meditation training in stress levels in secondary school teachers. 1999; 15(2):69-77.

Anon. The effects of meditation on selected measures of human potential. Dissertation Abstracts International 1982; 42((11-A)):4717.

Anon. Meditation-based treatment for binge-eating disorder. Http://Www.Clinicaltrials.Gov 2003.

Anon. Meditation or education for Alzheimer caregivers or meditation for Alzheimer caregivers. Http://Www.Clinicaltrials.Gov 2007.

Anon. Mindfulness meditation as a rehabilitation strategy for persons with schizophrenia. Http://Wwwclinicaltrialsgov 2009.

Anthony Jr W. An evaluation of meditation as a stress reduction technique for persons with spinal cord injury. Dissertation Abstracts International 1986; 46(11):3251.

Arcari P. Efficacy of a workplace smoking cessation program: mindfulness meditation vs cognitive-behavioral interventions. Boston College, 1996.

Arch JJ, Craske MG. Mechanisms of mindfulness: emotion regulation following a focused breathing induction. Behav Res Ther 2006; 44(12):1849-58.

Berghmans C, Tarquinio C, Kretsch M. Impact of the therapeutic approach of mindfulness-based stress reduction (MBSR) on psychic health (stress, anxiety, depression) in students: A controlled and randomized pilot study: Impact de l'approche therapeutique de pleine conscience mindfulness-based stress reduction (MBSR) sur la sant psychique (stress, anxiety, depression) chez des etudiants : une etude pilote controle et randomise. 2010; 20(1):11-5.

Blom KC, Baker B, Irvine J et al. The harmony study: Hypertension analysis of stress reduction using mindfulness meditation and yoga. J. Clin. Hypertens. 2011; 13(4):A141.

Brach AW. Clinical applications of meditation: A treatment outcome evaluation study of an intervention for binge eating among the obese that combines formal meditation and contingent formal and informal meditation. Dissertation Abstracts International 1992; 52(7-B):3898.

Britton Willoughby B. Meditation and depression. Dissertation Abstracts International 2007; 68(5-B):3387.

Broota A, Dhir R. Efficacy of two relaxation techniques in depression. Journal of Personality and Clinical Studies 1990; 6(1):83-90.

Broota A, Sanghvi C. Efficacy of two relaxation techniques in examination anxiety. Journal of Personality and Clinical Studies 1994; 10(1-2):29-35.

Brown LL, Robinson SE. The relationship between meditation and/or exercise and three measures of self-actualization. Journal of Mental Health Counseling 1993; 15(1):85-93.

Butler LD, Spiegel D. Meditation and hypnosis for chronic depressed mood. Controlled-Trials.Com 2006.

Calderon R, Jr. Effects of nonpharmacological approaches on cholesterol levels in mild hypertensive African Americans: A pilot study of the Transcendental Meditation program and a health education program. 2000.

Canter P, Gangadhar B. Possible antidepressant effects of yogic breathing during early stage alcohol detoxification. Focus on Alternative & Complementary Therapies 2006; 11(4):318-9.

Carlson CR, Bacaseta PE, Simanton DA. A controlled evaluation of devotional meditation and progressive relaxation. Journal of Psychology and Theology 1988; 16(4):362-8.

Carmody J, Olendzki B, Reed G, Andersen V, Rosenzweig P. A dietary intervention for recurrent prostate cancer after definitive primary treatment: results of a randomized pilot trial. Urology 2008; 72(6):1324-8.

Chan AS, Han YM, Cheung MC. Electroencephalographic (EEG) measurements of mindfulness-based Triarchic body-pathway relaxation technique: a pilot study. Appl Psychophysiol Biofeedback 2008; 33(1):39-47.

Chang J, Midlarsky E, Lin P. Effects of meditation on music performance anxiety. Medical Problems of Performing Artists 2003; 18(3):126-30.

Chhabra AK. The effect of self-aware meditation on stress in Indian immigrants living in the United States. Dissertation Abstracts International: Section B: The Sciences and Engineering 2011; 71(10-B):6435.

Chu L. The benefits of meditation vis-a-vis emotional intelligence, perceived stress and negative mental health. Stress & Health: Journal of the International Society for the Investigation of Stress 2010; 26(2):169-80.

Cohen-Katz J, Wiley S, Capuano T, Baker DM, Deitrick L, Shapiro S. The effects of mindfulness-based stress reduction on nurse stress and burnout: a qualitative and quantitative study, part III. Holist Nurs Pract 2005; 19(2):78-86.

Colby F. An analogue study of the initial carryover effects of meditation, hypnosis, and relaxation using naive college students. Biofeedback & Self Regulation 1991; 16(2):157-65.

Comer James F. Meditation and progressive relaxation in the treatment of test anxiety. Dissertation Abstracts International 1978; 38(12-B):6142-3.

Cooper S, Oborne J, Newton S et al. Do breathing exercises (buteyko and pranayama) help to control asthma: a randomised controlled trial [abstract]. European Respiratory Society Annual Congress 2002 2002; abstract P1929.

Cooper SE, Oborne J, Newton S et al. The effect of two breathing exercises (Buteyko and Pranayama) on the ability to reduce inhaled corticosteroids in asthma: a randomised controlled trial [abstract]. American Thoracic Society 99th International Conference 2003; B023 Poster 924.

Cropley M, Ussher M, Charitou E. Acute effects of a guided relaxation routine (body scan) on tobacco withdrawal symptoms and cravings in abstinent smokers. 2007; 102(6):989-93.

Curiati JA, Bocchi E, Freire JO et al. Meditation reduces sympathetic activation and improves the quality of life in elderly patients with optimally treated heart failure: a prospective randomized study. J Altern Complement Med 2005; 11(3):465-72.

da Silva GD, Lorenzi-Filho G, Lage LV. Effects of yoga and the addition of Tui Na in patients with fibromyalgia. J Altern Complement Med 2007; 13(10):1107-13.

De Jong-Meyer R, Parthe T, Projektgruppe. The influence of mindfulness exercises and decentring on rumination and specificity of autobiographical memory: Einfluss von achtsamkeitsbung und dezentrierung auf rumination und spezifitñt autobiographischererinnerungen. 2009; 38(4):240-9.

De La Arias JF, Justo CF, Manas I. Results of a program on mindfulness on the emotional situation of university students: Efectos de un programa de entrenamiento en conciencia plena (mindfulness)en el estado emocional de estudiantes universitarios. 2010; (19):31-52.

de la Fuente Arias M, Justo CF, Granados MS. Effects of a meditation program (mindfulness) on the measure of alexithymia and social skills: Efectos de un programa de meditacion (mindfulness) en la medida de la alexitimia y las habilidades sociales. 2010; 22(3):369-75.

de la Fuente M, Franco C, Salvador M. Reduction of blood pressure in a group of hypertensive teachers through a program of mindfulness meditation: Reduccion de la presion arterial en un grupo de docentes hipertensos mediante un programa de entrenamiento en conciencia plena (mindfulness). 2010; 18(3):533-52.

Deberry S. The Effects Of Meditation-Relaxation On Anxiety And Depression In A Geriatric Population. Psychotherapy 1982; 19(4):512-21.

Deberry S, Davis S, Reinhard KE. A comparison of meditation-relaxation and cognitive/behavioral techniques for reducing anxiety and depression in a geriatric population. J Geriatr Psychiatry 1989; 22(2):231-47.

DeBlassie PA. Christian meditation: A clinical investigation. Dissertation Abstracts International 1981; 42(3-B):1167.

Delgado LC, Guerra P, Perakakis P, Viedma MI, Robles H, Vila J. Human values education and mindfulness meditation as a tool for emotional regulation and stress prevention for teachers: An efficiency study: Eficacia de un programa de entrenamiento en conciencia plena (mindfulness) y valores humanos como herramienta de regulacion emocional y prevencion del estres para profesores. 2010; 18(3):511-33.

Delgado LC, Guerra P, Perakakis P, Viedma MaI, Robles H, Vila J. Eficacia de un programa de entrenamiento en conciencia plena (mindfulness) y valores humanos como herramienta de regulacion emocional y prevencion del estres para profesores. Behavioral Psychology/Psicologia Conductual: Revista Internacional Clinica y De La Salud 2010; 18(3):511-32.

Diner MD. The differential effects of meditation and systematic desensitization on specific and general anxiety. Dissertation Abstracts International 1978; 39(4-B):1950.

Downey N. Mindfulness training: The effect of process and outcome instructions on the experience of control and the level of mindfulness among older women. Educational Gerontology 1991; 17(2):97-109.

Duncan L, Weissenburger D. Effects of a Brief Meditation Program on Well-being and Loneliness. TCA Journal 2003; 31(1):4-14.

Duraiswamy G, Thirthalli J, Nagendra HR, Gangadhar BN. Yoga therapy as an add-on treatment in the management of patients with schizophrenia--a randomized controlled trial. Acta Psychiatr Scand 2007; 116(3):226-32.

Ellett L, Freeman D, Garety PA. The psychological effect of an urban environment on individuals with persecutory delusions: the Camberwell walk study. Schizophr Res 2008; 99(1-3):77-84.

English EH, Baker TB. Relaxation training and cardiovascular response to experimental stressors. Health Psychology 1983; 2(3):239-59.

Erisman SM, Roemer L. A preliminary investigation of the effects of experimentally induced mindfulness on emotional responding to film clips. Emotion 2010; 10(1):72-82.

Evans S, Cousins L, Tsao JC, Sternlieb B, Zeltzer LK. Protocol for a randomized controlled study of Iyengar yoga for youth with irritable bowel syndrome. Trials 2011; 12:15.

Evans S, Cousins L, Tsao JC, Subramanian S, Sternlieb B, Zeltzer LK. A randomized controlled trial examining Iyengar yoga for young adults with rheumatoid arthritis: a study protocol. Trials 2011; 12:19.

Faber MJ, Bosscher RJ, Chin A Paw MJ, van Wieringen PC. Effects of exercise programs on falls and mobility in frail and pre-frail older adults: A multicenter randomized controlled trial. Arch Phys Med Rehabil 2006; 87(7):885-96.

Fang W, Weidong W, Rongrui Z et al. Clinical observation on physiological and psychological effects of Eight-Section Brocade on type 2 diabetic patients. 2008; 28(2):101-5.

Fjellman-Wiklund A, Stenlund T, Steinholtz K, Ahlgren C. Take charge: Patients' experiences during participation in a rehabilitation programme for burnout. J Rehabil Med 2010; 42(5):475-81.

Franco C, Sola MadM, Justo E. Reduccion del malestar psicoligico y de la sobrecarga en familiares cuidadores de enfermos de Alzheimer mediante la aplicacion de un programa de entrenamiento en mindfulness (conciencia plena). Revista Espanola De Geriatria y Gerontologia 2010; 45(5):252-8.

Franco Justo C. Reducing stress levels and anxiety in primary-care physicians through training and practice of a mindfulness meditation technique: Reduccion de los niveles de estres y ansiedad en medicos de Atencion Primaria mediante la aplicacion de un programa de entrenamiento en conciencia plena (mindfulness). 2010; 42(11):564-70.

Franco Justo C. Reduccion de la percepcion del estres en estudiantes de magisterio mediante la praíctica de la meditacion fluir. Apuntes De Psicologia 2009; 27(1):99-109.

Frisvold MH. The "midlife study": Mindfulness as an intervention to change health behaviors in midlife women. University of Minnesota, 2009.

Fukushima M, Kataoka T, Hamada C, Matsumoto M. Evidence of Qi-gong energy and its biological effect on the enhancement of the phagocytic activity of human polymorphonuclear leukocytes. Am J Chin Med 2001; 29(1):1-16.

Galani K, Vyas SN, Dave AR. A clinical study on role of of "Saptasamo yoga and darvyadi yamak malahara" In the management of ekakushtha (psoriasis). AYU 2009; 30(4):415-20.

Garcia-Trujillo MR, De Rivera JLG. Physiological changes induced by meditation and deep relaxation: Cambios Fisiologicos Durante Los Ejercicios De Meditacion Y Relajacion Profunda. 1992; 13(6-7):57-63.

Geisler M. Transcendental meditation as a therapeutic tool for drug users. Zeitschrift Fr Klinische Psychologie 1978; 7(4):235-55.

Gilmore JV. Relative effectiveness of meditation and autogenic training for the self-regulation of anxiety. Dissertation Abstracts International 1985; 45(8-B):2686.

Gordon L, Morrison EY, McGrowder DA et al. Changes in clinical and metabolic parameters after exercise therapy in patents with type 2 diabetes. 2008; 4(4):427-37.

Gordon LA, Morrison EY, McGrowder DA et al. Effect of exercise therapy on lipid profile and oxidative stress indicators in patients with type 2 diabetes. 2008; 8.

Greene YN, Hiebert B. A comparison of mindfulness meditation and cognitive self-observation. Canadian Journal of Counselling 1988; 22(1):25-34.

Griffiths TJ, Steel DH, Vaccaro P, Karpman MB. The effects of relaxation techniques on anxiety and underwater performance. International Journal of Sport Psychology 1981; 12(3):176-82.

Gross CR, Kreitzer MJ, Reilly-Spong M, Winbush NY, Schomaker EK, Thomas W. Mindfulness meditation training to reduce symptom distress in transplant patients: rationale, design, and experience with a recycled waitlist. Clin Trials 2009; 6(1):76-89.

Gururaja D, Harano K, Toyotake I, Kobayashi H. Effect of yoga on mental health: Comparative study between young and senior subjects in Japan. Int J Yoga 2011; 4(1):7-12.

Heeren A, Philippot P. Changes in ruminative thinking mediate the clinical benefits of mindfulness: Preliminary findings. Mindfulness 2011; 2(1):8-13.

Heffner KL, Talbot NL, Krasner MS, Moynihan JA. Pain in older men is associated with interleukin (IL)-6 change across time following a mindfulness-based stress reduction intervention. Brain Behav. Immun. 2011; 25:S205.

Hillemeier MM, Downs DS, Feinberg ME et al. Improving women's preconceptional health: findings from a randomized trial of the Strong Healthy Women intervention in the Central Pennsylvania women's health study. Womens Health Issues 2008; 18(6 Suppl):S87-96.

Hong PY, Lishner DA, Han KH, Huss EA. The positive impact of mindful eating on expectations of food liking. Mindfulness 2011; 2(2):103-13.

Hui PN, Wan M, Chan WK, Yung PM. An evaluation of two behavioral rehabilitation programs, qigong versus progressive relaxation, in improving the quality of life in cardiac patients. J Altern Complement Med 2006; 12(4):373-8.

Humphrey CW. A stress management intervention with forgiveness as the goal (Meditation, mind-body medicine). Dissertation Abstracts International : Section B: the Sciences and Engineering 1999; 60(4-B):1855.

Innes KE, Selfe TK, Alexander GK, Taylor AG. A new educational film control for use in studies of active mind-body therapies: acceptability and feasibility. J Altern Complement Med 2011; 17(5):453-8.

Innes KE, Selfe TK, Vishnu A. Association of fructosamine to indices of dyslipidemia in older adults with type 2 diabetes. Diabetes Metab. Syndr. Clin. Res. Rev. 2010.

Jones Roger C. A comparison of aerobic exercise, anaerobic exercise and meditation on multidimensional stress measures. Dissertation Abstracts International 1981; 42(6-B):2504-5.

Kabat-Zinn J, Wheeler E, Light T et al. Part II: Influence of a mindfulness meditation-based stress reduction intervention on rates of skin clearing in patients with moderate to severe psoriasis undergoing phototherapy (UVB) and photochemo-therapy (PUVA). [References]. Constructivism in the Human Sciences 2003; 8(2):85-106.

Kaviani A, Hatami N, ShafiAbadi A. The impact of mindfulness-based cognitive therapy on the quality of life in non-clinically depressed people. Advances in Cognitive Science 2008; 10(4).

Kember P. The Transcendental Meditation technique and postgraduate academic performance. British Journal of Educational Psychology 1985; 55(2):164-6.

Khasky AD, Smith JC. Stress, relaxation states, and creativity. Percept Mot Skills 1999; 88(2):409-16.

Khianman B, Pattanittum P, Thinkhamrop J, Lumbiganon P. Relaxation therapy for preventing and treating preterm labour. 2008; (4).

Khumar SS, Kaur P, Kaur S. Effectiveness of Shavasana on depression among university students. Indian Journal of Clinical Psychology 1993; 20(2):82-7.

Kiken LG, Shook NJ. Looking up: Mindfulness increases positive judgments and reduces negativity bias. Social Psychological and Personality Science 2011; 2(4):425-31.

Kim TS, Park JS, Kim MA. The relation of meditation to power and well-being. Nurs Sci Q 2008; 21(1):49-58.

Kligler B, Homel P, Blank AE, Kenney J, Levenson H, Merrell W. Randomized trial of the effect of an integrative medicine approach to the management of asthma in adults on disease-related quality of life and pulmonary function. Altern Ther Health Med 2011; 17(1):10-5.

Kolsawalla MB. An experimental investigation into the effectiveness of some yogic variables as a mechanism of change in the value-attitude system. Journal of Indian Psychology 1978; 1(1):59-68.

Koole SL, Govorun O, Cheng CM, Gallucci M. Pulling yourself together: Meditation promotes congruence between implicit and explicit self-esteem. Journal of Experimental Social Psychology 2009; 45(6):1220-6.

Kova-ii-ì T, Kova-ii-ì M. Impact of relaxation training according to Yoga in Daily Life-« system on perceived stress after breast cancer surgery. 2011; 10(1):16-26.

Kozasa EH, Santos RF, Rueda AD, Benedito-Silva AA, De Ornellas FL, Leite JR. Evaluation of Siddha Samadhi Yoga for anxiety and depression symptoms: a preliminary study. Psychol Rep 2008; 103(1):271-4.

Krueger RC. The comparative effects of Zen focusing and muscle relaxation training on selected experiential variables. Dissertation Abstracts International 1980; 41(4-A):1405.

Kubose SK. An experimental investigation of psychological aspects of meditation. Psychologia: An International Journal of Psychology in the Orient 1976; 19(1):1-10.

Kulkarni R, Nagarathna R, Nagendra HR, An H. Measures of heart rate variability in women following a meditation technique. International Journal of Yoga 2010; 3(1):6-9.

Kulmatycki L, Burzyäski Z. Yoga nidra and Benson's meditative relaxation and anxiety level, anger and depression emotions: Relaksacja joga nidry i medytacji Bensona a poziom leku oraz emocje gniewu i depresji. 2007; 21(3):23-8.

Kyizom T, Singh S, Singh KP, Tandon OP, Kumar R. Effect of pranayama & yoga-asana on cognitive brain functions in type 2 diabetes-P3 event related evoked potential (ERP). Indian J Med Res 2010; 131:636-40.

Labelle LE, Campbell TS, Carlson LE. Mindfulness-based stress reduction in oncology: Evaluating mindfulness and rumination as mediators of change in depressive symptoms. Mindfulness 2010; 1(1):28-40.

Laitinen J. Meditation--relaxation: Mietiskely - rentoutuminen. 1975; 91(19):1136-41.

Lee EN, Kim YH, Chung WT, Lee MS. Tai chi for disease activity and flexibility in patients with ankylosing spondylitis--a controlled clinical trial. Evid Based Complement Alternat Med 2008; 5(4):457-62.

Lee JH, Kim YM, Choi YM, Lee GC. The effect of meditation on problem solving ability and self-perception. Journal of the Korean Neuropsychiatric Association 1997; 36(4):723-31.

Lee LY, Lee DT, Woo J. Effect of Tai Chi on state self-esteem and health-related quality of life in older Chinese residential care home residents. J Clin Nurs 2007; 16(8):1580-2.

Lee MS, Kang C-W, Lim H-J, Lee M-S. Effects of Qi-training on anxiety and plasma concentrations of cortisol, ACTH, and aldosterone: A randomized placebo-controlled pilot study. 2004; 20(5):243-8.

Lee W, Bang H. The effects of mindfulness-based group intervention on the mental health of middle-aged Korean women in community. Stress & Health: Journal of the International Society for the Investigation of Stress 2010; 26(4):341-8.

Leung RW, Alison JA, McKeough ZJ, Peters MJ. A study design to investigate the effect of short-form Sun-style Tai Chi in improving functional exercise capacity, physical performance, balance and health related quality of life in people with Chronic Obstructive Pulmonary Disease (COPD). Contemp Clin Trials 2011; 32(2):267-72.

Li M, Chen K, Mo Z. Use of qigong therapy in the detoxification of heroin addicts. Altern Ther Health Med 2002; 8(1):50-4, 56-9.

Lin MR, Hwang HF, Wang YW, Chang SH, Wolf SL. Community-based tai chi and its effect on injurious falls, balance, gait, and fear of falling in older people. Phys Ther 2006; 86(9):1189-201.

Lu CF, Liao JC, Liu CY, Liu HY, Chang YH. Meditation therapy in the treatment of anxiety disorders. Taiwanese Journal of Psychiatry 1998; 12(4):343-51.

Luethcke CA, McDaniel L, Becker CB. A comparison of mindfulness, nonjudgmental, and cognitive dissonance-based approaches to mirror exposure. Body Image 2011; 8(3):251-8.

Maloney R, Altmaier E. An initial evaluation of a mindful parenting program. J Clin Psychol 2007; 63(12):1231-8.

Marfurt S. Reducing stress in women recovering from substance abuse. Texas Woman's University, 2006.

Mariano C. A 16-week tai chi programme prevented falls in healthy older adults. Evid Based Nurs 2008; 11(2):60.

Maybery DJ, Graham D. The influence of physical and mental training on plasma beta-endorphin level and pain perception after intensive physical exercise. 2001; 17(2):121-7.

McMillan TM, Robertson IH, Brock D, Chorlton L. Brief mindfulness training for attentional problems after traumatic brain injury: A randomised control treatment trial. Neuropsychological Rehabilitation 2002; 12(2):117-25.

Mirabel-Sarron C, Dorocant ES, Sala L, Bachelart M, Guelfi J-D, Rouillon F. Mindfulness based cognitive therapy (MBCT): A pilot study in bipolar patients: Mindfulness based cognitive therapy (MBCT) dans la prevention des rechutes thymiques chez le patient bipolaire I : une etude pilote. Ann. Med.-Psychol. 2009; 167(9):686-92.

Miro DJ. A comparative evaluation of relaxation training strategies utilizing EMG biofeedback. Dissertation Abstracts International 1981; 42(3-B):1183-4.

Mohan A, Sharma R, Bijlani RL. Effect of meditation on stress-induced changes in cognitive functions. J Altern Complement Med 2011; 17(3):207-12.

Monk-Turner E. The benefits of meditation: Experimental findings. The Social Science Journal 2003; 40(3):465-70.

Moretti-Altuna G. The effects of meditation versus medication in the treatment of Attention Deficit Disorder with Hyperactivity [dissertation]. 1987.

Moynihan JA, Klorman R, Chapman BP et al. Mindfulness to improve elders' immune and health status. Brain Behav. Immun. 2010; 24:S13.

Mustata S, Cooper L, Langrick N, Simon N, Jassal SV, Oreopoulos DG. The effect of a Tai Chi exercise program on quality of life in patients on peritoneal dialysis: a pilot study. Perit Dial Int 2005; 25(3):291-4.

Nakamura Y, Lipschitz DL, Landward R, Kuhn R, West G. Two sessions of sleep-focused mind-body bridging improve self-reported symptoms of sleep and PTSD in veterans: A pilot randomized controlled trial. J Psychosom Res 2011; 70(4):335-45.

Nakamura Y, Lipschitz DL, Landward R, Kuhn R, West G. Two sessions of sleep-focused mind-reported symptoms of sleep and PTSD in veterans: A pilot randomized controlled trial. Journal of Psychosomatic Research 2011; 70(4):335-45.

NCT00558402 (2007). Meditation or Education for Alzheimer Caregivers Or Meditation for Alzheimer Caregivers: Stress & Physiology. Http://Www.Clinicaltrials.Gov 2007.

Paty J, Brenot P, Tignol J, Bourgeois M. [Evoked cerebral activity (contingent negative variation and evoked potentials) and modified states of consciousness (sleeplike relaxation, transcendential meditation)]. Ann Med Psychol (Paris) 1978; 136(1):143-69.

Rakhshaee Z. Effect of three yoga poses (cobra, cat and fish poses) in women with primary dysmenorrhea: a randomized clinical trial. J Pediatr Adolesc Gynecol 2011; 24(4):192-6.

Ramos NS, Hernandez SM, Blanca MJ. Effects of an integrated programme of mindfulness and emotional intelligence on cognitive strategies of emotional regulation: Efecto de un programa integrado de mindfulness e inteligencia emocional sobre las estrategias cognitivas de regulacion emocional. 2009; 15(2-3):207-16.

Rasmussen LB. Transcendental meditation and mild hypertension: Transcendental meditasjon og mild hypertensjon. 1998; 118(5):775.

Rediger JD, Summers L. Mindfulness training and meditation for mental health. Adv Mind Body Med 2007; 22(1):16-26.

Robins JL, McCain NL, Gray DP, Elswick RK Jr, Walter JM, McDade E. Research on psychoneuroimmunology: tai chi as a stress management approach for individuals with HIV disease. Appl Nurs Res 2006; 19(1):2-9.

Rogers CE, Keller C, Larkey LK, Ainsworth BE. A Randomized Controlled Trial to Determine the Efficacy of Sign Chi Do Exercise on Adaptation to Aging. Res Gerontol Nurs 2011; 1-13.

Rohini V, Pandey RS, Janakiramaiah N, Gangadhar BN, Vedamurthachar A. A comparative study of full and partial Sudarshan Kriya Yoga (SKY) in major depressive disorder. NIMHANS Journal 2000; 18(1-2):53-7.

Rosdahl D. The effect of mindfulness meditation on tension headaches and secretory immunoglobulin A in saliva. University of Arizona, 2003.

Sawada Y, Steptoe A. The effects of brief meditation training on cardiovascular stress responses. Journal of Psychophysiology 1988; 2(4):249-57.

Schneider RH, Alexander CN, Staggers F et al. Long-term effects of stress reduction on mortality in persons

Semple RJ. Does mindfulness meditation enhance attention? A randomized controlled trial. Mindfulness 2010; 1(2):121-30.

Shahar B, Britton WB, Sbarra DA, Figueredo AJ, Bootzin RR. Mechanisms of change in mindfulness-based cognitive therapy for depression: Preliminary evidence from a randomized controlled trial. International Journal of Cognitive Therapy 2010; 3(4):402-18.

Shapiro SL, Astin JA, Bishop SR, Cordova M. Mindfulness-Based Stress Reduction for Health Care Professionals: Results From a Randomized Trial. International Journal of Stress Management 2005; 12(2):164-76.

Sharma I, Azmi SA, Settiwar RM. Evaluation of the effect of pranayama in anxiety state. Alternative Medicine 1991; 3(4):227-35.

Shin T-B, Jin S-R. The qualitative study of "mindfulness group" toward the self-care and counseling practice of counselor interns. Bulletin of Educational Psychology 2010; 42(1):163-84.

Smith JC. Meditation as psychotherapy. Dissertation Abstracts International 1975; 36(6-B):3073.

Smith WP, Compton WC, West WB. Meditation as an adjunct to a happiness enhancement program. J Clin Psychol 1995; 51(2):269-73.

Spadaro K. Weight loss: exploring self-regulation through Mindfulness Meditation. University of Pittsburgh, 2008.

Sridevi K, Krishna Rao PV. Yoga practice and menstrual distress. Journal of the Indian Academy of Applied Psychology 1996; 22(1-2):47-54.

Stormer-Labonte M, Machemer P, Hardinghaus W. Ein meditatives Streewaltigungsprogramm bei psychosomatischen Patienten. Psychotherapie Psychosomatik Medizinische Psychologie 1992; 42(12):436-43.

Stevinson C. Preliminary results suggest that yoga can alleviate depression. Focus on Alternative & Complementary Therapies 2001; 6(1):27-8.

Strijk JE, Proper KI, van der Beek AJ, van Mechelen W. A process evaluation of a worksite vitality intervention among ageing hospital workers. Int J Behav Nutr Phys Act 2011; 8:58.

Szabo A, Mesko A, Caputo A, Gill T. Examination of exercise-induced feeling states in four modes of exercise. International Journal of Sport Psychology 1998; 29(4):376-90.

Tanay G, Lotan G, Bernstein A. Salutary Proximal Processes and Distal Mood and Anxiety Vulnerability Outcomes of Mindfulness Training: A Pilot Preventive Intervention.

Targ EF, Levine EG. The efficacy of a mind-body-spirit group for women with breast cancer: a randomized controlled trial. Gen Hosp Psychiatry 2002; 24(4):238-48.

Taylor DN. Effects of a behavioral stress-management program on anxiety, mood, self-esteem, and T-cell count in HIV positive men. Psychol Rep 1995; 76(2):451-7.

Telles S, Naveen KV. Effect of yoga on somatic indicators of distress in professional computer users. Med Sci Monit 2006; 12(10):LE21-2.

Tloczynski J, Malinowski A, Lamorte R. Rediscovering and reapplying contingent informal meditation. Psychologia: An International Journal of Psychology in the Orient 1997; 40(1):14-21.

Tloczynski J, Tantriella M. A comparison of the effects of Zen breath meditation or relaxation on college adjustment. Psychologia: An International Journal of Psychology in the Orient 1998; 41(1):32-43.

Travis F, Olson T, Egenes T, Gupta HK. Physiological patterns during practice of the Transcendental Meditation technique compared with patterns while reading Sanskrit and a modern language. Int J Neurosci 2001; 109(1-2):71-80.

van den Hout MA, Engelhard IM, Beetsma D et al. EMDR and mindfulness. Eye movements and attentional breathing tax working memory and reduce vividness and emotionality of aversive ideation. J Behav Ther Exp Psychiatry 2011; 42(4):423-31.

Vanfraechem-Raway R. [Fatigue. Relaxation therapy]. Arch Belg 1985; 43(11-12):511-7.

Vedamurthachar A, Janakiramaiah N, Hegde JM et al. Antidepressant efficacy and hormonal effects of Sudarshana Kriya Yoga (SKY) in alcohol dependent individuals. J Affect Disord 2006; 94(1-3):249-53.

Wang F, Wang W, Zhang R et al. Clinical observation on physiological and psychological effects of Eight-Section Brocade on type 2 diabetic patients. J Tradit Chin Med 2008; 28(2):101-5.

Warber SL, Ingerman S, Moura VL et al. Healing the heart: a randomized pilot study of a spiritual retreat for depression in acute coronary syndrome patients. Explore (NY) 2011; 7(4):222-33.

Weiner Donald E. The effects of mantra meditation and progressive relaxation on self-actualization, state and trait anxiety, and frontalis muscle tension. Dissertation Abstracts International 1977; 37(8-B):4174.

Wenger Ma, Bagchi Bk, Anand Bk. Experiments In India On "Voluntary" Control Of The Heart And Pulse. Circulation 1961; 24:1319-25.

Williams JMG, Alatiq Y, Crane C et al. Mindfulness-based Cognitive Therapy (MBCT) in bipolar disorder: Preliminary evaluation of immediate effects on between-episode functioning. 2008; 107(1-3):275-9.

Wolfson L, Whipple R, Derby C et al. Balance and strength training in older adults: intervention gains and Tai Chi maintenance. J Am Geriatr Soc 1996; 44(5):498-506.

Wood DT. The effects of progressive relaxation, heart rate feedback, and content-specific meditation on anxiety and performance in a class situation. Dissertation Abstracts International 1978; 39(6-A):3458.

Yan X, Shen H, Jiang H et al. External Qi of Yan Xin Qigong Induces apoptosis and inhibits migration and invasion of estrogen-independent breast cancer cells through suppression of Akt/NF-kB signaling. Cell Physiol Biochem 2010; 25(2-3):263-70.

Yan X, Shen H, Jiang H et al. External Qi of Yan Xin Qigong differentially regulates the Akt and extracellular signal-regulated kinase pathways and is cytotoxic to cancer cells but not to normal cells. Int J Biochem Cell Biol 2006; 38(12):2102-13.

Yan X, Shen H, Jiang H et al. External Qi of Yan Xin Qigong induces G2/M arrest and apoptosis of androgen-independent prostate cancer cells by inhibiting Akt and NF-kappa B pathways. Mol Cell Biochem 2008; 310(1-2):227-34.

Oktedalen O, Solberg EE, Haugen AH, Opstad PK. The influence of physical and mental training on plasma beta-endorphin level and pain perception after intensive physical exercise. Stress and Health: Journal of the International Society for the Investigation of Stress 2001; 17(2):121-7.

Zautra AJ, Fasman R, Davis MC, Craig AD. The effects of slow breathing on affective responses to pain stimuli: an experimental study. Pain 2010; 149(1):12-8.

Zika B. The effects of hypnosis and meditation on a measure of self-actualization. Australian Journal of Clinical & Experimental Hypnosis 1987; 15(1):21-8.

Appendix E. Evidence Tables

Evidence Table E1. Study characteristics for included studies

Author, year	Study location	Study setting	Recruitment (start year–end year)	Total duration of study (including training and participants followup)	Inclusion criteria	Exclusion criteria
Barrett, 2012[1]	USA	outpatient (community based)	not mentioned	5 months	> 50yo, >1 cold in last years or >=1 cold on average for past several years	previous meditation training, moderate exercise, <24 on MMSE, >14 patients on PHQ9 depression screen, immunodeficiency, autoimmune, malignant disease, allergy to egg or influenza vaccine
Borman, 2006[2]	United States		NR	3 months (12 weeks after post treatment assessment)	Age: 18–65 HIV-infected ≥6 months Clean and sober from drug/alcohol abuse for ≥6 months Ability to read, write, and comprehend English	Cognitive impairment Dementia Active psychosis Type 1 diabetes mellitus Cancer Asthma Chronic hepatitis Chronic fatigue syndrome Initiated the practice of a new alternative/ complementary therapy in past 3 months Practice of other forms of mantram repetition such as the rosary, chanting, or TM Loss of family, loved one, or significant other in past 3 months Acute infection or a change in highly active anti-retroviral therapy (HAART) defined as 3 or more antiretroviral drugs with at least one being a protease-inhibitor or non-nucleoside transcriptase inhibitor Score ≤ 25 on Mini-Mental Status Exam

Author, year	Study location	Study setting	Recruitment (start year–end year)	Total duration of study (including training and participants followup)	Inclusion criteria	Exclusion criteria
Brewer, 2009[3]	United States	Outpatient	NR	Variable depending on treatment arm: 9 weeks for Mindfulness, 12 weeks for CBT. Measures taken at baseline, weekly, and post-intervention.	Age: at least 18 years Understands English Meet DSM criteria for abuse or dependence of ETOH or cocaine for the last year	Current psychotic disorder, or at risk of suicide or homicide Cognitive impairment On beta blocker medication
Brewer, 2011[4]	United States	Outpatient	NR	4 week treatment and up to 17 weeks after treatment initiation	Age:18–60 years Smoked 10+ cigarettes per day Had fewer than 3 months of smoking abstinence in the past year Reported interest in quitting smoking	Had a serious or unstable medical condition in the past 6 months Currently use psychoactive medications met DSM-IV criteria for other substance dependence in the past year
Castillo-Richmond, 2000[5]	United States	Outpatient		NR	Age:>20 Self-identified as African American and residing in Los Angeles Have high normal blood pressure, stage I hypertension or stage II hypertension	Candidates were excluded if they had evidence of complications due to CVD or other life-threatening or disabling illnesses
Chiesa, 2012[6]	Italy	outpatient			> age 18, currently depressed, 8 weeks of antidepressant, HAMD>=8	psychosis, bipolar, substance abuse, svr physical/neurological problem, concurrent psychotherapy or meditation

E-3

Author, year	Study location	Study setting	Recruitment (start year–end year)	Total duration of study (including training and participants followup)	Inclusion criteria	Exclusion criteria
Delgado, 2010[7]	Spain	University	NR	Study was conducted 5 weeks	Age: 18–24 years High scores in the Penn State Worry Questionnaire	Participants were screened to guarantee that none suffered from Generalized Anxiety Disorder No participant was undergoing psychological or pharmacological treatment No participant had auditory or cardiovascular problems
Elder, 2006[8]	United States	Outpatient	July 2003–December 2003	6 months	Age:21–80 Diabetic with baseline HbA1cof 6.0–8.0 during the recruitment year (2003)[1] Patients able to comply with a 3-month trial period without anti-hyperglycemic agents	Psychotic disorder or hx of hospitalization for depression Serious medical condition Pregnant or nursing women Patients undergoing warfarin or systemic gluticosteriod treatment Any medical condition which would preclude treatment with herbal supplements Living outside study area
Garland, 2010[9]	United Kingdom	Inpatient	2008–	10 weeks (pre-post-test design)	Age:18 and older ETOH dependent adults Resident in a substance abuse treatment center for at least 18 months	Active psychosis or suicidality Scored < 16 on the AUDIT

Author, year	Study location	Study setting	Recruitment (start year–end year)	Total duration of study (including training and participants followup)	Inclusion criteria	Exclusion criteria
Gaylord, 2011[10]	United States	Outpatient	2006–2009	3 months post-primary outcome assessment	IBS diagnosis according to Rome II criteria and physician diagnosis; Female Age: 18–75 Ability to understand English Willingness to document bowel symptoms and medication use regularly and complete the assessments Willingness to attend eight weekly sessions plus one additional half-day session of either mindfulness training or SG	Diagnosis of mental illness with psychosis A history of inpatient admission for psychiatric disorder within the past 2 years A history or current diagnosis of inflammatory bowel disease or gastrointestinal malignancy Active liver or pancreatic disease Uncontrolled lactose intolerance; Celiac disease; A history of abdominal trauma or surgery involving gastrointestinal resection Pregnancy
Gross, 2010[11]	United States	Outpatient	NR	1 year	Age:18 and older Ability to read and write English Functioning solid-organ transplant (i.e., kidney, kidney/pancreas, pancreas, lung, liver, heart or heart-lung) Willingness to attend classes Patients were at least 6 months post-transplant	Having serious preexisting mental health issues Previously taken MBSR Medically unstable or on dialysis

Author, year	Study location	Study setting	Recruitment (start year–end year)	Total duration of study (including training and participants followup)	Inclusion criteria	Exclusion criteria
Gross, 2011[12]	United States	Study involved multiple settings: Outpatient center, center for spirituality and healing, and home	2007–2008	Up to 5 months	Age: 18–65 years Ability to read and speak English Diagnosis of primary chronic insomnia	Persons with medical conditions, mental disorders, or different sleep disorders suspected of being directly related to the insomnia Persons using prescription or nonprescription sleep aids prior to enrollment. They could be included if willing to discontinue use for the duration of the study Persons who would not accept the possibility of being randomized to pharmacotherapy
Herbert, 2001[13]	United States	Unclear	NR	12 months	Age: 20–65 Female Stage 1 or 2 breast cancer Able to function > 50% of the time (as assessed by the Eastern Cooperative Oncology Group) Willingness to accept randomization Willingness to be contacted by phone	Current chronic substance abuse (either drug or alcohol, e.g. >3 Drinks/day-3x/week) Major Depression Schizophrenia Organic brain syndrome Psychosis Cognitive impairment

Author, year	Study location	Study setting	Recruitment (start year–end year)	Total duration of study (including training and participants followup)	Inclusion criteria	Exclusion criteria
Jayadevappa, 2007[14]	United States	Authors don't mention the precise study setting, but they identified potential participants from the University of Pennsylvania Health Care System. It is possible that both inpatients and outpatients were recruited into the study.	NR	6 months	Age: >= 55 years Participants had to be in New York Heart Association class II or III Congestive Heart Failure and with a left ventricular ejection fraction of <.40. African American	Inability to verify heart failure diagnosis in medical record Cognitive impairment Inability/unwillingness to complete screening and intervention process Enrollment in other trials on Congestive Heart Failure
Jazaieri, 2012[15]	USA	outpatient	not mentioned	5 months	social anxiety disorder	current pharmacotherapy/psychotherapy, h/o medical disorders, head trauma, other psychiatric disorders, prior MBSR, regular current exercise
Kuyken, 2008[16]	United Kingdom	Outpatient	NR	15 months	Age: 18 or older 3 or more episodes of depression meeting DSM criteria Current use of a maintenance anti-depressant medication	Comorbid diagnoses of current substance dependence Disabling physical problem Organic brain damage Bipolar disorder or psychosis Persistent anti-social behavior

Author, year	Study location	Study setting	Recruitment (start year–end year)	Total duration of study (including training and participants followup)	Inclusion criteria	Exclusion criteria
Lee, 2006[17]	South Korea	NR	March 2003–August 2003	NR		Any history of substance abuse or dependency Psychiatric comorbidities Significant medical problems (such as diabetes mellitus, hypertension, tuberculosis, hepatitis, or pregnancy) Involvement in litigation or compensation
Lehrer, 1983[18]	United States	NR	NR	6 months	Anxious subjects were given the IPAT Anxiety Inventory and only accepted those whose scores were higher than 1 SD above the mean of the standardization group	All subjects were asked to refrain from alcohol, caffeine or other psychoactive substances for at least 24 hours prior to each testing session and each therapy session Subjects seriously physically ill Had previous training in any form of relaxation If subjects were taking any form of medication that could not be discontinued for the duration of the study
Malarkey, 2012[19]	USA	outpatient	not mentioned	8 weeks (they have 12 months outcomes not yet published)	CRP>3.0	CRP>10.0, psychiatric disorder other than depression, pregnancy, major life stressor in past 2 months, alcoholism, heavy smoking, drug use, vaccination or cold/illness in past month, BMI>40, exercising >30min /d, previous practice of mind-body technique
Miller, 2012[20]	USA	outpatient	not mentioned	6 months	35–65yo, DMII, BMI>27, HbA1c>7%	Insulin therapy, pregnancy, already in weight loss program
Moritz, 2006[21]	Canada	Outpatient	August 2000–March 2001	12 weeks	18 years of age or older Psychological distress	Already trained in or currently practices meditation/ stress reduction technique

Author, year	Study location	Study setting	Recruitment (start year–end year)	Total duration of study (including training and participants followup)	Inclusion criteria	Exclusion criteria
Morone, 2009[22]	United States	Pitt Center for Research on Healthcare	July 2007–	4 months total: measures at baseline, 8 weeks, 4 months	Age: 65 or older ability to understand English Intact cognition CLBP of at least 3 months duration CLBP of moderate intensity according to vertical verbal descriptor scale	Significant vision or hearing impairment, medical instability due to heart or lung disease, multiple recent falls, flags of more serious underlying disease (e.g. unexplained weight loss) Previous participation in a mindfulness meditation program Inability to stand independently Pain caused by an acute injury within the last 3 months
Mularski, 2009[23]	United States	Outpatient	NR	weeks	Cognitively intact patients with advanced and symptomatic COPD	Patients with cognitive impairment or those with medical record documentation or self-report of significant psychiatric disease Unwilling or unable to participate in the full 8-week program and evaluation
Murphy, 1986[24]	United States	Outpatient	NR	6 weeks	Age: 21-30 years High-volume drinkers according to a Drinking Habits Questionnaire, adapted from Cahalan's national drinking habits survey (Cahalan, Cisin, & Crossley, 1969) Male	No prior experience with meditation No prior experience in running

E-9

Author, year	Study location	Study setting	Recruitment (start year–end year)	Total duration of study (including training and participants followup)	Inclusion criteria	Exclusion criteria
Oken, 2010[25]	United States	Outpatient	NR	NR	Providing at least 12 hours per week of assistance for the person with progressive dementia Perceived Stress Scale score greater than 9	Unstable medical conditions Previous experience with similar types of stress-reduction classes Cognitive dysfunction with a score of less than 25 on the Modified Telephone Interview for Cognitive Status Medications that were not stable for at least 2 months Significant visual impairment (corrected binocular visual acuity worse than 20/50)
Paul-Labrador, 2006[26]	United States	Outpatient	NR		Age; 18 or older Cardiovascular Heart Disease (Myocardial infarction, Coronary artery bypass surgery, coronary angiography, angioplasty)	Unstable coronary syndromes Congestive heart failure greater than New York Heart Association class III Renal failure Acute myocardial infarction in the preceding 3 months Atrial fibrillation or a predominantly paced rhythm Prior TM or current stress management practice

Author, year	Study location	Study setting	Recruitment (start year–end year)	Total duration of study (including training and participants followup)	Inclusion criteria	Exclusion criteria
Pbert L, 2012[27]	Worcester, MA, USA	Primary and pulmonary care clinics at University of Massachusetts Memorial Health Care (UMMHC)	2006–2007	12 months	physician-documented asthma with an objective indicator of bronchial hyper-responsiveness (positive methacholine challenge test, >=12% improvement in forced expiratory volume in 1s (FEV1) or forced vital capacity (FVC) in response to bronchodilator, or 20% variability in diurnal peak expiratory flow (PEF) variation), or >=12% improvement in FEV1 in response to inhaled bronchodilator on spirometry at study entry, and met 2007 NIH/NHLBI criteria for mild, moderate or severe persistent asthma.	intermittent asthma (symptoms less than once/week, brief exacerbations, nocturnal symptoms <= twice/month, and normal lung function between episodes), smoked in the past year, other lung diseases, current treatment for symptomatic cardiovascular disease, history of a positive tuberculosis test, participated in MBSR and/or practicing meditation regularly.
Philippot, 2011[28]	Belgium	Outpatient	NR	Up to 3 months	Tinnitus experienced within the past 6 months A medical check-up by a physician specialized in hearing disorders Sufficient hearing capacity to follow instructions delivered during group sessions Significant psychological distress and impairment in everyday activities resulting from tinnitus	Tinnitus resulting from an organic condition that could benefit from a medical intervention Use of a tinnitus masking apparatus

Author, year	Study location	Study setting	Recruitment (start year–end year)	Total duration of study (including training and participants followup)	Inclusion criteria	Exclusion criteria
Piet, 2010[29]	Denmark	Outpatient	NR	12 months after end of treatment	Age:18–25 Participants with a primary diagnosis of social phobia according to DSM-IV criteria	Alcohol or drug dependence Psychosis, severe depression, bipolar disorder, cluster A and B personality disorders Current (but not previous) psycho-pharmacological or psychotherapeutic treatment
Plews-Ogan, 2005[30]	United States	Outpatient	NR	12 weeks	Adults with musculoskeletal pain for greater than 3 months	Prisoner status Cognitive impairment Lack of reliable transportation Being pregnant
Schmidt, 2010[31]	Germany	Outpatient	NR	8 weeks	Age: 18–70 Female Fibromyalgia Command of the German language	Evidence of suppressed immune functioning Participation in other clinical trials Life-threatening diseases
Schneider, 2012[32]	Milwaukee, WI	recruited from clinical database	March 1998–July 2007	Up to 9.3 years	AA; angiographic evidence of at least 1 coronary artery with >50% stenosis	Acute MI, stroke, or coronary revascularization within the previous 3 months, chronic heart failure with EF<20%, cognitive impairment, noncardiac life-threatening illness.
Segal, 2010[33]	Canada	Outpatient	NR	18 months	Age: 18–65 English speaking and the ability to provide informed consent Diagnosis of MDD according to DSM-IV criteria A score of 16 or higher on the Hamilton Rating Scale for Depression (HRSD) 2 or more previous episodes of MDD (to ensure that those randomized would have a minimum of 3 past episodes)	Substance use or dependence Current practice of meditation more than once per week or yoga more than twice per week. Current or planned pregnancy within the 6 months of acute-phase treatment Depression secondary to a concurrent medical disorder A trial of electroconvulsive therapy within the past 6 months

Author, year	Study location	Study setting	Recruitment (start year–end year)	Total duration of study (including training and participants followup)	Inclusion criteria	Exclusion criteria
Seyedalinaghi, 2012[34]	Iran	outpatient	Aug 2008–Mar 2010	14 months	HIV+, >18 years	substance abuse, psychosis, h/o PTSD, CD4<250, clinically symptomatic
Henderson[35]	United state	Outpatient	NR	24 months	Age: 20–65 Ability to understand English Maintain residence near clinic for two years Able to function normally >50% of the time (ECOG score 0,1,2) Having a working home telephone Willing to accept randomization Newly diagnosed stage I or II breast cancer w/in past 2 years	Current Alcohol/Substance abuse Past psychiatric or neurologic disorder that would limit participation in the study Previous diagnosis of cancer in past 5 years (except non-melanomic skin cancer)
Smith, 1976[36]	United States	University research setting	NR	6 months	Michigan State college student volunteers	No prior meditation experience Not receiving psychotherapy
Taub, 1994[37]	United States	Residential ETOH rehabilitation center	NR	18 months	Male, inner-city, transient severe alcoholics recruited through center	Severe brain damage Serious medical problems IQ below 80 Dx of psychosis Previous exposure to one of special therapies

Author, year	Study location	Study setting	Recruitment (start year–end year)	Total duration of study (including training and participants followup)	Inclusion criteria	Exclusion criteria
Wachholtz, 2008[38]	Canada	Unclear	NR	NR	Current diagnosis of DSM-IV SAD, generalized subtype, based on psychiatric interview and a structured clinical interview Reported at least moderately severe SAD symptoms as determined by a total score X50 on the clinician-rated Liebowitz Social Anxiety Scale (LSAS) Severity rating X4 on the Clinical Global Impression (CGI) Severity of Illness subscale at screening and baseline visits	Substance abuse in past 12 months Current suicide risk, Any form of psychotherapy in last 3 months Received CBT or meditation training in past 12 months Unsafe medical condition Hamilton Depression Rating Scale >14 Presence of other Axis I disorders Lifetime history of psychotic disorders or bipolar disorder
Whitebird, 2012[39]	United States	Outpatient	2007–2010	6 months	caregiver, >21yo, English speaking, no prior meditation program, >5 on stress scale	psych issue past 2 years, SI, antipsychotic or anticonvulsant meds
Wolever, 2012[40]	USA	outpatient	not mentioned	14 weeks	PSS>16; employees of a national health insurance agency	medication or pacemaker affecting heart rate; pregnancy; heavy tobacco use; major medical condition or psychological disorder, prior yoga or meditation experience

Author, year	Study location	Study setting	Recruitment (start year–end year)	Total duration of study (including training and participants followup)	Inclusion criteria	Exclusion criteria
Wong, 2011[41]	Hong Kong	Outpatient	2006–2006	10 months	Age: 18–65 Chronic pain for at least 3 months at mod-severe level on S pain score Not to receive other new treatments during intervention Ability to give written consent	Receiving concurrent treatment with therapies other than medications for pain or psychological symptoms Concurrent doctor diagnosed DSM-IV axis I disorder Illiterate patients Previous participation in an MBSR program or current practice of meditation/relaxation techniques including MBSR

Notes: NR = Not Reported; DX = Description; IQ = Intelligence Quotient; CVD = Cardiovascular Disease; Tx = Treatment; DSM = Diagnostic and Statistical Manual (of mental disorders); CGI = ETOH = Alcohol; TM = Transcendental Meditation; IBS = Inflammatory Bowel Disease; SG = Support Group; MDD = Major Depressive Disorder; COPD = Chronic Obstructive Pulmonary Disorder; LSAS = Liebowitz Social Anxiety Scale; CBT = Cognitive Behavioral Therapy; CGI = Clinical Global Impression

References for Evidence Table E1

1. Barrett B, Hayney MS, Muller D et al. Meditation or exercise for preventing acute respiratory infection: a randomized controlled trial. Ann Fam Med 2012; 10(4):337-46.

2. Bormann JE, Gifford AL, Shively M et al. Effects of spiritual mantram repetition on HIV outcomes: a randomized controlled trial. J Behav Med 2006; 29(4):359-76.

3. Brewer JA, Sinha R, Chen JA et al. Mindfulness training and stress reactivity in substance abuse: results from a randomized, controlled stage I pilot study. Subst Abus 2009; 30(4):306-17.

4. Brewer JA, Mallik S, Babuscio TA et al. Mindfulness training for smoking cessation: Results from a randomized controlled trial. Drug Alcohol Depend 2011.

5. Castillo-Richmond A, Schneider RH, Alexander CN et al. Effects of stress reduction on carotid atherosclerosis in hypertensive African Americans. Stroke 2000; 31(3):568-73.

6. Chiesa A, Mandelli L, Serretti A. Mindfulness-based cognitive therapy versus psycho-education for patients with major depression who did not achieve remission following antidepressant treatment: a preliminary analysis. J Altern Complement Med 2012; 18(8):756-60.

7. Delgado LC, Guerra P, Perakakis P, Vera MN, Reyes del Paso G, Vila J. Treating chronic worry: Psychological and physiological effects of a training programme based on mindfulness. Behav Res Ther 2010; 48(9):873-82.

8. Elder C, Aickin M, Bauer V, Cairns J, Vuckovic N. Randomized trial of a whole-system ayurvedic protocol for type 2 diabetes. Altern Ther Health Med 2006; 12(5):24-30.

9. Garland EL, Gaylord SA, Boettiger CA, Howard MO. Mindfulness training modifies cognitive, affective, and physiological mechanisms implicated in alcohol dependence: results of a randomized controlled pilot trial. J Psychoactive Drugs 2010; 42(2):177-92.

10. Gaylord SA, Palsson OS, Garland EL et al. Mindfulness training reduces the severity of irritable bowel syndrome in women: results of a randomized controlled trial. Am J Gastroenterol 2011; 106(9):1678-88.

11. Gross CR, Kreitzer MJ, Thomas W et al. Mindfulness-based stress reduction for solid organ transplant recipients: a randomized controlled trial. Altern Ther Health Med 2010; 16(5):30-8.

12. Gross CR, Kreitzer MJ, Reilly-Spong M et al. Mindfulness-based stress reduction versus pharmacotherapy for chronic primary insomnia: a randomized controlled clinical trial. Explore (NY) 2011; 7(2):76-87.

13. Hebert JR, Ebbeling CB, Olendzki BC et al. Change in women's diet and body mass following intensive intervention for early-stage breast cancer. J Am Diet Assoc 2001; 101(4):421-31.

14. Jayadevappa R, Johnson JC, Bloom BS et al. Effectiveness of transcendental meditation on functional capacity and quality of life of African Americans with congestive heart failure: a randomized control study Ethn Dis. 2007 Summer;17(3):595. Ethnicity & Disease 2007; 17(1):72-7.

15. Jazaieri H, Goldin PR, Werner K, Ziv M, Gross JJ. A Randomized Trial of MBSR Versus Aerobic Exercise for Social Anxiety Disorder. J Clin Psychol 2012.

16. Kuyken W, Byford S, Taylor RS et al. Mindfulness-based cognitive therapy to prevent relapse in recurrent depression. J Consult Clin Psychol 2008; 76(6):966-78.

17. Lee SH, Ahn SC, Lee YJ, Choi TK, Yook KH, Suh SY. Effectiveness of a meditation-based stress management program as an adjunct to pharmacotherapy in patients with anxiety disorder. J Psychosom Res 2007; 62(2):189-95.

18. Lehrer PM. Progressive relaxation and meditation: A study of psychophysiological and therapeutic differences between two techniques. Behav Res Ther 1983; 21(6):651-62.

19. Malarkey WB, Jarjoura D, Klatt M. Workplace based mindfulness practice and inflammation: A randomized trial. Brain Behav Immun 2012.

20. Miller CK, Kristeller JL, Headings A, Nagaraja H, Miser WF. Comparative Effectiveness of a Mindful Eating Intervention to a Diabetes Self-Management Intervention among Adults with Type 2 Diabetes: A Pilot Study. J Acad Nutr Diet 2012; 112(11):1835-42.

21. Moritz S, Quan H, Rickhi B et al. A home study-based spirituality education program decreases emotional distress and increases quality of life—a randomized, controlled trial. Altern Ther Health Med 2006; 12(6):26-35.

22. Morone NE, Rollman BL, Moore CG, Li Q, Weiner DK. A mind-body program for older adults with chronic low back pain: results of a pilot study. Pain Med 2009; 10(8):1395-407.

23. Mularski RA, Munjas BA, Lorenz KA et al. Randomized controlled trial of mindfulness-based therapy for dyspnea in chronic obstructive lung disease. J Altern Complement Med 2009; 15(10):1083-90.

24. Murphy TJ, Pagano RR, Marlatt GA. Lifestyle modification with heavy alcohol drinkers: effects of aerobic exercise and meditation. Addict Behav 1986; 11(2):175-86.

25. Oken BS, Fonareva I, Haas M et al. Pilot controlled trial of mindfulness meditation and education for dementia caregivers. J Altern Complement Med 2010; 16(10):1031-8.

26. Paul-Labrador M, Polk D, Dwyer JH et al. Effects of a randomized controlled trial of transcendental meditation on components of the metabolic syndrome in subjects with coronary heart disease. Arch Intern Med 2006; 166(11):1218-24.

27. Pbert L, Madison JM, Druker S et al. Effect of mindfulness training on asthma quality of life and lung function: A randomised controlled trial. 2012; 67(9):769-76.

28. Philippot P, Nef F, Clauw L, Romree M, Segal Z. A Randomized Controlled Trial of Mindfulness-Based Cognitive Therapy for Treating Tinnitus. Clin Psychol Psychother 2011.

29. Piet J, Hougaard E, Hecksher MS, Rosenberg NK. A randomized pilot study of mindfulness-based cognitive therapy and group cognitive-behavioral therapy for young adults with social phobia. Scand J Psychol 2010; 51(5):403-10.

30. Plews-Ogan M, Owens JE, Goodman M, Wolfe P, Schorling J. A pilot study evaluating mindfulness-based stress reduction and massage for the management of chronic pain. J Gen Intern Med 2005; 20(12):1136-8.

31. Schmidt S, Grossman P, Schwarzer B, Jena S, Naumann J, Walach H. Treating fibromyalgia with mindfulness-based stress reduction: results from a 3-armed randomized controlled trial. Pain 2011; 152(2):361-9.

32. Schneider RH, Grim CE, Rainforth MV et al. Stress Reduction in the Secondary Prevention of Cardiovascular Disease: Randomized, Controlled Trial of Transcendental Meditation and Health Education in Blacks. (1941-7705 (Electronic). 1941-7713 (Linking)).

33. Segal ZV, Bieling P, Young T et al. Antidepressant monotherapy vs sequential pharmacotherapy and mindfulness-based cognitive therapy, or placebo, for relapse prophylaxis in recurrent depression. Arch Gen Psychiatry 2010; 67(12):1256-64.

34. Seyed Alinaghi S, Jam S, Foroughi M et al. Randomized controlled trial of mindfulness-based stress reduction delivered to human immunodeficiency virus-positive patients in Iran: effects on CD4[sup]+[/sup] T lymphocyte count and medical and psychological symptoms. Psychosom Med 2012; 74(6):620-7.

35. Henderson VP, Clemow L, Massion AO, Hurley TG, Druker S, Hebert JR. The effects of mindfulness-based stress reduction on psychosocial outcomes and quality of life in early-stage breast cancer patients: a randomized trial. Breast Cancer Res Treat 2011.

36. Smith JC. Psychotherapeutic effects of transcendental meditation with controls for expectation of relief and daily sitting. J Consult Clin Psychol 1976; 44(4):630-7.

37. Taub E, Steiner SS, Weingarten E, Walton KG. Effectiveness of broad spectrum approaches to relapse prevention in severe alcoholism: A long-term, randomized, controlled trial of Transcendental Meditation, EMG biofeedback and electronic neurotherapy. Alcoholism Treatment Quarterly 1994; 11(1-2):187-220.

38. Koszycki D, Benger M, Shlik J, Bradwejn J. Randomized trial of a meditation-based stress reduction program and cognitive behavior therapy in generalized social anxiety disorder. Behav Res Ther 2007; 45(10):2518-26.

39. Whitebird RR, Kreitzer M, Crain AL, Lewis BA, Hanson LR, Enstad CJ. Mindfulness-Based Stress Reduction for Family Caregivers: A Randomized Controlled Trial. Gerontologist 2012.

40. Wolever RQ, Bobinet KJ, McCabe K et al. Effective and viable mind-body stress reduction in the workplace: a randomized controlled trial. J Occup Health Psychol 2012; 17(2):246-58.

41. Wong SY, Chan FW, Wong RL et al. Comparing the Effectiveness of Mindfulness-based Stress Reduction and Multidisciplinary Intervention Programs for Chronic Pain: A Randomized Comparative Trial. Clin J Pain 2011; 27(8):724-34.

Evidence Table E2. Participant characteristics for included studies

Author, Year	Total N at randomization	Target Population	Arm (n)	Women (%)	Mean Age, years (SD)	Race, n(%)	Education, n(%)	Mean Weight, (SD)	Mean BMI, (SD)
Henderson VP, 2011[1]	180	Women with early stage Breast Cancer	Overall (163)	163 (100)	49.8 ± 8.4	NR	NR	NR	NR
			Arm 1 MBSR (53)	53 (100)	NR	W:51(96) O: 2 (4)	HS:9 (17) C: 11 (21) GS: 12 (23) O: 21 (39)	NR	NR
			Arm 2 NEP (52)	52(100)	NR	W:48 (92) O: 4 (8)	HS:13 (25) C: 7 (14) GS: 10 (19) O: 22 (42)	NR	NR
			Arm 3 UC (58)	58(100)	NR	W:56 (97) O: 2 (3)	HS:15 (26) C: 10 (17) GS: 17 (29) O: 16 (28)	NR	NR
Wong SY-S, 2011[2]	100	Patients with chronic pain	Overall (99)	NR	47.9 (7.84)	NR	HS:53 C: 11 GS: 13 PE: 22	NR	NR
			Arm 1 MBSR (51)	NR	48.7 (7.84)	NR	HS:31 C: 4 GS: 6 PE: 10	NR	NR
			Arm 2 MPI (48)	NR	47.1 (7.82)	NR	HS:22 C: 7 GS: 7 PE: 12	NR	NR
Brewer, 2011[3]	88	Nicotine-dependent adults with interest in smoking cessation	Overall(87)	33(37.9)	45.9	W:43(49.4) B:34(39.1) L:9(10.3) O:1(1.1)	<HS:6(6.9) HS:31(35.6) C:25(28.7) O:25(28.7)	NR	NR
			Arm MT (41)	14(34.1)	46.5	W:24(58.5) B:15(36.6) L:2(4.9) O:0	<HS:2(4.9) HS:17(41.5) C:12(29.3) O:10(24.4)	NR	NR
			Arm FFS(46)	19(41.3)	45.3	W:19(41.3) B:19(41.3) L:7(15.2) O:1(2.2)	<HS:4(8.7) HS:314(30.4) C:213(28.3) O:15(32.6)	NR	NR

Author, Year	Total N at randomization	Target Population	Arm (n)	Women (%)	Mean Age, years (SD)	Race, n(%)	Education, n(%)	Mean Weight, (SD)	Mean BMI, (SD)
Gaylord SA, 2011[4]	97	Women with Irritable Bowel Syndrome	Overall (75)	75(100)	NR	NR	NR	NR	NR
			Arm 1 MG (36)	36(100)	44.72 (12.55)	W:29(81) B: 5 (14) O: 2 (6)	HS:0(0) C: 7(19) GS:19(53) O: 9(25) PE: 1(3)	NR	NR
			Arm 2 SG (39)	39(100)	40.89 (14.68)	W:25 (64) B: 8 (21) O: 6 (15)	HS:3 (8) C: 9 (23) GS:12 (30) O:14(36) PE:1(3)	NR	NR
Philippot P, 2011[5]	30	Patients with Tinnitus	Overall (25)	NR	60 (11.53)	NR	NR	NR	NR
			Arm 1 MG (13)	NR	60.92 (11.09)	NR	PE: 14.61(2.60)	NR	NR
			Arm 2 RG (12)	NR	59.75 (12.46)	NR	PE: 14.58(2.71)	NR	NR
Gross CR, 2011[6]	30	Adults Primary Chronic Insomnia	Overall (30)	NR	Range (19–65)	NR	NR	NR	NR
			Arm 1 MBSR (20)	15(75)	Median (47) Range (21–65)	W:20(100) B: 0 (0) L: 1 (5)	C: 18(90)	NR	NR
			Arm 2 PCT (10)	7(70)	Median (53.5) Range (29–59)	W:9(90) B: 1(10) L: 1(10)	C: 6 (60)	NR	NR
Schmidt S, 2010[7]	177	Women with Fibromyalgia	Overall (168)	168 (100)	NR	NR	NR	NR	NR
			Arm 1 MBSR (53)	53(100)	53.4 (8.7)	NR	HS:20.8 PE: 34.0 (9) PE: 41.5 (11)	NR	NR
			Arm 2 RG (56)	56(100)	51.9 (9.2)	NR	HS:30.4 PE: 28.6(:9) PE:39.3(11)	NR	NR
			Arm 3 WL (59)	59(100)	52.3 (10.9)	NR	HS:42.4 PE: 30.5(9) PE:25.4(11)	NR	NR

Author, Year	Total N at randomization	Target Population	Arm (n)	Women (%)	Mean Age, years (SD)	Race, n(%)	Education, n(%)	Mean Weight, (SD)	Mean BMI, (SD)
Segal ZV, 2010[8]	84	Patients with recurrent depression	Overall (84)	53 (63)	44.0 (11.0)	W:66 (79)	NR	NR	NR
			Arm 1 MBCT (26)	13 (50)	44.8 (9.4)	W:19 (73)	NR	NR	NR
			Arm 2 M-ADM (28)	20 (71)	45.8 (11.4)	W:24 (86)	NR	NR	NR
			Arm 3 P+Cl (30)	20 (67)	41.9 (11.6)	W:23 W:(77)	NR	NR	NR
Oken BS, 2010[9]	31	Caregivers of close relatives with Dementia	Overall (31)	NR	NR	NR	NR	NR	NR
			Arm 1 MM (10)	10	62.50 (11.61)	W:8 B:1 A:1	NR	NR	NR
			Arm 2 EDN (11)	11	67.09 (8.36)	W:10 B:0 A:1	NR	NR	NR
			Arm 3 RO (10)	10	63.80 (7.93)	W:10 B:0 A:0	NR	NR	NR
Gross CR, 2010[10]	150	Solid Organ Transplant Recipients	Overall (137)	NR	NR	NR	NR	NR	NR
			Arm 1 MBSR (71)	33 (46.5)	55 (11.3)	W:65(91) O: 9(8)	HS:3(4) C: 29(41) GS: 15(21) O: 24(34)	NR	NR
			Arm 2 HE (66)	29 (43.9)	52 (10.4)	W:62(94) O: 9(6)	HS:10(15) C: 24(36) GS: 11(17) O: 21(32)	NR	NR
Garland EL, 2010[11]	53	Alcohol Dependent Adults	Overall (53)	11 (20.8)	40.3 (9.4)	W:18(34.0) B: 32(60.4) O: 3(5.6)	NR	NR	NR
			Arm 1 MORE (27)	5 (18.5)	39.9 (8.7)	W:7(25.9) B: 17 (62.9) O: 3(11.1)	NR	NR	NR
			Arm 2 ASG (26)	6 (23.1)	40.7 (10.2)	W:11(42.3) B: 15 (57.7) O: 0(0)	NR	NR	NR
Delgado LC, 2010[12]	36	Patients with chronic worry	Overall (36)	36 (100)	Range 18–24	NR	NR	NR	NR
			Arm 1 MG (18)	18 (100)	NR	NR	NR	NR	NR
			Arm 2 RG (18)	18 (100)	NR	NR	NR	NR	NR

Author, Year	Total N at randomization	Target Population	Arm (n)	Women (%)	Mean Age, years (SD)	Race, n(%)	Education, n(%)	Mean Weight, (SD)	Mean BMI, (SD)
Morone NE, 2009[13]*	40	Community dwelling older adults with chronic low back pain	Overall (35)	NR	NR	NR	NR	NR	NR
			Arm 1 MM (16)	11	78 (7.1)	W:15 B:1	NR	NR	NR
			Arm 2 HE (19)	11	73 (6.2)	W:15 B:1 A:1	NR	NR	NR
Brewer, 2009[14]	36	Patients with ETOH and/or cocaine use disorders	Overall(36)	7(28)	38.2	W:16(64) B:6(24) L:3(12)	YD:13.2	NR	NR
			MT(21)	5(27.8)	35.6	W:10(55.6) B:6(33.3) L:2(11.1)	YD:13.1	NR	NR
			CBT(15)	2(28.6)	45	W:6(85.7) B:0 L:1(14.3)	YD:13.7	NR	NR
Mularski RA, 2009[15]	86	Patients Chronic obstructive lung disease	Overall (86)		67.4 (2.2)	O:(49)	O:>high school (47)	NR	28.5(4.6)
			Arm 1 MBBT (44)	1	70.6 (10.6)	O: 17 (38.6)	HS:21(47.7)	NR	26.1 (7.5)
			Arm 2 SG (42)	0	64.0 (9.1)	O: 25 (60.0)	HS:19 (45.2)	NR	31.0 (6.9)
Kuyken W, 2008[16]	123	Patients with depression	Overall (123)	NR	NR	NR	NR	NR	NR
			Arm 1 MBCT (61)	47 (77)	48.95 (10.55)	W:60(98)	HS:24 (39) C: 12 (20) No Ed: 9 (15) Some School 16 (26)	NR	NR
			Arm 2 M-ADM (62)	47 (76)	49.37 (11.84)	W:62(100)	HS:15 (24) C: 14 (23) No Ed: 17 (27) Some School 16 (26)	NR	NR
Koszycki D, 2007[17]	53	Patients with Generalized Social Anxiety Disorder	Overall (53)	NR	NR	NR	NR	NR	NR
			Arm 1 MBSR (26)	16	38.6 (15.7)	NR	NR	NR	NR
			Arm 2 CBGT (27)	12	37.6 (11.1)	NR	NR	NR	NR

Author, Year	Total N at randomization	Target Population	Arm (n)	Women (%)	Mean Age, years (SD)	Race, n(%)	Education, n(%)	Mean Weight, (SD)	Mean BMI, (SD)
Lee SH, 2006[18]	46	Patients with Generalized Anxiety Disorder or Panic Disorder with or without agoraphobia	Overall	NR	NR	NR	NR	NR	NR
			Arm 1 MM (24)	9 (37)	38.6 (7.4)	NR	YE:13.0 (2.3)	NR	NR
			Arm 2 EDN (22)	7 (32)	38.1 (9.7)	NR	YE: 13.5 (2.4)	NR	NR
Moritz S, 2006[19]	165	Patients with psychological distress	Overall (165)	NR	NR	NR	NR	NR	NR
			Arm 1 MBSR (54)	41 (76.0)	43.6	NR	C: 29 (54.0) GS: 9 (17.0)	NR	NR
			Arm 2 Spirituality (56)	53 (95.0)	44.6	NR	C: 23 (41.0) GS:10(18.0)	NR	NR
			Arm 3 Control (55)	44 (80.0)	43.9	NR	C: 20 (36.0) GS: 13(24.0)	NR	NR
Elder, 2006[20]	60	diabetic patients in primary care setting	Overall(60)	NR	NR	NR	NR	NR	NR
			Vedic/TM(30)	(50)	53.7(8.4)	NR	NR	247 (49)	NR
			Health Education(30)	(67)	53.3(12.0)	NR	NR	231 (67)	NR
Bormann JE, 2006[21]	93	Adults with HIV Infection	Overall (93)	18 (19.4)	42.9 (6.84)	W:48(51.6) B: 29 (31.2) L: 14 (15.1) O: 2 (2.2)	HS:29 (31.2) C: 24 (25.8) O: 40 (43.0)	NR	NR
			Arm 1 MP (46)	9 (19.6)	43.3 (6.56)	W:25 (54.3) B: 16 (34.8) L: 5 (10.9) AI:0(0)	HS:11 (23.9) C: 14 (30.4) O: 21 (52.5)	NR	NR
			Arm 2 ACG (47)	9 (19.1)	42.5 (7.17)	W:23(48.9) B:13 (27.7) L: 9 (19.1) AI: 2 (4.3)	HS:18 (38.3) C: 10 (41.7) O: 19 (47.5)	NR	NR
Paul-Labrador M, 2006[22]	103	Patients with Metabolic Syndrome	Overall (103)	NR	NR	NR	NR	NR	NR
			Arm 1 TM (52)	11 (21.0)	67.7 (9.0)	NR	NR	NR	28.3 (4.5)
			Arm 2 HE (51)	8 (16.0)	67.1 (10.5)	NR	NR	NR	28.3 (4.6)
Plews-Ogan M, 2005[23]	30	Patients with chronic musculoskeletal pain	Overall (30)	23	46.5	NR	YE:12	NR	NR
			Arm 1 MBSR (10)	NR	NR	NR	NR	NR	NR
			Arm 2 MS (10)	NR	NR	NR	NR	NR	NR
			Arm 3 SC (10)	NR	NR	NR	NR	NR	NR

Author, Year	Total N at randomization	Target Population	Arm (n)	Women (%)	Mean Age, years (SD)	Race, n(%)	Education, n(%)	Mean Weight, (SD)	Mean BMI, (SD)
Hebert JR, 2001[24]	172	Patients with breast cancer	Overall (157)	NR	NR	NR	NR	NR	NR
			Arm 1 SR (51)	51 (100)	NR	W:49(96.0) O: 2 (4.0)	HS:8 (16.0) C: 11 (22.0) GS: 13(25.0) O: 19 (37.0)	72.2 (13.9)	NR
			Arm 2 NE (50)	50 (100)	NR	W:47(94.0) O: 3(6.0)	HS:10 (20.0) C: 6 (12.0) GS:10(20.0) O: 24 (48.0)	70.6 (11.7)	NR
			Arm 3 UC (56)	56 (100)	NR	W:54(96.0) O: 2(4.0)	HS:13(23.0) C: 10 (18.0) GS:17(30.0) O: 16 (29.0)	74.3 (17.5)	NR
Castillo-Riachmond, 2000[25]	138	Hypertension (high normal blood pressure, stage I or stage II hypertension	Overall(60)	NR	NR	NR	NR	NR	NR
			TM Group(31)	NR	55.2	NR	NR	196.6	NR
			Health Education Group(29)	NR	52.5	NR	NR	194.2	NR
Murphy, 1986[26]	60	High-volume drinkers with no prior running or meditation experience	Meditation(14)	0	25	NR	NR	NR	NR
			Running(13)	0	24.9	NR	NR	NR	NR
			NT(16)	0	24.5	NR	NR	NR	NR
Smith JC, 1976[27]	139	Anxious college students	TM (49)	NR	Reported as 22 for whole group, not by arm	NR	NR	NR	NR
			PSI (51)	NR		NR	NR	NR	NR
			WL (39)	NR		NR	NR	NR	NR
Piet J, 2010[28]	26	Adults with social phobia	Overall (26)			NR	NR	NR	NR
			Arm 1 MBCT (14)	11 (79.0)	21.6	NR	NR	NR	NR
			Arm 2 CBGT (12)	7 (58.0)	22.1	NR	NR	NR	NR
Taub E, 1994[29]	Ambiguous. 457 "agreed to participate," 250 were counted as study subjects after completing one week of trial	Alcoholics In rehab	TM	0	44.3 Reported as whole group mean, no SD	NR	Whole group mean education reported as 10.7 years, no SD	NR	NR
			EMG	0		NR	NR	NR	NR
			NT	0		NR	NR	NR	NR

Author, Year	Total N at randomization	Target Population	Arm (n)	Women (%)	Mean Age, years (SD)	Race, n(%)	Education, n(%)	Mean Weight, (SD)	Mean BMI, (SD)
Lehrer PM, 1983[30]	61	Adults with anxiety	Overall	NR	NR	NR	NR	NR	NR
			Arm 1 M (only) (23)	NR	NR	NR	NR	NR	NR
			Arm 2 RL (19)	NR	NR	NR	NR	NR	NR
			Arm 3 WL (19)	NR	NR	NR	NR	NR	NR
Jayadevappa R, 2007[31]	23	African American patients with heart failure	Overall (23)	NR	NR	B: 23 (100)	NR	NR	NR
			Arm 1 TM (13)	(46.15)	64.4 (5.7)	B: 13 (100)	HS:(38.46) C: (7.69) GS: (23.08) O: (15.38) PE: (15.38)	NR	NR
			Arm 2 HE (10)	(80.00)	63.8 (8.9)	B: 10 (100)	HS:(20.00) C: (20.00) GS: (0) O: (50.00) PE: (10.00)	NR	NR
Miller, 2012[32]	68	Overweight DM	Overall						
	32	MB-EAT	Arm 1	63	53.9	W:(82) B: (19) A: (0)	C: (48) GS: (48)	NR	NR
	36	SC	Arm 2	64	54	W:(72) B: (24) A: (4)	C: (60) GS:(60)	NR	NR
Malarkey, 2012[33]	186	CRP>3.0	Overall						
	93	MBI-ld	Arm 1	88	51	NR	NR	NR	NR
	93	Educ	Arm 2	87	49	NR	NR	NR	NR
Whitebird, 2012[34]	78	Caregivers	Overall	88.5	56.8 (9.9)	W: (97.4) L: (1.3) AI: (1.3)	HS: (43.6) C: (34.6) GS: (21.8)	NR	NR
			MBSR (38)	86.8	57.2 (9.6)	W: (100) L: (0) AI: (0)	HS: (44.7) C: (31.6) GS: (23.7)	NR	NR
			Education and Support(40)	90	56.4 (10.2)	W: (95) L: (2.5) AI: (2.5)	HS: (42.5) C: (37.5) GS: (20)	NR	NR

Author, Year	Total N at randomization	Target Population	Arm (n)	Women (%)	Mean Age, years (SD)	Race, n(%)	Education, n(%)	Mean Weight, (SD)	Mean BMI, (SD)
Chiesa, 2012[35]	18	Depression	Overall (18)		NR	NR	HS:89 C:29 O:0	NR	NR
			MBCT (9)	78	NR	NR	HS:29 C:42 O:29	NR	NR
			Education (9)	71					
Barrett, 2012[36]	154	>50yo w/ colds	Overall						
	51	MBSR	Arm 1	82	60	W: (93) O: (6)	C: (71) GS: (71)	NR	NR
	51	Exercise	Arm 2	83	59	W: (92) O: (2)	C: (57) GS: (57)	NR	NR
Jazaieri, 2012[37]	56	SAD	Overall						
	31	MBSR	Arm 1	61	32.9	W: (42) L: (10) A: (45)	O: (16.4)	NR	NR
	25	AE	Arm 2	40	32.9	W: (40) L: (4) A: (44)	O: (16.8)	NR	NR
Wolever, 2012[38]	239	stressed employees	Overall	77	42.9	W: (78) B: (6) L: (6) A: (8)	C: (72) GS:(72)	NR	NR
	96		Arm 1	77		W: (85) B: (4) A: (5)	HS: (3) C: (53) GS: (22)	NR	NR
	90		Arm 2	73		W: (74) B: (10) A: (8)	HS: (2) C: (50) GS: (28)	NR	NR
Seyedalinaghi, 2012[39]	245		Overall	31%	35.1	NR	NR	NR	NR
	120	MBSR	Arm 1	35%	34.7	NR	NR	NR	NR
	125	Educ/Spprt	Arm 2	27%	35.6	NR	NR	NR	NR
Pbert L, 2012[40]	83	83	Overall	56 (67.5)	52.8	W: 76(93.8)	NR	NR	NR
	42	MBSR	Arm 1	27 (64.3)	51.93 (13.6)	W: 36(90.0) B: 1 (2.5) L: 5 (12.8) O: 3 (7.5)	HS: 6 (14.6) C: 14 (34.1) GS: 8 (19.5) SC: 13 (31.7)	NR	NR
	41	HLC	Arm 2	29 (70.7)	53.61 (13.7)	W: 40(97.6) B: 0 (0.0) L: 1 (2.6) O: 1 (2.4)	HS: 7 (17.5) C: 13 (32.5) GS: 4 (10.0) SC: 16 (40.0)	NR	NR

Author, Year	Total N at randomization	Target Population	Arm (n)	Women (%)	Mean Age, years (SD)	Race, n(%)	Education, n(%)	Mean Weight, (SD)	Mean BMI, (SD)
Schneider, 2012[41]	201	AA w/CAD	Overall						
	99		Arm 1 TM	41.4	59.9(10.7)	B: (100)	O: 11.3(2.7)	NR	NR
			Arm 2 HE	44.1	58.4(10.5)	B: (100)	O: 9.9(3.6)	NR	NR

Notes: MBSR=Mindfulness-based Stress Reduction; NEP=Nutrition Education Program; UC=Usual Supportive Care; MPI=Multidisciplinary Pain Intervention; MT=Mindfulness Training; FFS=Freedom From Smoking Treatment; MG=Mindfulness Group/Mindfulness Treatment Group; SG=Support Group; RG=Relaxation Treatment Group; UD=Undisclosed; YE=Years of Education; PCT=Pharmacotherapy; WL=Wait List; MBCT=Mindfulness-based cognitive therapy; M-ADM=Maintenance Antidepressant Monotherapy; P+Cl=Placebo plus Clinical Management; MM=Mindfulness Meditation; EDN=Education; RO-Respite Only; HE=Health Education; MBBT=Mindfulness Based Breathing Therapy; SP=Spiritual Meditation Group; IS=Internal Secular Meditation Group; ES=External Secular Meditation Group; RL=Progressive Muscle Relaxation Group; CBGT=Cognitive Behavioral Group Therapy; MP=Mantram Practice; ACG=Attention Control Group; TM=Transcendental Meditation; MS=Massage; SC=Standard Care; NE=Nutrition Education; SR=Mindfulness Stress Reduction; M(only)=Meditation Only; SH=Sleep Hygiene; SC=Stimulus Control; WL=Wait List Control; CSM=Corporate Stress Management; NA=Not Applicable; NR=Not Reported; HS=high school; C= college degree; GS= graduate degree; PE=primary education

References for Evidence Table E2

1. Henderson VP, Clemow L, Massion AO, Hurley TG, Druker S, Hebert JR. The effects of mindfulness-based stress reduction on psychosocial outcomes and quality of life in early-stage breast cancer patients: a randomized trial. Breast Cancer Res Treat 2011.

2. Wong SY, Chan FW, Wong RL et al. Comparing the Effectiveness of Mindfulness-based Stress Reduction and Multidisciplinary Intervention Programs for Chronic Pain: A Randomized Comparative Trial. Clin J Pain 2011; 27(8):724-34.

3. Brewer JA, Mallik S, Babuscio TA et al. Mindfulness training for smoking cessation: Results from a randomized controlled trial. Drug Alcohol Depend 2011.

4. Gaylord SA, Palsson OS, Garland EL et al. Mindfulness training reduces the severity of irritable bowel syndrome in women: results of a randomized controlled trial. Am J Gastroenterol 2011; 106(9):1678-88.

5. Philippot P, Nef F, Clauw L, Romree M, Segal Z. A Randomized Controlled Trial of Mindfulness-Based Cognitive Therapy for Treating Tinnitus. Clin Psychol Psychother 2011.

6. Gross CR, Kreitzer MJ, Reilly-Spong M et al. Mindfulness-based stress reduction versus pharmacotherapy for chronic primary insomnia: a randomized controlled clinical trial. Explore (NY) 2011; 7(2):76-87.

7. Schmidt S, Grossman P, Schwarzer B, Jena S, Naumann J, Walach H. Treating fibromyalgia with mindfulness-based stress reduction: results from a 3-armed randomized controlled trial. Pain 2011; 152(2):361-9.

8. Segal ZV, Bieling P, Young T et al. Antidepressant monotherapy vs sequential pharmacotherapy and mindfulness-based cognitive therapy, or placebo, for relapse prophylaxis in recurrent depression. Arch Gen Psychiatry 2010; 67(12):1256-64.

9. Oken BS, Fonareva I, Haas M et al. Pilot controlled trial of mindfulness meditation and education for dementia caregivers. J Altern Complement Med 2010; 16(10):1031-8.

10. Gross CR, Kreitzer MJ, Thomas W et al. Mindfulness-based stress reduction for solid organ transplant recipients: a randomized controlled trial. Altern Ther Health Med 2010; 16(5):30-8.

11. Garland EL, Gaylord SA, Boettiger CA, Howard MO. Mindfulness training modifies cognitive, affective, and physiological mechanisms implicated in alcohol dependence: results of a randomized controlled pilot trial. J Psychoactive Drugs 2010; 42(2):177-92.

12. Delgado LC, Guerra P, Perakakis P, Vera MN, Reyes del Paso G, Vila J. Treating chronic worry: Psychological and physiological effects of a training programme based on mindfulness. Behav Res Ther 2010; 48(9):873-82.

13. Morone NE, Rollman BL, Moore CG, Li Q, Weiner DK. A mind-body program for older adults with chronic low back pain: results of a pilot study. Pain Med 2009; 10(8):1395-407.

14. Brewer JA, Sinha R, Chen JA et al. Mindfulness training and stress reactivity in substance abuse: results from a randomized, controlled stage I pilot study. Subst Abus 2009; 30(4):306-17.

15. Mularski RA, Munjas BA, Lorenz KA et al. Randomized controlled trial of mindfulness-based therapy for dyspnea in chronic obstructive lung disease. J Altern Complement Med 2009; 15(10):1083-90.

16. Kuyken W, Byford S, Taylor RS et al. Mindfulness-based cognitive therapy to prevent relapse in recurrent depression. J Consult Clin Psychol 2008; 76(6):966-78.

17. Koszycki D, Benger M, Shlik J, Bradwejn J. Randomized trial of a meditation-based stress reduction program and cognitive behavior therapy in generalized social anxiety disorder. Behav Res Ther 2007; 45(10):2518-26.

18. Lee SH, Ahn SC, Lee YJ, Choi TK, Yook KH, Suh SY. Effectiveness of a meditation-based stress management program as an adjunct to pharmacotherapy in patients with anxiety disorder. J Psychosom Res 2007; 62(2):189-95.

19. Moritz S, Quan H, Rickhi B et al. A home study-based spirituality education program decreases emotional distress and increases quality of life—a randomized, controlled trial. Altern Ther Health Med 2006; 12(6):26-35.

20. Elder C, Aickin M, Bauer V, Cairns J, Vuckovic N. Randomized trial of a whole-system ayurvedic protocol for type 2 diabetes. Altern Ther Health Med 2006; 12(5):24-30.

21. Bormann JE, Gifford AL, Shively M et al. Effects of spiritual mantram repetition on HIV outcomes: a randomized controlled trial. J Behav Med 2006; 29(4):359-76.

22. Paul-Labrador M, Polk D, Dwyer JH et al. Effects of a randomized controlled trial of transcendental meditation on components of the metabolic syndrome in subjects with coronary heart disease. Arch Intern Med 2006; 166(11):1218-24.

23. Plews-Ogan M, Owens JE, Goodman M, Wolfe P, Schorling J. A pilot study evaluating mindfulness-based stress reduction and massage for the management of chronic pain. J Gen Intern Med 2005; 20(12):1136-8.

24. Hebert JR, Ebbeling CB, Olendzki BC et al. Change in women's diet and body mass following intensive intervention for early-stage breast cancer. J Am Diet Assoc 2001; 101(4):421-31.

25. Castillo-Richmond A, Schneider RH, Alexander CN et al. Effects of stress reduction on carotid atherosclerosis in hypertensive African Americans. Stroke 2000; 31(3):568-73.

26. Murphy TJ, Pagano RR, Marlatt GA. Lifestyle modification with heavy alcohol drinkers: effects of aerobic exercise and meditation. Addict Behav 1986; 11(2):175-86.

27. Smith JC. Psychotherapeutic effects of transcendental meditation with controls for expectation of relief and daily sitting. J Consult Clin Psychol 1976; 44(4):630-7.

28. Piet J, Hougaard E, Hecksher MS, Rosenberg NK. A randomized pilot study of mindfulness-based cognitive therapy and group cognitive-behavioral therapy for young adults with social phobia. Scand J Psychol 2010; 51(5):403-10.

29. Taub E, Steiner SS, Weingarten E, Walton KG. Effectiveness of broad spectrum approaches to relapse prevention in severe alcoholism: A long-term, randomized, controlled trial of Transcendental Meditation, EMG biofeedback and electronic neurotherapy. Alcoholism Treatment Quarterly 1994; 11(1-2):187-220.

30. Lehrer PM. Progressive relaxation and meditation: A study of psychophysiological and therapeutic differences between two techniques. Behav Res Ther 1983; 21(6):651-62.

31. Jayadevappa R, Johnson JC, Bloom BS et al. Effectiveness of transcendental meditation on functional capacity and quality of life of African Americans with congestive heart failure: a randomized control study Ethn Dis. 2007 Summer;17(3):595. Ethnicity & Disease 2007; 17(1):72-7.

32. Miller CK, Kristeller JL, Headings A, Nagaraja H, Miser WF. Comparative Effectiveness of a Mindful Eating Intervention to a Diabetes Self-Management Intervention among Adults with Type 2 Diabetes: A Pilot Study. J Acad Nutr Diet 2012; 112(11):1835-42.

33. Malarkey WB, Jarjoura D, Klatt M. Workplace based mindfulness practice and inflammation: A randomized trial. Brain Behav Immun 2012.

34. Whitebird RR, Kreitzer M, Crain AL, Lewis BA, Hanson LR, Enstad CJ. Mindfulness-Based Stress Reduction for Family Caregivers: A Randomized Controlled Trial. Gerontologist 2012.

35. Chiesa A, Mandelli L, Serretti A. Mindfulness-based cognitive therapy versus psycho-education for patients with major depression who did not achieve remission following antidepressant treatment: a preliminary analysis. J Altern Complement Med 2012; 18(8):756-60.

36. Barrett B, Hayney MS, Muller D et al. Meditation or exercise for preventing acute respiratory infection: a randomized controlled trial. Ann Fam Med 2012; 10(4):337-46.

37. Jazaieri H, Goldin PR, Werner K, Ziv M, Gross JJ. A Randomized Trial of MBSR Versus Aerobic Exercise for Social Anxiety Disorder. J Clin Psychol 2012.

38. Wolever RQ, Bobinet KJ, McCabe K et al. Effective and viable mind-body stress reduction in the workplace: a randomized controlled trial. J Occup Health Psychol 2012; 17(2):246-58.

39. SeyedAlinaghi S, Jam S, Foroughi M et al. Randomized controlled trial of mindfulness-based stress reduction delivered to human immunodeficiency virus-positive patients in Iran: effects on CD4^{+} T lymphocyte count and medical and psychological symptoms. Psychosom Med 2012; 74(6):620-7.

40. Pbert L, Madison JM, Druker S et al. Effect of mindfulness training on asthma quality of life and lung function: A randomised controlled trial. 2012; 67(9):769-76.

41. Schneider RH, Grim CE, Rainforth MV et al. Stress Reduction in the Secondary Prevention of Cardiovascular Disease: Randomized, Controlled Trial of Transcendental Meditation and Health Education in Blacks. (1941-7705 (Electronic). 1941-7713 (Linking)).

Evidence Table E3. Scales for anxiety (KQ1)

Scale	Brief Description	Reliability	Validity	Original Citation Date
General Anxiety				
Beck Anxiety Inventory	21-item self report measure to assess severity of anxiety symptoms within an adult psychiatric population. Respondents rate their experience of specific anxiety symptoms within the last week using a four-point Likert scale.	Excellent internal consistency, α range from .85 to .93	The BAI correlated significantly more strongly with a measure of anxiety (r =.48) than with a measure of depression (r = .25) in a psychiatric sample. Although the BAI shows moderate correlations with measures of depression, it has been found to discriminate between self-report and diary ratings of anxiety and depression better than the State-Trait Anxiety Inventory-Trait Version.	1988
BSI (18) Anxiety	The BSI-18 is an 18-item self-report inventory designed to measure psychological distress and psychiatric disorders in medical and community populations. Symptom scales include Somatization, Depression and Anxiety.[1]	In a systematic review of assessment instruments for screening cancer patients for emotional distress, the BSI 18 was found to have high reliability, defined as Cronback alpha of ≥ .80 [2]	In a systematic review of assessment instruments for screening cancer patients for emotional distress, the BSI 18 was found to have high validity, defined as an averaged sensitivity and specificity of ≥ .8	2001

Scale	Brief Description	Reliability	Validity	Original Citation Date
HAM-Anxiety (aka HARS)	The Hamilton Anxiety Rating Scale is a clinician-administered assessment of generalized anxious symptomatology (as opposed to specific phobic avoidance) among clinically anxious individuals. The clinician rates the severity of each overarching symptom cluster on a scale from 0 to 4. The scale was developed specifically to provide a measure of the severity of anxious symptomatology among already-diagnosed individuals.	Estimates for the internal consistency as ranging from adequate to good (.77 to .81)n in one study, to excellent α = .92 in another.	HARS scores have been found to correlate significantly with self-report measures of anxiety in clinical samples. In addition, individuals with anxiety disorders scored substantially higher on the HARS than did normal controls. However, the discriminant and discriminative validity of the HARS has been challenged; in particular, high correlations with measures of depression have been found (r = .78) and items on the scale failed to discriminate individuals with GAD from those with MDD.	1959
POMS - tension	The POMS is a self-report measure that contains 65 adjectives for which respondents rate the degree to which the adjective describes the way they have been feeling during the last week. Ratings range from 0 to 4. The POMS can be scored accoring to six factor-analytically derived mood states, one of which is Tension-Anxiety. The score for each scale is derived by summing the resposes to the relevant adjectives.[4]	Chronbach's alpha .63–.92 for subscales, .75–.92 for total score. Correlations between subscale and total scores in the POMS equal to or exceeding .84. [4]	The POMS tension scale correlated significantly with both the STAI State (r = .72) and Trait (r = .70) in a validation study of POMS in 1999***	1971

E-32

Scale	Brief Description	Reliability	Validity	Original Citation Date
SCL-90 anxiety and phobic anxiety[5]	The SCL-90 R is a self-report inventory, where each of the 90 symptoms listed is rated on a five-point scale of distress ranging from 0 to 4. In addition to three global distress indices (general severity index, positive symptom distress index, and positive symptom total), the SCL-90 R provides information on nine primary symptom dimensions. These include anxiety, depression, hostility, interpersonal sensitivity, obsessive-compulsive, paranoid ideation, phobic anxiety, psychoticism, and somatization.	Coefficent alpha estimates for the nine primary symptom dimensions range from .70 to .90	Factor-analytic studies have generally failed to identify nine primary symptom dimensions. The SCL-90-R is proably best thought of as a general screening device that measures global levels of psychopathology.	1997
STAI	The STAI consists of two 20-item self-report measures to assess state and trait levels of anxiety. Respondents indicate how they feel right now (state version) or how they generally feel (trait version) using four-point Likert scales. "Anxiety absent" items on each scale are reverse-scored, and the 20 items of each scale are then summed for a total score.	The manual reports good to excellent internal consistency for both scales (as between .86 and .95) in adult, college, high school student, and military recruit samples.	Convergent validity for the STAI-T has been demonstrated in significant correlations with other trait measures of anxiety in normal populations. In addition, individuals diagnosed with anxiety disorders scored significantly higher on the STAI-T than did nonclinical volunteer participants. Validity of STAI-S is supported by findings of elevated scores in an exam situation and score decreases from pre-to-post surgery. Several studies have suggested that the STAI does not discriminate well from measures of depression. STAI-T has also been found to be sensitive to change in treatment, as evidence by a review of treatment studies.	1983

Scale	Brief Description	Reliability	Validity	Original Citation Date
IPAT - Anxiety inventory**	The Institute for Personality & Ability Testing (IPAT) Anxiety Scale consists of 40 items, each of which has three possible responses along a most-to-least or true-false continuum. The first 20 items are considered to be covert or indirect indices of anxiety, while the latter 20 items are overt, manifest symptoms. The ratio of the covert to the overt score might be considered as an index of the degree to which individuals of equivalent anxiety level are aware of their anxiety.	Test-retest reliability: Correlation between two test administrations three weeks apart was .94.	The correlation between IPAT and Manifest Anxiety Scale (MAS) scores was .55, which was the only significant coefficient found in interrelationships among the IPAT, the Affective Affect Checklist (AACL) MAS, and clinical ratings.	1976
Worry				
Penn State Worry Questionnaire	The PSWQ is a 16-item self-report questionnaire that assesses an individual's general tendecy to worry excessively. Each item presents a statement and is followed by a five-point Likert-type response scale representing how typical the individual feels the statement is of him or her.	The PSWQ is associated with good to very good internal consistency (as ranging from .86 to .93) across clinical and college samples.	PSWQ is moderately correlated with two other worry measures, the Student Worry Scale (r = .59) and the Worry Domains Questionnaire (r = .67) Among student samples, the PSWQ is moderately correlated with measures of anxiety (rs range from .40 to .74) and less strongly correlated with depression (r = .36), but within GAD samples, these relationships are weaker, suggesting that worry is a distinct construct among a clinically anxious sample.	1990

Scale	Brief Description	Reliability	Validity	Original Citation Date
Thought/Emotion Suppression				
White Bear Inventory (thought suppression)	The WBSI is a 15-item self-report measure developed to assess the tendency to suppress thoughts.	In original research conducted by the WBSI developers on large groups of college students, alpha reliability coefficients ranged from .87 to .89[6]	Studies of the predictive validity of the thought suppression measure revealed that it is a useful construct for anticipating whether individuals will develop obsessive thoughts (but not compulsive behaviors), whether individuals who report wishing they were not depressed will in fact be depressed, and whether individuals who are exposed to emotion-producing thoughts will fail to habituate to them over time.	1994
Courtauld Emotional Control Scale- Anxiety (CECS)[7]	The Courtauld Emotional Control Scale is a 21-item questionnaire which measures suppression of affect. It is rated on a four-point scale (almost never–almost always) developed to measure the extent to which individuals report that they control their emotions of anger (e.g. I hide my annoyance), anxiety (e.g. I say what I feel) and depressed mood (e.g. I hide my unhappiness).	Each of the three subscales demonstrated good internal consistency in the original research, with α coefficients of .86, .88 and .88 for the anger, depression and anxiety subscales, respectively.[5]	Not Available	1983

E-35

Scale	Brief Description	Reliability	Validity	Original Citation Date
Social Anxiety				
Fear of Negative Evaluation	The FNE consists of 30 items referring to expectation and distress related to negative evaluation from others.	Internal consistency for the FNE was excellent, ranging from .94 to .96	The FNE has been shown to differentiate between individuals diagnosed with various anxiety disorders. Across three college samples, the FNE was significantly correlated with measures of anxiety (.60), social-evaluative anxiety (.47), social approval (.77) and less strongly with measures of locus of control (.18) and achievement anxiety (.28). the FNE has been shown to be one of the most sensitive social phobia treatment outcome measures following cognitive-behavioral group therapy.	1969
Liebowitz Social Anxiety-Fear	24-item clinician-rated scale to assess fear and avoidance of particular situations in people with social phobia. The LSAS consists of two subscales that measure difficulty with social interacction (11 items) and performance (13 items). Fear and avoidance are rated on separate four-point scales ranging from 0 to 3 to represent symptom severity during the past week.	Cronback's alpha for the LSAS total score was .96. The alpha coefficients range from .81 to .92 for the fear subscales, and .83 to .92 for the avoidance subscales. Total fear and total avoidance scores were highly correlated (.91) suggesting that these subscales may not adequately assess independent constructs, at least in clinical samples.	LSAS total score was significantly associated with a clinician severity rating from a structured clinical interview (.52) and a number of self-report measures of social anxiety (rs ranging from .49 to .73).	1987

Scale	Brief Description	Reliability	Validity	Original Citation Date
Social Interactions (fear) (SIAS)	The original version of the SIAS consists of 19 items, but many studies use a 20-item version that is identical except for the addition of one item. Items on the SIAS describe cognitive, affective, and behavioral reactions to interactional situations. Items are rated on a five-point scale ranging from 0 to 4.	High internal consistency across a variety of clinical, community and students samples with αs ranging from .86 to .94	Other measures of social anxiety have been shown to be significantly associated with the SAIS (.66 to .81). Somewhat smaller correlations emerged between measures of general anxiety and the SAIS (.45 to .58), depression and the SAIS (.47) and locus of control and SAIS (.30).	1998
Social phobia Scale (SPS)	SPS contains 20 items that are rated on a five-point scale ranging from 0 to 4. Items describe situations involving being observed by others while engaged in activies such as eating or writing. The SPS is scored by taking the sum of all of the items.	High internal consistency across a variety of clinical, community and student samples with αs ranging from .87 to .94	Other measures of social anxiety have been shown to be significantly associated with the SPS (.64 to .75). Somewhat smaller correlations emerged between measures of general anxiety and the SPS (.42 to .57), depression and the SPS (.54) and locus of control and the SPS (.31)	1998

Scale	Brief Description	Reliability	Validity	Original Citation Date
Positive Mood				
PANAS Postive Affect	The PANAS is a 20-item self-report measure specifically designed to assess the distinct dimensions of positive and negative affect. Respondents are asked to indicate on a 5-point Likert-type scale the extent to which they feel or have felt a list of adjectives over a specified time period.	Good to excellent internal consistency estimates, αs ranging from .88 to .90 for the Postive Affect scale; αs ranging from .84 to .87 for the Negative Affect scale.	The Negtive Affect scale was significantly correlated with measures of general psychiatric distress (r = .74), depression (r=.58)and state anxiety (r = .51), whereas the PA scale was negatively correlated with measures of depression (r=-.36) in a student sample. The two scales show very modest correlations (rs ranting from -.12 to -.23) with one another, supporting the discrimination between the two factors. Further, relatively more depressed individuals reported significantly lower scores on the PA scale than relative more anxious individuals, whereas the two groups did not differ significantly on the NA scale, suggesting discriminative validity of the scale.	1989

Sources: Except as noted in footnotes, all information in this section is from: Antony MM, Orsillo SM, Roemer L, editors. Practitioner's guide to empirically based measures of anxiety. New York: Kluwer Academic/Plenum Publishers; 2001.

1. Description from proprietary website, psychcorp.pearsonassessments.com
2. Vodermaier A, Linden W, Siu C. Screening for Emotional Distress in Cancer Patients: A Systematic Review of Assessment Instruments J Natl Cancer Inst. 2009 November 4; 101(21): 1464–1488.
3. Nezu AM, Ronan GF, Meadows EA McClure KS, editors. Practitioner's guide to empirically based measures of depression. New York: Kluwer Academic/Plenum Publishers; 2000.
4. Advanced Practice Nursing Data Collection Toolkit, McMaster University: http://fhsson.mcmaster.ca/apn/index.php?option=com_content&view=article&id=265:profile-of-mood-states-scale&catid=46:mental-health&Itemid=64
**POMs Source: Advanced Practice Nursing Data Collection Toolkit, McMaster University
5. Nezu AM, Ronan GF, Meadows EA McClure KS, editors. Practitioner's guide to empirically based measures of depression. New York: Kluwer Academic/Plenum Publishers; 2000.
6. Myers LB, Vetereb A, Derakshan N. Are suppression and repressive coping related? *Personality and Individual Differences* 2004 April 36(5): 1009–1013
7. Watson M and Greer S. Development of a questionnaire measure of emotional control. *Journal of Psychosomatic Research* 1983 21 (4): 299–305
8. SF-36® Health Survey Update John E. Ware, Jr., Ph.D. www.sf-36.org/tools/sf36.shtml
**Levitt EE and Persky H. Experimental evidence for the validity of the IPAT Anxiety Scale. Journal of Clinical Psychology, 18(4), 1962. pp. 458-461.
***Nyenhuis, David L. Yamamoto, Chie Luchetta, Tracy Terrien, Annette Parmentier, Angie ; Adult and geriatric normative data and validation of the Profile of Mood States. Journal of Clinical Psychology, Vol 55(1), Jan, 1999. pp. 79–86.

Evidence Table E4. Scales for depression (KQ1)

Test	Brief Description	Reliability	Validity	Original Citation Date
Beck Depression Inventory[1]	The Beck Depression Inventory (BDI) is a 21-item, self-report rating inventory that measures characteristic attitudes and symptoms of depression.	Internal consistency estimates yielded a mean coefficient alpha of 0.86 for psychiatric patients and 0.81 for non-psychiatric subjects	The concurrent validities of the BDI with respect to clinical ratings and the Hamilton Psychiatric Rating Scale for Depression (HRSD) were also high. The mean correlations of the BDI samples with clinical ratings and the HRSD were 0.72 and 0.73, respectively, for psychiatric patients. With nonpsychiatric subjects, the mean correlations of the BDI with clinical ratings and the HRSD were 0.60 and 0.74, respectively.	1961
Beck Depression Inventory II	The BDI-II is a 21-item self-report measure of depressive symptoms that was developed in concert with criteria for diagnosing depressive disorders contained in the DSM-IV. Items include a four-point scale ranging from 0 to 3, representing levels of severity of symptoms or, in the case of two items, changes in sleep or appetite patterns.	Alpha estimates for internal consistency were found to be .92 for a psychiatric outpatient sample, and .93 for college students.	There is a significant correlation with an earlier version of this inventory, the BDI-IA (.93). BDI-II was also found to correlate with the Hamilton Rating Scale for Depression (.71)	1996
Zung Self Rating Depression Scale	The Zung SDS is a 20-item self-report measure of depression. All items are rated on a 4-point scale with anchor points referring to the amount of time the item is currently experienced.	Internal consistency was high with alphas of .91 for family escorts, .88 for depressed clients, .93 for non-depressed clients.	In separate studies, correlations with the HRSD and BDI were found to be .80 and .54 respectively.	1965
BSI (18) depression	The BSI-18 is an 18-item self-report inventory designed to measure psychological distress and psychiatric disorders in medical and community populations. Symptom scales include Somatization, Depression and Anxiety.[2]	In a systematic review of assessment instruments for screening cancer patients for emotional distress, the BSI 18 was found to have high reliability, defined as Cronbach alpha of ≥ .80[3]	In a systematic review of assessment instruments for screening cancer patients for emotional distress, the BSI 18 was found to have high validity, defined as an averaged sensitivity and specificity of ≥ .8	2001

Test	Brief Description	Reliability	Validity	Original Citation Date
SCL-90 (depression and interpersonal sensitivity)	The SCL-90 R is a self-report inventory, where each of the 90 symptoms listed is rated on a five-point scale of distress ranging from 0 to 4. In addition to three global distress indices (general severity index, positive symptom distress index, and positive symptom total), the SCL-90 R provides information on nine primary symptom dimensions. These include anxiety, depression, hostility, interpersonal sensitivity, obsessive-compulsive, paranoid ideation, phobic anxiety, psychoticism, and somatization.	Coefficent alpha estimates for the nine primary symptom dimensions range from .70 to .90	Factor-analytic studies have generally failed to identify nine primary symptom dimensions. The SCL-90-R is probably best thought of as a general screening device that measures global levels of psychopathology.	1994
CES-D	The CES-D is a 20-item self-report measure of depressive symptoms. Each item provides a statement representing a symptom characteristic of depression, followed by a 4-point Likert-type response scale ranging from "rarely or none of the time" to "most all of the time."	Coefficient alpha estimates for internal consistency were found to be .85 for the general population and .90 for the patient sample.	CES-D scores were significantly and substantially different between psychiatric inpatient groups and the general population. Correlation with the HRSD was .44 and correlation with the Raskin Three-Area Scale was .54. Discriminant validity was also supported by the CES-D's negative correlation with the Radburn Positive Affect Scale. Note that this scale is intended for research purposes only, not for clinical use.	1977
POMS-depression	The POMS is a self-report measure that contains 65 adjectives for which respondents rate the degree to which the adjective describes the way they have been feeling during the last week. Ratings range from 0 to 4. The POMS can be scored according to six factor-analytically derived mood states, one of which is Depression-Dejection. the Depression-Dejection scale contains 15 adjectives and represents a mood of depression accompanied by a sense of personal inadequacy.	Internal consistency for the Depression scale was found to be .95 in two separate studies.	The POMS Depression scale has been found to correlate highly with other measures of depressive symptomatology. The r values regarding its association with the BDI and MMPI-D scale were found to be .61 and .65, respectively.	1992

Test	Brief Description	Reliability	Validity	Original Citation Date
SCID and SCID-relapse	The Structured Clinical Interview For DSI-IV Axis I Disorders (SCID) is a semistructured interview designed to help clinicians and researchers make distinctions among various categories listed in the DSM-IV. There are both clinician and research versions of the SCID. The clinician version covers only diagnoses typically seen in clinical practice and exludes a majority of the subtypes and specifiers present in the research version. Note for SCID-relapse: The primary outcome measure was time to relapse/recurrence of DSM-IV major depressive episode, using the depression module of the SCID	Diagnostic agreement for diagnostic categories among different patient populations ranged from .61 for current diagnosis to .68 for lifetime diagnosis.	Because there are not 'gold standards' for determining psychiatric classification, validity of the SCID is heavily dependent upon the validity of the DSM-IV.	1995
HRSD (aka HAM-D)	The HSRD is a 21-item clinician-rated instrument that is completed following a thorough clinical interview. Each item presents a symptom of depression and is rated according to its severity as experienced by the patient during the past few days or week.	Most interrater reliability coefficients have been ≥.84	The validity of this instrument has been established by comparing HRSD scores to scores on numerous self-report and clinician-rated measures for depression. Comparisons with the BDI yielded correlations ranging from .21 to .82 with a median of .58 and comparisons with the Zung Self-Rating Depression Scale ranged from .38 to .62 with a median of .45.	1960, 1967
Institute for Personality and Ability Testing Depression Scale (IPAT)	The IPAT Depression Scale contains 36 items that assess thoughts and feelings related to depression. Respondents are asked to check one of three options for each item.	Coefficient alpha estimates for reliability range from .88 to .93, among a variety of populations including depressives, prisoners, alcoholics, narcotic addicts, college students and adult controls.	With regard to how well the test score correlates with depression, an obtained correlation of .88 between the scale and a "pure depression factor" was observed using 1904 normal and clinical cases.	1976

Sources: Except as noted in footnotes, information in this section is from: Nezu AM, Ronan GF, Meadows EA McClure KS, editors. Practitioner's guide to empirically based measures of depression. New York: Kluwer Academic/Plenum Publishers; 2000.

1. Source = Beck, AT. Psychometric properties of the Beck Depression Inventory: Twenty-five years of evaluation. Clinical Psychology Review 1988; 8:77-100.
2. Source = description from proprietary website, psychcorp.pearsonassessments.com
3. Source = Vodermaier A, Linden W, Siu C. Screening for Emotional Distress in Cancer Patients: A Systematic Review of Assessment Instruments J Natl Cancer Inst. 2009 November 4; 101(21): 1464–1488.

Evidence Table E5. Scales for stress (KQ1)

Test	Brief Description	Reliability	Validity	Original Citation Date
KQ1 Stress				
Perceived Stress Scale (10 & 14 item) (PSS)	It is a measure of the degree to which situations in one's life are appraised as stressful. Items were designed to tap how unpredictable, uncontrollable, and overloaded respondents find their lives. The scale also includes a number of direct queries about current levels of experienced stress. The PSS was designed for use in community samples with at least a junior high school education.	Coefficient alpha reliability for the PSS was .84, .85, and .86 in each of three samples in the originally published research, two large groups of university students and a smaller sample of smoking cessation program participants from the community.	The PSS is correlated in the expected manner with a range of self-report and behavioral criteria. Moreover, the PSS is more closely related to a life-event impact score, which is to some degree based on the respondent's appraisal of the event, than to the more objective measure of the number of events occurring within a particular timespan. The PSS also proved to be a better predictor of health and health-related outcomes than either of the two life-event scales examined (Number of Life Events and Impact of Life Events). Finally, the PSS, although highly correlated with depressive symptomatology, was found to measure a different and independently predictive construct.	1983
Life Stress Instrument (LSI)	Have not able to verified instrument			
BSI-18 Global Severity Index	The BSI-18 is an 18-item self-report inventory designed to measure psychological distress and psychiatric disorders in medical and community populations. Symptom scales include Somatization, Depression and Anxiety.[2]	In a systematic review of assessment instruments for screening cancer patients for emotional distress, the BSI 18 was found to have high reliability, defined as Cronbach alpha of ≥ .80[3]	In a systematic review of assessment instruments for screening cancer patients for emotional distress, the BSI 18 was found to have high validity, defined as an averaged sensitivity and specificity of ≥ .8	2001

Test	Brief Description	Reliability	Validity	Original Citation Date
Brief Symptom Inventory (53) Global Psychiatric Symptoms (BSI-53)	The BSI is a 53-item self-report inventory. Each of the symptoms contained is rated on a five-point scale of distress ranging from 0 to 4. In addtion to three global distress indices (general severity index, positive symptom distress index, and positive symptom total), the BSI provides information on nine primary symptom dimensions: anxiety, depression, hostility, interpersonal sensitivity, obsessive-compulsive, paranoid ideaion, phobic anxiety, psychoticism, and somatization.	estimates for the coefficient alpha of the primary symptom dimensions range from .71 to .85.	Several of the BSI scales have been found to correlate with related constructs measured using the MMPI. Nevertheless, the same lack of specificity noted for the primary symptom dimensions associed with the SCL 90-R is likely to be found for the BSI. Similar to the SCL-90, the BSI is probably best thought of as a general screening device that measures gloabl levels of psychopathology.	1993
PANAS Negative Affect	The PANAS is a 20-item self-report measure specifically designed to assess the distrinct dimensions of positive and negative affect. Respondents are asked to indicate on a 5-point Likert-type scale the extent to which they feel or have felt a list of adjectives over a specified time period.	Good to excellent internal consistency estimates, αs ranging from .88 to .90 for the Postive Affect scale; αs ranging from .84 to .87 for the Negative Affect scale.	The Negtive Affect scale was significantly correlated with measures of general psychiatric distress (r = .74), depression (r=.58) and state anxiety (r = .51) in a student sample. The two scales (positive and negative affect) show very modest correlations (rs ranting from –.12 to –.23) with one another, supporting the discrimination between the two factors. Further, relatively more depressed individuals reported significantly lower scores on the PA scale than relative more anxious individuals, whereas the two groups did not differ significantly on the NA scale, suggesting discriminative validity of the scale.	1989

Test	Brief Description	Reliability	Validity	Original Citation Date
SCL-90 General Severity Index	The SCL-90 R is a self-report inventory, where each of the 90 symptoms listed is rated on a five-point scale of distress ranging from 0 to 4. In addition to three global distress indices (general severity index, positive symptom distress index, and positive symptom total), the SCL-90 R provides information on nine primary symptom dimensions. These include anxiety, depression, hostility, interpersonal sensitivity, obsessive-compulsive, paranoid ideation, phobic anxiety, psychoticism, and somatization.	Coefficent alpha estimates for the nine primary symptom dimensions range from .70 to .90	Factor-analytic studies have generally failed to identify nine primary symptom dimensions. The SCL-90-R is probably best thought of as a general screening device that measures global levels of psychopathology.	1994
SF-36 Mental Health Subscale*	The SF-36 is a multipurpose, 36-item survey that measures eight domains of health: physical functioning, role limitations due to physical health, bodily pain, general health perceptions, vitality, social functioning, role limitations due to emotional problems, and mental health. It yields scale scores for each of these eight health domains, and two summary measures of physical and mental health: the Physical Component Summary (PCS) and Mental Component Summary (MCS).	The reliability of the eight scales and two summary measures has been estimated using both internal consistency and test-retest methods. With rare exceptions, published reliability statistics have exceeded the minimum standard of 0.70 recommended for measures used in group comparisons in more than 25 studies. Reliability estimates for physical and mental summary scores usually exceed 0.90.	Studies of validity generally support the intended meaning of high and low SF-36 scores as documented in the original user's manuals. Because of the widespread use of the SF-36 across a variety of applications, evidence from many types of validity research is relevant to these interpretations. Studies to date have yielded content, concurrent, criterion, construct, and predictive evidence of validity.	1993

E-44

Test	Brief Description	Reliability	Validity	Original Citation Date
POMS - Total Mood Disturbance	The POMS is a self-report measure that contains 65 adjectives for which respondents rate the degree to which the adjective describes the way they have been feeling during the last week. Ratings range from 0 to 4. The POMS can be scored accoring to six factor-analytically derived mood states, one of which is Tension-Anxiety. The score for each scale is derived by summing the resposes to the relevant adjectives. Source = Nezu et al for this general description.	Chronbach's alpha .63–.92 for subscales, .75–.92 for total score. Correlations between subscale and total scores in the POMS equal to or exceeding .84. **	Factorial validity of the 6 mood factors reported. Please see user's manual for more information**	1971

Sources

PSS sources: description from proprietary website: www.mindgarden.com/products/pss.htm and
PSS data from: Cohen S, Kamarck T and Mermelstein R. A Global Measure of Perceived Stress: Journal of Health and Social Behavior Dec 1983, Vol. 24, No. 4
BSI-18= description from proprietary website, psychcorp.pearsonassessments.com
BSI-53= Nezu AM, Ronan GF, Meadows EA McClure KS, editors. Practitioner's guide to empirically based measures of depression. New York: Kluwer Academic/Plenum Publishers; 2000.
PANAS=Antony MM, Orsillo SM, Roemer L, editors. Practitioner's guide to empirically based measures of anxiety. New York: Kluwer Academic/Plenum Publishers; 2001.
SCL-90=Antony MM, Orsillo SM, Roemer L, editors. Practitioner's guide to empirically based measures of anxiety. New York: Kluwer Academic/Plenum Publishers; 2001.
SF-36® Health Survey Update John E. Ware, Jr., Ph.D. www.sf-36.org/tools/sf36.shtml
POMs Source: Advanced Practice Nursing Data Collection Toolkit, McMaster University:
http://fhsson.mcmaster.ca/apn/index.php?option=com_content&view=article&id=265:profile-of-mood-states-scale&catid=46:mental-health&Itemid=64

Evidence Table E6. Scales for attention (KQ2)

Test	Brief Description	Reliability	Validity	Original Citation Date
KQ2: Attention				
Attentional Network	The Attention Network Test (ANT) is a tool used to assess the efficiency of the three attention networks—alerting, orienting, and executive control.	Split-half reliabilities of reaction time-based attention network scores were low for alerting (rweighted .20), and orienting (rweighted .32) and moderate high for executive control (rweighted .65).	Analysis of the variance structure of the ANT indicated that power to find significant effects was variable across networks and dependent on the statistical analysis being used. Both analysis of variance (significant interaction observed in 100% of 15 studies) and correlational analyses (multiple significant inter-network correlations observed) suggest that the networks measured by the ANT are not independent.	2002

Test	Brief Description	Reliability	Validity	Original Citation Date
Stroop Color Word Interference Test	The Stroop Color and Word Test is based on the observation that individuals can read words much faster than they can identify and name colors. The cognitive dimension tapped by the Stroop is associated with cognitive flexibility, resistance to interference from outside stimuli, creativity, and psychopathology—all of which influence the individual's ability to cope with cognitive stress and process complex input. It measures cognitive processing and provides valuable diagnostic information on brain dysfunction and cognition. The test-taker reads color words or names ink colors from different pages as quickly as possible within a time limit. The test yields three scores based on the number of items completed on each of the three stimulus sheets. An Interference score is useful in determining the individual's cognitive flexibility, creativity, and reaction to cognitive pressures.	The reliability of the Stroop scores is highly consistent across different versions of the test. In all cases, experimenters have looked at test-retest reliabilities covering periods from 1 minute to 10 days. Jensen reported reliabilities of .88, .79, and .71 for the three Raw scores. Golden (1975b) reported reliabilities of .89, .84, and .73 (N = 450) for the group version of the test, and reliabilities of .86, .82, and .73 (N = 30) for the individual version.	There appear to be no other valid measures of the same phenomenon.	1935

Sources
ATN SOURCE: MacLeod JW, Lawrence MA, McConnell MM
Eskes GA, Klein RM and Shore DI. Appraising the ANT: Psychometric and Theoretical Considerations of the Attention Network Test. *Neuropsychology*
2010, 24(5): 637–651.
Stroop Test description downloaded from proprietary website: www4.parinc.com/Products/Product.aspx?ProductID=STROOP
Stroop Data from: Golden CJ and Freshwater SM. The Stroop Color and Word Test: A Manual for Clinical and Expermimental Uses. 2002 Stoelting Co

Evidence Table E7. Scales for substance abuse (KQ3)

Test	Brief Description	Reliability	Validity	Original Citation Date
KQ3				
Alcohol				
Penn Alcohol Craving Scale	The PACS is a five-item, self-report measure that includes questions about the frequency, intensity, and duration of craving, the ability to resist drinking, and asks for an overall rating of craving for alcohol for the previous week. Each question is scaled from 0 to 6	The PACS proved to have excellent internal consistency	Construct validity of the PACS was demonstrated via its convergence with two commonly used measures for assessing craving, the Obsessive Compulsive Drinking Scale and the Alcohol Urge Questionnaire. Lack of correlation between PACS scores and several other noncraving, self-report measures indicates that the PACS also had good discriminant validity. Additional analyses revealed that there were significant differences in craving scores during the initial 3 weeks of the trial among those who did and those who did not relapse during weeks	1999

E-48

Test	Brief Description	Reliability	Validity	Original Citation Date
Attention (dot probe)	This task, which was developed by MacLeod, Mathews, and Tata (1986), is based on the fact that individuals tend to respond faster to a probe stimulus (e.g. a small dot) that is presented in an attended rather than unattended area of a visual display In a typical version of this task, a series of word pairs is presented briefly on a computer screen, with one member of the word pair above the other. In critical trials, one word of each pair is threat related and the other neutral. When the word pair disappears, occasionally a small dot appears in the position formerly occupied by one of the words. Participants are asked to push a button as quickly as possible when the dot appears. Attention allocation to threat is measured indirectly by the reaction times to the dot: fast reactions to dots that replace threat words and slow reactions to dots that replace neutral words indicate an attentional bias to threat.	Estimates of both internal consistency and retest reliability over one week lead to the conclusion that the dot probe task is a completely unreliable measure of attentional allocation in non-clinical samples. This unreliability may explain the inconsistent findings for the dot probe task as reported in the literature.		1986

Test	Brief Description	Reliability	Validity	Original Citation Date
Impaired Response Inhibition Scale for Alcohol (IRISA)	The preliminary version of the IRISA was a self-reported instrument of 28 items designed to assess the degree of impairment of response inhibition over drinking behavior. All the items were taken directly from phrases and expressions used by alcohol-dependent patients in recovery, from the authors' clinical experience, or from the scientific literature about alcohol dependence and drinking response inhibition. Each item has a response option based on a 4-point Likert scale (0 5yes, always; 1 5yes, usually; 2 5no, not usually; 3 5no, never).	Psychometric properties of this version of the IRISA scale showed excellent internal consistency (Cronbach's α: 0.96), and good test–retest reliability (intraclass correlation coefficient: 0.81).	Psychometric properties of this version of the IRISA scale showed satisfactory convergent, discriminant, and predictive validity. The IRISA has a good correlation with alcohol craving, the severity of alcoholism, and alcohol consumption during the recovery process.	2007
Weekly diary	The Substance Use Calendar was administered at baseline (past month) and weekly during treatment and measured in standardized drinks/day for alcohol (1 oz) and grams/day for cocaine (30).	Participant self-reports of drug use	n/a	REFID 1331, 2009

Test	Brief Description	Reliability	Validity	Original Citation Date
Daily diary	The daily diary used in this study was a non-standardized diary method designed to meet the needs of the study design. "Daily journals were distributed weekly to all subjects with instructions to supply daily information on 15 behavioral variables, including three variables concerned with alcohol intake (type and amount of alcohol consumed, and the amount of time spent drinking). Behavioral variables not concerned with alcohol intake served as distracter items and included the monitoring of mood, sleep and eating habits, smoking behavior, and other drug intake. The daily journal was devised to camouflage the dependent measure of alcohol consumption.	were verified by random breathalyzer for alcohol	n/a	REFID 5506, 1986
	and urine toxicology screens for drug use (approximately every 2 weeks). One hundred percent			
Sleep				
Pittsburgh Sleep Quality Index (PSQI)	The PSQI was created after observation that most patients with psychiatric disorders also have sleep disorders. The questionnaire has nineteen individual items which are used to generate seven composite scores. The results give numbers in seven categories: subjective sleep quality, sleep latency, sleep duration, habitual sleep efficiency, sleep disturbances, use of sleeping medication, and daytime dysfunction	of the breathalyzer and 98.4% (62/63) of	Validity analyses showed high correlations between PSQI and sleep log data and lower correlations with polysomnography data. A PSQI global score >5 resulted in a sensitivity of 98.7 and specificity of 84.4 as a marker for sleep disturbances in insomnia patients versus controls.	1989

Test	Brief Description	Reliability	Validity	Original Citation Date
Insomnia Severity Index (ISI)	The ISI is a 7-item self-report questionnaire assessing the nature, severity, and impact of insomnia. The usual recall period is the "last month" and the dimensions evaluated are: severity of sleep onset, sleep maintenance, and early morning awakening problems, sleep dissatisfaction, interference of sleep difficulties with daytime functioning, noticeability of sleep problems by others, and distress caused by the sleep difficulties. A 5-point Likert scale is used to rate each item (e.g., 0 = no problem; 4 = very severe problem), yielding a total score ranging from 0 to 28.	the urine specimens were consistent with selfreports	Convergent validity was supported by significant correlations between total ISI score and measures of fatigue, quality of life, anxiety, and depression.	1991
Epworth Sleepiness Scale (ESS)	The ESS is a simple, self-administered questionnaire which is shown to provide a measurement of the subject's general level of daytime sleepiness. Subjects are asked to rate on scale of 0–3 how likely they would be to doze off or fall asleep in the eight situations, based on their usual way of life in recent times. asked, nonetheless, to estimate how each might affect him.	Total ESS scores are reliable in a test-retest sense over a period of months (rho = 0.82, n = 87, p < 0.001). There is a high level of internal consistency within the ESS, as assessed by Cronbach's alpha statistic (alpha = 0.88 – 0.74 in 4 different groups of subjects).	ESS scores were significantly correlated with sleep latency measured during the multiple sleep latency test and during overnight polysomnography. In patients with obstructive sleep apnea syndrome ESS scores were significantly correlated with the respiratory disturbance index and the minimum Sa02 recorded overnight.	2006

Test	Brief Description	Reliability	Validity	Original Citation Date
Diary (Total Sleep Time. Wake After Sleep Onset)	Sleep diaries are detailed day-by-day reports of sleeping and waking activities. They are widely used in clinical and research settings to gather information about sleep/wake patterns. Subjects are asked to record on a daily basis actual sleep times as well as the occurrence of such symptoms as sleepwalking, nocturnal arousals, or sleep attacks; ingestion of medications, caffeine, and alcohol; and day timeactivities. Information may be recorded for as little as 24 hours or for as long as several weeks.	In one study of the reliability of sleep diaries, the percentage agreement between the subjective data recorded in the sleep diaries and polysomnographic data was accetpable (kappa = .87) The sleep diary is a reliable instrument for collecting data about sleep/wake patterns, but should be used with caution when collecting data from subjects who are likely to take frequent daytime naps.	Sensitivity and specificity in the same study were also high (92.3% and 95.6%).	
Actigraphy (Total Sleep Time. Wake After Sleep Onset)		Activity-based sleep-wake monitoring or actigraphy has gained a central role as a sleep assessment tool in sleep medicine. It is used for sleep assessment in clinical sleep research, and as a diagnostic tool in sleep medicine. This update indicates that according to most studies, actigraphy has reasonable validity and reliability in normal individuals with relatively good sleep patterns.Furthermore, actigraphy is sensitive in detecting sleep changes associated with drug treatments and non-pharmacologic interventions.		

Sources

Penn Alcohol Craving Scale Source: Flannery BA, Volpicelli J R , Pettinati H M. Psychometric properties of the Penn Alcohol Craving Scale. Alcoholism: Clinical and Experimental Research (1999) Volume: 23, Issue: 8

Dot Probe Attention Source: Schmulke SC. Unreliability of the Dot Probe Task. Eur. J. Pers. 19: 595–605 (2005)

IRISA Source: Guardia J, Trujols J, Burguete T, Luquero E, Cardús M. Impaired Response Inhibition Scale for Alcoholism (IRISA): Development and Psychometric Properties of a New Scale for Abstinence-Oriented Treatment of Alcoholism. Alcoholism: Clinical and Experimental Research Volume 31, Issue 2, pages 269–275, February 2007

PSQI Data Source: Backhause J, Junghanns K, Broocks A, Riemann D, Hohagen F. Test–retest reliability and validity of the Pittsburgh Sleep Quality Index in primary insomnia. Journal of Psychosomatic Research Volume 53, Issue 3, Pages 737–740, September 2002

PSQI Test description from public information website, Sleepdex: www.sleepdex.org/pittsburgh.htm

Insomnia severity index source: Morin CM; Belleville G; Bélanger L; Ivers H. The insomnia severity index: psychometric indicators to detect insomnia cases and evaluate treatment response. SLEEP 2011;34(5):601–608.

ESS reliability data form the official website of the Epworth Sleepiness Scale by Dr. Murray Johns: http://epworthsleepinessscale.com/about-epworth-sleepiness/

ESS Validity Data from: Johns M. A New Method For Measuring Daytime Sleepiness: The Epworth Sleepiness Scale. Sleep 1991. 14 (6)540-545

Sleep diary source: Rogers AE, Caruso CC, and Aldrich MS. Reliability of Sleep Diaries for Assessment of Sleep/Wake Patterns. Nursing Research, Nov/Dec 1993;42 (6):368–391

Actigraphy source: Sadeh A.The role and validity of actigraphy in sleep medicine: An update. Sleep Medicine Reviews, Vol 15(4), Aug, 2011. pp. 259–267.

Evidence Table E8. Scales for well-being (KQ1)

Test	Brief Description	Reliability	Validity	Original Citation
Well-Being				
Quality of Well Being Scale	The Quality of Well-Being (QWB-SA) survey is a preference-weighted measure of general health status. It combines three scales of functioning with a measure of symptoms/problems to produce a point-in-time expression of well-being that runs from 0 (death) to 1.0 (asymptomatic full function).		This self-administered survey had acceptable performance in older adults.	
QOL-Enjoyment/Satisfaction	The Quality of Life Enjoyment and Satisfaction Questionnaire (Q-LESQ), a measure of the degree of enjoyment and satisfaction experienced by participants with various mental and medical disorders in areas of daily functioning. Fourteen items are used to assess an overall quality of life score. Each item is scored on a 5-point Likert scale from 1 (not at all or never) to 5 (frequently or all the time) with higher scores indicating greater satisfaction	Test-retest reliability has been reported as .74. In this study, Cronbach's alpha was .92.	Validity has been reported using correlations with the Clinical Global Impressions Severity of Illness Rating (r = −.64), the Hamilton Rating Scale for Depression (r = −.66) and the Beck Depression Inventory (r = −.67).	

Test	Brief Description	Reliability	Validity	Original Citation
Sense of Coherence	The SOC scale consists of 29 five-facet items; respondents are asked to select a response, on a seven-point semantic differential scale with two anchoring phrases, There are 11 comprehensibility. 10 manageability and 8 meaningfulness items. The published scale allows for the possibility of using a short form of 13 of the 29 items. Unless 'SOC-13' is noted, reference IX always to SOC-29.	In 26 studies using SOC-29 the Cronbach alpha measure of internal consistency has ranged from 0.82 to 0.95. The alphas of 16 studies using SOC-13 range from 0.74 to 0.91.	The systematic procedure used in scale construction and examination of the final product by many colleagues points to a high level of content, face and consensual validity. The few data sets available point to a high level of construct validity.Criterion validity is examined by presenting correlational data between the SOC and measures in four domains: a global orientation to oneself and one's environment (19 r's); stressors (11 r's); health, illness and wellbeing (32 r's); attitudes and behavior (5 r's). The great majority of correlations are statistically significant.	1987
QOL-VAS	Operationally a VAS is usually a horizontal line, 100 mm in length, anchored by word descriptors at each end. The patient marks on the line the point that they feel represents their perception of their current state. The VAS score is determined by measuring in millimetres from the left hand end of the line to the point that the patient marks.			

Test	Brief Description	Reliability	Validity	Original Citation
QOL/Mental Health				
WHOQOL – Psychological	The WHOQOL-100 assesses individuals' perceptions of their position in life in the context of the culture and value systems in which they live and in relation to their goals, expectations, standards and concerns. It was developed collaboratively in some 15 cultural settings over several years and has now been field tested in 37 field centres. It is a 100-question assessment that currently exists in directly comparable forms in 29 language versions. It yields a multi-dimensional profile of scores across domains and sub-domains (facets) of quality of life. More recently, the WHOQOL-BREF, an abbreviated 26 item assessment has been developed.	Cronbach alpha values for each of the six domain scores ranged from .71 to .86, demonstrating good internal consistency	Confirmatory factor analysis showed adequate construct validity for the WHOQOL: multiple sample analysis for all domains displayed appropriate CFIs above 0.9 in all cases	1998
QOL (general for chronically ill)	The Quality of Life Profile for the Chronically Ill (PLC) is an HRQoL inventory especially designed for patients with chronic conditions It consists of 40 items and 6 subscales: physical functioning, ability to relax and enjoy life, positive affect, negative affect, social contact, and social integration. Scores of the 6 subscales can be summed to a total score.		The inventory is well validated and was used in an earlier MBSR investigation with fibromyalgia patients	1996

Test	Brief Description	Reliability	Validity	Original Citation
SF-36 (including Vitality subscale)	The SF-36 is a multipurpose, 36-item survey that measures eight domains of health: physical functioning, role limitations due to physical health, bodily pain, general health perceptions, vitality, social functioning, role limitations due to emotional problems, and mental health. It yields scale scores for each of these eight health domains, and two summary measures of physical and mental health: the Physical Component Summary (PCS) and Mental Component Summary (MCS).	The reliability of the eight scales and two summary measures has been estimated using both internal consistency and test-retest methods. With rare exceptions, published reliability statistics have exceeded the minimum standard of 0.70 recommended for measures used in group comparisons in more than 25 studies (Tsai, Bayliss, & Ware, 1997); most have exceeded 0.80 (McHorney et al., 1994; Ware et al., 1993). Reliability estimates for physical and mental summary scores usually exceed 0.90 (Ware et al., 1994).	Studies of validity generally support the intended meaning of high and low SF-36 scores as documented in the original user's manuals (Ware et al., 1993; Ware et al., 1994). Because of the widespread use of the SF-36 across a variety of applications, evidence from many types of validity research is relevant to these interpretations. Studies to date have yielded content, concurrent, criterion, construct, and predictive evidence of validity.	

Test	Brief Description	Reliability	Validity	Original Citation
SF-12 Mental component	The SF-12v2 is the most recent subset scale of the SF-36 health-related quality of life measure [4]. It includes 12 items, measures 8 domains of health, and is used to calculate 2 component scores, the Physical Component Summary Score (PCS) and the Mental Component Summary Score (MCS).	Both Mental Component Summary Scores (MCS) and Physical Component Summary Scores (PCS) were shown to have high internal consistency reliability (a[.80). PCS showed high test-retest reliability (ICC = .78) while MCS demonstrated moderate reliability (Intraclass correlation coefficient = .60). Prior research had demonstrated an Internal consistency reliability alpha coefficient of .89 for the Physical component score (PCS) and .86 for Mental Component Score (MCS)	PCS had high convergent validity for EQ-5D items (except selfcare) and physical health status (r[.56). MCS demonstrated moderate convergent validity on EQ-5D and mental health items (r[.38). PCS distinguish between groups with different physical and work limitations. Similarly, MCS distinguished between groups with and without cognitive limitations. The MCS and PCS showed perfect dose response when variations in scores were examined by participant's chronic condition status. Conclusions Both component scores showed adequate reliability and validity with the 2003–2004 MEPS and should be suitable for use in a variety of proposes within this database. Keywords SF-12 MEPS Medical expenditure panel survey Validity Reliability	[44] Solas for missing data analysis 2.0.

Notes: AHRQ = Agency for healthcare research and quality; ANOVA = Analysis of variance; BPN-DPN = Brief pain inventory modified for patients with diabetic peripheral neuropathy; DSM-IV Diagnostic

Quality of Well being Scale Source: Jayadevappa R, Johnson JC, Bloom BS et al. Effectiveness of transcendental meditation on functional capacity and quality of life of African Americans with congestive heart failure: arandomized control study. Ethn Dis. 2007 Winter;17(1):72-7.

QOL Enjoyment/Satisfaction Scale Source: Bormann JE, Gifford AL, Shively M et. al. Effects of spiritual mantram repetition on HIV outcomes: a randomized controlled trial. J Behav Med. 2006 Aug;29(4):359-76.

Sense of Coherence source: Antonovsky A. The structure and properties of the sense of coherence scale. Social Science & Medicine Volume 36, Issue 6, March 1993, Pages 725–733

QOL-VAS source: Gould D, Kelly D, Goldstone L, Gammon J. Examining the validity of pressure ulcer risk assessment scales:developing and using illustrated patient simulations to collect the data. Journal of Clinical Nursing, 10, 697-706

QOL general for chronically ill patients information taken directly from : Schmidt S, Grossman P, Schwarzer B et. al. Treating fibromyalgia with mindfulness-based stress reduction: results from a 3-armed randomized controlled trial. Pain. 2011 Feb;152(2):361-9.

WHOQOL SOURCE:WHOQOL Manual DIVISION OF MENTAL HEALTH AND PREVENTION OF SUBSTANCE ABUSE WORLD HEALTH ORGANIZATION 1998. Downloaded from www.who.int/mental_health/evidence/who_qol_user_manual_98.pdf

User Manual SF-12 Data Source:Cheak-Zamora NC, Wyrwich KW,McBride TD. Reliability and validity of the SF-12v2 in the medical expenditure panel survey. Qual Life Res (2009) 18:727–735

Evidence Table E9. Scales for pain (KQ4)

Test	Brief Description	Reliability	Validity	Original Citation Date
KQ 4 Pain				
Numeric Rating Scale 0–10 (sensation and/or unpleasantness)	The NRS is an 11 point verbally administered scale that measures pain intensity and pain unpleasantness.[1,2] NRS is one of the simplest and most frequently used instruments to measure pain intensity in children and adults.[1]	ICC for pain intensity =0.85 (95%CI:0 .73–0.92). For pain distress was 0.77 (95% CI: 0.58–0.87).[4] Cronbach's alpha = 0.888 Test-retest reliability r= 0.72–0.78.[3]	Convergent validity NRS compared to VRS r = 0.90 to 0.92[3]; construct validity r = 0.72 to 0.85; discriminant validity r =0.65 to 0.70[3]	n/a
IBS Abdominal Pain Severity				
Pain Perception Scale (Sensory and Affective)	PPS is a subscale for assessing sensory and affective pain dimensions from the original scale—Schmerzempfindungsskala (original article in German).[5,9] It allows multifaceted and standardized quantification of pain.[9] This questionnaire consists of 2 scales: sensory and affective pain, with 14 and 10 items respectively.[5]			1995
SF-36 Bodily Pain Subscale	The Short Form (SF) Bodily Pain Scale is a validated subscale of the Medical Outcomes Study SF-36 questionnaire. It includes 2 items that assesses intensity of pain and how much pain has interfered with work[6]	Cronbach's α coefficients>0.7[10] Cronbach's α coefficients =0.86.[7] test-retest reliability (ICC)=0.90[7]	Studies of validity generally support the intended meaning of high and low SF-36 scores as documented in the original user's manuals. Because of the widespread use of the SF-36 across a variety of applications, evidence from many types of validity research is relevant to these interpretations. Studies to date have yielded content, concurrent, criterion, construct, and predictive evidence of validity.	1992

E-59

Test	Brief Description	Reliability	Validity	Original Citation Date
McGill Pain Questionnaire (current pain score)	The MPQ provides a measure of the subjective pain experience, across sensory, affective, and evaluative dimensions of acute and chronic pain.[15,19] The SF-MPQ is an interviewer administered short form of the MPQ consisting of 15 descriptors (11 sensory; 4 affective)[16,18] The MPQ provides a measure of the subjective pain experience, across sensory, affective, and evaluative dimensions of acute and chronic pain.[15,19] The SF-MPQ is an interviewer administered short form of the MPQ consisting of 15 descriptors (11 sensory; 4 affective)[16,18]	test–retest reliability (relative reliability) for total, sensory and affective scores were respectively, 0.75, 0.76 and 0.62 (musculoskeletal pain) and 0.93, 0.95 and 0.79 (rheumatic pain)[14]	Concurrent validity of 2 of the primary metrics of the MPQ(VAS and TS) at predicting pain-related disability = (R^2=0.373)[15]	1975
Fibromyalgia Impact Questionnaire	The fibromyalgia impact questionnaire (FIQ) is a 20 item self administered scale that assesses physical functioning, well-being and fibromyalgia symptoms among patients.[20]	Cronbach [alpha]) of the SF-MPQ =0.90 and 0.85 (Hispanics and non-Hispanic Whites respectively)[15]	Construct validity—correlation coefficients between KFIQ score and FM symptoms as assessed by VAS, KHAQ, and TPC were 0.43–0.58, 0.44, and 0.60, respectively[20]	1991
Roland Morris Disability Questionnaire	Intra class Correlation Coefficient of 0.91[22] The ICC was 0.94 for the intra-observer score and 0.95 for inter-observer score[25] Spearman's correlation coefficient for intraobserver and interobserver reliability was r = 0.88 & 0.86 respectively,[25] internal consistency (α = 0.860)[26] and test-retest reliability (ICC = 0.972)[26]	Construct validity testing revealed a moderate correlation with the NRS (r = 0.418)[26]		1983

Notes: ICC = Intra-class Correlation Coefficient; VRS = Verbal Rating Scale (VDS); FPS= Faces Pain Scale; VAS = Visual Analog Scale; TS-SF-MPQ total score (TS); KHAQ = Korean health assessment questionnaire; FM = fibromyalgia; SF-36 = 36 Item Short Form Health Survey; TPC= tender point count
* In German, English version not found.

References for Evidence Table E9

1. Pagé, M. Gabrielle Katz, Joel Stinson, Jennifer Isaac, Lisa Martin-Pichora, Andrea L. Campbell, Fiona ; Validation of the numerical rating scale for pain intensity and unpleasantness in pediatric acute postoperative pain: Sensitivity to change over time. The Journal of Pain, Vol 13(4), Apr, 2012. pp. 359-369

2. Zhou, Yinghua Petpichetchian, Wongchan Kitrungrote, Luppana .Psychometric properties of pain intensity scales comparing among postoperative adult patients, elderly patients without and with mild cognitive impairment in China. International Journal of Nursing Studies, Vol 48(4), Apr, 2011. pp. 449-457.

3. Good Marion , Catherine Zauszniewski, Jaclene A. Anderson, Gene Cranston Stanton-Hicks, Michael Grass, Jeffrey A. Sensation and Distress of Pain Scales: Reliability, validity, and sensitivity.; Journal of Nursing Measurement, Vol 9(3), Win, 2001. pp. 219-238

4. Wood, Bradley M. Nicholas, Michael K. Blyth, Fiona Asghari, Ali Gibson, Stephen ;Assessing pain in older people with persistent pain: The NRS is valid but only provides part of the picture.; The Journal of Pain, Vol 11(12), Dec, 2010. pp. 1259-1266.

5. Laederach-Hofmann, Kurt Truniger, Clemens Mussgay, Lutz Jürgensen, Ralph; Sensory and affective components in the use of pain words in patients suffering from angina pectoris due to coronary artery disease or syndrome X. ; Zeitschrift für Klinische Psychologie und Psychotherapie: Forschung und Praxis, Vol 30(3), 2001. pp. 182-188

6. Krebs, Erin E. Bair, Matthew J. Damush, Teresa M. Tu, Wanzhu Wu, Jingwei Kroenke, Kurt ; Comparative responsiveness of pain outcome measures among primary care patients with musculoskeletal pain Medical Care, Vol 48(11), Nov, 2010. pp. 1007-1014. [Journal Article]

7. Pinar, Rukiye; Reliability and construct validity of the SF-36 in Turkish cancer patients. Quality of Life Research: An International Journal of Quality of Life Aspects of Treatment, Care & Rehabilitation, Vol 14(1), Feb, 2005. pp. 259-264.

8. Herr, K. A., Spratt, K., et al Pain intensity assessment in older adults: use of experimental pain to compare psychometric properties and usability of selected pain scales with younger adults. Clin J Pain 20: 207-219, (2004).

9. Geissner E. The Pain Perception Scale—a differentiated and change-sensitive scale for assessing chronic and acute pain]. Rehabilitation (Stuttg). 1995 Nov;34(4):XXXV-XLIII. [Article in German]

10. Hoopman, Rianne Terwee, Caroline B. Devillé, Walter Knol, Dirk L. Aaronson, Neil K. Evaluation of the psychometric properties of the SF-36 health survey for use among Turkish and Moroccan ethnic minority populations in the Netherlands. ; Quality of Life Research: An International Journal of Quality of Life Aspects of Treatment, Care & Rehabilitation, Vol 18(6), Aug, 2009. pp. 753-764

11. Ware, J. E., & Sherbourne, C. D. (1992). The MOS 36-item shortform health survey (SF-36). I. Conceptual framework and item selection. Medical Care, 30, 473–483.

14. Strand, Liv Inger Ljunggren, Anne Elisabeth Bogen, Baard Ask, Tove Johnsen, Tom Backer ;The Short-Form McGill Pain Questionnaire as an outcome measure: Test-retest reliability and responsiveness to change. ; European Journal of Pain, Vol 12(7), Oct, 2008. pp. 917-925

15. Zinke, Jennifer L. Lam, Chow S. Harden, R. Norman Fogg, Louis; Examining the cross-cultural validity of the English short-form McGill Pain Questionnaire using the matched moderated regression methodology; The Clinical Journal of Pain, Vol 26(2), Feb, 2010. pp. 153-162. [Journal Article]

16. Melzack R. The short-form McGill Pain Questionnaire. Pain. 1987;30:191–197.

17. The McGill Pain Questionnaire: major properties and scoring methods Pain, 1 (1975), pp. 275–299

18. Burckhardt, Carol S. Jones, Kim D; Adult Measures of Pain: Short-Form McGill Pain Questionnaire (SF-MPQ). Arthritis & Rheumatism: Arthritis Care & Research, Vol 49(5,Suppl), Oct, 2003. Special issue: Patient Outcomes in Rheumatology: A Review of Measures. pp. S98-S99.

19. Katz, Joel Melzack, Ronald ;The McGill Pain Questionnaire: Development, psychometric properties, and usefulness of the long form, short form, and short form-2.; In: Handbook of pain assessment (3rd ed.). Turk, Dennis C. (Ed.); Melzack, Ronald (Ed.); New York, NY, US: Guilford Press, 2011. pp. 45-66.

20. Bae, Sang-Cheol Lee, Ji-Hyun ;Cross-cultural adaptation and validation of the Korean fibromyalgia impact questionnaire in women patients with fibromyalgia for clinical research.; Quality of Life Research: An International Journal of Quality of Life Aspects of Treatment, Care & Rehabilitation, Vol 13(4), Jun, 2004. pp. 857-861

21. Burckhardt CS, Clark SR, Bennett RM. The fibromyalgia impact questionnaire: Development and validation. J Rheumatol 1991; 18: 728–733.

22. Brouwer, S. Kuijer, W. Dijkstra, P. U. Göeken, L. N. H. Groothoff, J. W. Geertzen, J. H. B; Reliability and stability of the Roland Morris Disability Questionnaire: Intra class correlation and limits of agreement.. ; Disability and Rehabilitation: An International, Multidisciplinary Journal, Vol 26(3), Feb, 2004. pp. 162-165

23. Bergner M, Bobbitt RA, Carter WB, Gilson BS. Sickness impact profile: development and final revision of health status measure. Medical Care 1981; 19: 787 – 805.

24. Roland M, Morris R. A study of the natural history of back pain,part I: development of a reliable and sensitive measure of disabilityin low back pain. Spine 1983; 8: 141 – 144.

25. Nusbaum, L. Natour, J. Ferraz, M. B. Goldenberg, J. Translation, adaptation and validation of the Roland-Morris questionnaire-Brazil Roland-Morris.; Brazilian Journal of Medical and Biological Research, Vol 34(2), Feb, 2001. pp. 203-210

26. Monticone, Marco Baiardi, Paola Nava, Tiziana Rocca, Barbara Foti, Calogero ;The Italian version of the Sickness Impact Profile-Roland Scale for chronic pain: Cross-cultural adaptation, reliability, validity and sensitivity to change. Disability and Rehabilitation: An International, Multidisciplinary Journal, Vol 33(15-16), 2011. pp. 1299-1305.

Evidence Table E10. KQ1 outcomes—difference in differences—MBSR for anxiety

Improvement In Scale	Author, year	Outcome	Arm	N1	Mean	SD	T2	P Value	Δ-Δ Calc	ΔΔ %	T3	P Value	Δ-Δ Calc	ΔΔ %
Nonspecific Active Control														
	Henderson VP, 2011[1]	Beck Anxiety Inv	MBSR	53			4 Mos				24 Mos			
	Henderson VP, 2011[1]	Beck Anxiety Inv	Nutrition education	47			4 Mos				24 Mos			
Lower	Gaylord SA, 2011[2]	BSI-18 Anxiety Subscale	Modified MBSR	36	55.0	9.8	8 Wks				3 Mos			
Lower	Gaylord SA, 2011[2]	BSI-18 Anxiety Subscale	SG	39	54.8	10.6	8 Wks	0.2	-2.22	-4.0	3 Mos	0.02	-3.75	-6.8
Lower	Schmidt S, 2010[3]	STAI trait	MBSR	53	51.6	9.2	8 Wks				16 Wks			
Lower	Schmidt S, 2010[3]	STAI trait	AC	56	49.8	10.9	8 Wks	Ns	-2.15	-4.2	16 Wks	0.02	-2.38	-4.6
Lower	Gross CR, 2010[4]	STAI	MBSR	71	36.4	(31.8, 40.9)	8 Wks				6 Mos			
Lower	Gross CR, 2010[4]	STAI	HE	66	35.5	(30.9, 40.1)	8 Wks	Ns	-3.3	-9.1	6 Mos	Ns	-2.2	-6.0
Lower	Whitebird, 2012[5]	STAI state	MBSR	38	40	12.7	8 Wks				6 Mos			
Lower	Whitebird, 2012[5]	STAI state	Education/ Support	40	47.4	14.6	8 Wks		-0.1	-0.3	6 Mos	0.98	0.9	2.2
Lower	Chiesa, 2012[6]	Beck Anxiety Inv	MBCT	9	20.66	18.37	8 Wks							
Lower	Chiesa, 2012[6]	Beck Anxiety Inv	Education	9	16.67	7.11	8 Wks	0.44	-9.1	-44.0				
Specific Active Control														
Lower	Wong SY-S, 2011[7]	STAI state	MBSR	51	48.2	12.3	8 Wks				6 Mos			
Lower	Wong SY-S, 2011[7]	STAI state	Pain A.control	48	46.8	9.7	8 Wks	Ns	-1.4	-2.9	6 Mos	0.19	-1.49	-3.1
Lower	Wong SY-S, 2011[7]	STAI trait	MBSR	51	45.0	9.5	8 Wks				6 Mos			
Lower	Wong SY-S, 2011[7]	STAI trait	Pain A.control	48	46.8	9.7	8 Wks	Ns	0.19	0.4	6 Mos	0.61	1.24	2.8
Lower	Wong SY-S, 2011[7]	POMS - tension	MBSR	51	12.5	8.5	8 Wks				6 Mos			

Improvement In Scale	Author, year	Outcome	Arm	N1	Mean	SD	T2	P Value	Δ-Δ Calc	Δ Δ %	T3	P Value	Δ-Δ Calc	Δ Δ %
Lower	Wong SY-S, 2011[7]	POMS - tension	Pain A.control	48	11.8	7.3	8 Wks	Ns	-1.44	-11.5	6 Mos	0.21	-1.45	-11.6
Lower For Δ	Gross CR, 2011[8]	STAI state	MBSR	18	33.94	11.3	8 Wks				5 Mos			
Lower For Δ	Gross CR, 2011[8]	STAI state	Drug	9	31.16	12.7	8 Wks	Ns	-1.24	-3.7	5 Mos	Ns	-2.21	-6.5
Lower	Moritz S, 2006[9]	POMS - tension	MBSR	54	12.7	1	8 Wks							
Lower	Moritz S, 2006[9]	POMS - tension	Spirituality	56	14.3	1	8 Wks	0.007	4.9	38.6				
Lower	Barrett, 2012[10]	STAI state	MBSR	51	32.2	8.1	9 Wks				5 Mos			
Lower	Barrett, 2012[10]	STAI state	Exercise	47	30.7	9.1	9 Wks	Ns	-1	-3.1	5 Mos	Ns	-0.9	-2.8
Lower	Jazaieri, 2012[11]	Liebowitz SAS	MBSR	31	86.82	20.91	8 Wks				5 Mos			
Lower	Jazaieri, 2012[11]	Liebowitz SAS	Exercise	25	87.38	16.06	8 Wks	Ns	-5.35	-6.2	5 Mos	Ns	1.26	1.5

Notes: MBSR = Mindfulness-based Stress Reduction; SG = Support Group; AC = Active Control; HE = Health Education

References for Evidence Table E10

1. Henderson VP, Clemow L, Massion AO, Hurley TG, Druker S, Hebert JR. The effects of mindfulness-based stress reduction on psychosocial outcomes and quality of life in early-stage breast cancer patients: a randomized trial. Breast Cancer Res Treat 2011.
2. Gaylord SA, Palsson OS, Garland EL et al. Mindfulness training reduces the severity of irritable bowel syndrome in women: results of a randomized controlled trial. Am J Gastroenterol 2011; 106(9):1678-88.
3. Schmidt S, Grossman P, Schwarzer B, Jena S, Naumann J, Walach H. Treating fibromyalgia with mindfulness-based stress reduction: results from a 3-armed randomized controlled trial. Pain 2011; 152(2):361-9.
4. Gross CR, Kreitzer MJ, Thomas W et al. Mindfulness-based stress reduction for solid organ transplant recipients: a randomized controlled trial. Altern Ther Health Med 2010; 16(5):30-8.
5. Whitebird RR, Kreitzer M, Crain AL, Lewis BA, Hanson LR, Enstad CJ. Mindfulness-Based Stress Reduction for Family Caregivers: A Randomized Controlled Trial. Gerontologist 2012.
6. Chiesa A, Mandelli L, Serretti A. Mindfulness-based cognitive therapy versus psycho-education for patients with major depression who did not achieve remission following antidepressant treatment: a preliminary analysis. J Altern Complement Med 2012; 18(8):756-60.
7. Wong SY, Chan FW, Wong RL et al. Comparing the Effectiveness of Mindfulness-based Stress Reduction and Multidisciplinary Intervention Programs for Chronic Pain: A Randomized Comparative Trial. Clin J Pain 2011; 27(8):724-34.
8. Gross CR, Kreitzer MJ, Reilly-Spong M et al. Mindfulness-based stress reduction versus pharmacotherapy for chronic primary insomnia: a randomized controlled clinical trial. Explore (NY) 2011; 7(2):76-87.

9. Moritz S, Quan H, Rickhi B et al. A home study-based spirituality education program decreases emotional distress and increases quality of life—a randomized, controlled trial. Altern Ther Health Med 2006; 12(6):26-35.

10. Barrett B, Hayney MS, Muller D et al. Meditation or exercise for preventing acute respiratory infection: a randomized controlled trial. Ann Fam Med 2012; 10(4):337-46.

11. Jazaieri H, Goldin PR, Werner K, Ziv M, Gross JJ. A Randomized Trial of MBSR Versus Aerobic Exercise for Social Anxiety Disorder. J Clin Psychol 2012.

Evidence Table E11. KQ1 outcomes—difference in differences—other mindfulness for anxiety

Improvement In Score	Author, year	Outcome	Arm	N1	Mean	SD	T2	P Value	Δ-Δ Calc	ΔΔ %	T3	P Value	Δ-Δ Calc	ΔΔ %
Nonspecific Active Control														
Lower For Δ	Pipe TB, 2009[1]	SCL-90 anxiety	MBSR	15			4 Wks							
Lower For Δ	Pipe TB, 2009[1]	SCL-90 anxiety	Educ	17			4 Wks	0.33	−0.27					
Lower	Lee SH, 2006[2]	STAI state	Meditation	21	24.7	14.6	8 Wks							
Lower	Lee SH, 2006[2]	STAI state	HE	20	28.6	11.7	8 Wks	<.05	−5.7	−23.1				
Lower	Lee SH, 2006[2]	STAI trait	Meditation	21	32.8	10.8	8 Wks							
Lower	Lee SH, 2006[2]	STAI trait	HE	20	40.3	11.5	8 Wks	<.05	−5.1	−15.5				
Lower	Lee SH, 2006[2]	HAM-A	Meditation	21	16.6	1.3	8 Wks							
Lower	Lee SH, 2006[2]	HAM-A	HE	20	15.9	5.6	8 Wks	<.05	−7.1	−42.8				
Lower	Lee SH, 2006[2]	SCL-90R anxiety subscale	Meditation	21	13.7	8.1	8 Wks							
Lower	Lee SH, 2006[2]	SCL-90R anxiety subscale	HE	20	16.3	8.8	8 Wks	<.05	−4.1	−29.9				
Specific Active Control														
Lower	Philippot P, 2011[3]	STAI (not specified)	modified MBCT	13	45.13	12.5	6 Wks				3 Mos			
Lower	Philippot P, 2011[3]	STAI (not specified)	Relaxation	12	44.22	10.7	6 Wks	Ns	−3.81	−8.4	3 Mos	Ns	−6.18	−14.0
Lower	Delgado LC, 2010[4]	STAI (Trait)	MM	15	29.7	10.7	5–6 Wks							
Lower	Delgado LC, 2010[4]	STAI (Trait)	Relaxation	17	31.6	11.6	5 Wks	Ns	1.3	4.4				
Lower	Piet J, 2010[5]	BAI	MBCT	14	12.3	7.3	8 Wks							
Lower	Piet J, 2010[5]	BAI	GCBT	12	17.9	5.6	12 Wks	Ns	3.28	26.6				

Notes: MBSR = Mindfulness-based Stress Reduction; HE = Health Education; Educ = Education; GCBT = Group Cognitive Behavioural Therapy; MM = Mindfulness Meditation

References for Evidence Table E11

1. Pipe TB, Bortz JJ, Dueck A, Pendergast D, Buchda V, Summers J. Nurse leader mindfulness meditation program for stress management: a randomized controlled trial. J Nurs Adm 2009; 39(3):130-7.

2. Lee SH, Ahn SC, Lee YJ, Choi TK, Yook KH, Suh SY. Effectiveness of a meditation-based stress management program as an adjunct to pharmacotherapy in patients with anxiety disorder. J Psychosom Res 2007; 62(2):189-95.

3. Philippot P, Nef F, Clauw L, Romree M, Segal Z. A Randomized Controlled Trial of Mindfulness-Based Cognitive Therapy for Treating Tinnitus. Clin Psychol Psychother 2011.

4. Delgado LC, Guerra P, Perakakis P, Vera MN, Reyes del Paso G, Vila J. Treating chronic worry: Psychological and physiological effects of a training programme based on mindfulness. Behav Res Ther 2010; 48(9):873-82.

5. Piet J, Hougaard E, Hecksher MS, Rosenberg NK. A randomized pilot study of mindfulness-based cognitive therapy and group cognitive-behavioral therapy for young adults with social phobia. Scand J Psychol 2010; 51(5):403-10.

Evidence Table E12. KQ1 outcomes—difference in differences—TM anxiety

Improvement In Scale	Author, year	Outcome	Arm	N1	Mean	SD	T2	P Value	Δ-Δ Calc	ΔΔ %	T3	P Value	Δ-Δ Calc	ΔΔ %
TM = All Nonspecific Active Control														
Lower	Paul-Labrador M, 2006[1]	STAI Trait	TM	52	14.4	10.1	16 Wks							
Lower	Paul-Labrador M, 2006[1]	STAI Trait	HE	51	17.8	11.7	16 Wks	Ns	0.4	2.8				
Lower	Smith JC, 1976[2]	STAI Trait	TM	19	47.0	14.9	6 Mos							
Lower	Smith JC, 1976[2]	STAI Trait	AC	22	47.9	9.3	6 Mos	Ns	-1.14	-2.4				
Other Mantra														
Lower For Δ	Lehrer PM, 1983[3]	IPAT Anxiety Inventory (Full Scale Sten Score)	CSM	23	8.9	21.0	6 Wks				6 Mos			
Lower For Δ	Lehrer PM, 1983[3]	IPAT Anxiety Inventory (Full Scale Sten Score)	PMR	19	8.9	16.0	6 Wks	Ns	0.77	8.7	6 Mos			
Lower For Δ	Lehrer PM, 1983[3]	SCL-90 Anxiety subscale	CSM	23	1.6	21.0	6 Wks				6 Mos			
Lower For Δ	Lehrer PM, 1983[3]	SCL-90 Anxiety subscale	PMR	19	1.5	16.0	6 Wks	Ns	0.26	16.3	6 Mos			
Lower For Δ	Lehrer PM, 1983[3]	STAI Trait	CSM	23	54.2	21.0	6 Wks				No F/U			
Lower For Δ	Lehrer PM, 1983[3]	STAI Trait	PMR	19	52.1	16.0	6 Wks	Ns	3.06	5.6	No F/U			
Lower For Δ	Lehrer PM, 1983[3]	STAI State	CSM	23	43.3	21.0	6 Wks				No F/U			
Lower For Δ	Lehrer PM, 1983[3]	STAI State	PMR	19	41.6	16.0	6 Wks	Ns	9.24	21.3	No F/U			
Lower	Bormann JE, 2006[4]	STAI Trait	Mantra	46	44.1	11.1	10 Wks				22 Wks			
Lower	Bormann JE, 2006[4]	STAI Trait	AC	47	44.9	10.4	10 Wks	Ns	-2.7	-6.1	22 Wks	0.15	-1.0	-2.3

*(adjusted for baseline scores)

Notes: MBSR = Mindfulness-based Stress Reduction; AC = Active Control; HE = Health Education; PMR = Progressive Muscle Relaxation; CSM = Clinically Standardized Meditation; MM = Mindfulness Meditation; TM = Transcendental Meditation

References for Evidence Table E12

1. Paul-Labrador M, Polk D, Dwyer JH et al. Effects of a randomized controlled trial of transcendental meditation on components of the metabolic syndrome in subjects with coronary heart disease. Arch Intern Med 2006; 166(11):1218-24.

2. Smith JC. Psychotherapeutic effects of transcendental meditation with controls for expectation of relief and daily sitting. J Consult Clin Psychol 1976; 44(4):630-7.

3. Lehrer PM. Progressive relaxation and meditation: A study of psychophysiological and therapeutic differences between two techniques. Behav Res Ther 1983; 21(6):651-62.

4. Bormann JE, Gifford AL, Shively M et al. Effects of spiritual mantram repetition on HIV outcomes: a randomized controlled trial. J Behav Med 2006; 29(4):359-76.

Evidence Table E13. KQ1 outcomes—difference in differences—thought emotion suppression for anxiety

Improvement In Scale	Author, year	Outcome	Arm	N1	Mean	SD	T2	P Value	Δ-Δ Calc	Δ Δ %	T3	P Value	Δ-Δ Calc	Δ Δ%
*** Worry Aspect Of Anxiety ***														
Lower	Delgado LC, 2010[1]	Penn State Worry Questionnaire	MM	15	67.0	4.1	5 Wks							
Lower	Delgado LC, 2010[1]	Penn State Worry Questionnaire	Relaxation	17	66.7	3.6	5 Wks	Ns	-0.2	-0.3				
Thought/ Emotion Suppression														
Lower	Garland EL, 2010[2]	WhiteBear Suppression Inventory (thought suppression)	MORE	18	53.6	8.7	10 Wks							
Lower	Garland EL, 2010[2]	WhiteBear Suppression Inventory (thought suppression)	ASG	19	50.9	11.2	10 Wks	0.04	-6.1	-11.4				
Lower	Henderson VP, 2011[3]	Courtald emotional control (emotion suppresion)	MBSR	53	15.1	0.6	4 Mos				24 Mos			
Lower	Henderson VP, 2011[3]	Courtald emotional control (emotion suppresion)	Nutrition education	47	16.6	0.6	4 Mos	Ns	-0.8	-5.3	24 Mos	Ns	0.8	5.3

Notes: MBSR = Mindfulness-based Stress Reduction; MM = Mindfulness Meditation; MORE = Mindfulness-oriented Recovery Enhancement; ASG = Alcohol-dependence Support Group

References for Evidence Table E13

1 Delgado LC, Guerra P, Perakakis P, Vera MN, Reyes del Paso G, Vila J. Treating chronic worry: Psychological and physiological effects of a training programme based on mindfulness. Behav Res Ther 2010; 48(9):873-82.

2 Garland EL, Gaylord SA, Boettiger CA, Howard MO. Mindfulness training modifies cognitive, affective, and physiological mechanisms implicated in alcohol dependence: results of a randomized controlled pilot trial. J Psychoactive Drugs 2010; 42(2):177-92.

3 Henderson VP, Clemow L, Massion AO, Hurley TG, Druker S, Hebert JR. The effects of mindfulness-based stress reduction on psychosocial outcomes and quality of life in early-stage breast cancer patients: a randomized trial. Breast Cancer Res Treat 2011.

Evidence Table E14. KQ1 outcomes—difference in differences—social anxiety

Improvement In Scale	Author, year	Outcome	Arm	N1	Mean	SD	T2	P Value	Δ-Δ Calc	Δ Δ %
Lower	Piet J, 2010[1]	Liebowitz Social Anxiety Scale (fear+avoidance)	MBCT	14	59.29	19.78	8 wks			
Lower	Piet J, 2010[1]	Liebowitz Social Anxiety Scale (fear+avoidance)	GCBT	11	71.37	19.56	12 wks	Ns	4.2	7.0
Lower	Piet J, 2010[1]	Social Phobia Scale	MBCT	14	35.21	13.22	8 wks			
Lower	Piet J, 2010[1]	Social Phobia Scale	GCBT	12	35.06	12.16	12 wks	Ns	1.0	3.0
Lower	Piet J, 2010[1]	Fear of Negative Evaluation-Brief Version	MBCT	14	46.05	7.99	8 wks			
Lower	Piet J, 2010[1]	Fear of Negative Evaluation-Brief Version	GCBT	12	49.32	7.92	12 wks	Ns	-1.9	-4.1
Lower	Piet J, 2010[1]	Social Interaction Scale	MBCT	14	44.52	13.87	8 wks			
Lower	Piet J, 2010[1]	Social Interaction Scale	GCBT	12	48.67	15.79	12 wks	Ns	4.3	9.6
Lower	Koszycki D, 2007[2]	Liebowitz Social Anxiety- Fear	MBSR	26	40.80	7.90	8 wks			
Lower	Koszycki D, 2007[2]	Liebowitz Social Anxiety- Fear	CBGT	27	37.30	7.60	12 wks	Ns	2.4	5.9
Lower	Koszycki D, 2007[2]	Liebowitz Social Anxiety- Avoidance	MBSR	26	39.10	8.90	8 wks			
Lower	Koszycki D, 2007[2]	Liebowitz Social Anxiety- Avoidance	CBGT	27	34.30	8.60	12 wks	Ns	3.1	7.9
Lower	Koszycki D, 2007[2]	Social Phobia Scale	MBSR	26	34.00	14.00	8 wks			
Lower	Koszycki D, 2007[2]	Social Phobia Scale	CBGT	27	33.30	13.20	12 wks	Ns	8.5	25.0
Lower	Koszycki D, 2007[2]	Social Interaction Scale	MBSR	26	44.60	10.60	8 wks			
Lower	Koszycki D, 2007[2]	Social Interaction Scale	CBGT	27	46.10	8.90	12 wks	Ns	5.4	12.1

Notes: MBSR = Mindfulness-based Stress Reduction; GCBT = Group Cognitive Behavioural Therapy

References for Evidence Table E14

1. Piet J, Hougaard E, Hecksher MS, Rosenberg NK. A randomized pilot study of mindfulness-based cognitive therapy and group cognitive-behavioral therapy for young adults with social phobia. Scandinavian Journal of Psychology 2010; 51(5):403-10.

2. Koszycki D, Benger M, Shlik J, Bradwejn J. Randomized trial of a meditation-based stress reduction program and cognitive behavior therapy in generalized social anxiety disorder. Behav Res Ther 2007; 45(10):2518-26.

Evidence Table E15. KQ1 outcomes—difference in differences—MBSR for depression

Improvement In Scale	Author, year	Outcome	Arm	N1	Mean	SD	T2	P Value	Δ-Δ Calc	ΔΔ%	T3	P Value	Δ-Δ Calc	ΔΔ%
Nonspecific Active Control														
	Henderson VP, 2011[1]	BDI	MBSR	53			4 Mos				24 Mos			
	Henderson VP, 2011[1]	BDI	Nutrition education	52			4 Mos				24 Mos			
Lower	Henderson VP, 2011[1]	SCL-90R Depression	MBSR	53	0.6	0.07*	4 Mos	<0.05	-0.32	-49.2	24 Mos			
Lower	Henderson VP, 2011[1]	SCL-90R Depression	Nutrition education	52	0.5	0.07*	4 Mos				24 Mos		-0.09	-13.8
Lower	Gaylord SA, 2011[2]	BSI-18 Depression subscale	Modified MBSR	36	55.1	10.5	8 Wks				3 Mos			
Lower	Gaylord SA, 2011[2]	BSI-18 Depression subscale	SG	39	54.8	11.3	8 Wks	0.725	-0.71	-1.3	3 Mos	0.205	-2.44	-4.4
Lower	Schmidt S, 2010[3]	CES-D	MBSR	53	25.2	9.6	8 Wks				16 Wks			
Lower	Schmidt S, 2010[3]	CES-D	AC	56	22.9	10.3	8 Wks		0.03	0.1	16 Wks		-3.12	-12.4
Lower	Gross CR, 2010[4]	CES-D	MBSR	71	13.2	(9.8, 17.8)	8 Wks				12 Mos			
Lower	Gross CR, 2010[4]	CES-D	HE	66	11.6	(8.6, 15.7)	8 Wks		-3.80	-28.8	12 Mos	0.1	-4.20	-31.8
Lower	Malarkey, 2012[5]	CES-D	MBI-ld	93	16.7	0.5	8 Wks							
Lower	Malarkey, 2012[5]	CES-D	Education	93	16.3	0.5	8 Wks	NS						
Lower	Whitebird, 2012[6]	CES-D	MBSR	38	17.9	8.9	8 Wks				6 Mos			
Lower	Whitebird, 2012[6]	CES-D	Education/ Support	40	19.2	11.8	8 Wks		-5.2	-29.1	6 Mos	0.07	-1.9	-10.6
Specific Active Control														
Lower	Wong SY-S, 2011[7]	POMS-D	MBSR	51	15.3	13.7	8 Wks				6 Mos			
Lower	Wong SY-S, 2011[7]	POMS-D	Pain A.control	48	15.3	11.7	8 Wks	Ns	-1.63	-10.7	6 Mos	Ns	-1.96	-12.8
Lower	Wong SY-S, 2011[7]	CES-D	MBSR	51	35.8	8.9	8 Wks				6 Mos			

E-71

Improvement In Scale	Author, year	Outcome	Arm	N1	Mean	SD	T2	P Value	Δ-Δ Calc	ΔΔ%	T3	P Value	Δ-Δ Calc	ΔΔ%
Lower	Wong SY-S, 2011[7]	CES-D	Pain A.control	48	35.7	6.5	8 Wks	Ns	-0.83	-2.3	6 Mos	Ns	-0.24	-0.7
Lower For Δ	Gross CR, 2011[8]	CES-D	MBSR	18	10.9	7.9	8 Wks				5 Mos			
Lower For Δ	Gross CR, 2011[8]	CES-D	drug	9	13.7	12.1	8 Wks		2.76	25.4	5 Mos		4.58	42.2
Lower	Koszycki D, 2007[9]	Interpersonal sensitivity	MBSR	26	112.0	11.8	8 Wks							
Lower	Koszycki D, 2007[9]	Interpersonal sensitivity	CBGT	27	111.9	13.4	12 Wks		4.30	3.8				
Lower	Koszycki D, 2007[9]	BDI	MBSR	26	15.1	10.4	8 Wks							
Lower	Koszycki D, 2007[9]	BDI	CBGT	27	15.8	12	12 Wks		0.80	5.3				
Lower	Moritz S, 2006[10]	POMS - D	MBSR	54	22.7	1.8*	8 Wks							
Lower	Moritz S, 2006[10]	POMS - D	Spirituality	56	26.9	1.8*	8 Wks		7.20	31.7				
Lower	Jazaieri, 2012[11]	BDI II	MBSR	31	13.94	11.46	8 Wks				5 Mos			
Lower	Jazaieri, 2012[11]	BDI II	AE	25	16.4	7.84	8 Wks	Ns	-3.2	-22.8	5 Mos	Ns	-2.0	-14.2
Lower	Wolever, 2012[12]	CES-D	Mindfulness	96	20.1	0.91	12 Wks							
Lower	Wolever, 2012[12]	CES-D	Vinyana yoga	90	18.45	0.94	12 Wks	Ns	-1.7	-8.5				

Notes: MBSR = Mindfulness-based Stress Reduction; SG = Support Group; AC = Active Control; HE = Health Education; CBGT = Cognitive Behavioural Group Therapy

References for Evidence Table E15

1. Henderson VP, Clemow L, Massion AO, Hurley TG, Druker S, Hebert JR. The effects of mindfulness-based stress reduction on psychosocial outcomes and quality of life in early-stage breast cancer patients: a randomized trial. Breast Cancer Res Treat 2011.

2. Gaylord SA, Palsson OS, Garland EL et al. Mindfulness training reduces the severity of irritable bowel syndrome in women: results of a randomized controlled trial. Am J Gastroenterol 2011; 106(9):1678-88.

3. Schmidt S, Grossman P, Schwarzer B, Jena S, Naumann J, Walach H. Treating fibromyalgia with mindfulness-based stress reduction: results from a 3-armed randomized controlled trial. Pain 2011; 152(2):361-9.

4. Gross CR, Kreitzer MJ, Thomas W et al. Mindfulness-based stress reduction for solid organ transplant recipients: a randomized controlled trial. Altern Ther Health Med 2010; 16(5):30-8.

5. Malarkey WB, Jarjoura D, Klatt M. Workplace based mindfulness practice and inflammation: A randomized trial. Brain Behav Immun 2012.

6. Whitebird RR, Kreitzer M, Crain AL, Lewis BA, Hanson LR, Enstad CJ. Mindfulness-Based Stress Reduction for Family Caregivers: A Randomized Controlled Trial. Gerontologist 2012.

7. Wong SY, Chan FW, Wong RL et al. Comparing the Effectiveness of Mindfulness-based Stress Reduction and Multidisciplinary Intervention Programs for Chronic Pain: A Randomized Comparative Trial. Clin J Pain 2011; 27(8):724-34.

8. Gross CR, Kreitzer MJ, Reilly-Spong M et al. Mindfulness-based stress reduction versus pharmacotherapy for chronic primary insomnia: a randomized controlled clinical trial. Explore (NY) 2011; 7(2):76-87.

9. Koszycki D, Benger M, Shlik J, Bradwejn J. Randomized trial of a meditation-based stress reduction program and cognitive behavior therapy in generalized social anxiety disorder. Behav Res Ther 2007; 45(10):2518-26.

10. Moritz S, Quan H, Rickhi B et al. A home study-based spirituality education program decreases emotional distress and increases quality of life—a randomized, controlled trial. Altern Ther Health Med 2006; 12(6):26-35.

11. Jazaieri H, Goldin PR, Werner K, Ziv M, Gross JJ. A Randomized Trial of MBSR Versus Aerobic Exercise for Social Anxiety Disorder. J Clin Psychol 2012.

12. Wolever RQ, Bobinet KJ, McCabe K et al. Effective and viable mind-body stress reduction in the workplace: a randomized controlled trial. J Occup Health Psychol 2012; 17(2):246-58.

Evidence Table E16. KQ1 outcomes—difference in differences—other meditation for depression

Improvement In Scale	Author, year	Outcome	Arm	N1	Mean	SD	T2	P Value	Δ-Δ Calc	Δ Δ%	T3	P Value	Δ-Δ Calc	Δ Δ%
Nonspecific Active Control														
Lower	Oken BS, 2010[1]	CESD	MM	8	15.8	7.7	7–10 Wks							
Lower	Oken BS, 2010[1]	CESD	Education	11	16.9	10.0	7–10 Wks		-1.60	-10.1				
Lower	Oken BS, 2010[1]	CESD	Respite only	9	14.5	7.7	7–10 Wks							
Lower	Lee SH, 2006[2]	BDI	Meditation	21	14.2	10.6	8 Wks							
Lower	Lee SH, 2006[2]	BDI	HE	20	16.2	9.7	8 Wks	Ns	-4.30	-30.3				
Lower	Lee SH, 2006[2]	SCL-90R depression subscale	Meditation	21	15.5	9.8	8 Wks							
Lower	Lee SH, 2006[2]	SCL-90R depression subscale	HE	20	20.8	14.0	8 Wks	Ns	-2.70	-17.4				
Lower	Chiesa, 2012[3]	HAM-D	MBCT	9	16.11	7.01	8 Wks							
Lower	Chiesa, 2012[3]	HAM-D	Education	9	14.14	4.98	8 Wks	0.04	-8.31	-51.6				
Specific Active Control														
Lower	Philippot P, 2011[4]	BDI	MBCT	13	12.3	8.4	6 Wks				18 Wks			
Lower	Philippot P, 2011[4]	BDI	Relaxation	12	15.2	7.7	6wks		-1.07	-8.7	18 Wks		0.38	3.1
Lower	Delgado LC, 2010[5]	BDI	MM	15	9	6.2	5 Wks							
Lower	Delgado LC, 2010[5]	BDI	PMR/Relaxation	17	9.8	8.6	5 Wks		-1.20	-13.3				
MBCT Vs Specific Active Control														
Lower	Kuyken W, 2008[6]	BDI-II	MBCT	61	18.5	10.9	3 Mos				15 Mos			
Lower	Kuyken W, 2008[6]	BDI-II	Antidepressant	62	20.1	12.9	3 Mos		-2.71	-14.6	15 Mos		-2.77	-15.0
Lower	Piet J, 2010[7]	BDI-II	MBCT	14	13.1	6.7	8 Wks							
Lower	Piet J, 2010[7]	BDI-II	GCBT	12	19.5	9.0	14 Wks		3.18	24.3				

Notes: MBSR = Mindfulness-based Stress Reduction; HE = Health Education; PMR = Progressive Muscle Relaxation; MM = Mindfulness Meditation; MBCT = Mindfulness Based Cognitive Therapy; GCBT = Group Cognitive Behavioural Therapy

References for Evidence Table E16

1. Oken BS, Fonareva I, Haas M et al. Pilot controlled trial of mindfulness meditation and education for dementia caregivers. J Altern Complement Med 2010; 16(10):1031-8.

2. Lee SH, Ahn SC, Lee YJ, Choi TK, Yook KH, Suh SY. Effectiveness of a meditation-based stress management program as an adjunct to pharmacotherapy in patients with anxiety disorder. J Psychosom Res 2007; 62(2):189-95.

3. Chiesa A, Mandelli L, Serretti A. Mindfulness-based cognitive therapy versus psycho-education for patients with major depression who did not achieve remission following antidepressant treatment: a preliminary analysis. J Altern Complement Med 2012; 18(8):756-60.

4. Philippot P, Nef F, Clauw L, Romree M, Segal Z. A Randomized Controlled Trial of Mindfulness-Based Cognitive Therapy for Treating Tinnitus. Clin Psychol Psychother 2011.

5. Delgado LC, Guerra P, Perakakis P, Vera MN, Reyes del Paso G, Vila J. Treating chronic worry: Psychological and physiological effects of a training programme based on mindfulness. Behav Res Ther 2010; 48(9):873-82.

6. Kuyken W, Byford S, Taylor RS et al. Mindfulness-based cognitive therapy to prevent relapse in recurrent depression. J Consult Clin Psychol 2008; 76(6):966-78.

7. Piet J, Hougaard E, Hecksher MS, Rosenberg NK. A randomized pilot study of mindfulness-based cognitive therapy and group cognitive-behavioral therapy for young adults with social phobia. Scand J Psychol 2010; 51(5):403-10.

Evidence Table E17. KQ1 outcomes—difference in differences—other meditation for depression

Improvement In Scale	Author, year	Outcome	Arm	N1	Mean	SD	T2	P Value	Δ-Δ Calc	ΔΔ%	T3	P Value	Δ-Δ Calc	ΔΔ%
Lower	Segal ZV, 2010[1]	SCID Relapse Rate	MBCT	26	0	0	600 Days							
Lower	Segal ZV, 2010[1]	SCID Relapse Rate	Antidepressant	28	0	0	600 Days		−0.08	n/a				
Lower	Kuyken W, 2008[2]	SCID Relapse Rate	MBCT	61							15 Mos			
Lower	Kuyken W, 2008[2]	SCID Relapse Rate	Antidepressant	62							15 Mos	0.21	−0.13	N/A
Lower	Kuyken W, 2008[2]	HAM-D	MBCT	61	5.6	4.3	3 Mos				15 Mos			
Lower	Kuyken W, 2008[2]	HAM-D	Antidepressant	62	5.8	4.7	3 Mos		−1.78	−31.7	15 Mos	0.02	−1.50	−26.7
Lower	Lee SH, 2006[3]	HAM-D	Meditation	21	13.5	5.9	8 Wks							
Lower	Lee SH, 2006[3]	HAM-D	HE	20	14.7	5.2	8 Wks	<0.05	−3.20	−23.7				

Notes: MBCT = Mindfulness Based Cognitive Therapy; HE = Health Education

References for Evidence Table E17

1. Segal ZV, Bieling P, Young T et al. Antidepressant monotherapy vs sequential pharmacotherapy and mindfulness-based cognitive therapy, or placebo, for relapse prophylaxis in recurrent depression. Arch Gen Psychiatry 2010; 67(12):1256-64.
2. Kuyken W, Byford S, Taylor RS et al. Mindfulness-based cognitive therapy to prevent relapse in recurrent depression. J Consult Clin Psychol 2008; 76(6):966-78.
3. Lee SH, Ahn SC, Lee YJ, Choi TK, Yook KH, Suh SY. Effectiveness of a meditation-based stress management program as an adjunct to pharmacotherapy in patients with anxiety disorder. J Psychosom Res 2007; 62(2):189-95.

Evidence Table E18. KQ1 outcomes—difference in differences—mantra for depression

Improvement In Scale	Author, year	Outcome	Arm	N1	Mean	SD	T2	P Value	Δ-Δ Calc	Δ Δ%	T3	P Value	Δ-Δ Calc	Δ Δ%
TM Vs Nonspecific Active Control														
Lower	Paul-Labrador M, 2006[1]	CES-D	TM	52	6.8	7.1	16 Wks							
Lower	Paul-Labrador M, 2006[1]	CES-D	HE	51	12.2	10.7	16 Wks		1.30	19.1				
Lower	Schneider, 2012[2]	CES-D	TM	99	13.8	9.9					5.4 yrs (avg)			
Lower	Schneider, 2012[2]	CES-D	HE	102	17.8	11.7					5.4 yrs (avg)	0.2	−0.9	−6.8
Higher For Δ	Jayadevappa R, 2007[3]	CES-D	TM	13	14.8	6.4	3 Mos				6 Mos			
Higher For Δ	Jayadevappa R, 2007[3]	CES-D	HE	10	14.1	12.1	3 Mos		6.83	46.1	6 Mos	0.85	7.25	49.0
Other Mantra (1 Specific Active Control & 1 Nonspecific Active Control)														
Lower	Bormann JE, 2006[4]	CES-D	Mantra	46	18.4	11.0	10 Wks				22 Wks			
Lower	Bormann JE, 2006[4]	CES-D	AC	47	22.3	11.6	10 Wks		0.3	1.6	22 Wks	0.07	3.7	20.1
Lower For Δ	Lehrer PM, 1983[5]	SCL-90 Depression	CSM	23	1.8		6 Wks				6 Mos			
Lower For Δ	Lehrer PM, 1983[5]	SCL-90 Depression	Progressive Relaxation	19	1.7		6 Wks		0.5	27.8	6 Mos		0.14	7.8

Notes: AC = Active Control; HE = Health Education; CSM = Clinically Standardized Meditation; TM = Transcendental Meditation

References for Evidence Table E18

1. Paul-Labrador M, Polk D, Dwyer JH et al. Effects of a randomized controlled trial of transcendental meditation on components of the metabolic syndrome in subjects with coronary heart disease. Arch Intern Med 2006; 166(11):1218-24.

2. Schneider RH, Grim CE, Rainforth MV et al. Stress Reduction in the Secondary Prevention of Cardiovascular Disease: Randomized, Controlled Trial of Transcendental Meditation and Health Education in Blacks. (1941-7705 (Electronic). 1941-7713 (Linking)).

3. Jayadevappa R, Johnson JC, Bloom BS et al. Effectiveness of transcendental meditation on functional capacity and quality of life of African Americans with congestive heart failure: a randomized control study Ethn Dis. 2007 Summer;17(3):595. Ethnicity & Disease 2007; 17(1):72-7.

4. Bormann JE, Gifford AL, Shively M et al. Effects of spiritual mantram repetition on HIV outcomes: a randomized controlled trial. J Behav Med 2006; 29(4):359-76.

5. Lehrer PM. Progressive relaxation and meditation: A study of psychophysiological and therapeutic differences between two techniques. Behav Res Ther 1983; 21(6):651-62.

Evidence Table E19. KQ1 outcomes—difference in differences—stress

Improvement In Scale	Author, year	Outcome	Arm	N1	Mean	SD	T2	P Value	Δ-Δ Calc	Δ Δ%	T3	P VALUE	Δ-Δ Calc	Δ Δ%
Nonspecific Active Control														
Lower	Oken BS, 2010[1]	PSS	MM	8	18.5	8.5	7–10 Wks							
Lower	Oken BS, 2010[1]	PSS	Education	11	18.6	7.5	7–10 Wks	Ns	-2.6	-14.1				
Lower	Oken BS, 2010[1]	PSS	Respite only	9	17.3	4.9	7–10 Wks							
Lower	Garland EL, 2010[2]	PSS 10 item	MORE	18	15.6	4.7	10 Wks							
Lower	Garland EL, 2010[2]	PSS 10 item	ASG	19	16.0	7.6	10 Wks	0.03	-3.3	-21.2				
Lower For	Mularski RA, 2009[3]	PSS	MBBT	20	14.1		8 Wks							
Lower For	Mularski RA, 2009[3]	PSS	SG	29	13.7		8 Wks	Ns	-0.2	-1.4				
Lower	Bormann JE, 2006[4]	PSS 10 item	Mantra	46	16.6	7.4	10 Wks				22 Wks			
Lower	Bormann JE, 2006[4]	PSS 10 item	AC	47	17.6	6.5	10 Wks	Ns	-0.2	-1.2	22 Wks	0.89	-0.5	-3.0
Lower	Paul-Labrador M, 2006[5]	Life Stress Ins Q	TM	52	1.7	1.8	16 Wks							
Lower	Paul-Labrador M, 2006[5]	Life Stress Ins Q	HE	51	2.3	2.5	16 Wks	Ns	0.1	5.9				
Lower	Malarkey, 2012[6]	PSS 10 item	MBI-ld	93	19.7	0.3	8 Wks							
Lower	Malarkey, 2012[6]	PSS 10 item	Education	93	19.8	0.3	8 Wks	Ns						
Lower	Whitebird, 2012[7]	PSS 10 item	MBSR	38	21.2	4.7	8 Wks							
Lower	Whitebird, 2012[7]	PSS 10 item	Education/Support	40	21.2	7.5	8 Wks		-4.1	-19.3	6 Mos	0.01	-2.7	-12.7
Lower	Pbert L, 2012[8]	PSS 10 item	MBSR	41	17.3	1.1	10 Wks							
Lower	Pbert L, 2012[8]	PSS 10 item	HLC	41	15.8	1.1	10 Wks	0.055	-2.8	-16.2	12 Mos	0.001	-4.5	-26.0
Higher For Δ	Jayadevappa R, 2007[9]	PSS 14 item	TM	13	32.0	8.5	3 Mos				6 Mos			
Higher For Δ	Jayadevappa R, 2007[9]	PSS 14 item	HE	10	35.9	7.5	3 Mos	Ns	0.28	0.9	6 Mos	0.75	0.4	1.3
Specific Active Control														
Lower	Barrett, 2012[10]	PSS 10 item	MBSR	51	13	4.7	9 Wks				5 Mos			
Lower	Barrett, 2012[10]	PSS 10 item	Exercise	47	11.4	6	9 Wks	Ns	0.1	0.8	5 Mos	Ns	-0.2	-1.5
Lower	Jazaieri, 2012[11]	PSS 4 item	MBSR	31	10	2.4	8 Wks							
Lower	Jazaieri, 2012[11]	PSS 4 item	AE	25	10.17	3.01	8 Wks	Ns	-1.76	-17.6				
Lower	Wolever, 2012[12]	PSS 10 item	Mindfulness	96	24.72	0.38	12 Wks							
Lower	Wolever, 2012[12]	PSS 10 item	Vinyana yoga	90	24.93	0.4	12 Wks	Ns	-0.67	-2.7				

Notes: AC = Active Control; HE = Health Education; MM = Mindfulness Meditation; TM = Transcendental Meditation; MORE = Mindfulness-oriented Recovery Enhancement; ASG = Alcohol-dependence Support Group; MBBT = Mindfulness-based Breathing Therapy

References for Evidence Table E19

1. Oken BS, Fonareva I, Haas M et al. Pilot controlled trial of mindfulness meditation and education for dementia caregivers. J Altern Complement Med 2010; 16(10):1031-8.

2. Garland EL, Gaylord SA, Boettiger CA, Howard MO. Mindfulness training modifies cognitive, affective, and physiological mechanisms implicated in alcohol dependence: results of a randomized controlled pilot trial. J Psychoactive Drugs 2010; 42(2):177-92.

3. Mularski RA, Munjas BA, Lorenz KA et al. Randomized controlled trial of mindfulness-based therapy for dyspnea in chronic obstructive lung disease. J Altern Complement Med 2009; 15(10):1083-90.

4. Bormann JE, Gifford AL, Shively M et al. Effects of spiritual mantram repetition on HIV outcomes: a randomized controlled trial. J Behav Med 2006; 29(4):359-76.

5. Paul-Labrador M, Polk D, Dwyer JH et al. Effects of a randomized controlled trial of transcendental meditation on components of the metabolic syndrome in subjects with coronary heart disease. Arch Intern Med 2006; 166(11):1218-24.

6. Malarkey WB, Jarjoura D, Klatt M. Workplace based mindfulness practice and inflammation: A randomized trial. Brain Behav Immun 2012.

7. Whitebird RR, Kreitzer M, Crain AL, Lewis BA, Hanson LR, Enstad CJ. Mindfulness-Based Stress Reduction for Family Caregivers: A Randomized Controlled Trial. Gerontologist 2012.

8. Pbert L, Madison JM, Druker S et al. Effect of mindfulness training on asthma quality of life and lung function: A randomised controlled trial. 2012; 67(9):769-76.

9. Jayadevappa R, Johnson JC, Bloom BS et al. Effectiveness of transcendental meditation on functional capacity and quality of life of African Americans with congestive heart failure: a randomized control study Ethn Dis. 2007 Summer;17(3):595. Ethnicity & Disease 2007; 17(1):72-7.

10. Barrett B, Hayney MS, Muller D et al. Meditation or exercise for preventing acute respiratory infection: a randomized controlled trial. Ann Fam Med 2012; 10(4):337-46.

11. Jazaieri H, Goldin PR, Werner K, Ziv M, Gross JJ. A Randomized Trial of MBSR Versus Aerobic Exercise for Social Anxiety Disorder. J Clin Psychol 2012.

12. Wolever RQ, Bobinet KJ, McCabe K et al. Effective and viable mind-body stress reduction in the workplace: a randomized controlled trial. J Occup Health Psychol 2012; 17(2):246-58.

Evidence Table E20. KQ1 outcomes—difference in differences—distress

Improvement In Scale	Author, year	Outcome	Arm	N1	Mean	SD	T2	P Value	Δ-Δ Calc	ΔΔ%	T3	P Value	Δ-Δ Calc	ΔΔ%
Nonspecific Active Control														
Lower	Gaylord SA, 2011[1]	BSI 18 Gen sx	MBSR	36	57.1	8.3	8 Wks				5.5 Mos			
Lower	Gaylord SA, 2011[1]	BSI 18 Gen sx	SG	39	56.2	9.7	8 Wks	0.15	-2.08	-3.6	5.5 Mos		-2.97	-5.2
Lower	Garland EL, 2010[2]	BSI 53	MORE	18	42.7	36.4	10 Wks							
Lower	Garland EL, 2010[2]	BSI 53	ASG	19	46.7	33.0	10 Wks	0.48	-8.2	-19.2				
Lower	Seyedalinaghi, 2012[3]	SCL-90R	MBSR	85	109.32	64.81	8 Wks				14 Mos			
Lower	Seyedalinaghi, 2012[3]	SCL-90R	Education/ Support	86	109.23	59.16	8 Wks		-12.01	-11.0	14 Mos		5.4	4.9
Specific Active Control														
Lower	Delgado LC, 2010[4]	PANAS-N	MG	15	23.2	6.5	5 Wks							
Lower	Delgado LC, 2010[4]	PANAS-N	Relax group	17	23.4	9.0	5 Wks	Ns	1.2	5.2				
Lower	Moritz S, 2006[5]	POMS: total mood disturbance	MM	54	85.8	4.5*	8 Wks				12 Wks			
Lower	Moritz S, 2006[5]	POMS: total mood disturbance	Spirituality	56	94.4	4.4*	8 Wks	0.034	20.4	23.8	12 Wks		9.3	10.8
Higher	Moritz S, 2006[5]	SF36 Mental Health subscale	MM	54	48.7	2.4*	8 Wks							
Higher	Moritz S, 2006[5]	SF36 Mental Health subscale	Spirituality	56	45.0	2.3*	8 Wks	0.034	-10.9	-22.4				
Lower	Piet J, 2010[6]	SCL 90 GSI	MBCT	14	0.9	0.5	14 Wks							
Lower	Piet J, 2010[6]	SCL 90 GSI	CBGT	12	1.3	0.5	14 Wks	Ns	0.12	13.2				
Nonspecific Active Control (Tm)														
More (-) For Δ	Jayadevappa R, 2007[7]	SF36 Mental Health subscale	TM	13	73.3	28.9	3 Mos				6 Mos			
More (-) For Δ	Jayadevappa R, 2007[7]	SF36 Mental Health subscale	HE	10	71.7	18.3	3 Mos		-10	-13.6	6 Mos	0.56	-8.41	-11.5

*se

Notes: MBSR = Mindfulness-Based Stress Reduction; HE = Health Education; MM = Mindfulness Meditation; TM = Transcendental Meditation; MORE = Mindfulness-Oriented Recovery Enhancement; ASG = Alcohol-Dependence Support Group; CBGT = Cognitive Behavioural Group Therapy; MBCT = Mindfulness-Based Cognitive Therapy; MG = Mindfulness Group

References for Evidence Table E20

1. Gaylord SA, Palsson OS, Garland EL et al. Mindfulness training reduces the severity of irritable bowel syndrome in women: results of a randomized controlled trial. Am J Gastroenterol 2011; 106(9):1678-88.

2. Garland EL, Gaylord SA, Boettiger CA, Howard MO. Mindfulness training modifies cognitive, affective, and physiological mechanisms implicated in alcohol dependence: results of a randomized controlled pilot trial. J Psychoactive Drugs 2010; 42(2):177-92.

3. SeyedAlinaghi S, Jam S, Foroughi M et al. Randomized controlled trial of mindfulness-based stress reduction delivered to human immunodeficiency virus-positive patients in Iran: effects on CD4[sup]+[/sup] T lymphocyte count and medical and psychological symptoms. Psychosom Med 2012; 74(6):620-7.

4. Delgado LC, Guerra P, Perakakis P, Vera MN, Reyes del Paso G, Vila J. Treating chronic worry: Psychological and physiological effects of a training programme based on mindfulness. Behav Res Ther 2010; 48(9):873-82.

5. Moritz S, Quan H, Rickhi B et al. A home study-based spirituality education program decreases emotional distress and increases quality of life—a randomized, controlled trial. Altern Ther Health Med 2006; 12(6):26-35.

6. Piet J, Hougaard E, Hecksher MS, Rosenberg NK. A randomized pilot study of mindfulness-based cognitive therapy and group cognitive-behavioral therapy for young adults with social phobia. Scand J Psychol 2010; 51(5):403-10.

7. Jayadevappa R, Johnson JC, Bloom BS et al. Effectiveness of transcendental meditation on functional capacity and quality of life of African Americans with congestive heart failure: a randomized control study Ethn Dis. 2007 Summer;17(3):595. Ethnicity & Disease 2007; 17(1):72-7.

Evidence Table E21. KQ1 outcomes—difference in differences—QOL/mental health

Improvement In Scale	Author, year	Outcome	Arm	N1	Mean	SD	T2	P Value	Δ-Δ Calc	Δ Δ%	T3	P Value	Δ-Δ Calc	Δ Δ%
Higher	Wong SY-S, 2011[1]	SF-12 mental component	MBSR	51	40.6	11.2	8 Wks				5 Mos			
Higher	Wong SY-S, 2011[1]	SF-12 mental component	Pain control	48	39.3	9.2	8 Wks	Ns	-0.34	-0.8	5 Mos	Ns	-0.48	-1.2
Higher For Δ	Gross CR, 2011[2]	SF-12 mental component	MBSR	18	45.1	9.7	8 Wks				5 Mos			
Higher For Δ	Gross CR, 2011[2]	SF-12 mental component	PCT	9	45.2	8.8	8 Wks	Ns	0.54	1.2	5 Mos			
Higher	Gross CR, 2010[3]	SF-12 mental component	MBSR	71	45.7	41.6, 49.9 CI	8 Wks				1 Year			
Higher	Gross CR, 2010[3]	SF-12 mental component	HE	66	46.6	42.4, 50.7 CI	8 Wks		2.3	5.0	1 Year	0.29	2.3	5.0
Higher For Δ	Mularski RA, 2009[4]	VR-36 mental summary score	MBBT	20	50.9		8 Wks							
Higher For Δ	Mularski RA, 2009[4]	VR-36 mental summary score	SG	29	49.8		8 Wks	Ns	4.2	8.3				
Higher	Kuyken W, 2008[5]	WHOQL-Psychological	MBCT	61	17.8	3.8	3 Mos				15 Mos			
Higher	Kuyken W, 2008[5]	WHOQL-Psychological	Antidepressant	62	18.0	3.6	3 Mos		1.64	9.2	15 Mos	0.01	1.48	8.3
Higher	Moritz S, 2006[6]	SF-36 Mental component	MBSR	54	31.7	1.5 *	8 Wks				12 Wks			
Higher	Moritz S, 2006[6]	SF-36 Mental component	Spirituality	56	29.6	1.5 *	8 Wks	0.029	-7.3	-23.0	12 Wks	Ns	-3.9	-12.3
Higher	Plews-Ogan M, 2005[7]	SF -12 mental component	MBSR	6	42.4	38.4, 46.2*	8 Wks				12 Wks			
Higher	Plews-Ogan M, 2005[7]	SF -12 mental component	Massage	9	38.9	35.6, 42.2*	8 Wks	Ns	-4.6	-10.8	12 Wks	Ns	7.8	18.4
Higher	Whitebird, 2012[8]	SF 12-MH	MBSR	38	36.6	8.8	8 Wks				6 Mos			
Higher	Whitebird, 2012[8]	SF 12-MH	Education/ Support (NSAC)	40	40.4	11.9	8 Wks		10.4	28.4	6 Mos	<.001	8.9	24.3
Higher	Pbert L, 2012[9]	Asthma QOL-Emot	MBSR	41	5.2	0.21*	10 Wks				12 Mos			
Higher	Pbert L, 2012[9]	Asthma QOL-Emot	HLC (NSAC)	41	5.37	0.21*	10 Wks	0.19	0.32	6.2	12 Mos	0.002	0.81	15.6

Improvement In Scale	Author, year	Outcome	Arm	N1	Mean	SD	T2	P Value	Δ-Δ Calc	Δ Δ%	T3	P Value	Δ-Δ Calc	Δ Δ%
Higher	Barrett, 2012[10]	SF12-MH	MBSR	51	50.9	8.6	9 Wks	Ns	1	2.0	5 Mos	Ns	2.2	4.3
Higher	Barrett, 2012[10]	SF12-MH	Exercise (SAC)	47	52.3	6.6	9 Wks				5 Mos			

*se

Notes: MBSR = Mindfulness-based Stress Reduction; MBBT = Mindfulness-based Breathing Therapy ; HE = Health Education; MBCT = Mindfulness-based Cognitive Therapy; SG = Support Group; PCT = Pharmacotherapy

References for Evidence Table E21

1. Wong SY, Chan FW, Wong RL et al. Comparing the Effectiveness of Mindfulness-based Stress Reduction and Multidisciplinary Intervention Programs for Chronic Pain: A Randomized Comparative Trial. Clin J Pain 2011; 27(8):724-34.

2. Gross CR, Kreitzer MJ, Reilly-Spong M et al. Mindfulness-based stress reduction versus pharmacotherapy for chronic primary insomnia: a randomized controlled clinical trial. Explore (NY) 2011; 7(2):76-87.

3. Gross CR, Kreitzer MJ, Thomas W et al. Mindfulness-based stress reduction for solid organ transplant recipients: a randomized controlled trial. Altern Ther Health Med 2010; 16(5):30-8.

4. Mularski RA, Munjas BA, Lorenz KA et al. Randomized controlled trial of mindfulness-based therapy for dyspnea in chronic obstructive lung disease. J Altern Complement Med 2009; 15(10):1083-90.

5. Kuyken W, Byford S, Taylor RS et al. Mindfulness-based cognitive therapy to prevent relapse in recurrent depression. J Consult Clin Psychol 2008; 76(6):966-78.

6. Moritz S, Quan H, Rickhi B et al. A home study-based spirituality education program decreases emotional distress and increases quality of life—a randomized, controlled trial. Altern Ther Health Med 2006; 12(6):26-35.

7. Plews-Ogan M, Owens JE, Goodman M, Wolfe P, Schorling J. A pilot study evaluating mindfulness-based stress reduction and massage for the management of chronic pain. J Gen Intern Med 2005; 20(12):1136-8.

8. Whitebird RR, Kreitzer M, Crain AL, Lewis BA, Hanson LR, Enstad CJ. Mindfulness-Based Stress Reduction for Family Caregivers: A Randomized Controlled Trial. Gerontologist 2012.

9. Pbert L, Madison JM, Druker S et al. Effect of mindfulness training on asthma quality of life and lung function: A randomised controlled trial. 2012; 67(9):769-76.

10. Barrett B, Hayney MS, Muller D et al. Meditation or exercise for preventing acute respiratory infection: a randomized controlled trial. Ann Fam Med 2012; 10(4):337-46.

Evidence Table E22. KQ1 outcomes—difference in differences—well being

Improvement In Scale	Author, year	Outcome	Arm	N	Mean	SD	T2	P Value	Δ-Δ Calc	ΔΔ%	T3	P Value	Δ-Δ Calc	ΔΔ%
Higher	Henderson VP, 2011[1]	Sense of Coherence: Meaningfulness subscale	MBSR	50	45.4	1.0*	4 Mos				24 mos			
Higher	Henderson VP, 2011[1]	Sense of Coherence: Meaningfulness subscale	Nutrition education	50	45.2	1.0*	4 Mos	Ns	3.10	6.8	24 mos	Ns	1.90	4.2
More (-) For Δ	Jayadevappa R, 2007[2]	Quality of Well Being Scale	TM	13	0.6	0.2	3 Mos				6 mos			
More (-) For Δ	Jayadevappa R, 2007[2]	Quality of Well Being Scale	HE	10	0.6	0.3	3 Mos	Ns	−0.13	−21.0	6 mos	0.95	−0.12	−19.4
Higher	Chiesa, 2012[3]	Psychological General Well-being index	MBCT	9	45.88	16.15	8 Wks							
Higher	Chiesa, 2012[3]	Psychological General Well-being index	Education (NSAC)	9	52.83	22.17	8 Wks	0.05	25.06	54.6				
Higher	Barrett, 2012[4]	PANAS-P	MBSR	51	36.2	6.5	9 Wks				5 Mos			
Higher	Barrett, 2012[4]	PANAS-P	Exercise (SAC)	47	36.7	6.2	9 Wks	Ns	0.3	0.8	5 Mos	Ns	0.6	1.7
Higher	Jazaieri, 2012[5]	SWLS	MBSR	31	14	4.26	8 Wks				5 Mos			
Higher	Jazaieri, 2012[5]	SWLS	AE (SAC)	25	14	6.3	8 Wks	Ns	1.43	10.2	5 Mos	Ns		

*se

Notes: MBSR = Mindfulness-based Stress Reduction; HE = Health Education; TM = Transcendental Meditation

References for Evidence Table E22

1. Henderson VP, Clemow L, Massion AO, Hurley TG, Druker S, Hebert JR. The effects of mindfulness-based stress reduction on psychosocial outcomes and quality of life in early-stage breast cancer patients: a randomized trial. Breast Cancer Res Treat 2011.

2. Jayadevappa R, Johnson JC, Bloom BS et al. Effectiveness of transcendental meditation on functional capacity and quality of life of African Americans with congestive heart failure: a randomized control study Ethn Dis. 2007 Summer;17(3):595. Ethnicity & Disease 2007; 17(1):72-7.

3. Chiesa A, Mandelli L, Serretti A. Mindfulness-based cognitive therapy versus psycho-education for patients with major depression who did not achieve remission following antidepressant treatment: a preliminary analysis. J Altern Complement Med 2012; 18(8):756-60.

4. Barrett B, Hayney MS, Muller D et al. Meditation or exercise for preventing acute respiratory infection: a randomized controlled trial. Ann Fam Med 2012; 10(4):337-46.

5. Jazaieri H, Goldin PR, Werner K, Ziv M, Gross JJ. A Randomized Trial of MBSR Versus Aerobic Exercise for Social Anxiety Disorder. J Clin Psychol 2012.

Evidence Table E23. KQ1 outcomes—difference in differences—positive mood

Improvement In Scale	Author, year	Outcome	N1	Arm	Mean	SD	T2	P Value	Δ-Δ Calc	ΔΔ%	T3	P Value	Δ-Δ Calc	ΔΔ%
Higher	Gross CR, 2010[1]	SF-36 vitality	63	MBSR	44.4	40.5, 48.3 CI	8 wks				1 year			
Higher	Gross CR, 2010[1]	SF-36 vitality	59	HE	44.4	40.5, 48.3 CI	8 wks		0.3	0.7	1 year	0.29	4.7	10.6
Higher	Delgado LC, 2010[2]	PANAS positive mood	15	MM	30.2	4.8	5 wks							
Higher	Delgado LC, 2010[2]	PANAS positive mood	17	PMR/ Relaxation	28.5	7.9	5 wks	Ns	0	0.0				
Higher	Moritz S, 2006[3]	SF-36 vitality	54	MBSR	29.1	2.3	8 wks							
Higher	Moritz S, 2006[3]	SF-36 vitality	56	Spirituality	23.8	2.3	8 wks	0.024	−13.1	−45.0				
Lower For Δ	Jayadevappa R, 2007[4]	SF-36 vitality	13	TM	66.7	14.9	3 mos				6 mos			
Lower For Δ	Jayadevappa R, 2007[4]	SF-36 vitality	10	HE	56.3	17.7	3 mos	Ns	−1.6	−2.4	6 mos	0.82	0.7	1.0

Notes: MBSR = Mindfulness-based Stress Reduction; HE = Health Education; TM = Transcendental Meditation; MM = Mindfulness Meditation; PMR = Progressive Muscle Relaxation

References for Evidence Table E23

1. Gross CR, Kreitzer MJ, Thomas W et al. Mindfulness-based stress reduction for solid organ transplant recipients: a randomized controlled trial. Altern Ther Health Med 2010; 16(5):30-8.

2. Delgado LC, Guerra P, Perakakis P, Vera MN, Reyes del Paso G, Vila J. Treating chronic worry: Psychological and physiological effects of a training programme based on mindfulness. Behav Res Ther 2010; 48(9):873-82.

3. Moritz S, Quan H, Rickhi B et al. A home study-based spirituality education program decreases emotional distress and increases quality of life—a randomized, controlled trial. Altern Ther Health Med 2006; 12(6):26-35.

4. Jayadevappa R, Johnson JC, Bloom BS et al. Effectiveness of transcendental meditation on functional capacity and quality of life of African Americans with congestive heart failure: a randomized control study Ethn Dis. 2007 Summer;17(3):595. Ethnicity & Disease 2007; 17(1):72-7.

Evidence Table E24. KQ3 outcomes—difference in differences—substance use

Improvement In Scale	Author, year	Outcome	Arm	N1	Mean	SD	T2	P Value	Δ-Δ Calc	ΔΔ%	T3	P Value	Δ-Δ Calc	Δ Δ%
Lower	Brewer, 2011[1]	Smoking (Cigs/Day)	MT	33	17.8		4 wks				17wks			
Lower	Brewer, 2011[1]	Smoking (Cigs/Day)	FFS	38	15.0		4 wks	0.008	-4.2	-23.6	17 wks			
Higher	Brewer, 2011[1]	7 Day Cig Abstinence (%)	MT	33	0.0		4 wks				17 wks			
Higher	Brewer, 2011[1]	7 Day Cig Abstinence (%)	FFS	38	0.0		4 wks	0.06	21	n/a	17 wks	0.012	25	n/a
Lower	Garland EL, 2010[2]	Penn Alcohol Craving Scale	MORE (mindfulness)	18	4.7	5.5	10 wks							
Lower	Garland EL, 2010[2]	Penn Alcohol Craving Scale	ASG	19	4.9	4.4	10 wks	0.31	1.6	34.0				
Lower	Garland EL, 2010[2]	Impaired Alcohol Response Inhibition Scale	MORE (mindfulness)	18	7.8	5.5	10 wks							
Lower	Garland EL, 2010[2]	Impaired Alcohol Response Inhibition Scale	ASG	18	6.2	4.9	10 wks	0.35	-2	-25.6				
Lower	Brewer, 2009[3]	% Days Of Cocaine Use*	MT	17	6.0		9 wks							
Lower	Brewer, 2009[3]	% Days Of Cocaine Use*	CBT	7	0.0	0	12 wks	ns	-0.6					
Lower	Brewer, 2009[3]	% Days Of Alcohol Use*	MT	17	6.0		9 wks							
Lower	Brewer, 2009[3]	% Days Of Alcohol Use*	CBT	7	0.0	0	12 wks	ns	18.3					
Lower	Castillo-Richmond, 2000[4]	Smoking (Cigs/Day)	TM	31	1.4	4.6	6.8 mos							
Lower	Castillo-Richmond, 2000[4]	Smoking (Cigs/Day)	HE	29	0.7	3.7	6.8 mos	0.35	-0.67	-48.9				
Lower	Murphy, 1986[5]	Alcohol Consumption (Ml / Wk)	Meditation	14	275		7–10 wks				11–16 wks			
Lower	Murphy, 1986[5]	Alcohol Consumption (Ml / Wk)	Running	13	314		7–10 wks	ns	99.3	36.1	11–16 wks			
Higher	Taub E, 1994[6]	% Days Abstinent From Etoh	TM	35	26.2		1–6 mos				13–18 mos			
Higher	Taub E, 1994[6]	% Days Abstinent From Etoh	BF	24	21.3		1–6 mos	ns	-1.2	-4.6	13–18 mos			

Improvement In Scale	Author, year	Outcome	Arm	N1	Mean	SD	T2	P Value	Δ-Δ Calc	ΔΔ%	T3	P Value	Δ-Δ Calc	Δ Δ%
Higher	Taub E, 1994[6]	% Days Abstinent From Etoh	Neurotherapy	28	28.1		1-6 mos	ns	13.8	19.2	13-18 mos			
Lower	Schneider, 2012[7]	EToh drinks/wk	TM								5.4 yrs avg			
Lower	Schneider, 2012[7]	EToh drinks/wk	HE								5.4 yrs avg	0.46	0.615	
Lower	Schneider, 2012[7]	Cigarettes	TM								5.4 yrs avg			
Lower	Schneider, 2012[7]	Cigarettes	HE								5.4 yrs avg	0.16	-0.61	

Notes: MT = Mindfulness Training; FFS = American Lung Association's Freedom From Smoking; MORE = Mindfulness-oriented Recovery Enhancement; ASG = Alcohol-dependence Support Group; CBT= Cognitive Behavioral Therapy; TM = Transcendental Meditation; HE = Health Education; BF = Biofeedback

References for Evidence Table E24

1. Brewer JA, Mallik S, Babuscio TA et al. Mindfulness training for smoking cessation: Results from a randomized controlled trial. Drug Alcohol Depend 2011.

2. Garland EL, Gaylord SA, Boettiger CA, Howard MO. Mindfulness training modifies cognitive, affective, and physiological mechanisms implicated in alcohol dependence: results of a randomized controlled pilot trial. J Psychoactive Drugs 2010; 42(2):177-92.

3. Brewer JA, Sinha R, Chen JA et al. Mindfulness training and stress reactivity in substance abuse: results from a randomized, controlled stage I pilot study. Subst Abus 2009; 30(4):306-17.

4. Castillo-Richmond A, Schneider RH, Alexander CN et al. Effects of stress reduction on carotid atherosclerosis in hypertensive African Americans. Stroke 2000; 31(3):568-73.

5. Murphy TJ, Pagano RR, Marlatt GA. Lifestyle modification with heavy alcohol drinkers: effects of aerobic exercise and meditation. Addict Behav 1986; 11(2):175-86.

6. Taub E, Steiner SS, Weingarten E, Walton KG. Effectiveness of broad spectrum approaches to relapse prevention in severe alcoholism: A long-term, randomized, controlled trial of Transcendental Meditation, EMG biofeedback and electronic neurotherapy. Alcoholism Treatment Quarterly 1994; 11(1-2):187-220.

7. Schneider RH, Grim CE, Rainforth MV et al. Stress Reduction in the Secondary Prevention of Cardiovascular Disease: Randomized, Controlled Trial of Transcendental Meditation and Health Education in Blacks. (1941-7705 (Electronic). 1941-7713 (Linking)).

Evidence Table E25. KQ3 outcomes—difference in differences—eating

Improvement In Scale	Author, year	Outcome	Arm	N1	mean	SD	T2	P Value	Δ-Δ Calc	Δ Δ %	T3	P Value	Δ-Δ Calc	Δ Δ %
Lower	Hebert JR, 2001[1]	Total energy (Kcal/d)	Mindfulness (SRC)	56	1884	549	4 Mos				12 Mos			
Lower	Hebert JR, 2001[1]	Total energy (Kcal/d)	NEP	50	1991	674	4 Mos	ns	103.1	5.5	12 Mos	Ns	65.1	3.5
Lower	Hebert JR, 2001[1]	Total fat (% energy)	Mindfulness (SRC)	56	34.5	7.4	4 Mos				12 Mos			
Lower	Hebert JR, 2001[1]	Total fat (% energy)	NEP	50	34	8.6	4 Mos	<.05	6.6	19.1	12 Mos	<0.05	3.9	11.3
Lower	Miller, 2012[2]	Energy(kcal)	MB-EAT	27	1851	129	12 Wks				6 Mos			
Lower	Miller, 2012[2]	Energy(kcal)	SC (SAC)	25	2019	131	12 Wks	NR	276	14.9	6 Mos	0.2198	192	10.4
Lower	Schneider, 2012[3]	Diet	TM						NR/NS					
Lower	Schneider, 2012[3]	Diet	HE (NSAC)						NR/NS					

Notes: SRC = Stress Reduction Clinic; NEP = Nutrition Education Program

References for Evidence Table E25

1. Hebert JR, Ebbeling CB, Olendzki BC et al. Change in women's diet and body mass following intensive intervention for early-stage breast cancer. J Am Diet Assoc 2001; 101(4):421-31.
2. Miller CK, Kristeller JL, Headings A, Nagaraja H, Miser WF. Comparative Effectiveness of a Mindful Eating Intervention to a Diabetes Self-Management Intervention among Adults with Type 2 Diabetes: A Pilot Study. J Acad Nutr Diet 2012; 112(11):1835-42.
3. Schneider RH, Grim CE, Rainforth MV et al. Stress Reduction in the Secondary Prevention of Cardiovascular Disease: Randomized, Controlled Trial of Transcendental Meditation and Health Education in Blacks. (1941-7705 (Electronic). 1941-7713 (Linking)).

Evidence Table E26. KQ3 outcomes—difference in differences—sleeping

Improvement In Scale	Author, year	Outcome	Arm	N1	Mean	SD	T2	P Value	Δ-Δ Calc	Δ-Δ %	T3	P Value	Δ-Δ Calc	ΔΔ %
Higher	Gross CR, 2011[1]	Total sleep time - actigraphy (hrs)	MBSR	18	6.3	0.6	6–8 Wks							
Higher	Gross CR, 2011[1]	Total sleep time - actigraphy (hrs)	drug	9	6.4	0.6	6–8 Wks		−0.68	−10.7				
Lower	Gross CR, 2011[1]	Wake after sleep onset-actigraphy (min)	MBSR	18	57.2	24.8	6–8 Wks							
Lower	Gross CR, 2011[1]	Wake after sleep onset-actigraphy (min)	drug	9	61.2	38.3	6–8 Wks		10.71	18.7				
Higher	Gross CR, 2011[1]	Total sleep time - DIARY (hrs)	MBSR	17	6.3	0.7	8 Wks				5 Mos			
Higher	Gross CR, 2011[1]	Total sleep time - DIARY (hrs)	drug	9	6.2	0.9	8 Wks		−0.4	−6.3	5 Mos			
Lower	Gross CR, 2011[1]	Wake after sleep onset-DIARY (min)	MBSR	18	46.6	21.3	6–8 Wks				5 Mos			
Lower	Gross CR, 2011[1]	Wake after sleep onset-DIARY (min)	drug	9	72.2	42.5	6–8 Wks		24.86	53.3	5 Mos			
Lower For Δ	Gross CR, 2011[1]	PSQI	MBSR	18	11.5	1.9	8 Wks				5 Mos			
Lower For Δ	Gross CR, 2011[1]	PSQI	drug	9	11.7	3.6	8 Wks		−1.69	−14.7	5 Mos		−0.12	−1.0
Lower For Δ	Gross CR, 2011[1]	Insomnia severity Index	MBSR	18	16.4	3.0	8 Wks				5 Mos			
Lower For Δ	Gross CR, 2011[1]	Insomnia severity Index	drug	9	18.6	3.8	8 Wks		2.55	15.5	5 Mos		2.69	16.4
Lower	Schmidt S, 2010[2]	PSQI	MBSR	53	11.3	3.4	8 Wks				16 Wks			
Lower	Schmidt S, 2010[2]	PSQI	AC	56	11.4	4.2	8 Wks		−0.02	−0.2	16 Wks		−0.18	−1.6
Lower	Oken BS, 2010[3]	Epworth Sleepiness Scale	Meditation	8	4.7	2.8	7–10 Wks							
Lower	Oken BS, 2010[3]	Epworth Sleepiness Scale	Education	11	6.6	4.8	7–10 Wks		0.6	12.8				
Lower	Oken B.S., 2010[3]	Epworth Sleepiness Scale	Respite only	9	7.1	4.7	7–10 Wks							

Improvement In Scale	Author, year	Outcome	Arm	N1	Mean	SD	T2	P Value	Δ-Δ Calc	Δ-Δ %	T3	P Value	Δ-Δ Calc	ΔΔ %
Lower	Oken BS, 2010[3]	PSQI	Meditation	8	8.7	3.4	7–10 Wks							
Lower	Oken BS, 2010[3]	PSQI	Education	11	8.0	2.7	7–10 Wks		0.3	3.4				
Lower	Oken BS, 2010[3]	PSQI	Respite only	9	9.5	3.7	7–10 Wks							
Lower	Gross CR, 2010[4]	PSQI	MBSR	71	8.3	(6.9, 10.1)	8 Wks				12 Mos			
Lower	Gross CR, 2010[4]	PSQI	HE	66	7.2	(6.0, 8.8)	8 Wks		-2	-24.1	12 Mos	0.02	-2.5	-30.1
Lower	Malarkey, 2012[5]	PSQI	MBI-ld	93	8.7	0.3	8 Wks		NR/NS					
Lower	Malarkey, 2012[5]	PSQI	Education (NSAC)	93	8.4	0.3	8 Wks	Ns	NR/NS					
Lower	Barrett, 2012[6]	PSQI	MBSR	51	5.1	2.6	9 Wks				5 mos			
Lower	Barrett, 2012[6]	PSQI	Exercise (SAC)	47	4.6	3.1	9 Wks	Ns	-0.09	-1.8	5 Mos	Ns	-0.02	-0.4
Lower	Wolever, 2012[7]	PSQI	Mindfulness	96	8.07	0.34	12 Wks							
Lower	Wolever, 2012[7]	PSQI	Vinyana Yoga (SAC)	90	7.69	0.35	12 Wks	Ns	0.12	-1.5				

Notes: PSQI = Pittsburgh Sleep Quality Index; MBSR = Mindfulness-based Stress Reduction; HE = Health Education; AC = Active Control

References for Evidence Table E26

1. Gross CR, Kreitzer MJ, Reilly-Spong M et al. Mindfulness-based stress reduction versus pharmacotherapy for chronic primary insomnia: a randomized controlled clinical trial. Explore (NY) 2011; 7(2):76-87.

2. Schmidt S, Grossman P, Schwarzer B, Jena S, Naumann J, Walach H. Treating fibromyalgia with mindfulness-based stress reduction: results from a 3-armed randomized controlled trial. Pain 2011; 152(2):361-9.

3. Oken BS, Fonareva I, Haas M et al. Pilot controlled trial of mindfulness meditation and education for dementia caregivers. J Altern Complement Med 2010; 16(10):1031-8.

4. Gross CR, Kreitzer MJ, Thomas W et al. Mindfulness-based stress reduction for solid organ transplant recipients: a randomized controlled trial. Altern Ther Health Med 2010; 16(5):30-8.

5. Malarkey WB, Jarjoura D, Klatt M. Workplace based mindfulness practice and inflammation: A randomized trial. Brain Behav Immun 2012.

6. Barrett B, Hayney MS, Muller D et al. Meditation or exercise for preventing acute respiratory infection: a randomized controlled trial. Ann Fam Med 2012; 10(4):337-46.

7. Wolever RQ, Bobinet KJ, McCabe K et al. Effective and viable mind-body stress reduction in the workplace: a randomized controlled trial. J Occup Health Psychol 2012; 17(2):246-58.

Evidence Table E27. KQ4 outcomes—difference in differences—pain severity

Improvement In Scale	Author, year	Outcome	Arm	N1	Mean	SD	T2	P Value	Δ-Δ Calc	Δ-Δ%	T3	P Value	Δ-Δ Calc	Δ Δ%
Lower	Wong SY-S, 2011[1]	NRS Pain Intensity	MBSR	51	6.5	1.5	8 Wks				8 Mos			
Lower	Wong SY-S, 2011[1]	NRS Pain Intensity	MPI	48	6.8	1.3	8 Wks		0.04	0.6	8 Mos	0.869	−0.05	−0.8
Lower	Gaylord SA, 2011[2]	Abd Pain Severity	MM	36	54.5	22.8	10 Wks				5.5 Mos			
Lower	Gaylord SA, 2011[2]	Abd Pain Severity	SG	39	53.3	28.1	10 Wks	0.013	−16.68	−30.6	5.5 Mos	0.015	−15.57	−28.5
Lower	Schmidt S, 2010[3]	Pps Affective	MBSR	53	35.5	9.4	8 Wks				16 Wks			
Lower	Schmidt S, 2010[3]	Pps Affective	AC	56	34.7	8.7	8 Wks	0.18	−1.43	−4.0	16 Wks		−2.11	−5.9
Lower	Schmidt S, 2010[3]	Pps Sensory	MBSR	53	22.3	6.1	8 Wks				16 Wks			
Lower	Schmidt S, 2010[3]	Pps Sensory	AC	56	22.8	6.6	8 Wks	0.6	−1.28	−5.7	16 Wks		−0.21	−0.9
Higher	Gross CR, 2010[4]	SF36 Bodily Pain	MBSR	63	43.2	(39.6, 46.7)	8 Wks				1 Year			
Higher	Gross CR, 2010[4]	SF36 Bodily Pain	HE	59	45.5	(42.0, 49.1)	8 Wks		2.20	5.1	1 Year	0.92	2.30	5.3
Higher	Morone NE, 2009[5]	SF36 Bodily Pain	MM	16	39.6	(38.2, 41.2)	8 Wks				6 Mos			
Higher	Morone NE, 2009[5]	SF36 Bodily Pain	HE	19	40.2	(38.6, 41.7)	8 Wks		3.40	8.6	6 Mos		1.50	3.8
Lower	Morone NE, 2009[5]	MPQ (Current Pain)	MM	16	3.0		8 Wks				6 Mos			
Lower	Morone NE, 2009[5]	MPQ (Current Pain)	HE	19	4.4		8 Wks		0	0.0	6 Mos		0.10	3.3
Higher	Moritz S, 2006[6]	SF36 Bodily Pain	MBSR	54	56.8	3.4*	8 Wks							
Higher	Moritz S, 2006[6]	SF36 Bodily Pain	Spirituality	56	56.0	3.3*	8 Wks		−3.30	−5.8				
Higher	Moritz S, 2006[6]	SF36 Bodily Pain	Control	55	51.8	3.3*	8 Wks							
Lower	Plews-Ogan M, 2005[7]	NRS Unpleasantness	MBSR	6	6.6	(6.07, 7.15)	8 Wks				12 Wks			
Lower	Plews-Ogan M, 2005[7]	NRS Unpleasantness	Massage	9	7.2	(6.54, 7.69)	8 Wks		2.12	31.9	12 Wks		1.48	22.3

Improvement In Scale	Author, year	Outcome	Arm	N1	Mean	SD	T2	P Value	Δ-Δ Calc	Δ-Δ%	T3	P Value	Δ-Δ Calc	Δ Δ%
Lower For Δ	Jayadevappa R, 2007[8]	SF36 Bodily Pain	TM	13	67.8	23.5	3 Mos				6 Mos			
Lower For Δ	Jayadevappa R, 2007[8]	SF36 Bodily Pain	HE	10	78.3	24.8	3 Mos		1.45	2.1%	6 Mos	0.08	−12.5	−18.4
Lower	Wolever, 2012[9]	Avg pain x 1 wk	Mindfulness	96	2.52	0.22	12 Wks							
Lower	Wolever, 2012[9]	Avg pain x 1 wk	Vinyana yoga (SAC)	90	2.64	0.23	12 Wks		0.28	11.1				

*se

References for Evidence Table E27

1. Wong SY, Chan FW, Wong RL et al. Comparing the Effectiveness of Mindfulness-based Stress Reduction and Multidisciplinary Intervention Programs for Chronic Pain: A Randomized Comparative Trial. Clin J Pain 2011; 27(8):724-34.

2. Gaylord SA, Palsson OS, Garland EL et al. Mindfulness training reduces the severity of irritable bowel syndrome in women: results of a randomized controlled trial. Am J Gastroenterol 2011; 106(9):1678-88.

3. Schmidt S, Grossman P, Schwarzer B, Jena S, Naumann J, Walach H. Treating fibromyalgia with mindfulness-based stress reduction: results from a 3-armed randomized controlled trial. Pain 2011; 152(2):361-9.

4. Gross CR, Kreitzer MJ, Thomas W et al. Mindfulness-based stress reduction for solid organ transplant recipients: a randomized controlled trial. Altern Ther Health Med 2010; 16(5):30-8.

5. Morone NE, Rollman BL, Moore CG, Li Q, Weiner DK. A mind-body program for older adults with chronic low back pain: results of a pilot study. Pain Med 2009; 10(8):1395-407.

6. Moritz S, Quan H, Rickhi B et al. A home study-based spirituality education program decreases emotional distress and increases quality of life—a randomized, controlled trial. Altern Ther Health Med 2006; 12(6):26-35.

7. Plews-Ogan M, Owens JE, Goodman M, Wolfe P, Schorling J. A pilot study evaluating mindfulness-based stress reduction and massage for the management of chronic pain. J Gen Intern Med 2005; 20(12):1136-8.

8. Jayadevappa R, Johnson JC, Bloom BS et al. Effectiveness of transcendental meditation on functional capacity and quality of life of African Americans with congestive heart failure: a randomized control study Ethn Dis. 2007 Summer;17(3):595. Ethnicity & Disease 2007; 17(1):72-7.

9. Wolever RQ, Bobinet KJ, McCabe K et al. Effective and viable mind-body stress reduction in the workplace: a randomized controlled trial. J Occup Health Psychol 2012; 17(2):246-58.

Evidence Table E28. KQ4 outcomes—difference in differences—pain interference

Improvement In Scale	Author, year	Outcome	Arm	N1	Mean	SD	T2	P Value	Δ-Δ Calc	Δ-Δ%	T3	P Value	Δ-Δ Calc	ΔΔ%
Lower	Schmidt S, 2010[1]	FIQ	MBSR	53	5.8	1.4	8 Wks		M		16 Wks			
Lower	Schmidt S, 2010[1]	FIQ	AC	56	5.5	1.7	8 Wks		-0.52	-8.9	16 Wks	0.36	-0.44	-7.5
Lower	Morone NE, 2009[2]	RMDQ	MM	16	8.9	(7.8, 10.0)	8 Wks				6 Mos			
Lower	Morone NE, 2009[2]	RMDQ	HE	19	11.4	(10.3, 12.7)	8 Wks		1	11.2	6 Mos		0	0.0

Notes: MBSR = Mindfulness-based Stress Reduction; AC = Active Control; MM = Mindfulness Meditation

References for Evidence Table E28

1. Schmidt S, Grossman P, Schwarzer B, Jena S, Naumann J, Walach H. Treating fibromyalgia with mindfulness-based stress reduction: results from a 3-armed randomized controlled trial. Pain 2011; 152(2):361-9.

2. Morone NE, Rollman BL, Moore CG, Li Q, Weiner DK. A mind-body program for older adults with chronic low back pain: results of a pilot study. Pain Med 2009; 10(8):1395-407.

Evidence Table E29. KQ4 outcomes—difference in differences—weight

Improvement In Scale	Author, year	Outcome	Arm	N1	Mean	SD	T2	N2	P Value	Δ-Δ Calc	Δ Δ%	T3	P Value	Δ-Δ Calc	Δ Δ%
Lower For Δ	Elder, 2006[1]	Weight (lb)	TM	26	246.1	49	6 Mos	26	0.26 Δ-Δ	-4.4	-1.8				
Lower For Δ	Elder, 2006[1]	Weight (lb)	HE	28	228.6	67	6 Mos	28							
Lower For Δ	Hebert JR, 2001[2]	Weight (kg)	MBSR	50	72.2	13.9	4 Mos	49				12 mos			
Lower For Δ	Hebert JR, 2001[2]	Weight (kg)	Nutrition	49	70.6	11.7	4 Mos	41		1.2	1.7	12 mos		0.3	0.4
Lower For Δ	Castillo-Richmond, 2000[3]	Weight (lb)	TM	31	196.6	33.6	7 Mos	31							
Lower For Δ	Castillo-Richmond, 2000[3]	Weight (lb)	HE	29	194.2	40.4	7 Mos	29	0.48 Δ-Δ	2.32	1.2				
Lower	Miller, 2012[4]	Weight(kg)	MB-EAT	27	106.04	3.66	12 Wks					6 Mos			
Lower	Miller, 2012[4]	Weight(kg)	SC	25	103.38	3.8	12 Wks		NR	-1.19	1.1	6 Mos	0.07	-1.27	-1.2
Lower	Schneider, 2012[5]	BMI	TM									5.4 yrs (avg)			
Lower	Schneider, 2012[5]	BMI	HE									5.4 yrs (avg)	0.94	0.074	

Notes: TM = Transcendental Meditation; HE = Health Education; MBSR = Mindfulness-based Stress Reduction

References for Evidence Table E29

1. Elder C, Aickin M, Bauer V, Cairns J, Vuckovic N. Randomized trial of a whole-system ayurvedic protocol for type 2 diabetes. Altern Ther Health Med 2006; 12(5):24-30.

2. Hebert JR, Ebbeling CB, Olendzki BC et al. Change in women's diet and body mass following intensive intervention for early-stage breast cancer. J Am Diet Assoc 2001; 101(4):421-31.

3. Castillo-Richmond A, Schneider RH, Alexander CN et al. Effects of stress reduction on carotid atherosclerosis in hypertensive African Americans. Stroke 2000; 31(3):568-73.

4. Miller CK, Kristeller JL, Headings A, Nagaraja H, Miser WF. Comparative Effectiveness of a Mindful Eating Intervention to a Diabetes Self-Management Intervention among Adults with Type 2 Diabetes: A Pilot Study. J Acad Nutr Diet 2012; 112(11):1835-42.

5. Schneider RH, Grim CE, Rainforth MV et al. Stress Reduction in the Secondary Prevention of Cardiovascular Disease: Randomized, Controlled Trial of Transcendental Meditation and Health Education in Blacks. (1941-7705 (Electronic). 1941-7713 (Linking)).

Evidence Table E30. Sponsors and AEs for included studies

Author, year	Key Question (KQ)	Study Sponsor Details	Adverse Events
Henderson VP, 2011[1]	KQ1	The BRIDGES Study was funded by grant DAMD17-94-J-4475 from the US Army Medical Research and Materiel Command. Dr. Massion was supported by a Career Development Award, grant # DAMD17-94-J-4261 from the U.S. Army Medical Research and Materiel Command. Dr. He'bert was supported by the Established Investigator Award in Cancer Prevention and Control K05 CA136975 from the Cancer Training Branch of the National Cancer Institute.	Not addressed
Wong SY-S, 2011[2]	KQ1, K Q4	Funded by The Health and Health Services Research Fund was established and granted by the Food and Health Bureau, Hong Kong SAR Government, Hong Kong.	Not addressed
Brewer, 2011[3]	KQ3	This study was funded by the following grants: NIDA K12-DA00167, P50-DA09241, K05-DA00457, K05-DA00089, UL1 DE019586-02, and the U.S. Veterans Affairs New England Mental Illness Research, Education, and Clinical Center (MIRECC). The NIDA and VA had no further role in study design; in the collection, analysis and interpretation of data; in the writing of the report; or in the decision to submit the paper for publication.	No serious adverse events were reported in either treatment group (p. 75, results section).
Gaylord SA, 2011[4]	KQ1, KQ4	This study was supported by Grant # R21 AT003619 from the National Institutes of Health, National Center for Complementary, and Alternative Medicine Grant.	"The diaries were analyzed for adverse events and differences in abdominal pain between the treatment groups (MG vs. SG) during the treatment period." (p. 1682, data analysis). However, data on adverse events was not addressed in the Results or Discussion section.
Philippot P, 2011[5]	KQ1	This research was supported by a grant from the Fonds National de la Recherche Scientifique de Belgique (grant no. 8.4505.00). Data collection was supported by the UCL Psychology Department Consulting Center.	Not addressed

Author, year	Key Question (KQ)	Study Sponsor Details	Adverse Events
Gross CR, 2011[6]	KQ1, KQ3	Supported by a faculty development grant from the Academic Health Center, University of Minnesota to Drs. Gross & Kreitzer and by also the National Institutes of Health, National Center for Research Resources (grant M01 RR00400, Dr. Seaquist, PI).	"There were no unexpected, serious adverse events related to the interventions in this trial. One PCT patient was switched from eszopiclone to controlled-release zolpidem during the first month of treatment because of persistent complaints of an extremely unpleasant after-taste. Other side effects reported in the PCT arm included excessive sleepiness, headache, and dizziness. No adverse events related to MBSR were reported." (p. 83)
Schmidt S, 2010[7]	KQ1, KQ3, KQ4	This study was supported by the Samueli Institute, Alexandria, VA, and by the Manfred Köhnlechner Stiftung, Munich, Germany.	Not addressed
Segal ZV, 2010[8]	KQ1	This study was funded by grant R01 066992 (Dr Segal) from the National Institute of Mental Health.	Not addressed
Oken BS, 2010[9]	KQ1, KQ2, KQ3	This project was supported in part by NIH (U19 AT002656, P30 AG008017, K24 AT05121, and UL1 RR024140) and the Oregon Partnership for Alzheimer's Research Oregon Tax Check-Off Grant.	Not addressed
Gross CR, 2010[10]	KQ1, KQ3, KQ4	Funding sources: National Institutes of Health, National Institute of Nursing Research grant R01 NR008585, and National Center for Research Resources grant M01 RR00400.	"Because benefits were obtained with no evidence of adverse events, these findings suggest that clinicians should consider recommending MBSR to transplant recipients who..." (p. 36)
Garland EL, 2010[11]	KQ1, KQ3	One author was supported by Grant Number T32AT003378 from the National Center for Complementary and Alternative Medicine, a Francisco Varela Research Grant from the Mind & Life Institute, Boulder, CO, and an Armfield-Reeves Innovation Grant from the UNC School of Social Work, Chapel Hill, NC. Another author was supported by Award Number KL2RR025746 from the National Center for Research Resources.	Not addressed
Delgado LC, 2010[12]	KQ1	We thank the Junta de Andalucía and the Spanish Ministry of Science and Education for their support to the present research (HUM-388, SEJ2004-07956, and PSI2008-04372).	Not addressed

Author, year	Key Question (KQ)	Study Sponsor Details	Adverse Events
Morone NE, 2009[13]	KQ4	During the time of this work Dr. Morone was funded by the NIH Roadmap Multidisciplinary Clinical Research Career Development Award Grant (1KL2RR024154-04) from the National Institutes of Health (NIH). This publication was also made possible by Grant Number UL1RR024153 from the National Center for Research Resources (NCRR), a component of the NIH and NIH Roadmap for Medical Research.	"There were no adverse events reported." (p. 1401)
Brewer, 2009[14]	KQ3	This study was funded by the following grants: NIDA K12-DA00167 (J.A.B.), P50-DA09241 (B.J.R.), R37-DA15969 (K.M.C.), T32-DA007238 (J.A.B.), K05-DA00457 (K.M.C.), K05-DA00089 (B.J.R.), P50-DA16556 (R.S.), K02-DA17232 (R.S.), R01 DA020908 (M.N.P.), RL1 AA017539 (M.N.P.), the U.S. Veterans Affairs New England Mental Illness Research, Education, and Clinical Center (MIRECC) (B.J.R.), and a Varela grant from the Mind and Life Institute (J.A.B.).	"No side effects or adverse events were noted." (p. 310, Results – Substance Use Outcomes)
Mularski RA, 2009[15]	KQ1	This study was supported by the VET-HEAL program, cooperation between the Veterans Health Administration and the Samueli Institute of Information Biology. Dr. Karl Lorenz was supported by a VA HSR&D Career Development Award.	Not addressed
Kuyken W, 2008[16]	KQ1	This trial was registered (ISRCTN12720810) and was funded by the UK Medical Research Council (TP 72167).	"No adverse events were recorded through the oversight of the Trial Steering Committee." (p. 971)
Koszycki D, 2007[17]	KQ1	This study was funded in part by a grant from the University (Ottawa) Medical Research Fund.	Not addressed
Lee SH, 2006[18]	KQ1	No funding sources listed.	Not addressed
Moritz S, 2006[19]	KQ1, KQ4	This study was funded by Alberta Health and Wellness, the Alberta Medical Association and the George Family Foundation. Hude Quan, PhD, is supported by an Alberta Heritage Foundation for Medical Research Population Health Investigator Award and a Canadian Institute of Health Research New Investigator Award. None of the study funders had any involvement in design and conduct of the study; collection, management, analysis, and interpretation of the data; and preparation, review, or approval of the manuscript.	Not addressed

Author, year	Key Question (KQ)	Study Sponsor Details	Adverse Events
Elder, 2006[20]	KQ4	This research was supported by a grant (R21 AT01324) from the National Center for Complementary and Alternative Medicine, National Institutes of Health.	"No significant study-related adverse events were reported. Table 5 describes the results of serologic monitors [hematocrit, WBC, platelets, creatinine, BUN, AST]. The results suggest no significant hepatic, renal, or hematologic toxicities related to any component of the Vedic protocol." (p. 30)
Bormann JE, 2006[21]	KQ1	This study was conducted with core support from the National Center of Complementary and Alternative Medicine, National Institutes of Health (NCCAM/NIH) grant # R21AT01159-01A1 and with indirect support from the Office of Research and Development, Health Services Research and Development Service, Department of Veterans Affairs and the Health Services Research Unit of the VA San Diego Healthcare System; San Diego Veterans Medical Research Foundation; University of California San Diego (UCSD) General Clinical Research Center (#1637), National Institutes of Health/National Center for Research Resources (M01RR008); UCSD Center for AIDS Research (CFAR 5P30 AI 36214) and the UCSD Antiretroviral Research Center (AVRC); San Diego State University School of Nursing's Institute of Nursing Research (#900521); and Sigma Theta Tau International Honor Society-Gamma Gamma Chapter.	Not addressed
Paul-Labrador M, 2006[22]	KQ1	This study was supported by grants R01 AT00226, 1-P50-AA0082-02, 1-R15-HL660242-01, and R01-HL51519-08 from the National Center for Alternative and Complementary Medicine, National Institutes of Health; and General Clinical Research Centers grant MO1-RR00425 from the National Center for Research Resources.	"No adverse events were reported [in TE or HE groups]." (p. 1220)
Plews-Ogan M, 2005[23]	KQ1, KQ4	This study was supported in part by Grant 1D12HP00040-03: Academic Administrative Units in Primary Care, Department of Health and Human Services and in part by the John W. Kluge Foundation.	Not addressed
Hebert JR, 2001[24]	KQ3, KQ4	This work was supported by grand DAMD17-94-J-4475 from the US Army Medical Research and Materiel Command.	Not addressed
Castillo-Richmond, 2000[25]	KQ3, KQ4	This study was supported by National Heart, Lung, and Blood Institute grants HL-51519 to Drs Schneider, Alexander, and Myers and HL-51519-S2 to Dr Castillo-Richmond.	Not addressed
Murphy, 1986[26]	KQ3	This research was supported by a grant from the Alcoholism and Drug Abuse Institute, University of Washington.	Not addressed

Author, year	Key Question (KQ)	Study Sponsor Details	Adverse Events
Smith JC, 1976[27]	KQ1	The author gratefully acknowledges the assistance and cooperation of Maharishi International University and the Kast Lansing, Michigan, chapter of the Students' International Meditation Society. (The present article is based on the author's dissertation submitted to Michigan State University in partial fulfillment of the requirements for the PhD degree.)	Not addressed
Piet J, 2010[28]	KQ1	Funding support not mentioned.	Not addressed
Taub E, 1994[29]	KQ3	This work was supported in part by Public Health Service Grant AA 01279.	Not addressed
Lehrer PM, 1983[30]	KQ1	This research was supported in part by a General Research Support Grant from Rutgers Medical School.	Not addressed
Jayadevappa R, 2007[31]	KQ, KQ4	This study was sponsored by the National Institutes of Health–National Center for Complementary and Alternative Medicine (P50-AT00082-05 developmental research grant).	Not addressed
Miller, 2012[32]	4	National Institute of Diabetes and Digestive and Kidney Diseases	Not evaluated
Malarkey, 2012[33]	1, 3	National Center For Complementary & Alternative Medicine, National Center for Research Resources, which is now at the National Center for Advancing Translational Sciences	Not evaluated
Whitebird, 2012[34]	1	National Center for Complementary and Alternative Medicine	Not evaluated
Chiesa 2012,[35]	1	Not reported	Not evaluated
Barrett, 2012[36]	1, 3	National Institutes of Health (NIH), National Center for Complementary and Alternative Medicine, and a grant from the Clinical and Translational Science Award (CTSA) Program of the National Center for Research Resources, National Institutes of Health.	Not evaluated
Jazaieri, 2012[37]	1	NIMH and NCCAM	Not evaluated
Wolever, 2012[38]	1, 3, 4	Aetna, Inc. and eMindful, Inc.	Not evaluated
Seyedalinagh, 2012[39]	1	Tehran University of Medical Sciences and two research training fellowships	Not evaluated
Pbert, 2012[40]	1	National Center for Complementary and Alternative Medicine	Not evaluated
Schneider, 2012[41]	1, 3, 4	National Institutes of Health-National Heart, Lung and Blood Institute.	Not evaluated

References for Evidence Table E30

1. Henderson VP, Clemow L, Massion AO, Hurley TG, Druker S, Hebert JR. The effects of mindfulness-based stress reduction on psychosocial outcomes and quality of life in early-stage breast cancer patients: a randomized trial. Breast Cancer Res Treat 2011.

2. Wong SY, Chan FW, Wong RL et al. Comparing the Effectiveness of Mindfulness-based Stress Reduction and Multidisciplinary Intervention Programs for Chronic Pain: A Randomized Comparative Trial. Clin J Pain 2011; 27(8):724-34.

3. Brewer JA, Mallik S, Babuscio TA et al. Mindfulness training for smoking cessation: Results from a randomized controlled trial. Drug Alcohol Depend 2011.

4. Gaylord SA, Palsson OS, Garland EL et al. Mindfulness training reduces the severity of irritable bowel syndrome in women: results of a randomized controlled trial. Am J Gastroenterol 2011; 106(9):1678-88.

5. Philippot P, Nef F, Clauw L, Romree M, Segal Z. A Randomized Controlled Trial of Mindfulness-Based Cognitive Therapy for Treating Tinnitus. Clin Psychol Psychother 2011.

6. Gross CR, Kreitzer MJ, Reilly-Spong M et al. Mindfulness-based stress reduction versus pharmacotherapy for chronic primary insomnia: a randomized controlled clinical trial. Explore (NY) 2011; 7(2):76-87.

7. Schmidt S, Grossman P, Schwarzer B, Jena S, Naumann J, Walach H. Treating fibromyalgia with mindfulness-based stress reduction: results from a 3-armed randomized controlled trial. Pain 2011; 152(2):361-9.

8. Segal ZV, Bieling P, Young T et al. Antidepressant monotherapy vs sequential pharmacotherapy and mindfulness-based cognitive therapy, or placebo, for relapse prophylaxis in recurrent depression. Arch Gen Psychiatry 2010; 67(12):1256-64.

9. Oken BS, Fonareva I, Haas M et al. Pilot controlled trial of mindfulness meditation and education for dementia caregivers. J Altern Complement Med 2010; 16(10):1031-8.

10. Gross CR, Kreitzer MJ, Thomas W et al. Mindfulness-based stress reduction for solid organ transplant recipients: a randomized controlled trial. Altern Ther Health Med 2010; 16(5):30-8.

11. Garland EL, Gaylord SA, Boettiger CA, Howard MO. Mindfulness training modifies cognitive, affective, and physiological mechanisms implicated in alcohol dependence: results of a randomized controlled pilot trial. J Psychoactive Drugs 2010; 42(2):177-92.

12. Delgado LC, Guerra P, Perakakis P, Vera MN, Reyes del Paso G, Vila J. Treating chronic worry: Psychological and physiological effects of a training programme based on mindfulness. Behav Res Ther 2010; 48(9):873-82.

13. Morone NE, Rollman BL, Moore CG, Li Q, Weiner DK. A mind-body program for older adults with chronic low back pain: results of a pilot study. Pain Med 2009; 10(8):1395-407.

14. Brewer JA, Sinha R, Chen JA et al. Mindfulness training and stress reactivity in substance abuse: results from a randomized, controlled stage I pilot study. Subst Abus 2009; 30(4):306-17.

15. Mularski RA, Munjas BA, Lorenz KA et al. Randomized controlled trial of mindfulness-based therapy for dyspnea in chronic obstructive lung disease. J Altern Complement Med 2009; 15(10):1083-90.

16. Kuyken W, Byford S, Taylor RS et al. Mindfulness-based cognitive therapy to prevent relapse in recurrent depression. J Consult Clin Psychol 2008; 76(6):966-78.

17. Koszycki D, Benger M, Shlik J, Bradwejn J. Randomized trial of a meditation-based stress reduction program and cognitive behavior therapy in generalized social anxiety disorder. Behav Res Ther 2007; 45(10):2518-26.

18. Lee SH, Ahn SC, Lee YJ, Choi TK, Yook KH, Suh SY. Effectiveness of a meditation-based stress management program as an adjunct to pharmacotherapy in patients with anxiety disorder. J Psychosom Res 2007; 62(2):189-95.

19. Moritz S, Quan H, Rickhi B et al. A home study-based spirituality education program decreases emotional distress and increases quality of life—a randomized, controlled trial. Altern Ther Health Med 2006; 12(6):26-35.

20. Elder C, Aickin M, Bauer V, Cairns J, Vuckovic N. Randomized trial of a whole-system ayurvedic protocol for type 2 diabetes. Altern Ther Health Med 2006; 12(5):24-30.

21. Bormann JE, Gifford AL, Shively M et al. Effects of spiritual mantram repetition on HIV outcomes: a randomized controlled trial. J Behav Med 2006; 29(4):359-76.

22. Paul-Labrador M, Polk D, Dwyer JH et al. Effects of a randomized controlled trial of transcendental meditation on components of the metabolic syndrome in subjects with coronary heart disease. Arch Intern Med 2006; 166(11):1218-24.

23. Plews-Ogan M, Owens JE, Goodman M, Wolfe P, Schorling J. A pilot study evaluating mindfulness-based stress reduction and massage for the management of chronic pain. J Gen Intern Med 2005; 20(12):1136-8.

24. Hebert JR, Ebbeling CB, Olendzki BC et al. Change in women's diet and body mass following intensive intervention for early-stage breast cancer. J Am Diet Assoc 2001; 101(4):421-31.

25. Castillo-Richmond A, Schneider RH, Alexander CN et al. Effects of stress reduction on carotid atherosclerosis in hypertensive African Americans. Stroke 2000; 31(3):568-73.

26. Murphy TJ, Pagano RR, Marlatt GA. Lifestyle modification with heavy alcohol drinkers: effects of aerobic exercise and meditation. Addict Behav 1986; 11(2):175-86.

27. Smith JC. Psychotherapeutic effects of transcendental meditation with controls for expectation of relief and daily sitting. J Consult Clin Psychol 1976; 44(4):630-7.

28. Piet J, Hougaard E, Hecksher MS, Rosenberg NK. A randomized pilot study of mindfulness-based cognitive therapy and group cognitive-behavioral therapy for young adults with social phobia. Scand J Psychol 2010; 51(5):403-10.

29. Taub E, Steiner SS, Weingarten E, Walton KG. Effectiveness of broad spectrum approaches to relapse prevention in severe alcoholism: A long-term, randomized, controlled trial of Transcendental Meditation, EMG biofeedback and electronic neurotherapy. Alcoholism Treatment Quarterly 1994; 11(1-2):187-220.

30. Lehrer PM. Progressive relaxation and meditation: A study of psychophysiological and therapeutic differences between two techniques. Behav Res Ther 1983; 21(6):651-62.

31. Jayadevappa R, Johnson JC, Bloom BS et al. Effectiveness of transcendental meditation on functional capacity and quality of life of African Americans with congestive heart failure: a randomized control study Ethn Dis. 2007 Summer;17(3):595. Ethnicity & Disease 2007; 17(1):72-7.

32. Miller CK, Kristeller JL, Headings A, Nagaraja H, Miser WF. Comparative Effectiveness of a Mindful Eating Intervention to a Diabetes Self-Management Intervention among Adults with Type 2 Diabetes: A Pilot Study. J Acad Nutr Diet 2012; 112(11):1835-42.

33. Malarkey WB, Jarjoura D, Klatt M. Workplace based mindfulness practice and inflammation: A randomized trial. Brain Behav Immun 2012.

34. Whitebird RR, Kreitzer M, Crain AL, Lewis BA, Hanson LR, Enstad CJ. Mindfulness-Based Stress Reduction for Family Caregivers: A Randomized Controlled Trial. Gerontologist 2012.

35. Chiesa A, Mandelli L, Serretti A. Mindfulness-based cognitive therapy versus psycho-education for patients with major depression who did not achieve remission following antidepressant treatment: a preliminary analysis. J Altern Complement Med 2012; 18(8):756-60.

36. Barrett B, Hayney MS, Muller D et al. Meditation or exercise for preventing acute respiratory infection: a randomized controlled trial. Ann Fam Med 2012; 10(4):337-46.

37. Jazaieri H, Goldin PR, Werner K, Ziv M, Gross JJ. A Randomized Trial of MBSR Versus Aerobic Exercise for Social Anxiety Disorder. J Clin Psychol 2012.

38. Wolever RQ, Bobinet KJ, McCabe K et al. Effective and viable mind-body stress reduction in the workplace: a randomized controlled trial. J Occup Health Psychol 2012; 17(2):246-58.

39. SeyedAlinaghi S, Jam S, Foroughi M et al. Randomized controlled trial of mindfulness-based stress reduction delivered to human immunodeficiency virus-positive patients in Iran: effects on CD4^{+} T lymphocyte count and medical and psychological symptoms. Psychosom Med 2012; 74(6):620-7.

40. Pbert L, Madison JM, Druker S et al. Effect of mindfulness training on asthma quality of life and lung function: A randomised controlled trial. 2012; 67(9):769-76.

41. Schneider RH, Grim CE, Rainforth MV et al. Stress Reduction in the Secondary Prevention of Cardiovascular Disease: Randomized, Controlled Trial of Transcendental Meditation and Health Education in Blacks. (1941-7705 (Electronic). 1941-7713 (Linking)).

Evidence Table E31. Meditation intervention descriptions

Meditation Intervention	Description
Mindfulness Based Stress Reduction (MBSR)	A program devised of various formal and informal practices to cultivate moment to moment awareness. Practices include Hatha yoga and body scan to cultivate awareness of the body, and sitting meditation (including awareness of the breath, body, and mental state).
Mindfulness Based Cognitive Therapy (MBCT)	A program that integrates components of cognitive-behavioral therapy and mindfulness-based stress reduction (MBSR). The program was originally developed to prevent depression relapse. In addition to MBSR techniques to help individuals focus on the present moment, MBCT includes education about depression and the link between thoughts, feelings and bodily sensations so that individuals can learn to observe these thoughts, feelings, and sensations that may contribute to depression without rumination.
Transcendental Meditation (TM)	A meditation technique whereby a person uses a mantra and repeatedly directs the mind to the mantra as the mind strays. With continual repetition of the mantra the actual mantra becomes secondary and the meditator becomes increasingly self-aware and in state of "restful alertness."
Vipassana	A meditation technique to practice awareness of present moment experiences through several focal points: observation and awareness of the body, feelings, mind, and thought content.
Zen	A meditation technique that generally focuses on regulating awareness to the present moment. This generally includes the breath and counting from 1 to 10 with each exhalation.
Sahaj yoga	A form of meditation consisting of silent self-affirmations and breathing techniques that lead to a state of thoughtless awareness (alertness without unnecessary mental activity)
Meditation-Based Stress Management Program	A training program comprised of meditation, exercise, stretching, muscle buildup and relaxation, and hypnotic suggestion.
Modified MBCT	A program based on the original manual for MBCT but modified for individuals with tinnitus. The content on depression, which was not relevant to this population was excluded, and the number of sessions were reduced from 8 to 6 with adaptation to dealing with tinnitus rather than depression
Mindfulness Training Program	A mindfulness training program comprised of guided meditation with attention to body position, emotional state, interoceptive consciousness, and acceptance.
Mindfulness meditation program based on MBSR and MBCT adapted for caregivers	A program that includea didactics on stress, relaxation, and meditation, as well as meditation and mindfulness exercises (awareness of breathing, awareness of body sensation, awareness of cognitive and emotional experience), mindful movement and mindful awareness during other activities.
Mindfulness-Oriented Recovery Enhancement (MORE)	An MBCT-adapted meditation program for alcohol dependence. The program involves mindful breathing and walking meditations, and exercises relating mindfulness principles to addiction-specific issues.
Mindfulness-Based Breathing Therapy (MBBT)	A program that combines the standard MBSR program with relaxation response training with a focus on a breath-centered approach.
Mindfulness-Based Stress and Pain Management Program	A mindfulness program based largely on MBSR but tailored to an irritable bowel syndrome (IBS) population by having them focus on IBS related-symptoms (e.g., focusing on sensations in the abdominal area)
Mindfulness Meditation Program for Stress Management	A condensed 4-week version of the traditional MBSR course (8 weeks), which taught the core MBSR components.
Mindfulness Training for Smoking Cessation	A program based on a previous mindfulness training manual for drug relapse prevention and adapted for smoking cessation. The focus was on present moment awareness and acceptance of cravings. Mindfulness practices included breath awareness meditation, walking meditation, and body scan, loving-kindness meditation, and mindfulness of daily activities.
Spirituality-Teaching Program	A program that teaches concepts related to spirituality and also includes breathing and visualization exercises, self-awareness using the senses, practices of gratitude, and acceptance and loving kindness meditation.

Meditation Intervention	Description
Adaptation of Mindfulness–Based Relapse Prevention Program (MBRP)	A program based on MBRP with several modifications. The sessions after the first session were delivered in 2 four-week modules that could be completed in either order. A session was added that specifically focused on working with anger as a trigger for stress and drug use, the yoga meditation was removed, and sessions were shortened to 1 hour.
Clinically Standardized Meditation (CSM)	A mantra-based meditation technique whereby subjects repeat a mantra in their minds for 20 minutes at a time (Carrington, 1978)
Mantra Meditation with variations	A program in which participants were taught the basic CSM (Clinically Standardized Meditation) technique (Carrington, 1978) in addition to several other mantra meditation variations. These included 'mini-meditations', a meditation with open eyes with a neutral gaze at a surface, a meditation on a candle flame with and without a mantra, counting of the breaths with a focus on air movement, and a breathing-paced meditation where subjects say the first syllable of their mantra on the inhalation and the second syllable during exhalation.
Spiritual mantra meditation	A program in which participants were provided with a manual with a list of various spiritual mantrams of various traditions in order to choose a mantram. They were also provided with methods to enhance mantram repitition, such as practicing "one-pointed attention and mindfulness while engaging in one task at a time, and intentionally slowing down mentally and behaviorally while using a mantram". The course book also provided mantram meditation exercises.

www.ingramcontent.com/pod-product-compliance
Lightning Source LLC
Chambersburg PA
CBHW081715170526
45167CB00009B/3586